Chinese Acupuncture and Moxibustion

For Churchill Livingstone

Publisher: Mary Law
Project editor: Dinah Thom
Copy editor: Ruth Swan
Production controller: Mark Sanderson
Design: Design Resources Unit
Sales Promotion Executive: Hilary Brown

Chinese Acupuncture and Moxibustion

Managing Editor

Qiu Mao-liang MD
Professor at Nanjing College of TCM

Vice-Managing Editor

Zang Shan-chen MD
Professor at Shandong College of TCM

Members of Editorial Board
Yu Zhong-quan MD
Professor at Chengdu College of TCM
Zhou Xing-xiao MD
Professor at Shanghai College of TCM
Gao Zhen-wu MD
Professor at Zhejiang College of TCM

Managing Translator
Li Liang-yu MD
Lecturer at Nanjing College of TCM

Consultant Language Editor and Subject Adviser
Richard Bertschinger BA BAc DipAc(China) CertEd MTAcS
General Acupuncture Practitioner

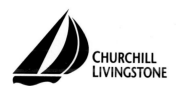

CHURCHILL
LIVINGSTONE

EDINBURGH LONDON MADRID MELBOURNE NEW YORK AND TOKYO 1993

CHURCHILL LIVINGSTONE
An imprint of Harcourt Brace and Company Limited

Distributed in the United States of America by
Redwing Book Company, 44 Linden Street, Brookline,
Massachusetts 021460

This edition of Acupuncture and Moxibustion is published by
arrangement with Shanghai Scientific and Technical Publishers.

First published 1993
   Reprinted 1996
   Reprinted 1998

ISBN 0-443-04223-3

British Library of Cataloguing in Publication Data
A catalogue record for this book is available from the British
Library.

Library of Congress Cataloging in Publication Data
Chinese acupuncture and moxibustion/managing editor, Qiu Mao-Liang;
vice managing editor, Zang Shan-chen; Managing translator, Li Liang-yu;
English language editor and subject advisor, Richard Bertschinger.
      p.   cm.
   Includes bibliographical references and indexes.
   ISBN 0-443-04223-3
   1. Acupuncture.   2. Moxa.   I. Chiu, Mao-liang.   II. Li, Liang-yü.
   [DNLM: 1. Acupuncture.   2. Moxibustion.   WB 369 C5393]
RM184.C54226   1993
615.8′92—dc20
DNLM/DLC
for Library of Congress   92-49859
                                                                  CIP

The
publisher's
policy is to use
**paper manufactured
from sustainable forests**

Printed in China
CTPS/03

Contents

Subject Adviser's Preface

The importance of acupuncture and moxibustion to modern medicine cannot be denied. The theories of traditional Chinese medicine (TCM) permeate their clinical practice, and provide a worthy foundation for any natural philosophy of medicine. This authoritative manual is a translation of the standard textbook on acupuncture and moxibustion prepared for the main TCM colleges in China. It represents a pragmatic blend of East and West, incorporating all 365 classical points, but also new methods such as scalp-needling (which makes reference to modern neuro-physiology), point injection therapy (injecting Western drugs as well as Chinese herbal solutions into acupuncture points), and acupuncture anaesthesia.

The history of the book is interesting. As described in Dr Qiu Mao-liang's Introduction, TCM was born again in the mid-20th century following 100 or more years of decline. This renaissance was due to the need in China, following 20 years of warfare and disorder, for a cheap, practical and simply taught medicine which could serve the population undergoing the massive task of social and economic reconstruction.

In 1956 the first four colleges of Traditional Chinese Medicine were established in Beijing, Shanghai, Guangzhou and Chengdu. The 60s and 70s saw a great deal of research and the development of new techniques, especially in acupuncture.

In 1982, following nearly 30 years of experimentation and the publication of new editions of the ancient classical texts, a conference was convened in Nanjing to survey the education climate in traditional medicine. At the conference it was decided to produce a truly comprehensive and up-to-date set of textbooks, based upon a scientific approach, which would be systematically produced and cover all areas of traditional medicine. This manual is one of the textbooks that were written as part of that plan.

Acupuncture and moxibustion together form only one specialist area within a traditional medicine programme which includes herbal remedies (involving also the use of minerals and animal products), massage and manipulation, dietary therapy and therapeutic exercise (involving *gigong* or breathing therapy).

Five colleges of TCM, at Nanjing, Shandong, Zhejiang, Shanghai and Chengdu, were mainly involved in the preparation of this book which aims to provide a first text for all students. The work was based upon past textbooks dating back to the 1960s.

In editing the Chinese translation into English I have stayed true to the original Chinese, aiming only to improve on punctuation, paragraphing, word order, etc. However it is justifiable to broach the subject of terminology. More particularly, Phlegm and Wind have been the usual translations of *tan* and *feng*, but in this edition they have been replaced by the original transliterated Chinese words. This is because *tan* and *feng* (along with *yin*, *yang*, *qi*, etc.) are fundamental concepts in Chinese medicine; and the partial and narrow "wind" and "phlegm" ignore the richly adaptable nature of the Chinese language.

Tan is slippery and sticky but when unsubstantial may settle into the joints or obstruct the heart, so obviously Phlegm is an inadequate expression of this function.

Feng is a complex, multifaceted expression, combining the suggestion of environmental, climatic and seasonal change, although it may also be used to imply rapidly changing and altering symptoms within the body.

Traditionally *feng* occupied a more important position than it is accorded in contemporary Chinese medical texts. However, the idea of *feng* as a pathogenic force is still potent nowadays in TCM, but no modern Western physician can readily incorporate the idea of a "wind", which acts somewhat ethereally, blowing within the body, precipitating disease and bringing about pathogenic change.

In Chapter 3, "The Living Qi Penetrating all Nature", at the beginning of the *Plain Questions* section of the *Yellow Emperor's Book of Medicine*, it states: "*Feng* is the precursor of all disease." The idea of *feng* as a subtle and deeply influential factor in sickness is fundamental to Chinese medicine. To ridicule and isolate it as Wind— with suggestions of bowel, or intestinal gas, or of something which blows through the sky—is to do a fundamental injustice to the Chinese idea. *Feng* includes ideas of subtlety and all-pervasiveness; it identifies the all-enveloping environment which precipitates disease.

The terms *yin* and *yang* are no longer capitalised: they are frequently occurring medical terms and as such (along with the term *qi*) an understanding of their use quickly becomes second nature. The same applies to *jingluo* and *zangfu* and, to a lesser extent, to the six-fold division of *Taiyang, Shaoyang, Yangming, Taiyin, Jueyin* and *Shaoyin*.

Less importantly, Bi syndrome and Wei syndrome have been left as they are in the original Chinese translation; this also applies to the *yuan* and *luo*, Back-Shu, Jing-well points, etc. *Yuan* and *luo* are left in the Chinese as these groups of points are much more familiar in the West. All Chinese terms and phrases have been grouped with their original characters in the Glossary at the back of the book.

Lastly, as this is an acupuncture text, the names of the organs—heart, liver, spleen, etc.— have been given without the capitalisation which has become usual. This ensures that our idea of them is not set apart from a naturally intuitive grasp of their function. This a further development of the terminology used in my translation of *The Golden Needle and other Odes of Traditional Acupuncture*, Churchill Livingstone, 1991.

A summary of the modern scientific research which formed Appendix 6 of the original work is now included within the Introduction. This section summarises recent research into the actual nature of the jingluo and the propagation of a needling sensation along the meridians (PSM), morphological research into the meridians (as they correspond to the sensory conductive structures of the body), and also research into the conductive pathways of the acupuncture effect. It also outlines tentative conclusions as to the three basic mechanisms of acupuncture—analgesic, regulatory and immunological. References to the original research papers were omitted from the original Chinese, but may be found in such books as Alan Bensoussan's *The Vital Meridian*, Churchill Livingstone, 1991. The rearrangment and editing of this section has been done with the full agreement of Dr Qui Mao-liang.

The most commonly used points are identified in the lists and tables with an asterisk (*), as they are in the original, and in the schematic diagrams in the same chapter, they are identified as bold.

Montacute, 1993   Richard Bertschinger

Acknowledgements

My thanks go to the people who helped with part of the translation: Yi Sumei, Li Huilin, Yuan Jiashui and Li Wen.

I am indebted to Yue Qiaozhen for her help in completing this work.

Nanjing, 1993   Li Liang-yu

Introduction

Historical survey

The science of acupuncture and moxibustion takes the theories of Chinese medicine as its guide. It is a clinical discipline which aims at the prevention and treatment of disease by puncturing certain points on the body with acupuncture needles or by applying the heat of ignited moxa wool onto the body surface. It is an important component of TCM (traditional Chinese medicine), comprising the idea of the jingluo (or channels and collaterals), the idea of the acupoints (sensitive points on the body for treatment) and the main techniques of acupuncture and moxibustion all employed in clinical treatment.

Acupuncture and moxibustion have the special advantages of being indicated in a wide variety of conditions, of marked efficacy and of economy, convenience and safety, and they have been widely popular in China over thousands of years. They have made an immense contribution to the prosperity and development of the Chinese nation.

The development of acupuncture and moxibustion has been a long historical process following the drawn-out struggle of the Chinese labouring people, and their physicians, against disease. The origins of acupuncture and moxibustion are difficult to trace, but according to findings from ancient records, and the evidence of unearthed artifacts, the germination of their use can be dated back to an epoch before the creation of Chinese characters.

The primary chapter of the *Miraculous Pivot* (around second century BC to second century AD), entitled "On the 9 Needles and 12 Yuan-source Points" states, "I want to treat disease without using toxic drugs and not using any longer the *bian* stones. I apply fine needles to remove obstructions from the jingluo and regulate the circulation of blood and qi...". From this quotation it can be seen that *bian* (砭) stones were the medical instruments used prior to fine filiform needles.

It is also stated in the *Study on the Principles of Composition of Chinese Characters*, around the second century AD, that "the word *bian* connotes treating disease with acupuncture stones". And in the chapter on "Eastern Mountains" in the *Legends of Mountains and Seas* (around 300 BC) it is recorded that "Mount Gaoshi is rich in jade, and at its foot there are regions rich in acupuncture stones." Guo Pu, at a later date, noted "acupuncture stones that were called *bian* stones, used as implements in the treatment of boils".

In remote antiquity ancient peoples prayed when they suffered from disease and at the same time pounded certain parts of the body surface, instinctively, with pieces of stone. Unexpectedly, the disease was found to be alleviated and, after a long accumulation of such experience and practice, the therapeutic method of the *bian* stones finally came into being.

In 1963, at Toudaowa district, Duolun County (Inner Mongolia), a stone needle which had been fashioned by grinding was excavated in the Neolithic ruins, and it can be identified as a primitive acupuncture implement—the *bian* stone. Therefore the origin of the *bian* stone needle can be dated back to the Neolithic (10 000–4000 years ago) or perhaps even earlier.

Along with the invention of the technique of smelting, the making of the needles was gradually improved. However, stone and bone were not replaced by bronze, iron, gold or silver until the time when the canonical *Yellow Emperor's Book of Medicine* (or *Nei Jing*) appeared, around the second century BC. In this work, the *bian* stone needles had been replaced by therapy with metal needles. This has been again further improved into the present acupuncture technique with stainless steel needles.

The improvement of metal needles was proven by the excavation of a bronze acupuncture needle from the Bronze Age in Dalate County (Inner Mongolia) in 1978, and of nine needles for medical use, finely made of gold and silver, dating from a Western Han Dynasty tomb (206 BC–AD 24) in Mancheng County (Hebei Province) in 1968.

The treatment of moxibustion emerged only after the discovery and use of fire. Ancient peoples found that diseases and pain in certain parts of the body were alleviated by applying the heat of fire and, after the long accumulation of experience, treatment by ignited twigs was developed into treatment by moxibustion, with ignited moxa made from the plant *Artemisia vulgaris*. In the chapter "The Suitability of Dif-

fering Rules and Prescriptions" in the *Plain Questions* (Ch. 12 of the *Nei Jing*), it is stated that "abdominal pain or distension by the cold, are suitable for treatment by moxibustion"; and, during later generations, moxibustion was developed into various differing methods, following the progress of medicine.

The gradual reform and development of acupuncture and moxibustion instruments and materials, not only increased their indications, but also enhanced their therapeutic effect and vigorously promoted their academic and scientific development.

As far as the academic accomplishments of acupuncture and moxibustion are concerned, they are the result of a long historical process. In 1973, there were excavated several medical books, copied onto silk, from a Han Dynasty tomb in Hunan Province Tomb No. 3, Changsha City. Among them were two ancient books on the meridians, namely the *Moxibustion Classic on the Eleven Meridians of the Foot and Hand* and the *Moxibustion Classic on the Eleven Meridians of Yin and Yang*, which deal with the distribution of the eleven meridians, their pathological manifestations and moxibustion treatment. Textual research shows that these two books appeared earlier than the *Yellow Emperor's Book of Medicine* (i.e. at least 3rd century, perhaps even 4th century, BC) and from their content we can get a glimpse of the theory of the jingluo at an early stage. Even at this early date, there are mentioned over 450 prescriptions and over 200 separate items of materia medica.

The *Yellow Emperor's Book of Medicine* itself (the *Huangdi Nei Jing*) has fairly detailed descriptions of the jingluo, the acupoints, various methods of acupuncture and moxibustion, and precautions and contraindications to treatment. This is especially so in the *Miraculous Pivot* (or *Ling Shu*), the second part of the book, where the theories of acupuncture and moxibustion are particularly detailed and systematic in their presentation. This is why the *Miraculous Pivot* is also known as the "Canon of Acupuncture". It can be seen that, by this period, the study of acupuncture and moxibustion was already fully mature, laying a theoretical basis for its later academic and scientific growth and development.

Excluding the *Miraculous Pivot*, the earliest surviving treatise on acupuncture and moxibustion is the *Systematic Classic on Acupuncture and Moxibustion* compiled by the famous medical doctor Huangfu Mi of the Jin Dynasty in AD 256–260, through reference to the *Yellow Emperor's Book of Medicine* and the *Ming Tang Essentials of Points*, a work now unfortunately lost. In this classic the theories of the zangfu (or internal) organs, and meridians and collaterals are discussed, and the acupoints are described according to differing parts of the body—head, face, chest, abdomen, back, etc. Three hundred and forty nine points are summarized on the basis of the *Nei Jing* along with their locations, indications and methods of puncturing and manipulation, various other techniques, precautions and contraindications, and acupuncture and moxibustion prescriptions for commonly seen diseases. This book serves as a link between the *Yellow Emperor's Book of Medicine* and later generations of acupuncture and moxibustion literature.

During the Eastern Jin Dynasty (AD 317–420), the famous doctor Ge Hong wrote the book *Prescriptions for Emergencies* in which he described 109 prescriptions for acupuncture and moxibustion treatment, 99 of which specifically involve moxibustion. This attracted people's interest, and consequently moxibustion later developed greatly as a therapy.

Sun Simiao compiled *Prescriptions Worth a Thousand Gold Coin* around AD 650–652, during the Tang Dynasty, in which he explained the method of selection, and application, of the "ah shi points" (阿是穴).[1] He also designed and made the *Charts of Three Views* in which the twelve regular meridians and eight extra meridians were illustrated in various colours and shown separately anteriorly, posteriorly and laterally. He especially advocated moxibustion in the prevention of disease—making a great contribution to the preventive medicine of later generations. There was also Wang Tao who wrote *The Medical Secrets of An Official* in AD 752, in which a host of moxibustion methods, of varying schools, were recorded. This book played an active role in popularizing moxibustion therapy.

During the Sui (581–618) and Tang (618–907)

Dynasties the Imperial Medical Bureau responsible for medical education was established, and the department of acupuncture was one of the faculties of medical specialities, in which there were professors of acupuncture, assistant professors and instructors in charge of the the teaching work. This shows the great importance attached to acupuncture during that period.

Wang Weiyi wrote the book *An Illustrated Manual on Points for Acupuncture and Moxibustion on the New Bronze Figure* during the Northern Song Dynasty, and it was set up, inscribed, on stone tablets erected in the capital. These were intended for students to read and use to make rubbings from. Among these inscriptions were the locations of the 354 acupoints, with their related meridians and indications, all described and revised. The next year (AD 1027) two bronze figures, designed by Wang Weiyi, were manufactured. These were the earliest models for acupuncture and moxibustion learning and played an important role in the teaching of the jingluo and the acupoints.

Hua Shou of the Yuan Dynasty (1231–1368) did textual research on the pathways of jingluo, as well as their relationship with the acupuncture points, and held that the Ren and Du meridians, although extra meridians, yet had their own points and should be mentioned together with the twelve regular meridians. Accordingly, he identified fourteen meridians and wrote the book *An Exposition of the Fourteen Meridians* (published 1341) which systematically expounded the meridians' courses and their related acupoints, thus facilitating the study of the meridians for later generations.

In the Ming Dynasty (1368–1644) acupuncture and moxibustion reached their greatest period of flowering. Yang Jizhou, on the basis of the book *Secrets of Acupuncture And Moxibustion for Health Care* handed down in his family, collected all sorts of acupuncture and moxibustion works from past dynasties and, in combination with his practical experience, compiled the book *A Compendium of Acupuncture and Moxibustion* (1601) which has a rich and varied content. It is another complete summary of the science of acupuncture and moxibustion, following on the tradition of the *Yellow Emperor's Book of*

Medicine and Huang Fumi's *Systematic Classic of Acupuncture and Moxibustion*. The *Compendium of Acupuncture and Moxibustion* is still a main reference book for the study of acupuncture and moxibustion today.

During this time, there were many famous doctors specializing in this field, with books such as *A Classic of Effective Treatment* (1425) written by Chen Hui, *A Complete Collection of Acupuncture and Moxibustion* (1439) by Xu Feng, *An Exemplary Collection of Acupuncture and Moxibustion* (1529) by Gao Wu, *Questions and Answers Concerning Acupuncture and Moxibustion* (1532) by Wang Ji and *Research on the Eight Extra Meridians* (1578) by Li Shizhen; all formulating different views and schools of thought, but each exerting a tremendous influence upon the development of acupuncture and moxibustion.

In the Qing Dynasty (1644–1911), although there were books such as *A Golden Mirror of Medicine* (1742) by Wu Qian, with a chapter entitled *Essentials of Acupuncture and Moxibustion in Verse*, and the *Collection of Acupuncture and Moxibustion* (1874) written by Liao Runhong, they put forth few new ideas; and by the end of the Qing both acupuncture and moxibustion gradually began to decline.

The medical science of acupuncture and moxibustion has grown gradually, over several thousand years, but its development still suffered the mishaps of history. In 1822 the authorities of the Qing Dynasty declared an order abolishing acupuncture and moxibustion departments from the Imperial Medical College. This was on the pretext that "acupuncture with needles and moxibustion with burning moxa, are unsuitable for service to the emperor" and thereafter some doctors regarded herbal medication as superior to acupuncture. Following the Opium War in 1840, the aggressive attitude of the imperialists, with the establishment of missionary hospitals, medical colleges, and schools of western medicine, led to discrimination against TCM. This meant that TCM—including acupuncture and moxibustion—declined to a critical level.

However, because of their advantages of marked efficacy, economy and convenience, and because of the great need of the Chinese labouring people for medical care, acupuncture and moxibustion gained a chance to spread among the folk people in spite of later restriction by the Guo Ming Dang Government. At the same time, many high-minded people and acupuncturists made unremitting efforts to protect and develop acupuncture and moxibustion, setting up acupuncture and moxibustion associations and schools.

Acupuncture and moxibustion were also disseminated to foreign countries long ago. In the 6th century, they were both introduced into Korea and books such as Huang Fumi's *Systematic Classic of Acupuncture and Moxibustion* were taken there as textbooks.

In AD 562 Zhi Cong of Wu County in China brought the *Ming Tang Charts of Acupuncture and Moxibustion*, the *Systematic Classic of Acupuncture and Moxibustion* and other medical books to Japan. In AD 701 acupuncture and moxibustion were set up as specialties in Japanese medical education, and indeed colleges and schools of acupuncture and moxibustion have been in Japan up to the present time, deeply appreciated by the Japanese people.

At the end of the 17th century, acupuncture and moxibustion also spread to Europe, and centres involved in research into acupuncture and moxibustion have been established there—along with the holding of international conferences and seminars. In some provinces and cities in China international training centres of acupuncture and moxibustion have been established, to which large numbers of foreign students come to be trained as qualified acupuncturists.

Since the founding of the People's Republic of China, the Chinese Communist party has attached great importance to the inheritance and development of this legacy of TCM and pharmacology. This has brought new life to TCM and a rejuvenation of interest in acupuncture and moxibustion. Chinese medical colleges and hospitals, which include faculties and departments of acupuncture and moxibustion, and special research institutes, have been set up; and these have done a great deal, achieving successes in the teaching of this science, in clinical treatment and in scientific research.

In the thirty years or more since the founding

of the New China, a large number of acupuncture and moxibustion works have been published including a unified textbook of acupuncture and moxibustion for higher level students in the medical colleges, modern language versions of the classics, such as the *Yellow Emperor's Book of Medicine*, the *Classic of Medical Problems*, the *Systematic Classic of Acupuncture and Moxibustion* and the *Compendium of Acupuncture and Moxibustion*. Furthermore, over ten thousand monographs have been published in journals all over the country, and these have greatly enriched the science of acupuncture and moxibustion, and facilitated its study.

Recent research into the real nature of the jingluo

A great deal of very important research work has been done on the real nature of the jingluo (the meridians and collaterals which cross and crisscross the body): research into the phenomenon of the propagation of needling sensation along the meridians (PSM), the route of the PSM, the correlation between the viscera and the body surface, and the morphological basis of the meridians. These all lay a foundation for further research which will finally reveal the real nature of the jingluo.

1. RESEARCH INTO THE PROPAGATION OF NEEDLING SENSATION ALONG THE MERIDIANS

The phenomenon of a needling sensation—soreness, numbness, distension and heaviness—propagated along the course of the jingluo after the "de qi" or "arrival of qi" has been obtained, while the acupoint of a particular meridian is being punctured with a needle, is known as propagation of needling sensation along meridians (or PSM).

Similar phenomena have been noted in ancient medical literature, for example the *The History of Three Kingdoms: The Profile of Hua Tuo* (who lived during the Han Dynasty) records: "On giving needling, I tell the patient that

I'll direct the needling sensation to that place, and if it arrives, he tells me. The patient says, 'Yes, it arrives', I withdraw the needle and the case is cured." In the *Prescriptions Worth A Thousand Gold Coin: Acupuncture* (AD 652) there is a record of "conducting qi along the course of the meridian to drive out and eliminate disease".

These both indicate that by conducting the propagation of the needling sensation to the affected site, satisfactory therapeutic results could be obtained.

Modern research into PSM started in the early 50s and, since 1972, many surveys on PSM have been carried out by related units in more than 20 provinces, according to one method and one criterion. The Jing-well or *yuan* points are stimulated with a low-frequency electric impulse, and, if either the PSM can reach or pass beyond the elbow and knee joints in two meridians, or the PSM can reach or pass beyond the shoulder and hip joints in one meridian, in a tested subject, this person's PSM is considered positive. If the PSM should appear along the whole course of more than 6 meridians, this person's PSM is considered remarkable.

According to the analysis of surveys of 63 000 persons, the appearance rate of PSM in most units was 12–24%, and in half of the units the remarkable appearance rate was over 0.2%. PSM might also appear in persons of different nations, ages, sexes and in differing conditions of health. Such a survey was done among 203 Mozambicans, and 1.5% were found with a "remarkable" appearance rate, 30% with a less remarkable rate and a further 50.3% with a still less remarkable rate. All in all, an appearance rate of 81.8% revealed that the PSM phenomenon exists in persons of different races.

CHARACTERISTICS OF PSM

Route of the PSM. The route of PSM was found to be basically identical with the course of the meridians recorded in the *Miraculous Pivot*.[2] There were also other routes, longer or shorter, or newly appearing branches, compared to the classical routes recorded in the *Miraculous*

Pivot. Those in the limbs were generally identical with the classical ones, some of those in the trunks went astray from those classically recorded while many different routes were observed in the head and face. PSM was also found between externally-internally related or other meridians.

Speed of the PSM. The speed of the PSM is obviously slower than that of nerves. According to some reports, the speed of the somatic nervous propagation is 100 m/second, the speed of the autonomic nervous propagation is 1 m/second, while the speed of the PSM is 10 cm/second, much slower.

Biphasic and regurgitant PSM. The PSM in all the points on the body (except the Jing-well points in which the PSM is monoconcentric) generally travels biphasically upwards and downwards simultaneously from the point being stimulated, and the PSM stops as soon as the stimulation in the point stops. In some cases, the PSM "faded" and disappeared after the stop of the propagated sensation, but in others the PSM flowed back to the points being stimulated or to a place nearby and then disappeared.

Width and depth of the PSM. Most PSM are of thread and cord-like shape (2–5 mm in diameter), while some are tape-shaped to a width of 1–3 cm. The sensations are narrow at the distal end, gradually widening at the proximal end and into the body trunk. The PSM are superficial at the thin muscles and deep at the thick muscles, while in the trunk deep sensations travel within the body cavity and superficial ones travel within the subcutaneous somatic layer.

Properties of the PSM. The properties of the PSM vary with each individual and method of stimulation. There is often soreness, numbness and distension in the case of needling, a warm or hot flow in moxibustion, electrical numbness in the case of electroneedling, and a sensation of flowing water in point-injection therapy. There may be also itching or a sensation as of creeping ants or insects upon the skin.

The PSM can be blocked. The PSM can be blocked by possible surgical incisions, scars, tumours, lumps and abscesses on the pathway of the PSM, or by mechanical pressure, fluid injection, freezing or stimulatory cutaneous disturbance such as repeated rubbing back and forth with a soft brush, applied along the on-going course of the PSM.

Furthermore, PSM also appears to have the characteristic of being specific to individual points or diseases.

VISIBLE MERIDIAN PHENOMENON

When puncturing points there may be a milky or red linear discoloration along the course of the stimulated meridians, which may last for a few tens of seconds or even several hours.

Also there may be papules of belt-shape, linear skin eruptions looking like eczema, linear sweating, linear nervous dermatitis or flat mucus along the course of the meridians being stimulated.

LATENT PSM PHENOMENON

It is well recognized that the needling sensation reaching the affected site during treatment can enhance the therapeutic effect; but actually in many patients, after the needling sensation was felt, no PSM was observed and yet good therapeutic results were obtained, and this phenomenon is considered as "latent PSM". Research into this began in 1977.

In this research, electric impulses were applied to Jing-well points and no PSM was observed. Then percussion was applied to lines perpendicular to the course of the meridian and on the levels of different points above the *yuan* point of the meridian. On each line there would be a positively reactive spot which, whilst being percussed, would have a particular sensation of numbness and distension radiating to the Jing-well point. Then if these positive spots were linked together there would appear a line which was precisely identical with the classical course of the meridian. If the same method were applied to persons with a remarkable PSM, the same phenomenon could appear along the whole course of the tested meridian. The latent PSM could also be proved by only the percussion method without the primary electro-stimulation of the Jing-well point.

A survey among 200 patients showed latent PSM in 107 persons with a presence rate of 69%. Latent PSM was also observed in normal healthy subjects and a survey of 100 cases showed the presence rate of latent PSM was 94%, the unstable presence rate was 4%, and the absence rate was 2%. This indicates that in normal subjects latent PSM is more obvious than in patients, and that the universal existence of PSM among normal subjects is a normal physiological phenomenon—not a pathological phenomenon.

PSM can also be stimulated by applying the manipulative techniques of acupuncture, or electroneedling, or by applying heat along the meridian, or the injection of drugs along the course of the meridian.

CONNECTIONS BETWEEN THE PSM, THE SENSORY ORGANS AND THE ZANGFU

Any change in the functioning of the meridians will have a reaction at the corresponding zangfu organ of the related meridian. This is manifest most obviously in observing subjects with remarkable PSM.

When the PSM reached the cheek the subject felt soreness in the lower gums; when it reached the point Yingxiang (LI 20), soreness was observed in the nose; when it reached the lips, a sensation of "thickened lips" was felt; when it reached the eyes, blurred or brighter vision was observed; when it reached the ear, tinnitus was observed; when it reached the throat, dryness and a difficulty in speaking were observed; and when it reached the face, facial muscular twitching was observed and myoelectricity was recorded.

When the PSM reached the lung, the subject's ventilation capacity increased in volume; when puncturing a point on the Spleen meridian with the PSM reaching the abdomen, a burning hot sensation was felt by the subject; when puncturing a point on the Pericardium meridian, the PSM reached the cardiac region along the meridian, and a stuffiness in the chest was suddenly relieved; when the PSM reached the kidney region, soreness and a distending sensation was felt; and when it reached the vulva, the subject had a desire to pass urine.

THE RELATIONSHIP BETWEEN THE PSM AND DISEASE

When puncturing points with the PSM reaching a painful site, the analgesic effect was enhanced: for example, angina pectoris could be relieved by puncturing Neiguan (P 5), with the PSM reaching the chest; biliary colic could be relieved or even disappear when puncturing Yanglingquan (GB 34), with the PSM reaching the right hypochondrium; dysmenorrhoea could be relieved by puncturing Taichong (Liv 3), with the PSM reaching the lower abdomen. This proves the theory that the whole course of a meridian is amenable to treatment or, as it is also expressed, the therapeutic effect is achieved when the qi of the meridian reaches the affected site.

2. MORPHOLOGICAL RESEARCH INTO THE JINGLUO

According to records in the *Yellow Emperor's Book of Medicine*, the routes of the meridians can be classified into two systems: those circulating qi and blood inside the vessels and those circulating qi and blood outside the vessels.

The *ying* (营) or nutrient system corresponds to the blood system in modern medicine, while the *wei* (卫) or defensive qi circulating outside the vessels, corresponds to the sensory conductive structure of the body in modern medicine. This is an important field of study and the main route for research into the real nature of the jingluo. The task of research in this field is to further study the sensory conductive structure of the body—especially its physiology and pathology—as well as the function of the sensory nerves, all through adopting modern scientific method.

THE RELATIONSHIP BETWEEN THE JINGLUO AND THE NERVOUS SYSTEM

The statement in *Miraculous Pivot* that, "flicking the muscle region of the Meridian of the Hand Taiyang will have a reaction at the small finger",[3] indicates that the muscle region of the Meridian of the Hand Taiyang and the ulnar nerve are actually of the same tissue structure. It is also stated that, "the muscle region along the meridian of the Foot Shaoyang on the left side connects with that on the right, so that an injury on the left angle of the heel leads to paralysis of the right foot",[4] which is a similar principle to that of the "pyramidal decussation" of the motor nerves in the medulla oblongata. Furthermore, from pathological manifestations of the muscle region along the meridians, such as deviation of the mouth and cramp in the gastrocnemius muscles in cholera morbus, it can be seen that the muscles have a close relationship with the nerves.

Acupoints and meridians are also closely related to each other. Morphological observation on cadavers revealed that among 324 points, those points with an innervation of cranial and spinal nerves within a radius of 0.5 cm around them, are 323 (99%); those related to superficial cutaneous nerves are 304 (94%); those related to deep nerves are 155 (48%) and those related to both deep and superficial nerves are 137 (42%). This indicates a close relationship between the jingluo and the nervous system. Also the acupoints, and the nerves of their related zangfu organs, pertain to the same spinal segment or to within the same nerve segment as that to which the zangfu organ pertains. The externally-internally related meridians also pertain fundamentally to the same spinal segment.

A histochemical method was applied whilst observing tissue obtained from animals and human beings (during surgical operations). Deep or superficial connective tissue, tissue from the joint capsule of the knee joint, skeletal muscle, the visceral serous coating and tissue from the viscera was all used. The results of examining these section preparations revealed that, both in human beings and animals, innervation of the adrenergic (sympathetic) and cholinergic (parasympathetic) nerve-endings around the small blood vessels in the above mentioned connective tissue, can be observed under a microscope. However, the innervation of these nerve-endings is only at resistance vessels and of the double innervation type; and among the adrenergic and cholinergic nerves doubly innervating the same small vessel, some followed the same routes while others followed different routes.

These findings suggest that, regarding the idea which occurs both in the *Miraculous Pivot* and the *Plain Questions* that "the nutrient qi circulates in the vessels while the defensive qi circulates outside the vessels", the wei (defensive) qi travels along small vessels which may be the adrenergic and cholinergic nerves of the autonomic nervous system.

These closely combined two kinds of sympathetic postganglionic neurofibres and resistant vessels are conformable with the close relationship between the qi and blood, and the jingluo and vessels, which was recognized by the ancient doctors of the *Miraculous Pivot* through their clinical practice. Further, nowadays it is held by those involved in research that the autonomic nervous system is an important component in the true nature of the jingluo.

THE RELATIONSHIP BETWEEN THE JINGLUO AND THE BLOOD VESSELS

Ancient doctors had already observed a close relationship between meridians and blood vessels, and even a difference between arteries and veins.[5] It was noticed that "blood is clear and turbid", and also "he who has flourishing blood, qi and much yang qi, has slippery blood which would spurt out if the vessel were punctured. He who has accumulated yang qi, has blackish and turbid blood which cannot spurt out if the vessel is punctured". In the former case it is blood spurting from an artery, whilst in the latter the blood is from a vein.

Observation shows that among 309 points, 24 (7%) are just on an artery, while 262 (84%) are beside an artery; and, from the location of acupoints, it can be seen that the jingluo are closely related to the blood vessels. It has also been found that the vasculature of the arteries in the acupoint area has certain forms—regular convergences, radiating or perhaps less regular arrangements. Furthermore, in those with convergent arrangements, the points are often located in the centre of such arrangements.

THE RELATIONSHIP BETWEEN THE JINGLUO AND THE LYMPHATIC VESSELS

Research also found out that the meridians are related to the lymphatic plexus, or to the lymphatic vessels and lymph nodes. The Du, Ren and Dai meridians are related to the lymphatic plexus; the lung, stomach, heart, spleen and urinary meridians are almost completely conformable with the vasculature of the lymphatic vessels, and either deeply or superficially conformable with their corresponding distributions.

Observations were performed, according to TCM theory, on the lower limbs of 12 dead fetuses, by injecting ink into points of the three yin meridians near the toes (including the endings of their branches). It showed that the lymphatic vessels travel along the yin meridians, and meet or run close to each other at the place of the point Sanyinjiao (Sp 6), conforming with them in both distance and depth.

Finally, it was observed during some operations under acupuncture anaesthesia, by stimulating tissue directly, that stimulating the nerves would cause numbness, stimulating the blood vessels would often cause pain, whilst stimulating the muscles, tendons or periosteum often caused soreness and a sensation of distension.

THE RELATIONSHIP BETWEEN THE JINGLUO AND THE DERMO-RESISTANCE

Dermo-resistance estimation reveals that points on meridians are marked by low electric resistance and high electrical conductivity, and these are known as "eu-conductive points". It also shows that electrical conductivity is high at meridian points but low at non-meridian points, high at those with sufficient qi and blood but low at those with deficient qi and blood. This shows that the meridian points may be points of electrical conductivity and that the meridians are routes of an electrical current.

However, such research was objected to by arguments holding that the results were often affected by local sweating, humidity, temperature, pressure of the probe during testing, environmental, psychological and emotional factors, as the estimated value varied even in the same subject at different times of testing.

3. RESEARCH INTO THE CONDUCTIVE PATHWAY OF THE ACUPUNCTURE EFFECT

Research into the conductive pathway of the acupuncture effect is one particularly fruitful aspect of research into the jingluo.

THE AFFERENT PATHWAY

Experiments have proven that when a section of the pathway of a related nerve is blocked, cut or broken, the acupuncture effect disappears correspondingly. When the infraorbital nerve of an animal was cut, the effect of acupuncture in raising the blood pressure by puncturing Renzhong (Du 26) stopped; when the median nerve and brachial plexus were blocked, or the posterior cervical roots of the spinal cord (the 6th, 7th and 8th) were cut, it would directly influence the effect of needling Neiguan (P 6). This shows the effect of needling Renzhong may be imported via the infraorbital nerve, and the effect of needling Neiguan was most likely imported via the median nerve.

Experiments were made through observing changes in the bioelectricity of neurofilaments at acupoints in animals, in myoelectric changes on the arrival of qi during needling, and during localized trauma or when the spinal cord was cut. They all proved that acupuncture signals are imported through the peripheral nerves to the spinal cord, and through the lateral side of the anterior spinal cord to higher centres; a route which is closely related to the conductive pathways of pain and warmth. It was also found that the duration of the arrival of qi was largely related to the deep pathways of sensation, and that deep receptors were the main devices producing needling sensations.

Experiments proved that the main pathways of point Zusanli (St 36) were the somatic autonomic nerves. When only the saphenous nerve or the sciatic nerve was cut, or the conduction of only the sympathethic nerve fibres to the femoral artery and vein were blocked, it failed to make the inhibitive effect of the cortically-evoked potential disappear, whilst stimulating Zusanli by electroneedling.

If the above two experiments were combined, then this inhibitive effect disappeared in most of the animals, whilst a weak inhibition remained in a few animals. But when all somatic nerves at the upper part of the thigh were cut, and the sympathetic nervous conduction to the femoral arteries and veins and the obturator artery was blocked, the inhibitive effect of the cortically-evoked potential created applying electroneedling to Zusanli completely disappeared. This indicated that the impulses during electroneedling applied to the points were imported finally through the two pathways of the somatic nerves and the blood vessel sympathetic nerve plexus.

Some researchers hold that indications of points (especially those in the limbs) are mostly conformable with the segmental reflex connections, also that points have their own relative specificity, i.e. acupoints are actually the organic reactive spots on the body's surface of pathological and physiological conditions internally, and that the segmental connections of the somatic visceral nerves are their material basis.

THE EFFERENT PATHWAY

Quite a few researchers hold that some of the acupuncture effects operate through the autonomic nervous system. In cases where the animal's cervical sympathetic nerves and visceral macro-nerves were cut, or the transmission of the sympathetic nerves was blocked with a drug injection, the acupuncture effect when needling Renzhong (Du 26), Zusanli (St 36) or Gongsun (Sp 4) would no longer appear. Also when the animal's vagus nerve was cut, or the parasympathetic nerve blocked with a drug injection, previously observed effects, such as an accelerated heart rate when needling Zusanli, increased movement of the small intestine when needling Neiting (St 44), or a raising of the blood pressure when needling Suliao (Du 25) and Renzhong, were all much reduced or disappeared. This indicates that the autonomic nerves

might be the efferent pathway of the acupuncture effect.

THE RELATIONSHIP BETWEEN THE JINGLUO AND THE BRAIN

Scientific research in this aspect was done through a microelectrode technique in order to observe the electrical activity of the individual neurons. It found that a strong and painful stimulation can produce an electrical discharge from the brain cells, and that non-painful stimulation—such as stimulating certain points on the limbs of a cat or direct stimulation applied to the nerve trunk—could reduce the aforementioned reaction of an electric discharge. This indicates that acupuncture may remarkably reduce the reaction to pain and that such an effect is the result of the interaction of the needling sensation and the pain sensation. At the levels of the thalamus, brain stem and spinal cord, where there are interactions between the painful sensation and the efferent impulse of the needling, it is the needling impulse inhibiting the pain impulse which can be observed.

THE RELATIONSHIP BETWEEN THE NERVES AND HUMORAL COMPOSITION

This research concentrates on neurotransmitters and hormonal change. The acupuncture effect is manifest through changes in humoral composition.

Experiments were performed in which there was perfusion of the extremities in dogs, and cross-circulation in two cats. In the first case, they showed that electroneedling Zusanli (St 36) on the limbs of dogs could inhibit the vessel-dilating reaction of blood vessels on the opposite limbs to the bradykinin in some wounds and to histamine.

In the cross-circulation experiment between two cats, in 21 experiments, complete inhibition of the visceral macro-nervous cortically-evoked potential of cat B whilst cat A was stimulated with electroneedling, was observed in 7 experiments; partial inhibition was observed in 8 experiments; and no change in 6 experiments. This gives an inhibition rate of around 70%, indicating that humoral factors in the cat being needled acted on the cat which had no acupuncture stimulation, through the circulation of the blood between them.

THE RELATIONSHIP BETWEEN ACUPUNCTURE AND NEUROTRANSMITTERS

Experimental research has shown that increasing the content of 5-hydroxytryptamine (5 HT) with eutonyl could potentiate the analgesic effect of electroneedling, whilst reducing the content of 5 HT in the brain with para-chlorophenylamine (PCPA) could obviously decrease the 5 HT in the diencephalon and low brain stem; at the same time, the analgesic effect of electroneedling and morphine were also obviously weakened. This suggests that 5 HT plays an important role in acupuncture analgesia.

Injection of hemicholine (CH3) into the ventricles of the brain in order to reduce the biosynthesis of acetylcholine (ACh) in the brain, would obviously reduce the content of ACh in the brain but it also weakened the analgesic effect of acupuncture.

This suggests that both 5 HT and ACh, which are central neurotransmitters, play an important role in acupuncture analgesia.

Experimental research also showed that the effect of acupuncture is related to a monoamine substance which is similar in effect to morphine; when the monoamine substance had been consumed by the application of reserpine, the analgesic effect of neither morphine nor electroneedling would appear.

Injection of ACh into the ventricles of the brain can enhance the pain threshold, ACh plus electroneedling can also raise the pain threshold, which indicates in a marked manner that the two have a coordinating action.

Electroneedling stimulation on a rat's Shuigou (Du 26) and Chengjiang (Ren 24) points raised the skin pain threshold markedly and, at the same time, the true and pseudo-cholinesterase activity in the thalamus increased to a definite extent. This suggests that the increase of true cholinesterase activity might indicate an increase of ACh in the thalamus, whilst the increase of pseudo-cholinesterase activity might help in the regulation of the ACh content in the brain.

Most experimental research proved that 5 HT and catecholamine (CA) are contradictory to each other, and that their content change may directly affect the analgesic effect of acupuncture; 5 HT content increasing in the peripheral blood system can be observed in cases with a good analgesic effect. Furthermore, the increase in 5 HT content and the analgesic effect form a linear relationship. For example, in cases with a good analgesic effect the CA decreased remarkably.

Experiments also showed that the dopaminergic receptor blocking agent haloperidol applied to potentiate the analgesic effect of electroneedling, can clinically raise the effect of acupuncture analgesia remarkably.

Injection of noradrenaline into the brain ventricles has an analgesic effect which is weaker than that of 5 HT. There are some researchers who hold that noradrenaline can raise the pain threshold markedly and some who hold that the effect of noradrenaline in raising the threshold is of no statistical significance; however, if noradrenaline is injected whilst electroneedling, the threshold can be raised to a marked extent.

Scientists also found recently that, during acupuncture anaesthesia, the endorphins in the brains of animals increased significantly—which was also correlated with the analgesic effect.

The degradation of enkephalin, if delayed, may greatly prolong the analgesic effect of acupuncture.

THE RELATIONSHIP BETWEEN ACUPUNCTURE AND THE ENDOCRINE SYSTEM

The effect on the hypophysis-adrenocortical system. Acupuncture can strengthen the function of the adrenocortical system. It raises the content of cortisol and histamine in the blood and also markedly reduces the content of adrenolipoid, cholesterol and ascorbic acid; it increases the content of ribonucleic acid (RNA) and alkaline phosphatase, and markedly reduces the number of eosinophils in the blood. Acupuncture also influences the adrenocortical function by activating the anterior lobe of the hypophysis to release adrenocorticotropin.

The effect on the sympathetic nerve adrenal medulla system. Acupuncture can increase the numbers of adrenaline-producing cells in the adrenal medulla and the amount of noradrenaline; it can increase the size of cells and deepen the cytoplasmic reaction. Acupuncture applied to animals in shock can raise the blood sugar, lactic acid level and acetonic acid content in the blood markedly, and decrease the glycogen in the liver and muscles accordingly. If the sympathetic nerve chain at the lumbar region of the animal is removed, or the nervous conduction at the punctured site blocked, the original adrenaline-releasing effect will disappear totally. Thus the conclusion is that acupuncture, in releasing adrenaline, becomes operative through the whole nervous reflex arc.

The effect on the hypophysis-thyroid system. Clinical observation shows that needling Hegu (LI 4) and Tiantu (Ren 22) can promote the functional activity of thyroxine. This is the reason why acupuncture is effective in treating simple goitre. Needling or electroneedling can regulate blood sugar levels (decreasing those which are too high or raising those which are too low). This indicates that acupuncture also has an effect in regulating the thyroid function.

The effect on the hypophysis-sexual gland system. Acupuncture can strengthen the secretion of prolactin. Clinical observation shows that acupuncture can also treat infertility and secondary amenorrhoea, and restore normal ovulation and menstrual cycles.

Animal experiments show that, after needling, luteinization of the interstitial cells in the ovary of a rabbit and morphological changes in the sex organs can be observed. These might be caused by the action of gonadotrophin, released by the hypophysis and corpus luteum, acting through the central nervous system.

The effect on the posterior lobe of the hypophysis. Needling Suliao (Du 25) can raise low blood pressure, in a rabbit with shock, owing to acupuncture strengthening the function of the posterior lobe of the hypophysis. If the stem of the hypophysis is cut, the raising of low blood pressure disappears. Needling or electroneedling can also induce the formation and release of the antidiuretic hormone from the posterior lobe of the hypophysis.

4. THE CORRELATION BETWEEN THE VISCERA AND THE BODY SURFACE

The jingluo connect internally with the zangfu and externally with the limbs and joints. Disorders of the internal organs can be treated by needling points on the body surface, and, contrariwise, pathological changes within the internal organs may also affect the body surface—either via the jingluo, i.e. a tender or sensitive spot, or through a point of low electric resistance appearing on the body surface (including the auricle). Therefore research into the ways the internal organs affect the body surface is also one aspect of research into the jingluo, and such work is often done clinically.

For instance, tenderness often appears at Dannangxue (Extra 40) when the gallbladder is diseased, tenderness appears at Lanweixue (Extra 41) in cases of appendicitis, and tenderness appears at Zhongfu (Lu 1) in cases of lung diseases. Observations in recent years show that in cases of stomach disease a reaction may appear at Zusanli (St 36), Weishu (UB 21), Yanglingquan (GB 34) or Zhongwan (Ren 12); and that, in cases of liver disease, a reaction may appear at Yanglingquan, Ganshu (UB 18), Ququan (Liv 8) or Taichong (Liv 3).

These reactions can be classified into two kinds: one is a kind of hypersensitivity accompanied by tenderness, soreness or numbness, the other is a morphological change such as flaccidity, depression or reactive material appearing, such as nodes or rod-shaped prominences. Those appearing at Zusanli and Yanglingquan are rod-shaped, whilst at Weishu, Ganshu and Taichong, reactive morphological changes appear but only in severe cases and are mainly nodular. In deficiency cases there will often be flaccidity and depression appearing at the Back-Shu points.

Among 150 cases, reactions appeared in 149 cases, and in the 10 cases of the control group, without stomach and liver diseases, the reaction was negative. Observations also showed that the severity of the disease and the degree of the reaction were in a parallel relationship: functional diseases have milder point reactions generally while cancer cases have rather stronger reactions observed at their corresponding points.

Animal experiments showed that there exist certain connections between the stomach and the auricle. When the stomach was stimulated or diseased, the low electrical resistance at certain spots increased, suggesting that the sympathetic nerves of the ear and the vagus nerve of the stomach are involved.

Other experimental research showed that a headache may affect the electric conductivity of the auricular points "Head", "Forehead", "Occiput" or "Chin"; and that needling these points can lower and reduce this electric conductivity. Furthermore, the value of this electric activity is that, not only does it reflect the headache, but also it may be used as an objective index in detecting and judging the effects of ear acupuncture in treating such symptoms which facilitates the enhancement of its therapeutic effect.

Acupoints are places on the body surface into which the qi of the zangfu organs and jingluo pours, converges and gathers, and where needling produces a reaction such as the de qi. Study of the tissue structure and physiological function of acupoints may also, therefore, play an important part in research into the real nature of the jingluo.

The *Miraculous Pivot* points out that meridians mostly circulate in the deep tissues,[6] only a few of the jingluo circulate in the superficial portion of the body. Scientific research reveals that the de qi during acupuncture is produced from the deep tissue of these points. When needling the skin or a subcutaneous portion, usually pain, but not a needling sensation, is felt; or in a few cases soreness, numbness and distension (points on the head and auricle are exceptions). If the deep tissue of the points is blocked with procaine, the originally observed acupuncture effects no longer appear; but if only the skin or subcutaneous portion is blocked, the acu-

puncture effect is unaffected or only slightly influenced.

Most experiments show that the production of the de qi during needling originates from several receptors lying deep in the points. Research on limbs (to be amputated) with a uniquely designed concentric electrode "blue dot" method—for locating the needling sensations—was carried out on 14 points, including Zusanli (St 36). This was in order to observe the morphological structure of 44 spots where a needling sensation was felt, and to investigate whether what followed was soreness, numbness, distension, pain (not including the pain caused by stimulating the skin), soreness and distension, soreness-numbness, soreness-pain, distension-numbness, distension-pain, soreness-distension-pain or absence of needling sensation.

These 11 kinds of needling reactions were separately located in muscle, intermuscular connective tissue, tendon, periosteum, joint capsule, connective tissue in joint capsule, and subcutaneous connective tissue. It was found out that differing kinds of needling sensation could be produced in the same structure, and that the same needling sensation could appear in several different structures.

Generally, it was found that the needling sensation of body acupuncture forms in the deep tissues. However, the possibility of there being minute structures in the acupuncture points, which could be the morphological basis for the needling sensation, was also researched. It was found that nerve trunks, branches, sympathetic nerve-endings and free nerve ends, existed universally in all points and in very large numbers; and that, among these, the presence rate of nerve trunks, branches and sympathetic fibres was 100%, and of free endings over 54%. Among the 24 points located in the muscles, the presence rate was equal to that of needling sensation of any kind produced in the muscles. Also the presence rate of muscle spindles, which was secondary to that of the free endings, was found to be basically equal to that of needling sensation.

The presence rate of receptors, such as the tendon spindle, corpuscular lamellose and Krause end bulb was small, but the possibility of them being involved in the structure of needling sensation cannot be excluded completely. It was held that the blood vessels, nerve trunks and branches and the free endings and receptors, located mainly at the points, together form the morphological basis of needling sensation.

Observations on points on the Ren and Du meridians, chest, abdomen, back and lower back, showed that the distribution of these points and the innervation of nerve branches had a certain regularity, and that the receptors of needling sensation at these points were mainly free nerve-endings. Auricular points marked mainly by pain have their receptors for sensation mainly in the superficial nerve-endings. Morphological observations were made upon scalp points—such as Baihui (Du 20), Shangxing (Du 23), Yintang (Extra 2) and Sizhukong (SJ 23)—by making sections on a cadaver, and no receptors with cysts were found. Furthermore, it was hard to tell the difference between acupoints and non-acupoints, showing that the needling sensation might be produced by stimulating the receptors in the follicular nerve networks or the periosteum.

Research was carried out on limbs (before amputation) in order to study the tissue structure of the needling sensation at acupoints, in which stimulation was given to blood vessels, nerves, muscles, tendons and periosteum, and produced different kinds of sensations. Needling nerve trunks mostly caused numbness, stimulating tendons and periosteum mostly caused soreness, stimulating muscles mostly caused soreness and distension, whilst stimulating blood vessels mostly caused pain.

5. SOME OTHER TENTATIVE IDEAS

THE JINGLUO IN GENESIS AND STRUCTURE

According to this viewpoint the human structure is based on the somatome. Researchers held that the somatic nerve-segment to visceral connection is the basis of both the acupoints on the body surface and the meridional-visceral relation. This explains how pathological visceral changes may often be manifest on the correlated body surface, whilst functional changes on the body surface may also affect viscera of the same segment. And, from the distributing form of the acupoints, it can be seen that they are largely conformable with the segmental innervations; this is especially so on the trunk, abdomen and back.

It is held that the reason why acupuncture and moxibustion applied on points can treat diseases of the corresponding viscera, is that there are inner connections between genesis and structure in the organism. The acupoints might be the functional reactive points of visceral pathological and physiological states on the body surface, whilst the segmental connections between the somatic and visceral nerves might be the material basis for conduction along the jingluo.

There is still a great deal of clinical phenomena which cannot be explained by the assumption of nerve segment innervation, such as using the points Guangming (GB 37) and Taichong (Liv 3) in treating eye diseases, and Neiting (St 44) in treating pain in the nose. Therefore the viewpoint of genesis being adopted to explain the real nature of jingluo also is limited.

STUDIES INVOLVING BIOCYBERNETICS

The human body is considered an autocontrol system in biocybernetics. It is held that the jingluo are the control system of the human body, and that there are various kinds of regulatory and controlling processes in the body—such as the regulation of body temperature, blood pressure and blood sugar. All have an autoregulatory process. In this regard, the estimation of the balanced state of the jingluo can help in the diagnosis of disease, and regulating the balanced state of the jingluo will help in the treatment of disease. This implies that perhaps the theory of the jingluo and biocybernetic theory have much in common.

It is held that both acupuncture anaesthesia, and acupuncture and moxibustion treatments are a biocybernetic process, under specific conditions. But biocybernetic theory can only explain some of the physiological functions of the human body in a general way. For concrete and detailed problems it still lacks experimental evidence. Therefore this study is still at a period of conjecture.

THE "THIRD EQUILIBRIUM SYSTEM" ASSUMPTION

There are three balance structures in the human body known in modern physiology: the somatic nervous system, the autonomic nervous system and the endocrine system. The first two have fast reactions which are calculated in seconds, while the last is slower in reaction and calculated in minutes. Considering their speeds, it appears that there might exist an intermediate equilibrium system between the autonomic nervous system and the endocrine system, whose speed is slower than that of the nerves but faster than that of the endocrine system.

Therefore the researchers hold that there are four kinds of equilibrium systems in the human body with their speed and function as follows:

- 1st equilibrium system—the skeletal nerves, with a speed of 100m/second, for fast postural equilibrium,
- 2nd equilibrium system—the autonomic nerves, with a speed of 1m/second, for balance of visceral activities,
- 3rd equilibrium system—the jingluo, with a speed of 10cm/second, for balance between the body surface and the viscera,
- 4th equilibrium system—the endocrine system, with a speed calculated in minutes, for pan-somatic slow equilibrium.

The researchers hold that the activity of the jingluo is very like that of the nerves, and especially the autonomic nerves; but that their speed is far slower than that of the autonomic nerves, so they are called the "third structure"—considering they may or may not be part of the nervous system. Yet even if they are a branch of the nervous system they are a separated individual system.

Researchers hold that the third equilibrium system (of the jingluo) is a new field for future research by neurophysiologists. But others hold that, since research into the real nature of jingluo takes the PSM as their main goal, future research should be done on the basis of the courses of jingluo.

Clinically it is held that improvement in the real conditions of the circulation of the 12 regular meridians, 8 extra meridians and their correlatives should be taken as a prerequisite. Theoretically, modern scientific theories and methods should be widely employed to investigate and study thoroughly the conductive structures of sensation throughout the human body, especially the physiology, pathology and functions of the sensory nerves.

If new findings can be observed to explain the mechanism of, for example, the needling sensation at Dazhui (Du 14) reaching the lumbar and sacral regions, the needling sensation at Guanyuan (Ren 4) and Zhongji (Ren 3) reaching the private parts, and the needle-tip pointing in different directions enabling the needling sensation to radiate accordingly, that is, the physiology, pathology and especially the function of the nerves, related to their sensory conductivity, then it will help explain the mechanism of the radiation and propagation of needling sensation (PSM), which it is difficult for a nervous theory to explain. This would further help us to investigate the sensory structures of the body.

Finally, the combined analysis of results from both these theoretical and clinical studies may help us amass corresponding results in research with regard to understanding the real nature of the jingluo.

The basic mechanism of the acupuncture effect

By generalizing the indications of acupuncture and moxibustion, the effects of both on the organism can, very largely, be classified into three main aspects of function: analgesic, regulatory and immunological.

The mechanisms of acupuncture and moxibustion, and acupuncture anaesthesia (AA), have been researched into in a large number of ways, but they may be considered mainly in two possible ways, i.e. those concerning the jingluo, and those concerning the nervous and humoral systems. Only some mechanisms have been identified, whilst others require further study.

These three main areas of acupuncture and moxibustion research, analgesic, regulatory and immunological, are here briefly introduced.

1. THE ANALGESIC EFFECT

A large number of acupuncture studies and modern clinical experiments have proven that both acupuncture and moxibustion have a satisfactory analgesic effect. It can be observed in treating headache, flank pain, gastric pain, abdominal pain, lumbar pain, trigeminal pain, sciatica, dysmenorrhoea and postoperative pain. Acupuncture anaesthesia is based on, and developed from, good analgesic effects resulting from acupuncture treatment.

Research has shown that needling Neiguan (P 6), Zusanli (St 36), Sanyinjiao (Sp 6), Daheng (Sp 15), Qimen (Liv 14) and Tianshu (St 25) can raise the pain threshold in the abdomen. Experiments in animals have shown that needling Hegu (LI 4) and Neiting (St 44) bilaterally in 30 rabbits, in which the movement of the head caused by applying an electrode to the septum of the nose was taken as the index, caused local anaesthesia in 15 rabbits—making a success rate of 50%. The pain threshold was raised to differing degrees in the 15 rabbits, compared with the threshold before needling, but it did not produce total anaesthesia. This shows that acupuncture does not produce a total anaesthetic effect, but instead raises the pain threshold. It performs an analgesic effect which increases tolerance and reduces sensitivity to pain in the organism.

The manipulation conditioned reflex was taken as the index in research on monkeys, in which a reaction can be complete only with the mediation of a higher nervous system—which is similar to a sense of pain. This research confirmed the analgesic effect of acupuncture.

In many experiments on humans and animals, various kinds of pain-inducing and injuring factors have been applied, and numerous pain thresholds have been taken as indexes. The effect of acupuncture in raising the cutaneous threshold has been confirmed.

So how is it that acupuncture can remove pain? A great deal of research work has been done on the mechanisms of acupuncture analgesia. Descriptions in TCM such as: "the brain is the place where the *shen* (vitality) situates", "the qi comes out of the brain", "work on the *shen* (vitality) to make the qi circulate easier", and "pain disappears, along with the removal of all obstruction", together show that acupuncture can transfer or inhibit the activities of the *shen* and remove obstructions in the meridians, in order to achieve an analgesic effect.

The functions of both the peripheral and the central nervous systems in acupuncture analgesia have been carefully studied.

The peripheral nervous system

Direct electroneedling applied to nerves that conduct the sense of pain can cause a conductive block of the pain sensory fibres in such nerves and inhibit the reaction to an injurious stimulation of the cells within the posterior horns of the spinal cord grey matter. This indicates the possible mediation of the cells in laminae II, III, and IV, as it is known that the peripheral nerves are the afferent nerves of the acupuncture signal.

The central nervous system

A large amount of electro-physiological research has revealed a general condition of mediation at various levels of the central nervous system, for instance the spinal cord, the brain stem, and the thalamus, during analgesia.

Needling can cause postsynaptic inhibition in the posterior horns of the spinal cord. Acupuncture signals transmit along the lateral funiculus of the spinal cord and up to the medulla oblongata, activate the reticular structure, then descend along the posterior and lateral funiculus of the spinal cord and cause depolarization of the fine efferent fibres of the spinal cord, resulting in presynaptic inhibition, which partially blocks the efferent discharge of the fine fibres.

The function of the brain stem in acupuncture analgesia has been proven by the activity of the pain sensitive neurons of the midbrain reticular structure during electroneedling; electroneedling on nuclei of median raphe can not only raise the pain threshold in animals, but also strengthen the analgesic effect of acupuncture. Destroying the locus ceruleus can obviously strengthen the analgesic effect of acupuncture, but stimulating the locus ceruleus reduces the inhibitory effect of electroneedling.

Experiments show that, after receiving acupuncture signals, the grey matter around the aqueduct of the midbrain, the nuclei of the giant cells, and the median raphe at the medial aspect of the reticular structure of the brain stem, all issue descending impulses which inhibit the activity of the pain-transmitting neurons within the posterior horns of the spinal cord, and inhibit the discharge of the pain sensitive cells of the nuclei beside the fascicular thalamicus. These structures of the brain stem themselves may be controlled by structures such as the habenular nuclei.

So the conclusion of the research is that the para-nuclei of the fascicular thalamicus are an important site for the transmission of pain signals, and that needling exerts an inhibitory influence on this site, via highly positioned (the caudate nucleus and cortex) and lowly positioned (the nucleus of the median raphe) pathways. Researchers found that stimulating the caudate nucleus can raise the animal's pain threshold and increase the analgesic effect of electroneedling, but this kind of effect was reduced by destroying the caudate nucleus.

In summary, pain signals, after entering the central nervous system, reach the brain through a very long pathway in which the posterior horns of the spinal cord and the para-nuclei of the fascicular thalamicus are the two key positions. On the other hand, the caudate nuclei, the grey matter around the midbrain, the nuclei of the median raphe of the central nervous system, and the excitation of the descending inhibitory pathways, inhibit the transmission and reception of pain signals. Signals from needling, travelling via the spinal cord to the brain and through complex interactions can activate this inner analgesic system by ascending to inhibit the para-nuclei of the fascicular thalamicus and descending to inhibit the posterior horns of the spinal cord, both these mechanisms exerting an analgesic effect.

Research also holds that central neurotransmitters have an important function in acupuncture analgesia. Experiments in animals show that an increase or decrease of 5 HT content can increase or reduce the analgesic effect of acupuncture accordingly. Conversely catecholamine (CA) has just the opposite effect, because the analgesic effect of acupuncture can be strengthened by blocking the receptors of the CA transmitters.

Blocking the biosynthesis of ACh or the cholinergic receptors can also reduce the analgesic effect of acupuncture. During acupuncture analgesia the endorphins in the cerebral spinal fluid and the brain increase measurably.

Observations showed that the functions of the nervous system and the neurotransmitters are closely integrated. Acupuncture signals increase the content of morphine-like substances in the brain, and they, in turn, act on the grey matter around the aqueduct of the midbrain, thus exciting the nuclei of median raphe to release 5 HT via the descending fibres and inhibiting the posterior horns of the spinal cord.

It was also reported that needling can reduce the concentration of pain-inducing substances in the peripheral blood system, such as potassium ion, histamine and bradykinin.

Finally it is held that psychological factors have an influence on acupuncture analgesia, although these are not a decisive factor in influencing the analgesic effect.

The above shows that acupuncture analgesia is a very complex dynamic process, moving from the periphery to the centre, at differing levels, involving nerves, humoral factors, and pain-inducing or pain-reducing factors in the organism—all under the action of the acupuncture stimulation. Many aspects of these mechanisms of analgesia remain to be further studied and explained.

2. THE REGULATORY EFFECT

Acupuncture and moxibustion have an obvious regulatory effect on the organs and tissues of the various systems of the human body, thereby restoring their normal function. Only a few examples are given here:

THE REGULATORY EFFECT ON ORGANS AND TISSUES

It was reported that needling Shanzhong (Ren 17), Neiguan (P 6) and Zusanli (St 36), in 621 cases of coronary heart disease with angina pectoris, showed a total effective rate of 89%, a markedly effective rate of 48%, and a reduction rate of nitroglycerine intake of 94%.

In 578 cases of coronary heart disease, observation of an ECG before and after needling showed an effective rate of improvement of 53%. In 100 cases of coronary heart disease, observation under electrocardiograph showed the ECG, in 30 cases, to be markedly improved 1–20 minutes after needling—suggesting that needling can improve the coronary circulation.

Observation of an echocardiogram in 100 cases of coronary heart disease showed a very significant difference in the left ventricular posterior wall amplitude of vibration and in cardiac output, compared with that before needling. This indicates that needling may improve the function of the left ventricle in patients with coronary disease.

Observation of a rheo-encephalogram in 50 patients with coronary disease showed a very significant variation, compared with that before needling, indicating that needling may improve cerebral circulation in patients with coronary disease.

According to reports taking the ECG as an objective index, needling treatment given in 46 cases of cardiac arrhythmia showed a total effective rate of 87%, and a good effect was observed especially in cases with abnormal agitation. Reports showed that the effective rate of acupuncture treatment in premature heart beat (42 cases) was 85.7%. The researchers held that acupuncture has no obvious influence on the heart function in normal subjects, but has a favourable regulatory effect on the heart which is diseased.

Acupuncture and moxibustion have a biphasic regulatory function on blood pressure, i.e. they lower the hypertensive and raise the hypotensive. Reports show that acupuncture and moxibustion treatment applied in 230 cases of hypertension, showed an effective rate of 77%. In the treatment of 54 cases of hypertension with the "scarring moxibustion" method, hypertension was significantly relieved, and there was a significant difference observed in the blood viscosity and rheo-encephalogram readings, compared with those taken before moxibustion.

This shows that scarring moxibustion has the effect of improving blood viscosity and dilating the blood vessels to a certain extent. This would reduce the possible severe attacks of a stroke by lowering the blood pressure.

Experiments in animals also showed that acupuncture has an anti-hypertensive effect in various kinds of acute and chronic hypertension. A hypertensive state was caused in rabbits by injecting adrenaline; needling was then given to Zusanli (St 36) and Neiguan (P 6) and a lowering of the blood pressure was observed. The effect of acupuncture in regulating the blood pressure was fully proven by 160 cases of acupuncture treatment applied after shock—after needling Suliao (Du 25) and Neiguan (P 6), a rise in the blood pressure was observed in 87% cases.

Most researchers held that the raising of blood pressure was performed by the transmission of needling sensation through the points to the nerves, through which the impulse was transmitted to the central nervous system (mainly the brain stem and the reticular structure). Then it travelled on, via the autonomic system, especially the sympathetic nerves, to cause a reflex contraction of the small blood vessels of certain viscera, thereby increasing the peripheral resistance and strengthening the systolic function of the heart—all leading to an increase in the blood pressure.

Furthermore, the hormone vasopressin, from the posterior lobe of the pituitary gland, an antidiuretic and adrenocortical hormone, may be mediated in the action, which would further strengthen the effect of raising the blood pressure.

Most researchers held that the antihypertensive effect was produced during needling by its stimulating action on the vagus nerve, whereby ACh levels were increased and those of CA decreased. This caused a dilation of the small blood vessels and a consequent lowering of blood pressure.

The effects of acupuncture and moxibustion in treating diseases of the respiratory system showed results as follows. In 299 cases of asthma, applying moxibustion in summer onto Dazhui (Du 14) and Feishu (UB 13) caused pus to be formed by direct moxibustion. Treatment was given once every other day, with 3 treatments as one course (one course each summer). The effective rate was 70.6% with the markedly effective rate being 29.1%.

In treating 116 cases of bronchial asthma with acupuncture and moxibustion applied to Dazhui (Du 14), Feishu (UB 13), Tiantu (Ren 22), Gaohuang (UB 43), Zhongfu (Lu 1) and Qihu (St 13), 27 cases were cured (no attacks during 3 years), 50 cases obviously improved (frequency and severity of attacks reduced), whilst in 39 cases there was no effect. The researchers held that the occurrence of dyspnoea in bronchial asthma was caused by over-tension in the vagus nerve leading to spasm of the bronchi and increased tubular resistance. Acupuncture can reduce the tone of the vagus nerve and increase the excitation of the sympathetic nerves, thus relieving bronchial spasm, promoting contraction of the blood vessels of the bronchial mucous membrane and reducing fluid exudation, thereby reducing tubular resistance and improving ventilation.

Acupuncture and moxibustion have a good therapeutic effect in treating acute and chronic gastritis, gastric neuralgia, gastrospasm, ptosis of the stomach, and ulcers of the stomach and duodenum. A satisfactory effect has been observed in a hospital treating acute gastric perforations. Experiments in animals also showed that acupuncture had the effect of promoting the repair and healing of experimentally created gastric ulcers and gastric perforation. For example, electroneedling or needling the point Zusanli (St 36) promoted repair in cases of gastric ulcers or perforation.

So then, how did the needling exert an influence on the stomach? Many reports show that needling Zhongwan (Ren 12), Hegu (LI 4), Quchi (LI 11), Weishu (UB 21), Zusanli (St 36) and Chengshan (UB 57) relieves the spasm of the stomach, promotes the movement of the stomach in hypoperistalsis and makes gastric movement decrease in hyperperistalsis, or else facilitates the opening of the pylorus.

Experiments in 10 cases of malnutrition treated with needling Sifeng (Extra 23) showed a strengthening and regulatory action of acupuncture on the secretion of gastric acid. After needling, the pepsin level increased in all cases (before needling the pepsin was decreased); cases with a high level of gastric acid found it reduced after needling, whilst those with a low level of acid found it increased. The above evidence shows that acupuncture and moxibustion obviously have a regulatory effect on the stomach and gastric secretion, and this is the reason they can treat so many differing diseases of the stomach.

Needling the Lanweixue (Extra 41) in healthy subjects can strengthen the peristalsis of the appendix, manifest in its movement, increased tension, and evacuation.

The acupuncture effect on the gallbladder and biliary tract showed results as follows. In a hospital, electroneedling was applied with a dense sparse wave and an intensity up to the tolerance of the patients, on points Qimen (Liv 14) and Riyue (GB 24) for 60 minutes, and then 40 ml of magnesium sulphate (50%) was taken orally after the withdrawal of the needles. Treatment was given once a day, with 10 treatments making up one course.

The 522 cases in the electroneedling group were of 3 types—those stable, those with an acute attack, and those in shock. Clinical observation showed that the stone excretion rate was 35% in the stable group, 89% in the acute attack group, and 50% in the shock group, the total excretion rate being 78%. In the control group, only an oral intake of magnesium sulphate (50%) in 40 ml was prescribed, once a day; and, in the 73 cases with an acute attack, the excretion rate was 27%. Comparing the control group and the acute attack type within the electroneedling therapeutic group, the excretion rate of the needled group was measurably higher than that of the control group and the difference was significant.

Researchers also injected intravenously 20 ml of 50% Biligraphin (X-ray contrast medium), plus 100 ml 10% glucose, over one hour; 15 minutes later 5 mg morphine was injected subcutaneously to cause a spasm of the sphincter of Oddi at the biliary tract orifice. Then needling was given when the contrast was visualized in the biliary tract, and X-ray photographs were taken successively at fixed intervals. Points Juque (Ren 14), Yanglingquan (GB 34), Zusanli (St 36) and Burong (St 19) on the right side were used in the needling group whilst no needling was given in the control group. The methods of observation in the two groups were the same.

The results showed that, out of 4l cases in the needling group, there were 37 with significant change, and 4 without significant change, an effective rate of 90%; among the 14 cases of the control group, only 4 cases had any significant observable change, an effective rate of 28%. A marked difference was observed between the two groups.

The conclusions were, first, that needling Juque, Burong (on the right-hand side), Yanglingquan and Zusanli, obviously relieved the spasm of Oddi's sphincter of the biliary tract orifice and promoted the contraction of the common bile duct, the effect being stronger during manipulation of the needles, weaker during retention of the needles and disappearing after their withdrawal; second, that needling also promoted the secretion of bile and had a good analgesic effect which facilitated the discharge of the biliary stones. Furthermore it was suggested that by increasing the intensity of needling stimulation, the frequency of manipulation or the retention of the needles, the therapeutic effect could be enhanced.

Cholangiography was done (under a morphine injection) in patients with external drainage of the bile duct, which showed that 30 minutes after needling Qiuxu (GB 40), Yanglingquan (GB 34) and Riyue (GB 24), a regular contraction of the common bile duct appeared and peristalsis increased, obviously forcing the contrast medium through the sphincter of the orifice of the bile duct and into the duodenum. In another 2 cases of gallstones after operations of choledochostomy or cholecystotomy, after needling Qiuxu, Yanglingquan and Riyue the excretion of bile increased markedly, indicating that acupuncture has a significant regulatory or strengthening effect on the excretion and secretion of bile.

212 cases of acute viral hepatitis with jaundice treated with acupuncture were observed. The main points used were Taichong (Liv 3) angled towards Yongquan (K 1), and Zusanli (St 36). In the manual needling group, quick insertion and half an hour retention of the needles was applied and manipulation given every 5 minutes to strengthen the sensation. In the electroneedling group, the electrodes were applied separately on the main points for half an hour with dense-sparse waves: 177 cases were cured, 34 cases improved and in 1 case there was no effect.

Also reported were 55 cases of acute viral hepatitis treated with acupuncture and moxibustion, among which the type with jaundice were treated with Zusanli (St 36) and Yanglingquan (GB 34) angled towards Yinlingquan (Sp 9); and the type without jaundice with Zusanli, Yinlingquan and Sanyinjiao (Sp 6). Rapid insertion of the needles was used and strong stimulation given after the de qi; the needles were retained for 30–40 minutes and manipulation applied every 15 minutes. Treatments were given once a day until a cure was achieved. The type without jaundice were treated in combination with moxibustion.

The chief symptoms and signs, conditions of liver enlargement, liver function and depth of jaundice, were taken as criteria and all 55 cases were seen to be cured. This indicates that acupuncture and moxibustion have a good effect in reducing liver enlargement and enhancing its various functions.

Acupuncture and moxibustion also have a regulatory effect on kidney and bladder function, and a good effect in relieving nocturnal enuresis, incontinence of urine, retention of urine and dysuria. It was reported that Qihai (Ren 6), Guanyuan (Ren 4), Zhongji (Ren 3), Shuidao (St 38) and Sanyinjiao (Sp 6) were used with electroneedling in treating 100 cases of post-surgical retention of urine with the positive electrode on the points of the Ren Meridian and the negative electrode on the points of the lower limbs, for 15–30 minutes. In 61 cases under epidural anaesthesia there was an effective rate of 95%, while in 29 cases under spinal anaesthesia there was an effective rate of nearly 90%. This indicates that the treatment exerted a better effect in urinary retention after epidural anaesthesia applied during the operation than in the cases after an operation under spinal anaesthesia.

It was reported that acupuncture was also used as the main therapy in combination with herbal treatment in the treatment of some 29 cases of urinary stones. 15 cases were cured, in 5 cases there was some effect and in 9 cases no effect.

In one study acupuncture was applied to Shenshu (UB 23) in patients with an attack of nephritis. An obvious improvement of the diuretic function of the kidney was observed, along with a marked increase of phenolsulphonphthalein excretion, a decrease in or even disappearance of red and white cells in the urine, a lowering of blood pressure and relief of oedema.

Cyclic adenosine monophosphate (cAMP) is a key intermediate transmitter for cells reacting to any exogenous stimulation. It affects the cell's secretion, permeability and bio-synthesis, and conduction along the nerves, hormonal and auto-immune reactions, and is also related to the analgesic effect of acupuncture.

The influence of needling Fuliu (K 7) and Zhishi (UB 52) on changes in cAMP was observed, along with the creatinine level and volume of urine in normal subjects. An obvious rise in volume, and a change in the level of excretion of creatinine and cAMP in the urine was observed in 3 cases; there was a rise in the volume of urine and creatinine level in the urine in one case and a decrease following a rise in 3 cases. This suggested that needling Zhishi and Fuliu might have a regulatory effect on the renal activities.

The acupuncture effect on the renal diuretic function might be brought about on one hand, via the influence of a nervous reflex on the glomerular filtration rate, and, on the other, via the influence of the secretion of antidiuretic hormone on the reabsorption of the renal tubules. The mechanism influencing the content of protein in the urine might be related to acupuncture regulating the permeability of the capillaries. An acupuncture effect on the bladder may be achieved by regulating the tension of the bladder, by making the hypotense muscles contract and the hypertense relax. This is the reason why acupuncture may treat not only urinary retention but also nocturnal enuresis.

The effect of acupuncture and moxibustion on strengthening uterine contractions was also observed. Acupuncture and moxibustion were applied in 219 cases in order to hasten and induce childbirth. Among 134 cases where they were used for hastening childbirth the effective rate was 81%, among 85 cases where they were used for inducing labour the effective rate was 66%. One group used the distal points Hegu (LI 4), Sanyinjiao (Sp 6), Zusanli (St 36); one group used local points Zhibian (UB 54), Qugu (Ren 2) and Henggu (K 11); and one group used mixed points Zhibian, Hegu and Sanyinjiao.

It was held that the mechanism whereby uterine contractions were increased was marked by a reaction in the nervous system, in which, after needling the local points, the contractions increased rapidly and after removal of needles decreased at once. This has been proven also in animals. After needling the distal points (Hegu and Sanyinjiao) the reaction of the uterus was delayed—just as in the effects of oxytocin—coming about 20 minutes later, but the contractions were persistent and regular. This might be related to an increase in secretion of the posterior pituitary hormone.

Acupuncture also has a regulatory effect on nervous functions. Caffeine sodium benzoate was injected subcutaneously into a dog to cause excitation of the cerebral cortex and further reduce salivary secretion. Then electroneedling was applied and it was observed that salivary secretion was reduced even further, to nearly zero at the beginning, gradually restoring itself back to normal or even higher than the original amount later. This indicates that electroneedling has an obvious regulatory effect on the excitation and inhibition of the cerebral cortex.

Needling Shenmen (H 7), Yinxi (H 6), Tongli (H 5), Baihui (Du 20) and Daling (P 7) in patients with epilepsy could regulate the EEG in most patients with grand mal epilepsy, or lower the electric potential of pathological brain waves. This indicates that acupuncture and moxibustion can influence the process of nervous activity in the cerebral cortex, have a regulatory effect and restore a balance between excitation and inhibition.

THE REGULATORY EFFECT ON THE COMPOSITION OF THE BLOOD

Various kinds of stimulation (either exogenous or endogenous) on the organism often make a change in composition of the blood. Acupuncture and moxibustion have a regulatory effect on blood composition, with an obvious effect on the white cell count, red cell count, thrombocyte level, blood sedimentation rate, blood sugar and blood calcium levels.

It was reported that acupuncture and moxibustion were applied in treating 29 cases of leucocytopenia due to radioactive exposure. Initially the lowest white cell count was $650/mm^3$ and the highest $3800/mm^3$. The result was that 12 cases were cured (white cells increased to 5000–$7000/mm^3$), in 9 cases there was a marked effect (white cells 4000–$5000/mm^3$ or an increase of $2000/mm^3$), in 3 cases a poor effect (the increase was less than $2000/mm^3$ or white cells kept below $4000/mm^3$ after needling), and in 3 cases no effect or aggravation (these cases all with insufficiency of liver function). The effective rate was thus 90%.

It was reported that needling Dazhui (Du 14), Ganshu (UB 18) and Zusanli (St 36) for the treatment of tropic hypereosinophilic syndrome showed that, after needling, the eosinophil count decreased, and the effective rate was 100%.

It was reported that heavy thrusting and lifting during needling was applied to Hegu (LI 4) and Zusanli (St 36), on both sides, and the total leucocyte count was observed before and after needling. The result was that in 3 cases, with a total leucocyte count above $6000/mm^3$ before needling, a decrease was observed 3 hours after the needling; and in 5 cases, with a total leucocyte count below $6000/mm^3$ before needling, an increase was observed 3 hours after needling. Furthermore, the lower the total leucocyte count before needling, the more obvious the increase after needling, indicating that acupuncture had a regulatory effect, correcting the total leucocyte count and returning it to normal.

Research also showed that, by blocking with procaine the nerve trunks related to the points, or applying spinal anesthesia to inhibit the central nerves, no change in the quantity and quality of the leucocytes was observed after needling. Thus it was held that acupuncture can operate only when the efferent and afferent central nervous function and structure are complete.

Some people held that acupuncture operated through the way in which a stimulus is transmitted afferently via the peripheral angio-sympathetic nerve fibres and within the total environment of the nervous and endocrine system, i.e. through the mediation and under the influence of the pituitary and adrenal glands, and the autonomic nervous system, which all affected and regulated the formation and distribution of leucocytes.

Research during treatment of iron-deficiency anaemia with acupuncture and moxibustion showed that, after needling, the number of reticulocytes (immature red cells) in the peripheral blood system increased drastically. After an anaemic state was produced artificially in rabbits, needling was given to Geshu (UB 17) and Gaohuang (UB 43). Compared with those in the control group, the needling group were much more rapidly corrected and restored to normal. Needling was also applied in treating splenic panhaematopenia and hypercythaemia and certain therapeutic effects were observed. These indicate that acupuncture and moxibustion also have a regulatory effect on increasing and decreasing the number of erythrocytes.

In treating patients with inflammation who had an increased blood sedimentation rate with acupuncture and moxibustion, the symptoms were improved after needling and the blood sedimentation rate also returned to normal.

It was also reported that, in treating 8 cases of thrombocytosis after removal of the spleen, by needling Dazhui (Du 14), Zusanli (St 36), Neiguan (P 6), and Quchi (LI 11), the number of thrombocytes in all cases was reduced gradually to normal along with the needling.

In treating haemoptysis in pulmonary tuberculosis (109 cases) with plum-blossom needle tapping on the throbbing area of the carotid artery for 10–20 minutes, haemoptysis was stopped and this state maintained for 4–6 hours. Furthermore it was also held that an increase in thrombocytes was greatly significant in checking the blood loss; this indicates that acupuncture has an obvious and favourable regulatory effect on the increase and decrease of thrombocytes.

The treatment of 24 cases of diabetes by needling Pishu (UB 20), Geshu (UB 17) and Zusanli (St 36) showed that acupuncture has an effect in lowering the blood sugar. In 11 cases there was a marked effect, in 4 cases a good effect and in 4 cases some improvement, whilst in 5 cases there was no effect. The total effective rate was 79%.

The treatment of 30 cases of diabetes by needling Lieque (Lu 7), Qichong (St 30) and Taibai (Sp 3), during which the content of the blood sugar and the permeability of the blood vessels were estimated separately, showed that, after needling, the blood sugar decreased markedly while the capillary permeability was enhanced.

Reports show that needling Suliao (Du 25) had the effect of raising the blood sugar in patients with shock.

Observations on electroneedling applied in cases of hypoglycaemia caused by an injection of insulin, and hyperglycaemia caused by an injection of adrenaline in rabbits, showed a corresponding correction in the blood sugar level in both cases. Estimations of the secretion of insulin and adrenaline in cases of hypertension, both before and after needling or electroneedling, showed an increase in insulin secretion along with a decrease in blood sugar. It was held that the acupuncture had the effect of returning the blood sugar to a healthy state of balance, and that this effect might well be performed via the reflex action of the nerves on the secretion of insulin.

Reports also showed that acupuncture had the effect of increasing the blood calcium. Needling treatment was given in cases where there were spasms due to hypocalcinaemia (12 cases), once a day, for 10 minutes, with the needle retained. After 3 treatments, the blood calcium increased and the spasms disappeared, while the blood phosphate level decreased in all cases. The researchers held that needling intervertebral sites (particularly C5–C6) and the point Dazhu (UB 11) might affect the function of the parathyroid gland and regulate the metabolism of calcium and phosphate in the body.

Needling Sifeng (Extra 25), in cases of malnutrition complicated with rickets, showed an increase of serum calcium and phosphate, and a decrease in the activity of alkaline phosphatase, promoting the growth and development of the bones in affected infants. It was found that, in some units in cases differentiated as yang deficient, the blood lactic acid level was markedly higher than that in other patients. After needling, the blood lactic acid and potassium levels decreased markedly, although no obvious changes were observed in cases of yin deficiency.

This is the reason why acupuncture anaesthesia is particularly effective in cases of yang deficiency. It was held that the increase in the concentration of blood potassium led to a reduction in the excitation of the nerves and pain receptors, which might be related to the mechanism which produces acupuncture analgesia.

Research also found that, in 22 cases, 30 minutes after needling, the excretion of urinary sodium increased, that of blood sodium decreased and, simultaneously, the excretion of urinary potassium decreased while the blood potassium increased.

These results all show that acupuncture has a certain regulatory effect on the electrolytes in the blood, particularly influencing the blood calcium. It may be one of the reasons why acupuncture can be applied in treating spasms and contractions of the limbs, and rickets due to malnutrition.

Acupuncture can decrease the transaminase in the blood of hepatitis cases. In cardiovascular diseases, after needling, the serum cholesterol and beta-ester protein levels decreased and the blood viscosity reduced. In treating appendicitis with acupuncture, the activity of serum cholinesterase can be reduced, resulting in a decrease in ACh content in the blood. Acupuncture also had a regulatory effect on the lactic acid, pyruvic acid, citric acid and histamine levels. All such changes in the blood favour the improvement of the disease.

In short, acupuncture has the effect of returning to physiological balance various substantial elements in the blood, altering its chemical composition, affecting the blood amylase system and its electrolyte level. This is greatly significant for maintaining balance within the inner environment of the body.

The regulatory effect of acupuncture on the blood always goes along with an improvement in clinical manifestations. Observations show that the influence of acupuncture on the blood picture in normal subjects is not significant, and both temporary and irregular; but under pathological conditions, acupuncture has a significant favourable regulatory effect on the blood, returning it to physiological balance.

3. THE IMMUNOLOGICAL EFFECT

Acupuncture and moxibustion can strengthen the body's resistance and prevent illness, such as attacks of the common cold, the recurrence of malaria and asthma, etc. Acupuncture can treat diseases due to viruses, such as the common cold, mumps, icteric or non-icteric hepatitis; diseases due to bacteria, such as dysentery, enteritis and tetanus, and malaria due to parasites; and various acute and chronic inflammatory conditions, such as acute and chronic pharyngitis and laryngitis, appendicitis, gastritis, conjunctivitis, otitis media, mastitis, etc. Acupuncture and moxibustion have a favourable influence on the major pathological processes of inflammatory disease and are obviously effective in helping the subsidence of fever. All these results are achieved through a strengthening of the bodily resistance of the organism.

645 cases of acute bacillary dysentery with a positive result from stool culture were treated with needling at Qihai (Ren 6), Tianshu (St 25), Shangjuxu (St 37), Quchi (LI 11) and Hegu (LI 4). The reducing method was used, along with heavy lifting, gentle thrusting and rotation, and 30–60 minutes' retention of needles. Treatment was given 1–3 times a day, and 10 days treatment constituted 1 course. 596 cases were cured after 1 course of treatment with a curative rate of 92%.

Experimental research among 50 in-patients whilst observing 8 indexes—serum protein electrophoresis, serum total complement content, immunoglobulin content, plasma bactericidal power, antibody titration (specific), content of SIgA in stools, content of serum lysozyme and the phagocytic power of the hepatic reticuloendothelial system, showed that during acupuncture treatment the immunological power was strengthened continuously. The beneficial effect of acupuncture in treating acute bacillary dysentery was related to the strengthening of humoral immunological functions (both specific and non-specific) in the patients.

Observations during treatment with acupuncture of 33 cases of acute bacillary dysentery showed that all the cases were clinically cured, and also that, whilst before needling the cholinesterase activity of the whole blood was mostly lower than normal, after treatment in 64.7% cases it recovered its normal activity. Furthermore, whilst before needling the serum protein was decreased and the globulin level increased, after needling the serum proteins kept decreasing. Also the transformation rate of the lymphocytes was quite markedly lower than normal before needling, whilst after needling it was markedly higher. Thus it was held that acupuncture can regulate metabolism, both restoring the normal functioning of the organism when in a state of disorder and enhancing immunological functions.

Experiments made on 13 rabbits by needling Zusanli (St 36) on one side only, showed that, 2–3 hours after the needling, an increase in total leucocyte count was observed in 60% cases, an increase of neutrophils and decrease of lymphocytes in 36% cases, whilst 24 hours later they returned to nearly normal.

Needling Zusanli (St 36) and Hegu (LI 4) in 100 normal subjects revealed that the effective proportion of leucocytes phagocytizing *Staphylococcus aureus* increased from 48% to 71%, whilst no obvious changes were observed in the control group. This indicates that after needling the phagocytic function of the leucocytes was increased.

Observations made whilst needling Dazhui (Du 14) and Mingmen (Du 4) in male rats showed that acupuncture had the effect of activating and increasing the phagocytic activities of the hepatic reticulo-endothelial system. The most rapid increase was observed in the first week, whilst the speed of increase slowed down during the second week, proving that acupuncture had the effect of activating the phagocytic function of the reticulo-endothelial system.

Acupuncture can mobilize immunological physiological functions within the human body.

The serum opsonin is one of the immunological factors (non-specific) in the human body. After needling Zusanli (St 36) in rabbits, the serum opsonin promoting phagocytic index, the promoting phagocytic rate and the mean maximum number of phagocytes in phagocytizing bacteria, were all enhanced to a certain extent, compared with those recorded before needling. No increase was observed in the control group, indicating that acupuncture can mobilize an immunological function in the organism in order to fight against an invasion by exogenous pathogenic factors.

Experiments in animals showed that moxibustion can promote the production of agglutinin and haemolysin in rabbits. After moxibustion, the content of the IgG in the serum of the animals increased obviously, and the amount of the haemolytic plaque was markedly higher than that in the control group. This shows that moxibustion has a promoting effect on the immunological humoral system, which may be related to a strengthening in the production of antibodies and cell activity; the results also suggest that two moxa cones applied on Dazhui (Du 14) have a good effect.

Observation of changes in the immunological functions of the cells in 20 cases of hyperplasia of the mammary glands, both before and after needling, showed that acupuncture had the effect of promoting the formation of the E rosette and total E rosette.

Some reports mentioned that the sulphydryl group content, which is closely related to the defensive mechanism of the tissues, increased after needling.

What may be the mechanism behind this superior effect of acupuncture and moxibustion on the immunological system in the body?

In one experiment, turpentine oil was used to cause inflammation in rabbits' ears, and after needling Hegu (LI 4), the area and thickness of inflammation was much smaller and less common than that in the control group. This shows that acupuncture has a significant anti-inflammatory effect. But after cutting the posterior root of the spinal nerve or close to the superior cervical ganglion, acupuncture no longer exerted such an effect.

In this case it was held that the pathway of the acupuncture effect may be via the posterior roots innervated in the skin and muscles at the areas being punctured, leading to the spinal cord, and then to the lateral horns at the thoracic segment, the superior cervical ganglion, the fibres posterior to the ganglion and finally to the focal lesions on the rabbits' ears. It was held that acupuncture was effective mainly through the reflex reaction of the nerves.

In experiments on animals, in the needling group, the content of adrenocortico-lipoid, cholesterol and Vitamin C decreased, while that of ribonucleic acid (RNA), and alkaline phosphatase (AKP) increased. This indicates that the adrenocortical function was strengthened by needling. But if the nerve pathways were blocked or the adrenal glands on both sides were cut, no such effect would be observed after needling.

In short, this would seem to indicate that the effects of acupuncture and moxibustion on immunity are many-sided. The increased functional activity of the reticulo-endothelial system, and the increase of various specific and non-specific immunological antibodies in the organism, are all of great significance, and these effects may be related to nervous and humoral activities.

The above three main effects of acupuncture and moxibustion on the organism—analgesic, regulatory, and immunological—are interrelated and not separate from each other. The result of a functional regulation is the strengthening of the body's resistance (including both relief from pain and enhanced immunity); and the strengthening of the body's resistance is itself a manifestation of a functional regulation. The therapeutic effect of acupuncture and moxibustion in the clinic is mediated through many actions—for instance, in the last example, the anti-inflammatory effect of needling was probably a synthesized result of its effect on the autonomic nerves, local blood circulation, cellular immunity and the endocrine glands.

4. OTHER FACTORS

Acupuncture and moxibustion, similar to other

specialties of medicine, have their own scope of indication and are not universally indicated for every disease. In addition, the following aspects are especially worth mentioning and should be always borne in mind.

THE SPECIFICITY OF ACUPOINTS

Acupoints have their own relative specificity, e.g. Jingming (UB 1) can treat myopia in young patients but Zhiyin (UB 67) is without this effect; Zhiyin can correct malposition of the fetus but Jingming has no such effect; Sifeng (Extra 25) can be used in treating malnutrition and indigestion in children, but if Bafeng (Extra 42) is used the effect is poorer. Suliao (Du 25) can be used to raise the blood pressure in patients with shock; needling Quchi (LI 11) also has an effect in raising blood pressure, but it is not as good as Suliao. There are many other such examples, showing that acupoints have their own relative specificity.

THE METHODS OF MANIPULATION

Acupuncture effects vary with various kinds of needling methods, e.g. in treating shock, continuous manipulation of needles and retention of needles for one hour or more is required to achieve good therapeutic results; in treating acute bacillary dysentery, only applying a reducing method with a strong needling sensation and the needles retained for about 30 minutes can obtain a satisfactory result. In the above two cases, if the needles were withdrawn shortly after the needling sensation was achieved, it would be difficult to obtain good results.

In treating peripheral nerve paralysis, in its initial stages, mild stimulation applied after the needling sensation is achieved can exert a good effect, while strong stimulation or electroneedling applied for a long duration would often achieve an unsatisfactory effect.

During needling, attention should also be paid to the needling depth, whether reinforcing or reducing, the length of time the needle is retained, and the way the needle is manipulated—all

according with the differentiation of the particular syndrome. This is greatly significant in enhancing acupuncture's therapeutic effect.

CHOICE OF THE RIGHT TIME FOR TREATMENT

This is closely related to the therapeutic effect; e.g. in treating facial paralysis and hemiplegia after a stroke with acupuncture and moxibustion, if the treatment starts as early as possible after the attack the therapeutic result will be markedly enhanced, if it is 3–6 months later, or delayed even longer, the effect will be much poorer.

Another example: in treating malaria, if needling is given 2 hours before the attack the effect of acupuncture is usually good, but if the needling is given after the attack, the therapeutic effect will obviously be much poorer.

Furthermore, the quality of the material and thickness of the needle has also a certain relationship with the therapeutic effect, e.g. in applying warm needling, the temperature in silver needles is markedly higher than that in stainless steel needles and their clinical efficacy also differs.

Conclusion

Acupuncture and moxibustion have played an extremely important role in the health care of the Chinese people for several thousand years and more recently have been employed in clinical treatment and involved in research in more than one hundred countries throughout the world.

The above research into the acupuncture jingluo system has proven not only the objective existence of the transmission of the needling sensation along the course of the meridian, but also the pattern of its transmission, providing important clues to the real nature of the jingluo.

It also shows that acupuncture and moxibustion have the function of regulating the various systems of the organism and strengthening the body's resistance. Their therapeutic effect in treating cerebrovascular and cardiovascular diseases, calculi of the biliary tract, bacillary dysentery, etc. is confirmed by scientific methods (as shown above). Their mechanism of effect has been expounded by modern physiology, biochemistry, microbiology and immunology, and a large amount of statistical data and material accumulated in this respect.

Also it is shown that the mechanism of acupuncture analgesia may be understood from the aspects of both the peripheral and central nervous system, electrophysiology, and through the action of various neurotransmitters.

This unique science has become an imponent part of world medicine and will exert an active and wide influence in the future

The important task for all of us who are engaged in acupuncture and moxibustion practice today is to inherit and develop the legacies of TCM through teaching, clinical practice and research work under the guidance of its theories. We need further research into the real nature of the jingluo and the mechanism of acupuncture and moxibustion, so as to enrich and perfect this science. Provided we try our best to apply the viewpoint of dialectical materialism, and are courageous in our practice, we will certainly obtain subsequent achievements in this medical field so as to contribute further to the health care of mankind.

NOTES

1. These are painful points, literally "Ow! that's it! points".
2. *Miraculous Pivot*, Ch.10, "Meridians".
3. *Miraculous Pivot*, Ch.13 "Meridians and Muscles".
4. Ibid.
5. See *Miraculous Pivot*, Ch. 47, "Origins of the Zang", Ch. 78, "Discussion on the 9 Needles".
6. *Miraculous Pivot*, Ch. 10 "Meridians".

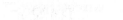

PART 1

JINGLUO AND ACUPOINTS

A general introduction to the jingluo 1

The theory of the *jingluo* (经络), or meridians and collaterals, results from the study of the course and distribution, physiological function and pathological change of the meridian and collateral system in the human body; and its interrelationship with the *zang* (脏), solid and *fu* (腑), hollow, internal organs, collectively known as the *zangfu*. The theory of the jingluo is an important component part of the theoretical system of TCM, and it has an especially close relationship with acupuncture and moxibustion, formed and developed, as it is, on the basis of long medical practice by the ancient physicians.

It has been the guiding principle of diagnosis and treatment in TCM ever since these ancient times.

Jingluo is a collective term in TCM. *Jing* (经), has the meaning of a "pathway", and the jing, or meridians, constitute the main trunks of the jingluo system, running longitudinally and interiorly within the body. The *luo* (络), on the other hand, are the collaterals, which represent a branching network, running transversely and superficially from, and interlocking with, the jing.

It is stated in the *Miraculous Pivot* that "the interior channels are the jing, the transverse branches are the luo, the sub-branches are the sub-collaterals".[1]

The jingluo connect interiorly with the zangfu and exteriorly with the body's surface and its extremities. They form a network which links the zangfu, tissues and other organs as one organic whole. They transport qi and blood which nourish yin and yang so that the normal functioning of the various organs is ensured and a relative equilibrium maintained.

Not only the differentiation of syndromes according to the jingluo, but also the selection of acupoints according to the course of the meridians, and the reinforcing and reducing methods of needling in the clinic, are all based on the theory of the jingluo.

It is recorded in the *Miraculous Pivot* that "the 12 meridians are the place where life and death are determined, disease is generated, treated and cared for; they are the place where beginners start and acupuncture masters end".[2] This shows the great importance of the jingluo in physiology, pathology, diagnosis and treatment.

The formation of the theory of jingluo

The jingluo theory was systematized by the ancient Chinese people during their long medical practice, and a preliminary theoretical system had been formed at the time of compilation of the *Nei Jing*, or *Yellow Emperor's Book of Medicine* (second century BC to second century AD).

According to analyses of records in medical literature and classics, the formation of the theory is generally considered to be related to the observation of the following aspects.

Transmission of the needling sensation

Needling may give rise to a reaction of soreness, numbness, heaviness and distension, which is known as "needling sensation" and transmits along a certain route to distant areas.

This is just as it states in the *Miraculous Pivot*, "if an acupoint is accurately punctured the needling sensation will transmit, just as people travel along streets and lanes".[3] Moxibustion will also give rise to a kind of hot or warm sensation, spreading from where the moxa is applied to distant areas.

On the basis of the long-term observation of these complex yet regular links and pathways, an outline of the distribution of the jingluo was put forward by the ancient physicians.

Generalization of the therapeutic effects of acupoints

Through the long-term practice of acupuncture and moxibustion, acupoints with similar indications were found, located regularly along certain lines.

For instance, acupoints located on the anterior border of the lateral aspect of the upper limbs are all indicated in syndromes of the head and face, and acupoints located on the anterior border of the medial aspect of the upper limbs—although very near the points mentioned above—are mainly indicated in syndromes of the throat, chest and lung. Acupoints with similar therapeutic effects were thus summarized and classified into separate categories, forming the lines of the jingluo.

Deduction from pathological manifestations on the body's surface

During clinical practice, tenderness, nodules, skin eruptions and discolorations were found in areas corresponding to zangfu organs, at the same time as pathological changes were occurring in that organ. Therefore the observation and analysis of pathological phenomena on the body's surface was also one of the ways in which the system of the jingluo was discovered.

The enlightenment of anatomy and physiology

Through anatomical practice the ancient physicians recognized, to a certain extent, the position, shape and physiological function of the various viscera in the human body. They found the distribution of many tubular and rope-like structures in the body, and their links with the four extremities, and also the circulation of the blood within some of the vessels. These observations gave enlightenment to the recognition of the jingluo.

The above different aspects show that there were different ways of discovering the existence of the jingluo, and that each could act as evidence, the one enlightening and supplementing the other. It is clear, according to the medical literature still surviving, that the formation of jingluo theory can be dated back at least two thousand years.

The composition of the jingluo system

The jingluo system consists of the jing (meridians), including 12 regular meridians and 8 extra meridians, and in addition 12 divergent meridians, 12 muscle regions and 12 cutaneous regions attached to the 12 regular meridians; and the luo (collaterals), meaning the 15 collaterals, including various other superficial collaterals and sub-collaterals.

The network of the jingluo is as follows (see Table 1.1).

THE 12 REGULAR MERIDIANS

The 12 meridians are the three yin meridians of the hand (lung, pericardium and heart), the three yang meridians of the hand (large intestine, sanjiao and small intestine), the three yang meridians of the foot (stomach, gallbladder and urinary bladder), and three yin meridians of the foot (spleen, liver and kidney).

They form the main part of the system of the jingluo and are therefore called the 12 regular meridians.

The complete name of each of the 12 regular meridians is composed of three parts: these identify it as either hand or foot, yin or yang, and linked to either a zang or fu organ.

The meridians that pertain to the zang organs are the yin meridians, mainly distributed on the medial (yin) aspect of the hands or feet. Those distributed on the medial aspect of the upper limbs are the three yin meridians of the hand, while those distributed on the medial aspect of the lower limbs are three yin meridians of the foot.

The meridians that pertain to the fu organs are the yang meridians, and they supply mainly the lateral (yang) aspect of the four limbs. Those supplying the lateral aspect of the upper limbs are the three yang meridians of the hand, while those supplying the lateral aspect of the lower limbs are the three yang meridians of the foot.

Furthermore both upper limbs and lower limbs are divided into the anterior, middle and posterior regions, which are supplied respectively by three yin (Taiyin, Shaoyin and Jueyin) and three yang (Yangming, Taiyang and Shaoyang) meridians. These names are determined by the inter-transforming relationship between yin and yang, and the exterior-interior relationship between the three yin and three yang meridians.

This then explains the nomenclature of the 12 regular meridians, for example the lung meridian of the hand Taiyin and the large intestine meridian of the hand Yangming.

Table 1.1   The network of meridians and collaterals

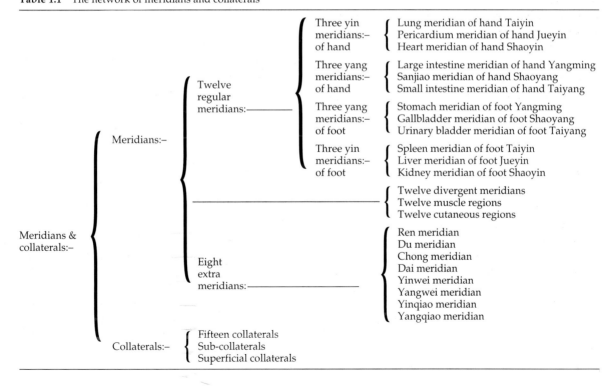

As regards the distribution of the 12 regular meridians on the body surface, they are placed symmetrically on left and right sides of the body—over the head, trunk and limbs. The medial aspect of the limbs is attributed to yin, the lateral to yang. Each limb is supplied by three yin and three yang meridians.

On the upper limbs, the anterior border of the medial aspect is supplied by the meridian of the hand Taiyin, the middle of the medial aspect by the meridian of the hand Jueyin, and the posterior border of the medial aspect by the meridian of the hand Shaoyin; whilst the anterior border of the lateral aspect is supplied by the meridian of the hand Yangming, the middle of the lateral aspect by the meridian of the hand Shaoyang, and the posterior border of the lateral aspect by the meridian of the hand Taiyang.

On the lower limbs, the anterior border of the lateral aspect is supplied by the meridian of the foot Yangming, the middle of the lateral aspect by the meridian of the foot Shaoyang, and the posterior border of the lateral aspect by the meridian of the foot Taiyang.

The distribution of the three yin meridians of the foot is as follows. Above the place where the foot Jueyin crosses the foot Taiyin (8 cun above the internal malleolus), the anterior, middle and posterior aspects of the lower limbs are supplied respectively by the meridians of the foot Taiyin, foot Jueyin and foot Shaoyin; below the place where the foot Jueyin and foot Taiyin meridians cross, the anterior is supplied by the foot Jueyin, the middle by the foot Taiyin and the posterior by the foot Shaoyin.

Among the 12 regular meridians, yin meridians pertain to zang organs and communicate with fu organs, while yang meridians pertain to fu organs and communicate with zang organs. Thus there is formed an exterior-interior relationship between yin and yang, zang and fu. This is as follows: the lung meridian of the hand Taiyin is exteriorly-interiorly related to the large intestine meridian of the hand Yangming, the stomach meridian of the foot Yangming is exteriorly-interiorly related to the spleen meridian of the foot Taiyin, and so on; the heart

meridian of the hand Shaoyin with the small intestine meridian of the hand Taiyang, the urinary bladder meridian of the foot Taiyang with the kidney meridian of foot Shaoyin, the pericardium meridian of the hand Jueyin with the Sanjiao meridian of the hand Shaoyang, and the gallbladder meridian of the foot Shaoyang with the liver meridian of the foot Jueyin.

Furthermore, there exist not only exterior-interior relationships between yin and yang meridians, via the "pertaining to" and "communicating with" relationships between the meridians and the zangfu, but also links between the exteriorly-interiorly related meridians via their collaterals in the limbs.

Thus six pairs of exteriorly-interiorly related meridians are formed, which are physiologically closely related, and which influence each other pathologically and assist each other therapeutically.

The 12 regular meridians also have their own courses and meeting-places as follows. The three hand yin meridians run from the chest to the hands, the three hand yang meridians from the hands to the head, the three foot yang meridians run from the head to the feet, the three foot yin meridians from the feet to the abdomen (chest).

Also they connect, or meet with each other, in the following fashion. Firstly, yin meridians meet yang meridians on the four limbs: the lung meridian of the hand Taiyin meets the large intestine meridian of hand Yangming at the index finger, the heart meridian of the hand Shaoyin meets the small intestine meridian of the hand Taiyang at the little finger, the pericardium meridian of the hand Jueyin meets the Sanjiao meridian of hand Shaoyang at the ring finger, the stomach meridian of the foot Yangming meets the spleen meridian of the foot Taiyin at the big toe, the urinary bladder meridian of the foot Taiyang travels obliquely from the little toe to the middle of the sole to meet the kidney meridian of the foot Shaoyin there, the gallbladder meridian of the foot Shaoyang travels obliquely on the dorsum of the foot to the hairy section of the big toe to meet the liver meridian of the foot Jueyin there.

Secondly, yang meridians meet yang meridians, bearing the same name, on the head and face: the large intestine meridian of the hand Yangming and the stomach meridian of the foot Yangming both pass by the side of the nose, the small intestine meridian of the hand Taiyang and the urinary bladder meridian of the foot Taiyang both supply the inner canthus, the Sanjiao meridian of the hand Shaoyang and the gallbladder meridian of the foot Shaoyang both supply the outer canthus.

Lastly, yin meridians meet yin meridians (the three yin meridians of the hands and feet) in the chest: the spleen meridian of the foot Taiyin meets the heart meridian of the hand Shaoyin at the heart, the kidney meridian of the foot Shaoyin meets the pericardium meridian of the hand Jueyin in the chest, the liver meridian of the foot Jueyin meets the lung meridian of the hand Taiyin in the lung.

Thus the 12 regular meridians link up with one another in a fixed order, supplying qi and blood inwardly to nourish the zangfu and other organs, and outwardly reaching into the muscles and flesh. They protect the body surface and nourish the whole organism. In this fashion, through these connecting meridians of the hands and feet, exteriorly and interiorly, yin and yang, a constant and cyclical flow of qi is maintained, circulating without a break.

Its order of circulation is shown in Table 1.2.

THE 8 EXTRA MERIDIANS

The 8 extra meridians are the Du (督), Ren (任), Chong (冲), Dai (带), Yinwei (阴维), Yangwei (阳维), Yinqiao (阴跷), and Yangqiao (阳跷). They are unlike the 12 regular meridians as none of them pertains to a zang or fu organ, or communicates with a zang or fu organ, and they are not exteriorly-interiorly related.

Among the 8 extra meridians, the Du, Ren and Chong meridians originate in the uterus and emerge from the perineum and are termed *yi yuan sanqi* (一源三岐) or "three branches from the same origin". The Du meridian runs along the midline of the back, up to the head and face; the Ren meridian runs along the front midline up to the chin; the Chong meridian, communicating with the kidney meridian of the foot Shaoyin, runs along either side of the abdomen, goes up and curves around the lips.

The Dai meridian originates below the hypochondriacal region and runs transversely around the waist like a belt.

The Yinwei meridian starts from the medial aspect of the foot and ascends along the medial aspect of the leg, up along the medial aspect of the thigh to meet with the Ren at the neck. The Yangwei meridian originates from the lateral aspect of the dorsum of the foot and ascends along

Table 1.2 The cyclical flow of qi in the twelve regular meridians

⟶ = pertaining to and communicative, <------> = exterior and interior relations

Zang organs (Yin meridians) (interior)	Fu organs (Yang meridians) (exterior)
Lung (Lu) ⟶ <------>	(LI) Large intestine
Spleen (Sp) ⟵ <------>	(St) Stomach
Heart (H) ⟶ <------>	(SI) Small intestine
Kidney (K) ⟵ <------>	(UB) Urinary bladder
Pericardium (P) ⟶ <------>	(SJ) Sanjiao
Liver (Liv) ⟵ <------>	(GB) Gallbladder

the lateral aspect of the leg up to the nape to meet the Du.

The Yinqiao meridian starts from the medial aspect of the heel, ascending along the kidney meridian of the foot Shaoyin to the inner canthus where it meets the Yangqiao. The Yangqiao meridian starts from the lateral aspect of the heel, ascends along the bladder meridian of foot Taiyang to the inner canthus where it meets with the Yinqiao, then further ascends along the bladder meridian of the foot Taiyang to the forehead and meets with the gallbladder meridian of the foot Shaoyang at the nape.

The 8 extra meridians crisscross with and are distributed among the 12 regular meridians.

They function mainly in two ways. Firstly, they strengthen the association between the 12 regular meridians. That is to say, the meridians which are near each other in distribution and similar to each other in function assume the responsibility of control and regulation concerning the qi and blood of their related meridians, harmonizing yin and yang.

The Du meets all yang meridians and is therefore described as "the sea of the yang meridians"; it functions in regulating the qi of all the yang meridians. The Ren meets all yin meridians and is known as "the sea of the yin meridians"; it functions in regulating the qi of all the yin meridians. The Chong relates to the Ren and Du and the foot Yangming and foot Shaoyin, and thus is termed "the sea of the 12 regular meridians" or "the sea of blood"; its function is to act as a reservoir for the qi and blood of the 12 regular meridians. The Dai passes around the waist as a girdle, functioning in binding up all the meridians of the feet running vertically up the trunk. The Yinwei and Yangwei connect with the yin and yang meridians and dominate respectively the interior and the exterior of the whole body. The Yinqiao and Yangqiao dominate motion (yang) and quietness (yin), and together control the movement of the lower limbs, waking and sleep.

Secondly, the 8 extra meridians store, supply and regulate the qi and blood of the 12 regular meridians. Therefore, when the qi and blood of the 12 regular meridians and zangfu organs are sufficient, the 8 extra meridians store them and then supply the qi and blood to meet the active demands of the body's functions.

The Chong, Dai, Yinqiao, Yangqiao, Yinwei and Yangwei share their points with other regular meridians, but the Ren and Du have their own acupoints and they are mentioned together with the 12 regular meridians as "the 14 meridians". The 14 meridians all have their own courses, pathological manifestations and acupoints. They constitute the main part of the network of the jingluo and provide the basis for acupuncture-moxibustion treatment and the prescription of herbal medicine according to the meridians.

The courses and distribution of the 14 meridians are shown in Figure 1.

THE 15 COLLATERALS

Each of the 12 regular meridians, as well as the Ren and Du meridians, has a collateral, and, along with the major collateral of the spleen, they are known collectively as "the 15 collaterals" — named after the respective *luo* (meaning in this case "connecting") points, from whence they derive.

The collaterals of the 12 regular meridians on the four limbs (below the elbow and knee joints) run to their exteriorly-interiorly related meridians. The collateral of the Ren branches off from the point Jiuwei (Ren 15) and disperses in the abdomen; the collateral of the Du branches off from point Changqiang (Du 1), dispersing in the head, and bilaterally joining the bladder foot Taiyang.

The major collateral of the spleen branches off from point Dabao (Sp 21), dispersing in the chest and hypochondrium. Among all the collaterals of the body, these 15 collaterals are the major ones, whilst those which run superficially are known as "superficial collaterals", and their minute branches are known as "minute collaterals" or "sub-collaterals", which are innumerable and spread all over the body.

The collaterals of the 12 regular meridians have the function of strengthening the relationship between the yin and yang, exteriorly-interiorly related meridians.

The collateral of the Ren links up with the

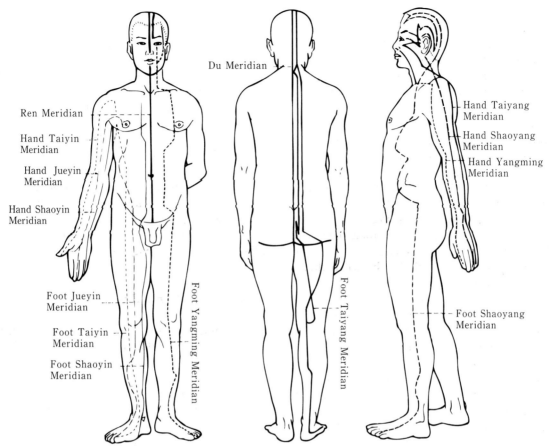

Fig. 1 Distribution of the 14 meridians of the hand and foot.
———— Taiyang and Shaoyin meridians of the hand and foot.
– – – – – Shaoyang and Jueyin meridians of the hand and foot.
- - - - - - Yangming and Taiyin meridians of the hand and foot.

meridional qi in the abdomen, the collateral of the Du meridian links up the qi of the meridians in the back, whilst the major collateral of the spleen links up the meridional qi along the lateral aspect of the chest. The minute collaterals, which are densely distributed, function mainly to transport qi and blood out to nourish the tissues and organs of the whole body.

THE 12 DIVERGENT MERIDIANS

The 12 divergent meridians branch off from the 12 regular meridians and run deep into the body. Most of them derive from the regular meridians in the regions of the limbs and then enter into the thoracic and abdominal cavities.

The divergent meridians of the yang meridians connect with the zangfu organs to which the yang meridians pertain, after entering the chest and abdomen, and then emerge at the back. The divergent meridians of the yang meridians connect with the yang meridians, but the divergent meridians of the yin meridians connect with the exteriorly-interiorly related yang meridians of the yin meridians; thus the 12 divergent meridians can be paired into "six convergences".

The divergent meridians of the bladder foot Taiyang and kidney foot Shaoyin, after branching off at the popliteal fossa, run to the kidney and bladder, ascend to emerge at the nape and finally converge with the urinary bladder meridian of the foot Taiyang. The divergent meridians of the gallbladder foot Shaoyang and liver foot

Jueyin branch off from the lower limbs, run up to the pubic region, enter and connect with the liver and gallbladder, ascend to connect with the eye and finally converge with the gallbladder foot Shaoyang.

The divergent meridians of the stomach foot Yangming and spleen foot Taiyin, after branching off from the thigh, enter and connect with the spleen and stomach, then run upward beside the nose and finally converge with the stomach foot Yangming. The divergent meridians of the small intestine hand Taiyang and heart hand Shaoyin, after branching off from the axillary fossa, enter and connect with the heart and small intestine, then run upward and emerge at the inner canthus and finally converge with the small intestine hand Taiyang.

The divergent meridians of the Sanjiao hand Shaoyang and pericardium hand Jueyin, after branching off from the regular meridians they pertain to, enter the chest and link up with the Sanjiao, then ascend and emerge behind the ear to finally converge with the Sanjiao hand Shaoyang. The divergent meridians of the large intestine hand Yangming and lung hand Taiyin, after branching off from the regular meridians they pertain to, enter and connect with the lung and large intestine, ascend and emerge at the supraclavicular fossa, to converge finally with the large intestine hand Yangming.

Through the course of their branching off, entering into, emerging and converging, the divergent meridians strengthen the connections between the zangfu organs. They make closer the relationship between the 12 regular meridians and other parts of the body, and widen the range of indications for the meridians and acupoints.

For instance, the divergent meridians of the yin meridians converge with their exteriorly-interiorly related yang meridians, thus strengthening the relation between the yin meridians and the head and face. This is why acupoints of the three hand yin meridians and the three foot yin meridians are indicated in diseases of the head and face, and sense organs—e.g. for headache, Taiyuan (Lu 9) and Lieque (Lu 7) can be selected, for toothache and disorders of the throat, Taixi (K 3) and Zhaohai (K 6) can be employed.

THE 12 MUSCLE REGIONS

The 12 muscle regions are the network in which the qi of the 12 regular meridians gathers at muscles, tendons and joints; they are peripheral connecting parts of the 12 regular meridians.

The distribution of the 12 muscle regions is basically the same as the courses and distribution of the 12 regular meridians, originating from the extremities of the limbs and ascending to the head and trunk. However, they run superficially, without entering into the internal organs but gathering at the joints and bones.

The three yang muscle regions of the foot start from the toes, ascend along the lateral aspect of the thigh and gather at the face. The three yin muscle regions of the foot start from the toes, ascend along the medial aspect of the thigh and knot at the genital region (abdomen). The three yang muscle regions of the hand start from the fingers, ascend along the lateral aspect of the arm and knot at the corner of the forehead. The three yin muscle regions of the hand start from the fingers, ascend along the medial aspect of the arm and knot at the chest.

Besides this, along their courses of distribution, the muscle regions also knot at the bones and joints of the ankle, popliteal area, knee, thigh, femur, wrist, elbow, arm, axilla, shoulder and neck. More especially, the muscle region of the foot Jueyin, as well as knotting at the genital region, gathers together the other muscle regions.

As it states in the *Plain Questions*, "The muscle regions possess the function mainly of connecting together all the bones and joints of the body and maintaining their normal range of motion".[4]

THE 12 CUTANEOUS REGIONS

The 12 cutaneous regions refer to sites through which the functional activities of the 12 regular meridians are manifest at the superficial portion of the body, and through which the qi and blood of the meridians is transferred to the body surface. The cutaneous regions are 12 distinct areas on the body surface, within the domains of the 12 regular meridians.

As stated in the *Plain Questions*, "the cutaneous regions are part of the meridian system located in the superficial layer of the body. The cutaneous regions are marked by the regular meridians."[5]

Since the cutaneous regions are the most superficial part of the body tissues, they bear the protective function of the organism.

The 12 regular meridians, 8 extra meridians, 15 collaterals, 12 divergent meridians, 12 muscle regions and 12 cutaneous regions constitute a single integral entity, making up the total network of the jingluo.

Origins and terminations, roots and branches, the major passages for the qi and the four seas

ORIGINS AND TERMINATIONS, ROOTS AND BRANCHES

As stated in the *Miraculous Pivot*,[6] the origins of the six foot meridians lie in the Jing-well points, at the extremities, while their terminations lie in certain parts of the head, chest and abdomen (see Table 1.3).

As further pointed out by Dou Hanqing in his *Lyric of the Standard Profundities* (see Appendix 2), the 12 regular meridians take the four limbs as their origins, and the head, chest and abdomen regions as their terminations. These are termed the *si gen* (四根) or "four origins" and *san jie* (三结) or "three terminations".

The *Miraculous Pivot* states that generally the *ben* (本) or roots of the 12 meridians are in the four limbs while their *biao* (标) or branches are in the head, face and trunk.[7] These cover a wider range than the origins and terminations (see Table 1.4).

Of course, origins and roots, terminations and branches are similar in location and meaning. Both the origins and the terminations are located in the lower half of the body, and both are where the meridian qi starts and originates; the terminations and branches are located in the upper half of the body, and both are sites where the meridian qi terminates.

The theory of "origins and terminations, roots and branches" is a supplementary description of the cyclical flow of the qi of the 12 regular meridians, which nourishes the whole body, as is described within the "Meridians" (Ch. 10), "Qi Character and Body Build" (Ch. 38) and "On Ying Qi Circulation" (Ch. 16) chapters in the *Miraculous Pivot*.

The theory of "origins and terminations, roots and branches" not only explains the close relationship between the four limbs and the head, but also emphasizes that the four limbs are the origin and root of the meridian qi.

Furthermore, the acupoints in these places can have a needling sensation induced more easily and quickly, regulating the functions of the zangfu and jingluo. This is why acupoints below the elbow and knee have a wider range of indications, involving symptoms at some distance—being indicated not only for local diseases, but also for disorders of the zangfu organs, head and face, and sense organs, which are far from these points.

THE MAJOR PASSAGES FOR THE QI AND THE FOUR SEAS

In the *Miraculous Pivot* it states that, "there

Table 1.3 Origin and termination of the six meridians of the foot

Meridian	Origin	Termination
Bladder meridian of foot Taiyang	Zhiyin (UB 67)	Mingmen (eye)
Stomach meridian of foot Yangming	Lidui (St 45)	the forehead (anterior site of ear)
Gallbladder meridian of foot Shaoyang	Qiaoyin (GB 44)	Chuanglong (in the ear)
Spleen meridian of foot Taiyin	Yinbai (Sp 1)	Dicang (St 4)
Kidney meridian of foot Shaoyin	Yongquan (K 1)	Lianquan (Ren 23)
Liver meridian of foot Jueyin	Dadun (Liv 1)	Yutang (Ren 18)

Table 1.4   Root and branch of the 12 regular meridians

Meridian	Root	Branch
3 Yang meridians of foot:		
Foot Taiyang	5 cun above the heel	Mingmen (eye)
Foot Shaoyang	around Foot-Qiaoyin (GB 44)	Chuanglong (in front of ear)
Foot Yangming	Lidui (St 45)	Renying (St 9)
3 Yin meridians of foot:		
Foot Shaoyin	3 cun above and below the internal malleolus	the Back-Shu points, and the two veins under the tongue
Foot Jueyin	5 cun above Xingjian (Liv 2)	the Back-Shu points
Foot Taiyin	4 cun anterior and superior to Zhongfeng (Liv 4)	Back-Shu points and tongue proper
3 Yang meridians of hand:		
Hand Taiyang	posterior to external malleolus	one cun above Mingmen
Hand Shaoyang	2 cun above the web-margin between fingers	from retroauricular upper angle down to outer canthus
Hand Yangming	from elbow joint up to Bieyang (SJ 4)	glabella and anterior site of the ear
3 Yin meridians of hand:		
Hand Taiyin	the area of the *cunkou* which is distal to the styloid process of the radius	axillary artery
Hand Shaoyin	small head of the ulna	the Back-Shu points
Hand Jueyin	2 cun above the palmar transverse crease of the wrist joint, between the two tendons	3 cun below the axilla

exists a major passage for the qi in the chest, a major passage for the qi in the abdomen, a major passage for the qi in the head and a major passage for the qi in the shins".[8] It illustrates that these *qi jie* (气街) or "major passages for the qi" are the main places where the meridional qi converges and passes through.

In the same chapter, it also states that "the qi in the head converges at the brain", showing how the 12 regular meridians all supply the face and openings in the skull. It also states, "the qi in the chest converges at the greater pectoral muscles and Back-Shu points, the qi in the abdomen converges at the Back-Shu points, the Chong meridian and the arteries beside the umbilicus",[9] showing how the qi of the 12 meridians and the zangfu converges at the chest, abdomen, and at sites along the spinal column.

Furthermore, in the same place, it states "the qi in the shins converges at a major passage for the qi", just as the qi of lower limbs usually converges at the major passage for the qi in the lower abdomen area (the area of Qichong, St 30).

Most locations of these major passages are also locations of the terminations, or branches, mentioned above, and, based upon this theory, points distributed on the head and trunk can be used in treating local or visceral disease, while a number of points can also be used in treating disease in the four limbs.

Also in the *Miraculous Pivot*, it states that there are four seas in the human body.[10] The brain is the sea of marrow, Shanzhong (Ren 17) is the sea of qi (in this case, the breath), the stomach is the sea of foodstuffs and the Chong meridian is the sea of the qi of the 12 meridians, also termed the sea of blood.

The locations of the four seas are similar to those of the major passages for the qi. The sea of marrow is in the head, the sea of qi in the chest, the sea of foodstuffs in the upper abdomen, and the sea of blood in the lower abdomen. Each has a connection with the other, and together the four seas are responsible for the circulation of qi, blood and body fluids throughout the body.

The sea of marrow in the brain is the origin of vitality. It acts as the commander, controlling the functional activities of the zangfu and the jingluo. The chest is the sea of qi, where the *zong qi* (宗气) or "pectoral qi" converges to promote the respiratory function of the lung and the circulation of blood through the heart. The stomach is the sea of foodstuffs where the *ying qi* (营气) or "nutrient qi" and *wei qi* (卫气) or "defensive qi" derive from and transform.

The Chong meridian originates in the uterus, travels up along with the kidney meridian of the foot Shaoyin to the place "below the umbilicus and between the kidneys, where the qi gushes"—as it is described in the *Classic on Difficult Questions*. The qi gushing between the kidneys is the original primary qi of the 12 regular meridians and it is termed *yuan qi* (原气) or "source qi". It takes the Sanjiao as the passage for its circulation, dispersing throughout the body, and is the motive force for the human body's vital activity.

Zong (pectoral) qi, *ying* (nutrient) qi, *wei* (defensive) qi and *yuan* (source) qi, together constitute the *zhen qi* (真气) or "genuine qi", which, when circulating in the jingluo, is known as *jing qi* (经气) or "meridional qi". In such a fashion, the theory of the four seas further defines the composition and origin of the qi of the meridians.

The physiological functions of the jingluo and the clinical application of jingluo theory

THE PHYSIOLOGICAL FUNCTIONS OF THE JINGLUO

The jingluo network, including the 8 extra meridians which communicate with the 12 regular meridians, the 12 muscle regions and cutaneous regions, is closely connected with the five zang and six fu organs, the four limbs and the bones, sense organs, orifices, skin, muscles and tendons. Thus it maintains a harmonious coordination between interior and exterior, upper and lower, within the body, and constitutes the organism as an integral organic whole. As it states in the *Miraculous Pivot*, "the 12 meridians pertain to the zangfu interiorly and link with the limbs, joints and superficial tissues exteriorly".[11]

The jingluo system has the function of transporting qi and blood in order to nourish the zangfu organs, skin, muscles, tendons and bones, to fight against exogenous pathogenic factors, and to defend the organism. Normal functioning of the various organs is thus ensured, and a relative equilibrium maintained.

The *Miraculous Pivot* says, "the jingluo transport blood and qi to adjust yin and yang, nourish the tendons and bones and improve joint function".[12] The *ying* qi flows inside the meridians and the *wei* qi runs outside the meridians. *Ying* and *wei* qi is distributed to all parts of the body, and thus the body's resistance is strengthened. As it states in the *Miraculous Pivot*, "harmonising the *wei* qi makes the muscles function normally and the skin and superficial tissues compact".[13]

THE CLINICAL APPLICATION OF JINGLUO THEORY

Explaining the transmission of pathological change

Under pathological conditions, when antipathogenic qi is weak and pathogenic factors invade, the jingluo are the pathways for the transmission of pathogens.

When the superficial portion of the body is affected by exogenous pathogens, the pathogens transmit from exterior to interior via the jingluo, and fevers, chills, headaches or general aching are seen at this early stage. Then the lung is affected via the relationship of "the lung dominating skin and hair" and symptoms of the lung, such as coughing, asthmatic breathing, stuffiness in the chest and chest pain ensue. As it states in the *Plain Questions*, "pathogens invade the body first via the skin and skin-pores, if not eliminated they transmit to sub-collaterals, if not eliminated they transmit to collaterals, then to meridians, then interiorly to the five zang organs and disperse in the intestines and stomach".[14]

Besides this, the jingluo are also pathways for the transmission of disease among the zangfu organs, and between the zangfu organs and the tissues and organs in the superficial portion of the body.

For example, heat in the heart transmits to the small intestine, liver disease may affect the stomach, and stomach disease can affect the spleen, which are all the result of the transmission of diseases among the zangfu via the jingluo. Liver disease may give rise to hypochondriacal pain, kidney disease can give rise to lumbar pain, upward disturbance of the heart fire may lead to ulcers on the tongue, or stomach heat lead to swelling and pain in the gums, and toothache, and these are all outward manifestations of disease in the internal organs reflected on the body surface, via the jingluo.

Guiding meridian classification on the basis of the differentiation of syndromes

Clinically the meridians involved in a disease can be classified according to the symptoms, the courses of the jingluo and the zangfu organs they pertain to and connect with.

For example, cases of headache can be differentiated according to the distribution of meridians on the head: an ache at the forehead is differentiated as a Yangming headache as the Yangming meridians are involved, at both sides of the head it is a Shaoyang headache as the Shaoyang meridians are involved, at the nape or posterior aspect of the head the Taiyang meridians are involved, and at the vertex the Jueyin meridian of the foot is involved. In cases of hypochondriacal or lower abdominal pain, the liver meridian is usually involved as it supplies the hypochondrium and lower abdomen.

Besides, in some diseases, obvious tenderness, nodules or sensitive reactions may occur, either along the courses of the involved meridians, or else at certain joints where the qi of the meridian converges. Alternatively, changes in skin morphology, skin temperature and skin electrical resistance may be observed. All these signs assist in making a diagnosis of certain diseases.

In an intestinal abscess, for instance, tenderness may occur at the point Shangjuxu (St 37) on the course of the stomach meridian of the foot Yangming. In chronic indigestion, abnormal changes may be observed at the point Pishu (UB 20, Back-Shu point of the spleen). Therefore, clinically, the method of palpating for tenderness, observing abnormal changes along the course of the involved meridian and at certain points, or a meridional electrometric method is often applied to assist as reference in making the diagnosis of disease.

Guiding acupuncture and moxibustion treatment

Acupuncture and moxibustion treatment aims at activating the circulation of the qi in meridians, regulating and restoring the normal functions of qi and blood and the zangfu organs so as to treat diseases by applying needling and moxibustion at acupoints.

The principles for selecting points are generally based on the correct differentiation of syndromes, selecting points along the course of the meridian in combination with local points, that is to say, when a certain meridian or zangfu organ is diseased, the distal points of the involved meridians or of the meridians pertaining to the involved zangfu organs are selected.

This is just as it is stated in the *Rhyme of the Four Major Points*: "for abdominal diseases Zusanli is needled, for lumbar and back disorders Weizhong is sought; for problems in the head and nape Lieque is selected, for disorders in the face and mouth Hegu will achieve good results".[15]

These are examples of selecting points along the course of the meridians and they are very widely employed in clinical practice. For instance, in stomach-ache Zusanli (St 36) and Liangqiu (St 34) are selected along the course of the stomach meridian, and in hypochondriacal pain the distal points Yanglingquan (GB 34) and Taichong (Liv 3) are selected along the involved meridians. In the case of a headache distal points are selected, on the upper limb Hegu (LI 4) and on the lower limb Neiting (St 44) along the Yangming meridians, which are usually involved in frontal headache.

Besides this, according to the relationship of the 12 cutaneous regions with the 12 regular meridians and the zangfu organs, cutaneous needles may be used to prick the skin superficially by tapping, and intradermal needles may be embedded in the skin to treat diseases of the zangfu organs and the jingluo. Also, according to the principle that blood stagnation should be treated by bleeding, pricking the collaterals to cause bleeding is used for treating some commonly seen diseases, e.g. bleeding point Taiyang (Extra 5) for congested, swollen or painful eyes, or bleeding Shaoshang (Lu 11) for a sore throat, or bleeding Weizhong (UB 40) for an acute lumbar sprain.

Furthermore, diseases of the muscle regions which manifest mainly as spasm, stiffness or convulsion are often treated by selecting local points, according to the principle of *yi tong wei shu* (以痛为输) or "tender spots can be used as acupoints".

The system of the jingluo possesses not only an important function physiologically, but also pathologically, and it forms an important theoretical basis for guiding the classification of the meridians involved according to the differentiation of syndromes, and for treatment by acupuncture and moxibustion in clinical practice.

As is stated in the *Miraculous Pivot*, "so important are the jingluo, that they determine life and death, the treatment of all disease and the regulation of deficiency and excess conditions. One must gain a thorough understanding of them!"[16]

NOTES

1. *Miraculous Pivot*, Ch.17, "Dimensions of the Meridians".
2. *Miraculous Pivot*, Ch. 11, "Other Meridians".
3. *Miraculous Pivot*, Ch. 4, "The Shape of Disease in the Zangfu according to the Evil Qi".
4. *Plain Questions*, Ch. 44, "Discussion on Wei Syndromes".
5. *Plain Questions*, Ch. 57, "Discussion on Skin Zones".
6. *Miraculous Pivot*, Ch. 5, "Origins and Terminations".
7. *Miraculous Pivot*, Ch. 52, "On Wei Qi Circulation".
8. Ibid.
9. Ibid.
10. *Miraculous Pivot*, Ch. 33, "Discussion on the Seas".
11. Ibid.
12. *Miraculous Pivot*, Ch. 47, "The Original Zang".
13. Ibid.
14. *Plain Questions*, Ch. 63, "Discussion on Contralateral Needling".
15. This rhyme is contained in many anthologies, including Book Three of Yang Jizhou's *Great Compendium* (1601).
16. *Miraculous Pivot*, Ch. 10, "Meridians".

A general introduction 2
to the acupoints

Acupoints are specific sites through which the qi of the zangfu organs and meridians is transported to the surface of the body. The Chinese characters for "acupoint", *shu-xue* (输穴) meant respectively "transportation" and "hole". In the medical literatures of past dynasties, the points where treatment was applied were called by other names, including "needling and moxibustion site", "joining", "confluence", "bone aperture", "qi point", as well as "acupoint".

In the *Miraculous Pivot* it states that acupoints are "the joining places and confluences, 365 in all ... and what is meant by the joining places? There are the places where the vital qi enters in and leaves, travelling to and fro."[1] Later it clarifies by stating "the joining and converging places, 365 in all, are the sites where the qi of the sub-channels is transported through and pours in".[2] This indicates that the jingluo and acupoints are closely related to each other.

The acupoints of the body are all separately assigned to a particular meridian, whilst the meridians each pertain to a certain zangfu. Thus the acupoints, the jingluo and the zangfu organs are combined into a completely interrelated system, in which neither component can be separated from the other.

The acupoints are the places where acupuncture and moxibustion are applied for the treatment of disease. In order to apply acupuncture and moxibustion correctly in the clinic and achieve a good therapeutic result, it is necessary to master the location of these points, their classification into meridians, and their indications.

The evolution and classification of the acupoints

Acupoints have been discovered and accumulated gradually, during the long struggle of the Chinese people against disease. Their evolution has undergone periods when they were not specifically located, not specifically named, and not in any specific system or classification.

Initially disease was treated by massaging, pounding, or applying needling and moxa to the local area of pain, i.e. "taking painful sites as the acupoints" (see end of Ch. 1). Then along with increasingly greater understanding of the sites where the therapy was applied, and the site's own therapeutic properties, the acupoints gained their definite locations and names. Later, through the efforts of generations of medical workers, generalizing and systematizing the points, and owing to the gradual formation of jingluo theory, the acupoints were no longer considered as isolated and scattered sites over the body surface. Thence the interrelationships between the acupoints, and the specific relationships between the points and the zangfu organs were recognized.

After repeated textual researches, the acupoints were finally classified, each into their separate meridians. Generally speaking, acupoints fall into the following three categories: acupoints of the 14 meridians, extraordinary points and ashi points.

Acupoints of the 14 meridians are also termed "regular points" or simply "points". They are distributed along the 12 regular meridians, and the Du and Ren meridians, and have common therapeutic indications for diseases of the meridians they pertain to. These points, totalling 361 in all, were found mainly before the Jin Dynasty (AD 265–420), and form the bulk of all acupoints.

The "extraordinary points" (or "extra points") are points with specific names and definite locations, but not as yet listed among the "acupoints of the 14 meridians" and thus termed "extra points". They have specific therapeutic effects in treating certain diseases, and a certain relationship with the jingluo system. Some of them have been progressively classified within the regular points.

Ashi points are also variously called "tender spots", "reactive points" and "unfixed points". They have no specific names or locations. Ashi points are places for acupuncture and moxibustion treatment where there is tenderness or a painful reaction, or nearby where disorder is located. Ashi points are often situated near affected sites, nevertheless they may also be far from affected sites.

The nomenclature of the acupoints

The naming of the acupoints is an important feature of the terminology of acupuncture and moxibustion. The *Supplementary Prescriptions Worth Their Weight in Gold Coin* states that "The names of the points have their meanings, and each is of profound significance".

Furthermore, the nomenclature of the acupoints not only has a significance in medicine, but also is part of the brilliant culture of ancient China. A knowledge of the significance of naming a particular point will help one memorize its location and action.

On the basis of the locations and actions of the points, they were named by the ancients in accordance with their observation of the natural world and their medical theories. In this respect, they chose to name the points by way of analogy.

Names based on the points' locations

Some points are named according to the anatomical terms of the sites where they are located: such as Wangu (SI 4, Wrist Bone), Rugen (St 18, Root of the Breast) and Jizhong (Du 6, Between Vertebrae).

Names based upon their therapeutic properties

Jingming (UB 1, Brightening the Eyes) and Guangming (GB 37, Bright Clear) are indicated for eye diseases. Shuifen (Ren 9, Water Division) and Shuidao (St 38, Water Passage) are for oedema. Feishu (UB 13, Lung Back-Shu), Xinshu (UB 15, Heart Back-Shu) and Ganshu (UB 18, Liver Back-Shu) are indicated for diseases of the zangfu organs.

Names based on theories of TCM

Some points are named according to their locations, or therapeutic properties, along with TCM theories, such as yin-yang, the zangfu, jingluo or qi and blood. For instance, Yangxi (LI 5, Stream on the Yang Aspect), Yangchi (SJ 4, Yang Pond) and Yanggu (SI 5, Yang Valley) are all situated on the lateral aspect of the upper limb, while Yinxi (H 6, Yin Cleft) lies on the medial aspect. Pohu (UB 42, Po-soul House) and Shentang (UB 44, Mind House) lie alongside Feishu (UB 13, Lung Back-Shu, the lung has the "will" to dominate the Po-soul) and Xinshu (UB 15, Heart Back-Shu, the heart houses the mind). There is also Sanyinjiao (Sp 6, Crossing point of the 3 Yin Meridians), Baihui (Du 20, Confluence of Various Meridians), Qihai (Ren 6, Sea of Qi) and Xuehai (Sp 10, Sea of Blood).

Names bearing analogy to geographical or geomorphological features

These include: mountain, mound, hill, wilderness, valley, stream, ravine, ditch, sea, river or marsh, pond and spring. Chengshan (UB 57, Supporting the Mountain), Daling (P 7, Big Mound), Shangqiu (Sp 5, The Shang Hill) and Shuigou (Du 26, Water Ditch) are some examples. Also there are names bearing analogy to astronomical or meteorological phenomena—the sun, moon, stars, etc.—in combination with the location of the points. For example, Shangxing (Du 23, Upper Star), Riyue (GB 24, Sun and Moon), and Taiyi (St 23, Grand Yi, which is the 2nd Heavenly Stem).

Names bearing analogy to animals and plants

These indicate features of the points. For instance, Dubi (St 35, Calf's Nose, at the knee joint), Jiuwei (Ren 15, Turtledove's Tail, at the junction of chest and abdomen), and Zanzhu (UB 2, Bamboo Tufts) at the ends of the eyebrow.

Names bearing analogy to architectural structures

These indicate the characteristics of the location or function of the point. For instance, door, house, gate or pass, pivot or hinge, hall, room, window, palace, courtyard, imperial palace, barn, well, etc.; Shenque (Ren 8, Palace of Vitality), Yintang (Extra 2, Seal Hall), Zhishi (UB 52, Will Chamber) and Kufang (St 14, Storehouse), are some examples.

The therapeutic properties of the acupoints

LOCAL AND ADJACENT THERAPEUTIC PROPERTIES OF THE POINTS

Local and adjacent therapeutic properties are a common feature of all the points.

Each point, located at a particular site, is able to treat disorders of this area and of nearby tissues and organs. For instance, points in the ocular area, such as Jingming (UB 1), Chengqi (St 1), Sibai (St 2) and Tongziliao (GB 1) are all indicated for eye diseases; points in the auricular region such as Tinggong (SI 19), Ermen (SJ 21) and Yifeng (SJ 17) are all indicated for ear diseases; and points in the gastric region such as Zhongwan (Ren 12), Jianli (Ren 11) and Liangmen (St 21) are all indicated for gastric diseases.

REMOTE THERAPEUTIC PROPERTIES OF THE POINTS

Remote therapeutic properties of the points are a basic feature of the points of the 14 meridians. For instance, those on the regular jingluo located on the limbs, especially those below the elbow and knee joints, are indicated not only for local disorders but also for disorders of the zangfu, and remote areas on the course of the meridians to which they pertain. In addition, some even have systemic therapeutic properties.

For instance, Hegu (LI 4) is indicated not only for disorders of the hand and wrist, but also for disorders of the neck, head and face, and fever seen in exogenous diseases as well. Zusanli (St 36) is indicated not only for disorders of the lower limbs, but also for regulating the functions of the whole digestive system, and it even has a major influence on the defensive system and immunity of the whole human body.

SPECIAL THERAPEUTIC PROPERTIES OF THE POINTS

Clinical practice has proved that needling some points can exert a biphasic regulatory effect under differing conditions of the organism. For example, in the case of diarrhoea, needling Tianshu (St 25) can check diarrhoea while, in case of constipation, needling the same point, Tianshu, can relieve constipation.

Besides this, there exists a relative specificity of the therapeutic properties of some points. For instance, Dazhui (Du 14) is used for subduing fever and Zhiyin (UB 67) for correcting malposition of the fetus.

The therapeutic properties of the points of the 14 meridians can be generalized as follows: points are indicated for disorders of the meridians to which they pertain, points of externally-internally related meridians are indicated for disorders of both related meridians, and adjacent points can be used in combination with the above, for treating local disorders.

The points of each meridian have specific yet common therapeutic properties which are shown as follows (see Tables 2.1, and 3.1–3.14 or Figure 2 (a–j).)

Specific points

Specific points are the points on the 14 meridians which have specific therapeutic properties and are grouped under special names which have a particular meaning.

THE FIVE SHU POINTS

Each of the 12 regular meridians has, below the

Table 2.1 Differing and common therapeutic properties of the points of the fourteen meridians

Meridian	Particular indications	Common indications of two	Common indications of the three
Three yin meridians of the hand			
Hand Taiyin	lung and throat diseases		
Hand Jueyin	heart and stomach diseases	{ mental disorders	{ diseases of the chest
Hand Shaoyin	heart diseases		
Three yang meridians of the hand			
Hand Yangming	anterior head, nose, mouth, tooth diseases		throat diseases,
Hand Shaoyang	lateral head and flank diseases	{ eye and ear disease	{ and febrile
Hand Taiyang	posterior head, scapular and mental diseases		diseases
Three yang meridians of the foot			
Foot Yangming	anterior head, mouth, tooth, throat and gastrointestinal diseases		eye, mental
Foot Shaoyang	lateral head, ear and flank diseases		{ and febrile
Foot Taiyang	posterior head, back, lumbar diseases (zangfu disease by the Back-Shu points)		diseases
Three yin meridians of the foot			
Foot Taiyin	spleen and stomach diseases		diseases of the external
Foot Jueyin	liver diseases		{ genitalia, gynaecological
Foot Shaoyin	kidney, lung and throat diseases		diseases
Ren and Du meridians			
Ren meridian	recapture yang from collapse, tonic		mental, zangfu organ
Du meridian	windstroke, coma, febrile diseases and diseases of the head and face		{ and gynaecological diseases

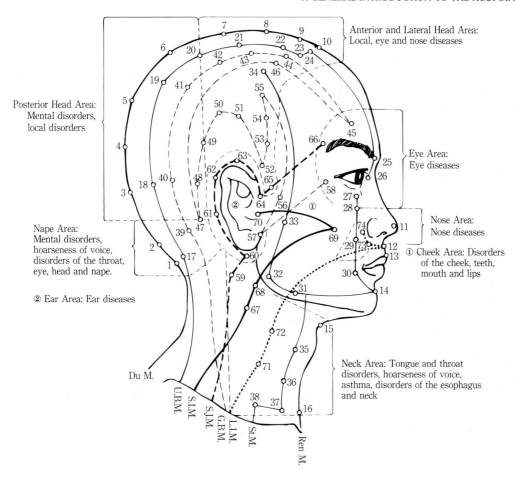

Fig. 2a On the head, face and neck: 1 Yamen, 2 Fengfu, 3 Naohu, 4 Qiangjian, 5 Houding, 6 Baihiu, 7 Qianding, 8 Xianhui, 9 Shangxing, 10 Shenting, 11 Suliao, 12 Shuigou, 13 Duiduan, 14 chengjiang, 15 Luangquan, 16 Tiantu, 17 Tianzhu, 18 Yuzhen, 19 Luoque, 20 Tongtian, 21 Chengguang, 22 Wuchu, 23 Quchai, 24 Meichong, 25 Zanzhu, 26 Jingming, 27 Chengqi, 28 Sibai, 29 Julio, 30 Dicang, 31 Daying, 32 Jiache, 33 Xiaguan, 34 Touwei, 25 Renying, 36 Shuiti, 37 Qishe, 38 Quepen, 39 Fengchi, 40 Naokong, 41 Chengling, 42 Zhengying, 43 Muchuang, 44 Joulinqi, 45 Yangbai, 46 Benshen, 47 Wangu, 48 Qiaoying, 49 Fubai, 50 Tianchong, 51 Shuaigu, 52 Qubin, 53 Xuanli, 54 Xuanlu, 55 Hanyan, 56 Kezhuren, 57 Tinghui, 58 Tongziliao, 59 Tianyou, 60 Yifeng, 61 Qimai, 62 Luxi, 63 Jiaosun, 64 Ermen, 65 Erheliao, 66 Sizhukong, 67 Tianchuang, 68 Tianrong, 69 Quanliao, 70 Tinggong, 71 Tianding, 72 Futu, 73 Kouheliao, 74 Yingxiang.

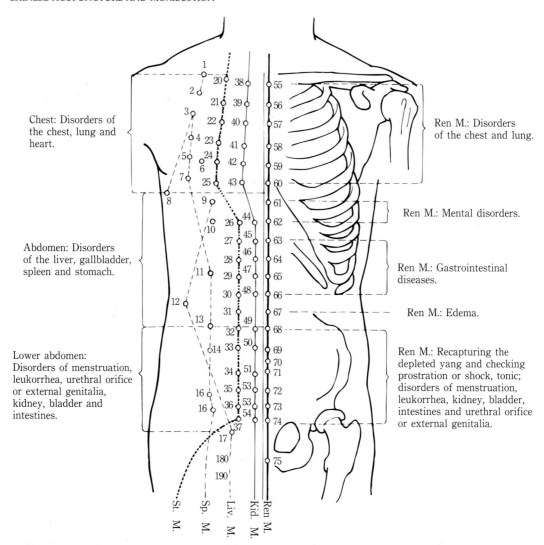

Chest: Disorders of the chest, lung and heart.

Abdomen: Disorders of the liver, gallbladder, spleen and stomach.

Lower abdomen: Disorders of menstruation, leukorrhea, urethral orifice or external genitalia, kidney, bladder and intestines.

Ren M.: Disorders of the chest and lung.

Ren M.: Mental disorders.

Ren M.: Gastrointestinal diseases.

Ren M.: Edema.

Ren M.: Recapturing the depleted yang and checking prostration or shock, tonic; disorders of menstruation, leukorrhea, kidney, bladder, intestines and urethral orifice or external genitalia.

St. M.   Sp. M.   Liv. M.   Kid. M.   Ren M.

Fig. 2b On the chest, hypochondrium and abdomen: 1 Yunmen, 2 Zhongfu, 3 Zhourong, 4 Xiongxiang, 5 Tianxi, 6 Tianchi, 7 Shidou, 8 Dabao, 9 Qimen, 10 Riyue, 11 Fuai, 12 Zhangmen, 13 Daheng, 14 Fujie, 15 Fushe, 16 Chongmen, 17 Jimai, 18 Yinlian, 19 Zuwuli, 20 Qihu, 21 Kufang, 22 Wuyi, 23 Yinchuang, 24 Ruzhong, 25 Rugen, 26 Burong, 27 Chengman, 28 Liangmen, 29 Guanmen, 30 Taiyi, 31 Huaroumen, 32 Tianshu, 33 Wailing, 34 Daju, 35 Shuidao, 36 Guilai, 37 Qichong, 38 Shufu, 39 Yuzhong, 40 Shencang, 41 Lingxu, 42 Shenfeng, 43 Bulang, 44 Youmen, 45 Futonggu, 46 Yindu, 47 Shiguan, 48 Shangqu, 49 Huangshu, 50 Zhongzhu, 51 Siman, 52 Qixue, 53 Dahe, 54 Henggu, 55 Xuanji, 56 Huagai, 57 Zigong, 58 Yutang, 59 Tanzhong, 60 Zhongting, 61 Jinwei, 62 Juque, 63 Shangwan, 64 Zhongwan, 65 Jianli, 66 Xiawan, 67 Shuifen, 68 Shenque, 69 Yinjiao, 70 Qihai, 71 Shimen, 72 Guanyuan, 73 Zhongji, 74 Qugu, 75 Huiyin.

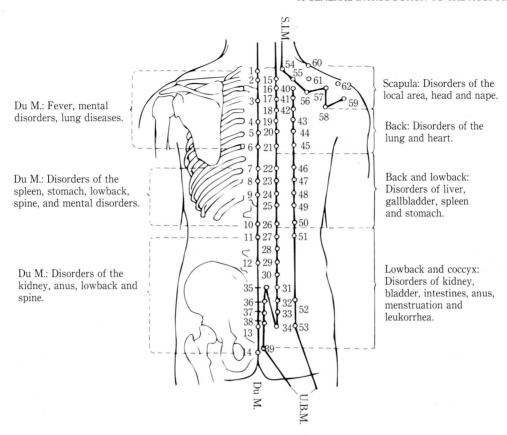

Du M.: Fever, mental disorders, lung diseases.

Du M.: Disorders of the spleen, stomach, lowback, spine, and mental disorders.

Du M.: Disorders of the kidney, anus, lowback and spine.

Scapula: Disorders of the local area, head and nape.

Back: Disorders of the lung and heart.

Back and lowback: Disorders of liver, gallbladder, spleen and stomach.

Lowback and coccyx: Disorders of kidney, bladder, intestines, anus, menstruation and leukorrhea.

Fig. 2c On the shoulder, back, lower back and coccyx: 1 Dazhui, 2 Taodao, 3 Shengzhu, 4 Shendao, 5 Lingtai, 6 Zhiyang, 7 Jinsuo, 8 Zhongshu, 9 Jizhong, 10 Xuanshu, 11 Mingmen, 12 Yaoyangguan, 13 Yaoshu, 14 Changqiang, 15 Dazhu, 16 Fengmen, 17 Feishu, 18 Jueyinshu, 19 Xinshu, 20 Dushu, 21 Geshu, 22 Ganshu, 23 Danshu, 24 Pishu, 25 Weishu, 26 Sanjiaoshu, 27 Shenshu, 28 Qihaishu, 29 Dachangshu, 30 Guanyuanshu, 31 Xiaochangshu, 32 Pangguangshu, 33 Zhonglushu, 34 Baihuanshu, 35 Shangliao, 36 Chiliao, 37 Zhongliao, 38 Xialiao, 39 Huiyang, 40 Fufen, 41 Pohu, 42 Gaohuang, 43 Shentang, 44 Yixi, 45 Geguan, 46 Hunmen, 47 Yanggang, 48 Yishe, 49 Weicang, 50 Huangmen, 51 Zhishi, 52 Baohuang, 53 Zhibian, 54 Jianzhongshu, 55 Jianwaishu, 56 Quyuan, 57 Bingfeng, 58 Tianzhong, 59 Naoshu, 60 Jianjing, 61 Tianliao, 62 Jugu.

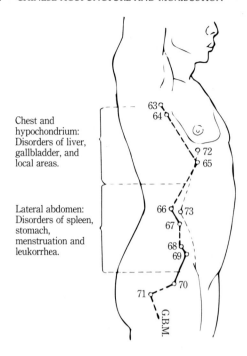

Chest and hypochondrium: Disorders of liver, gallbladder, and local areas.

Lateral abdomen: Disorders of spleen, stomach, menstruation and leukorrhea.

Fig. 2d   On the axilla, hypochondrium and lateral abdomen: 63 Yuanye, 64 Zhejin, 65 Riyue, 66 Jingmen, 67 Daimai, 68 Wushu, 69 Weidao, 70 Juliao, 71 Huantiao, 72 Qimen, 73 Zhangmen.

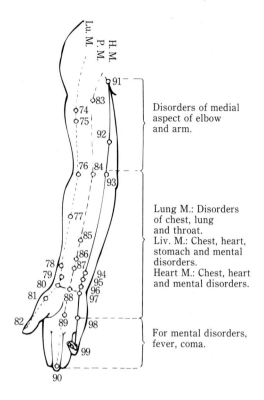

Disorders of medial aspect of elbow and arm.

Lung M.: Disorders of chest, lung and throat.
Liv. M.: Chest, heart, stomach and mental disorders.
Heart M.: Chest, heart and mental disorders.

For mental disorders, fever, coma.

Fig. 2e   On the medial aspect of the upper limb: 74 Tianfu, 75 Xiabai, 76 Chize, 77 Kongzui, 78 Lieque, 79 Jingqu, 80 Taiyuan, 81 Yuji, 82 Shaoshang, 83 Tianquan, 84 Quze, 85 Ximen, 86 Jianshi, 87 Neiguan, 88 Daling, 89 Laogong, 90 Zhongchong, 91 Jiquan, 92 Qingling, 93 Shaohai, 94 Lingdao, 95 Tongli, 96 Yinxi, 97 Shenmen, 98 Shaofu, 99 Shaochong.

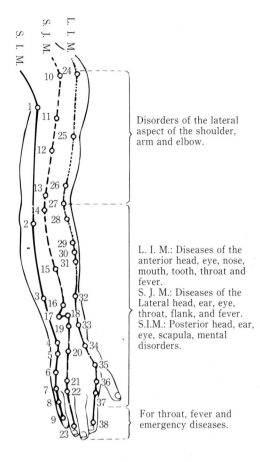

Disorders of the lateral aspect of the shoulder, arm and elbow.

L. I. M.: Diseases of the anterior head, eye, nose, mouth, tooth, throat and fever.
S. J. M.: Diseases of the Lateral head, ear, eye, throat, flank, and fever.
S.I.M.: Posterior head, ear, eye, scapula, mental disorders.

For throat, fever and emergency diseases.

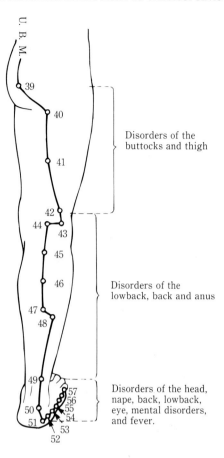

Disorders of the buttocks and thigh

Disorders of the lowback, back and anus

Disorders of the head, nape, back, lowback, eye, mental disorders, and fever.

Fig. 2f   On the lateral aspect of the upper limb: 1 Jianzhen, 2 Xiaohai, 3 Zhizheng, 4 Yanglao, 5 Yanggu, 6 Wangu, 7 Houxi, 8 Qiangu, 9 Shaoze, 10 Jianliao, 11 Naohui, 12 Xiaoluo, 13 Qinglengyuan, 14 Tianjing, 15 Sidu, 16 Sanyangluo, 17 Huizong, 18 Zhigou, 19 Waiguan, 20 Yangchi, 21 Zhongzhu, 22 Yemen, 23 Guanchong, 24 Jiangu, 25 Binao, 26 Shouwuli, 27 Zhouliao, 28 Quchi, 29 Shousanli, 30 Shanglian, 31 Xialian, 32 Wenliu, 33 Pianli, 34 Yangxi, 35 Hegu, 36 Sanjian, 37 Erjian, 38 Shangying.

Fig. 2g   On the posterior aspect of the lower limb: 39 Huiyan, 40 Chengfu, 41 Yinmen, 42 Fuxi, 43 Weiyan, 44 Weizhang, 45 Heyang, 46 Chengjin, 47 Chengshan, 48 Feiyang, 49 Fuyang, 50 Kunlun, 51 Pucan, 52 Shenmai, 53 Jinmen, 54 Jinggu, 55 Shugu, 56 Zutonggu, 57 Zhiyin.

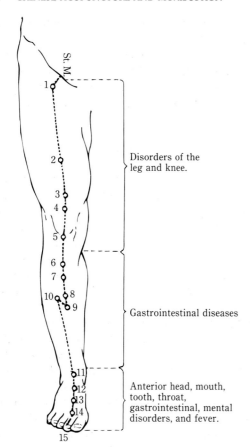

Disorders of the leg and knee.

Gastrointestinal diseases

Anterior head, mouth, tooth, throat, gastrointestinal, mental disorders, and fever.

Fig. 2h   On the anterior aspect of the lower limb: 1 Biguan, 2 Futu, 3 Yinshi, 4 Liangqui, 5 Dubi, 6 Zusanli, 7 Shangjuxu, 8 Tiaokou, 9 Xiajuxu, 10 Fenglong, 11 Jiexi, 12 Chongyang, 13 Xiangu, 14 Neiting, 15 Lidui.

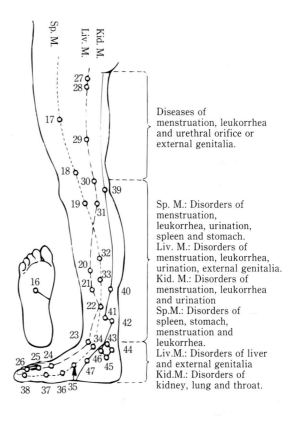

Diseases of menstruation, leukorrhea and urethral orifice or external genitalia.

Sp. M.: Disorders of menstruation, leukorrhea, urination, spleen and stomach.
Liv. M.: Disorders of menstruation, leukorrhea, urination, external genitalia.
Kid. M.: Disorders of menstruation, leukorrhea and urination
Sp.M.: Disorders of spleen, stomach, menstruation and leukorrhea.
Liv.M.: Disorders of liver and external genitalia
Kid.M.: Disorders of kidney, lung and throat.

Fig. 2i   On the medial aspect of the lower limb: 16 Yongquan, 17 Jimen, 18 Xuehai, 19 Yinlingquan, 20 Zhongdu, 21 Ligou, 22 Sanyinjiao, 23 Zhongfeng, 24 Taichong, 25 Xingjian, 26 Dadun, 27 Yinlian, 28 Zuwuli, 29 Yinbao, 30 Ququan, 31 Xiguan, 32 Diji, 33 Lougu, 34 Shangqiu, 35 Gongsun, 36 Taibai, 37 Dadu, 38 Yinbai, 39 Yingu, 40 Zhubin, 41 Jiaoxing, 42 Fuliu, 43 Taixi, 44 Dazhong, 45 Shuiquan, 46 Zhaohai, 47 Rangu.

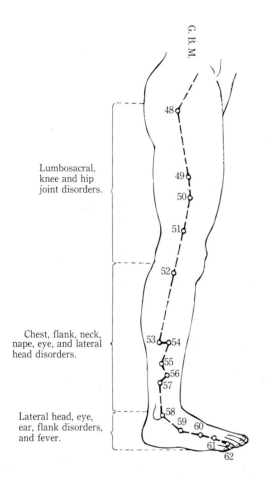

G.B.M.

48

Lumbosacral,
knee and hip
joint disorders.

49
50

51

52

Chest, flank, neck,
nape, eye, and lateral
head disorders.

53 54
55
56
57

Lateral head, eye,
ear, flank disorders,
and fever.

58
59 60
61
62

Fig. 2j On the lateral aspect of the lower limb: 48 Huantiao, 49 Fengshi, 50 Zhongdu, 51 Xiyangguan, 52 Yanglingquan, 53 Yangjiao, 54 Waiqiu, 55 Guangming, 56 Yangfu, 57 Xuanzhong, 58 Qiuxu, 59 Zulinqi, 60 Diwuhui, 61 Xiaxi, 62 Zuqiaoyin.

elbow or knee, five special points, namely the Jing-well, Ying-spring, Shu-stream, Jing-river and He-sea points, which are generally termed the "5 *Shu*" (五输). The 5 Shu points are situated, in the above order, from the distal extremities to the elbow or knee, according to the theory of Origins and Terminations, Roots and Branches (see Ch. 1).

The ancient physicians imagined the circulation of qi in the meridians to be like running water within the natural world. In this way they illustrated the coming and going of the flowing meridional qi, its relative depth and shallowness, and dissimilarity in function.

Thus the Jing-well point is situated at the place where the meridional qi starts to bubble up, the Ying-spring point where it starts to gush over, the Shu-stream point where it pours out, the Jing-river point where it is flowing abundantly, and finally the He-sea point where it reaches a confluence, like a river reaching the sea, and here the meridional qi most thrives.

YUAN POINTS AND LUO POINTS

Yuan (原), or source, points are located where the *yuan* qi passes through or accumulates. There is a *yuan* point for each of the 12 regular meridians. All occur at the extremities and are termed together the "12 *yuan* points".

On each of the six yang meridians there is a single *yuan* point, while on the yin meridians the *yuan* points overlap with the Shu-stream points of the 5 Shu points.

Each of the 12 regular meridians, at the place where the collateral branches off, has a *luo* (络) point, on the limbs, to link with its externally-internally related meridian. Each of the Du and Ren meridians, and the major collateral of the spleen has its *luo* point on the trunk (Jiuwei, Ren 15, on the abdomen, Changqiang, Du 1, at the coccyx, and Dabao, Sp 21, on the chest). These 15 points are similarly termed "the 15 *luo* points".

BACK-SHU AND FRONT-MU POINTS

Back-*Shu* (俞) points are specific points on the back where the qi of the respective zangfu organ is infused. The Front-*Mu* (募) points are specific points on the chest and abdomen where the qi of the respective zangfu organs is infused and converged. Both types of points are all situated on the trunk and closely related to the zangfu organs.

THE 8 INFLUENTIAL POINTS

The 8 Influential (会) points are sites where the qi or essence of the zang organs, fu organs, qi, blood, tendons, vessels, bone or marrow is converged. These points are situated on the trunk and limbs.

XI-CLEFT POINTS

Xi-Cleft (郄) points are sites where the qi and blood of the meridians is deeply converged. Each of the 12 regular meridians and the 4 extra meridians (Yinqiao, Yangqiao, Yinwei and Yangwei) has a Xi-Cleft point which is mostly situated on the limbs, below the elbow or knee joint. This amounts to 16 Xi-Cleft points in all.

LOWER HE-SEA POINTS

Lower He-Sea points (as distinct from the He-sea points among the 5 Shu points) are 6 points situated mainly near the knee joints on the lower limbs where the meridional qi of the hand and foot yang meridians, and the six fu organs, descends and converges at the three foot yang meridians.

THE 8 CONFLUENT POINTS OF THE 8 EXTRA MERIDIANS AND THE CROSSING POINTS

The 8 Confluent (交会) points refer to the 8 points on the limbs near the wrist and ankle joints where the regular meridians communicate with the 8 extra meridians.

The Crossing points are those at the intersection of two or more meridians; most of them are distributed on the trunk.

Methods of locating acupoints clinically

In clinical practice, the right or wrong location of an acupoint and the therapeutic result have a close relationship. In order to locate points precisely, it is necessary to master the following methods:

PROPORTIONAL MEASUREMENT

The earliest record of proportional measure-ments is found in the *Miraculous Pivot*, in the chapter entitled "Bone Measurements".[3] These measurements were then complemented and revised by later generations, and have been taken as the standards of measurement, applicable to any patient, of any sex, age or body weight.

The width or length of various portions of the human body is divided respectively into definite numbers of equal units, each unit being termed one *cun* (寸). These are then used as the proportional standard in locating points (obviously the length of the cun depends on the build of the individual patient), see Table 2.2.

In locating points clinically, the above mentioned lengths are often measured conveniently by the fingers, which are used to divide them into several equal divisions.

For example, when locating Jianshi (P 5), the length of 12 cun between the transverse carpal crease and transverse cubital crease is divided into two equal divisions and then the half near the wrist is further divided into two equal divisions, with the fingers of both hands, and Jianshi (located 3 cun above the wrist) can be accurately and rapidly located.

ANATOMICAL LANDMARKS

Anatomical landmarks on the body surface are employed in point location, and these landmarks fall into two categories.

Fixed landmarks. Fixed landmarks are those which do not change with body movement, such as the five sense organs, finger or nail, nipple or umbilicus.

Moving landmarks. Moving landmarks refer to those which appear only when a certain part of the body is kept in a specific position, such as a crease or fold of skin, a depression or prominence formed out of tendon and muscle, or a certain space within a joint.

Anatomical landmarks are used frequently in clinic in point location, for example, Shanzhong (Ren 17) is located at the midpoint between the two nipples and Houxi (SI 3) is located, when a loose fist is made, at the ulnar end of the palmar transverse crease.

Table 2.2   Commonly used standards in proportional measurement

Portion	Starting and ending points of measurement	Units	Direction	Remarks
head	from anterior hairline to posterior	12 cun	longi.	if anterior and posterior hairlines are indistinguishable, from glabella to Dazhui (Du 14) is 18 cun, glabella to anterior hairline is 3 cun, Dazhui to posterior hairline is 3 cun
	between the two mastoid processes	9 cun	trans.	for transverse measurement on head
chest and abdomen	from Tiantu (Ren 22) to xiphoid	9 cun	longi.	measurement on chest and costa is based on ribs (each rib as 1.6 cun)
	from xyphoid to the centre of umbilicus	8 cun		
	from centre of umbilicus to upper border of symphysis	5 cun		
	between the two nipples	8 cun	trans.	used for transverse measurement on chest and abdomen; distance between Quepen (St 12) on both sides can be used instead in women
back	from Dazhui to coccyx	21 vertebrae	longi.	it is based on the vertebrae—clinically, the inferior angle of scapula corresponds to T7, iliac spine corresponds to spinous process of L4
	between medial border of the scapula on both sides	6 cun	trans.	
upper limbs	between the end of axillary fold and transverse cubital crease	9 cun	longi.	used for proportional measurement in locating points of the three yin and three yang meridians of hand
	between the transverse cubital and carpal creases	12 cun		
lateral chest	from the end of axillary fold on lateral chest to tip of the 11th rib	12 cun	longi.	
lateral abdomen	from tip of 11th rib to the protuberance of great trochanter of femur	9 cun	longi.	
lower limbs	from the level of upper border of symphysis pubis to medial epicondyle of femur	18 cun	longi.	used for proportional measurement in locating points on the three yin meridians of foot
	from lower border of the medial condyle of tibia to tip of medial malleolus	13 cun		
	from prominence of greater trochanter to the middle of patella	19 cun	longi.	used for proportional measurement in locating points of the three yang meridians of the foot; the middle of patella corresponds to the level of Dubi (St 35) or Weizhong (UB 40)
	from gluteal transverse crease to middle of patella	14 cun		
	from middle of patella to tip of lateral malleolus	16 cun		
	tip of lateral malleous to sole	3 cun		

FINGER MEASUREMENT

This is the method in which the length and width of the patient's finger(s) is taken as the standard for point location, as there exists a certain proportion between the length and width of fingers and other parts of the body. Those of the doctor's can also be used after allowance has been made, by way of comparison, with those of the patient's.

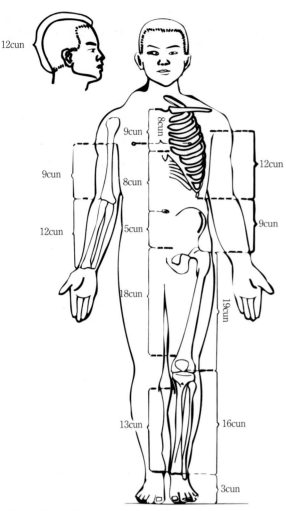

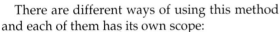

Fig. 3   Proportional measurements.

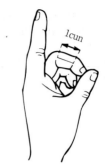

Fig. 4   Middle finger measurements.

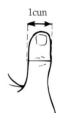

Fig. 5   Thumb measurement.

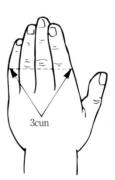

Fig. 6   Four-finger measurement.

There are different ways of using this method and each of them has its own scope:

Middle finger measurement. When the patient's middle finger is flexed, the distance between the two medial ends of the creases of the interphalangeal joints is taken as one cun. This method is employed for measuring longtitudinal distances in locating points of the yang meridians on the limbs, or for measuring transverse distances in point location on the back.

Thumb measurement. The width of the interphalangeal joint of the patient's thumb is taken as 1 cun. This method is also employed in

measuring longitudinal distances in point location on the limbs.

Four-finger measurement. The width of the four fingers (the index, middle, ring and little) when closed together, at the level of the dorsal skin crease of the proximal interphalangeal joint of the middle finger, is taken as 3 cun in point location.

SIMPLE WAYS OF LOCATING ACUPOINTS

There are some simple ways of locating points, convenient for point location in the clinic. For instance, Fengshi (GB 31) is located by asking the patient to stand upright with the hands close to the sides and the point is where the tip of the middle finger touches. Also Lieque (Lu 7) is located by asking the patient to cross the index fingers and thumbs of both hands, with the index finger of one hand placed on the styloid process of the radius of the other; the point is in the depression right under the tip of the index finger.

NOTES

1. *Miraculous Pivot*, Ch. 1, "On the 9 Needles and 12 Yuan-sources."

2. *Miraculous Pivot*, Ch. 3, "Explaining the Use of Small Needles".
3. *Miraculous Pivot*, Ch. 14, "Bone Measurements".

The jingluo and acupoints

The jingluo include the 12 regular meridians and the 8 extra meridians; each of them has a fixed course, which is internally related to the therapeutic indications of the points of that meridian.

Thus, knowing the course of the meridian will help in mastering the indications of the points, especially those below the elbow and knee. The 12 regular meridians and the Du and Ren meridians (out of the 8 extra meridians) have their own acupoints, while the Chong, Dai, Yinqiao, Yangqiao, Yinwei and Yangwei extra meridians share their points with the regular meridians and the Du and Ren.

Acupoints are specific places where acupuncture and moxibustion are applied for the treatment of disease, and their location and therapeutic indication form the basis of practical treatment in the clinic.

The 12 regular meridians

THE LUNG MERIDIAN OF THE HAND-TAIYIN (WITH 11 ACUPOINTS)

Course

The lung meridian of the hand Taiyin originates from the middle-jiao and runs downward to connect with the large intestine (1); it then winds back and goes along the upper orifice of the stomach (2). It passes through the diaphragm (3) and enters the lung (4), the organ it pertains to.

From the lung system (where the lung communicates with the throat) it comes out transversely (Zhongfu, Lu 1) (5); descending along the medial aspect of the upper arm it then passes in front of the heart meridian of the hand Shaoyin and the pericardium meridian of the hand Jueyin (6) and reaches the cubital fossa (7); then going continuously downward along the anterior border of the radial side on the medial aspect of the forearm (8) it enters the *cunkou* (寸口) (9), close to the radial artery at the wrist where the pulse is palpated; passing the thenar eminence (10), it goes along its radial border (11) and ends at the medial side of the tip of the thumb (12) (Shaoshang, Lu 11).

A branch proximal to the wrist emerges from Lieque (Lu 7) (13) and runs directly to the radial side of the tip of the index finger (Shangyang, LI 1), where it links with the large intestine hand Yangming.

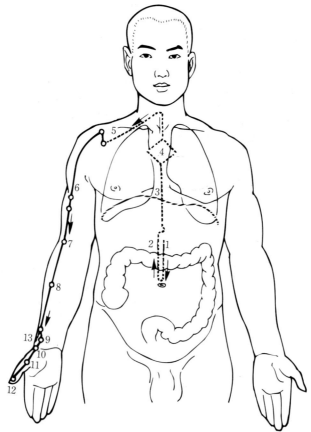

Fig. 7   The course of the lung meridian of the hand Taiyin.
——— Course of the involved meridian with points.
------- Course of the involved meridian without points.
○   Points of the involved meridian.
▲   Points of other meridians.

Chief pathological manifestations

Cough, asthmatic breathing, shortness of breath, haemoptysis, common cold, distension and fullness in the chest, congested and sore throat, pain in the supraclavicular fossa and the anterior border of the medial aspect of the arm, cold and pain in the shoulder and back.

Outline of therapeutic indications

Points on this meridian are indicated for diseases of the throat, chest and lung, and other diseases of areas the meridian supplies.

LU 1, ZHONGFU*

Front-Mu point of the lung, the Crossing point of the hand and foot Taiyin meridians.

Location. Latero-superior to the sternum at the lateral side and at the same level as the first intercostal space, 6 cun lateral to the Ren meridian (anterior midline), see Fig. 8.

Regional anatomy. The m. pectoralis and m. pectoralis minor, m. intercostales interni and externi; superolaterally, the axillary artery and vein, the thoracoacromial artery and vein; the intermediate supraclavicular nerve, the branches of the anterior thoracic nerve, and the lateral cutaneous branch of the 1st intercostal nerve.

Indications. Cough, asthmatic breathing, distension and fullness in the lung, pain in the chest, shoulder and back.

Method. Puncture obliquely or transversely 0.5–0.8 cun towards the lateral aspect of the chest. To avoid injuring the lung, never puncture deeply towards the medial aspect.

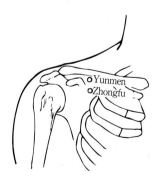

Fig. 8

Remarks. Under the manipulations mentioned in "Method", only routine methods of needling are introduced (except for contra-indicated points). Moxibustion methods will be dealt with later, (in Ch. 5 and in Part 3 under specific diseases). Only those with a special function are introduced in this chapter.

LU 2, YUNMEN

Location. Latero-superior to the sternum, 6 cun lateral to the Ren meridian, in the depression below the acromial extremity of the clavicle (see Fig. 8).

Regional anatomy. Lateral to the m. horasis; the cephalic vein, the thoracoacromial artery and vein, inferiorly the axillary artery; the intermediate and lateral supraclavicular nerve, the branches of the anterior thoracic nerve, and the lateral cord of the brachial plexus.

Indications. Cough, asthmatic breathing, pain in the chest and shoulder.

Method. Puncture obliquely and laterally 0.5–0.8 cun and, to avoid injuring the lung, never puncture deeply towards the medial aspect of the chest.

LU 3, TIANFU

Location. On the lateral aspect of the upper arm, 3 cun below the end of the axillary fold, on the radial side of the m. biceps brachii (see Fig. 9).

Regional anatomy. Lateral to the m. biceps brachii; the cephalic vein and branches of the brachial artery and vein; the lateral brachial cutaneous nerve at the place where the musculo-cutaneous nerve passes through.

Indications. Asthmatic breathing, epistaxis, goitre and pain in the medial aspect of the upper arm.

Method. Puncture perpendicularly 0.5–1 cun.

LU 4, XIABAI

Location. 1 cun below Tianfu and 5 cun above the cubital crease.

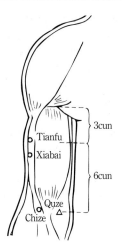

Fig. 9

Regional anatomy. Lateral to the m. biceps brachii; the cephalic vein and branches of the brachial artery and vein; the lateral brachial cutaneous nerve at the place where the musculocutaneous nerve passes through.

Indications. Cough, asthmatic breathing, dry vomiting, fullness in the chest and pain in the medial aspect of the upper arm.

Method. Puncture perpendicularly 0.5–1 cun.

LU 5, CHIZE*

The He-sea point.

Location. On the cubital crease, on the radial side of the tendon of the m. biceps brachii (see Fig. 9).

Regional anatomy. At the elbow joint, lateral to the tendon of the m. biceps brachii, at the head of the m. brachioradialis; the branches of the radial recurrent artery and vein, the cephalic vein; the lateral antebrachial cutaneous nerve, and directly inferior to the radial nerve.

Indications. Cough, asthmatic breathing, haemoptysis, hectic (tidal) fever, distension and fullness in the chest, congested and sore throat, infantile convulsion, vomiting and diarrhoea, spasmodic pain of the elbow and arm.

Method. Puncture perpendicularly 0.8–1.2 cun, or prick to cause bleeding.

LU 6, KONGZUI*

The Xi-Cleft point.

Location. On the line linking Taiyuan (Lu 9) and Chize (Lu 5), 7 cun above the transverse crease of the wrist (see Fig. 10).

Regional anatomy. The m. brachioradialis, lateral border of the upper end of the m. pronator teres and medial border of the m. extensor carpiradialis longus and brevis; the cephalic vein, the radial artery and vein; the lateral antebrachial cutaneous nerve and the superficial ramus of the radial nerve.

Indications. Cough, asthmatic breathing, haemoptysis, congested and sore throat, spasmodic pain of the elbow and arm and haemorrhoids.

Method. Puncture perpendicularly 0.5–1.0 cun.

LU 7, LIEQUE*

The *luo* point—one of the 8 Confluent Points of the 8 extra meridians communicating with the Ren meridian.

Location. Superior to the styloid process of the radius, 1.5 cun above the transverse crease of the wrist (see Fig. 10). A simple way of locating this point is when the index fingers and thumbs of both hands are crossed with the index finger of one hand placed on the styloid process of the radius of the other, the point lies in the depression just under the tip of the index finger (see Fig. 11).

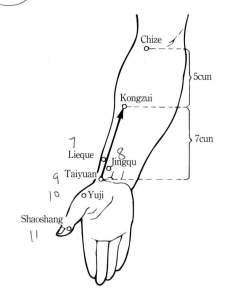

Fig. 10

Regional anatomy. Between the tendons of the m. brachioradialis and m. abductor pollicis longus, medial aspect of the tendon of the m. extensor carpiradialis longus; the cephalic vein, branches of the radial artery and vein; the mixed branches of the lateral antebrachial cutaneous nerve and the superficial ramus of the radial nerve.

Indications. Common cold, headache, neck rigidity, cough, asthmatic breathing, congested and sore throat, deviation of the mouth and eye, and toothache.

Method. Puncture upward obliquely 0.3–0.5 cun.

LU 8, JINGQU*

The Jing-river point.

Location. Medial to the styloid process of radius, 1 cun above the transverse crease of the wrist in the depression on the lateral side of the radial artery (see Fig. 10).

Regional anatomy. Lateral aspect of the tendon of the m. flexor carpi radialis, m. pronator quadratus; lateral to the radial artery and vein; the mixed branches of the lateral antebrachial cutaneous nerve and the superficial ramus of the radial nerve.

Indications. Cough, asthmatic breathing, pain in the chest, congested and sore throat and pain in the wrist.

Method. Avoid the radial artery, then puncture perpendicularly 0.3–0.5 cun.

Note. The **Systematic Classic of Acupuncture and Moxibustion** says moxibustion is contraindicated at this point.

LU 9, TAIYUAN*

The Shu-stream point, the *yuan* point, the Influential point of the vessels.

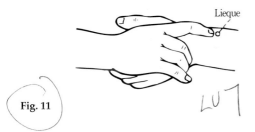

Lieque

Fig. 11

Location. At the radial end of the transverse crease of the wrist, in the depression at the lateral aspect of the radial artery (see Fig. 10).

Regional anatomy. Lateral aspect of the tendon of the m. flexor carpi radialis and medial aspect of the tendon of the m. abductor pollicis longus; the radial artery and vein; the mixed branches of the lateral antebrachial cutaneous nerve and the superficial ramus of the radial nerve.

Indications. Cough, asthmatic breathing, haemoptysis, pain in the chest, congested and sore throat, pain in the wrist and arm, and a disease without pulse.

Method. Avoid the radial artery and puncture perpendicularly 0.3– 0.5 cun.

LU 10, YUJI*

The Ying-spring point.

Location. At the midpoint of the first metacarpal bone, on the junction of the red and white skin (i.e. the junction of the dorsum and palm of the hand) (see Fig. 12).

Regional anatomy. The m. abductor pollicis brevis and m. opponeus pollicis; venules of the thumb draining to the cephalic vein; the mixed branches of the lateral antebrachial cutaneous nerve and the superficial ramus of the radial nerve.

Indications. Cough, haemoptysis, congested and sore throat, hoarseness of voice and fever.

Method. Puncture perpendicularly 0.5–0.8 cun.

LU 11, SHAOSHANG*

The Jing-well point.

Location. On the radial side of the thumb, about 0.1 cun beside the corner of the nail (see Fig. 12).

Regional anatomy. The arterial and venous network formed by the palmar digital proprial artery and veins; the terminal nerve network formed by the mixed branches of the lateral antebrachial cutaneous nerve and the superficial ramus of the radial nerve as well as the palmar digital proprial nerve of the median nerve.

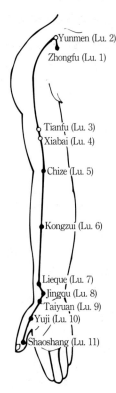

Fig. 12   Points on the lung meridian of hand Taiyin.
●   Frequently used points.
○   Ordinary points.

Indications.   Congested and sore throat, cough, epistaxis, fever, loss of consciousness and mania.
Method.   Puncture superficially 0.1 cun, or prick to cause bleeding.

THE LARGE INTESTINE MERIDIAN OF THE HAND YANGMING (WITH 20 ACUPOINTS)

Course

The large intestine meridian of the hand Yangming starts from the tip of the index finger (Shangyang, LI 1) (1), goes upward along the radial side of the index finger and passes through the interspace of the 1st and 2nd meta-carpal bones (Hegu, LI 4) and enters the depression between the tendons of the m. extensor pollicis longus and brevis (2); then following the lateral anterior aspect of the forearm (3), it reaches the lateral side of the elbow (4); from there it ascends along the lateral anterior aspect of the upper arm to the highest point of the shoulder (Jianyu, LI 15) (6), then along the anterior border of the acromion (7); it goes up to the 7th cervical vertebra (the confluence of the three yang meridians of the hand and foot, Dazhui, Du 14) (8), and descends to the supraclavicular fossa (9) to connect with the lung (10); it then passes through the diaphragm (11) and enters the large intestine (12), the organ to which it pertains.

Table 3.1   An outline of indications of points on the lung meridian

Point	Location	Indications	
		primary	secondary
		Chest: diseases of the chest and lung	
Zhongfu* (Lu 1)	chest	cough, asthmatic breathing, pain in the chest	
Yunmen (Lu 2)	chest	" "	
		Hand and arm: diseases of throat, chest and lung	
Tianfu (Lu 3)	upper arm	asthmatic breathing, epistaxis	
Xiabai (Lu 4)	upper arm	cough	
Chize* (Lu 5)	elbow	cough, haemoptysis, asthmatic breathing, fullness in chest	hectic fever, infantile convulsion
Kongzui* (Lu 6)	forearm	cough, haemoptysis, pain in the chest	
Lieque* (Lu 7)	forearm	cough, congested and sore throat	headache, deviation of the mouth
Jingqu* (Lu 8)	"	" "	
Taiyuan* (Lu 9)	wrist joint	" "	pulseless disease
Yuji* (Lu 10)	palm	haemoptysis, congested and sore throat	fever, hoarseness of voice
Shaoshang* (Lu 11)	tip of the thumb	congested and sore throat, cough	fever, coma, and mania

Note: *refers to a frequently used point. "Primary" refers to main diseases of this meridian and its connected zangfu organs, "secondary" refers to other diseases in which the point is also indicated.

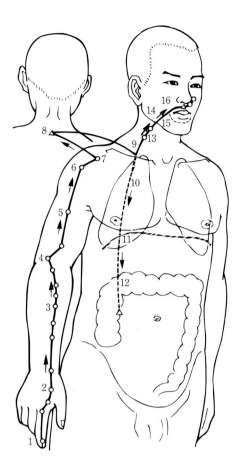

Fig. 13 The course of the large intestine meridian of the hand Yangming.

A branch from the supraclavicular fossa runs upward to the neck (13), passes through the cheek (14) and enters the gums of the lower teeth (15); then it curves around the upper lip and crosses the opposite meridian at the philtrum; from there the left meridian goes to the right and the right meridian to the left, to both sides of the nose (Yingxiang, LI 20) (16), where the large intestine meridian links with the stomach meridian of the foot Yangming.

Chief pathological manifestations

Abdominal pain, borborygmus, diarrhoea, constipation, dysentery, congested and sore throat, toothache, watery nasal discharge or epistaxis, pain, hotness and swelling, or coldness along the course of this meridian.

Outline of therapeutic indications

Points on this meridian are indicated in diseases of the head and face, five sense organs, pharynx and larynx, febrile diseases and other diseases of the areas the meridian supplies.

LI 1, SHANGYANG*

The Jing-well point.
Location. On the radial side of the index finger, about 0.1 cun beside the corner of the nail (see Fig. 14).
Regional anatomy. The arterial and venous network formed by the dorsal digital arteries and veins; the palmar digital proprial nerve derived from the median nerve and the lateral dorsal digital nerves of the radial nerve.
Indications. Deafness, toothache, congested and sore throat, swelling of the submandibular region, optic atrophy, numbness of the fingers, febrile diseases and loss of consciousness.
Method. Puncture superficially 0.1 cun or prick to cause bleeding.

LI 2, ERJIAN

The Ying-spring point.
Location. The point is located with the finger slightly flexed. It lies on the radial side of the index finger, in the depression distal to the metacarpal-phalangeal joint (see Fig. 14).

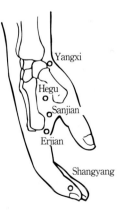

Fig. 14

Regional anatomy. The superficial and deep flexor tendons of the fingers; the dorsal digital and palmar digital proprial arteries and veins derived from the radial artery and vein; the dorsal digital nerve of the radial nerve and the palmar digital proprial nerve of the median nerve.

Indications. Blurred vision, epistaxis, toothache, deviation of the mouth, congested and sore throat and febrile diseases.

Method. Puncture perpendicularly 0.2–0.3 cun.

LI 3, SANJIAN*

The Shu-stream point.

Location. When a loose fist is made, the point is on the radial side of the index finger, in the depression proximal to the head of the second metacarpal bone (see Fig. 14).

Regional anatomy. Posterior to the small head of the second metacarpal bone, m. interossei dorsales and m. adductor pollicis; the dorsal venous network of the hand and the proper palmar digital arteries; the superficial ramus of the radial nerve.

Indications. Pain in the eyes, toothache, congested and sore throat, general feverishness, abdominal fullness and borborygmus.

Method. Puncture perpendicularly 0.5–0.8 cun.

LI 4, HEGU* (ALSO CALLED HUKOU)

The *yuan* point.

Location. On the dorsum of the hand, between the 1st and 2nd metacarpal bones, approximately in the middle of the 2nd metacarpal bone on the radial side (see Fig. 14).

A simple way of locating this point is to place in coincident position the transverse crease of the interphalangeal joint of the thumb, and the margin of the web between the thumb and the index finger of the other hand; then the point is where the tip of the thumb touches (see Fig. 15).

Regional anatomy. Between the 1st and 2nd metacarpal bones and dorsal muscle of the 1st metacarpal bone, the transverse head of the adductor muscle of the thumb deeply; the venous

network of the dorsum of the hand, the head of the cephalic vein; proximal to the point is the radial artery, running from the dorsum to the palm of the hand; the dorsal metacarpal nerve of the superficial ramus of the radial nerve, and deeply the palmar digital proprial nerve derived from the median nerve.

Indications. Headache, redness, swelling and pain in the eye, epistaxis, toothache, lockjaw, deviation of the mouth and eye, deafness, mumps, congestion and sore throat, febrile diseases, anhidrosis, hidrosis, abdominal pain, constipation, amenorrhoea and delayed labour.

Method. Puncture perpendicularly 0.5–1.0 cun.

Note. In the *Classic of Magical Effective Treatment* this point is contraindicated for pregnant women.

LI 5, YANGXI*

The Jing-river point.

Location. On the radial side of the dorsal carpal transverse crease. When the thumb is tilted upward it is in the depression between the tendons of the m. extensor pollicis longus and brevis (see Fig. 14).

Regional anatomy. Between the tendons of the m. extensor pollicis longus and brevis; the cephalic vein, the radial artery and its dorsal carpal branch; the superficial ramus of the radial nerve.

Indications. Headache, redness, swelling and pain in the eye, deafness, tinnitus, congested and sore throat and pain in the wrist.

Method. Puncture perpendicularly 0.5–0.8 cun.

LI 6, PIANLI*

The *luo* point.

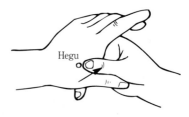

Fig. 15

Location. On the line joining Yangxi (LI 5) and Quchi (LI 11), 3 cun above Yangxi (LI 5) (see Fig. 16).

Regional anatomy. Distal end of the radius, between the tendon of the m. extensor carpi radialis and the tendon of the m. abductor pollicis longus; the cephalic vein; palmarly the lateral antebrachial cutaneous nerve and the superficial ramus of the radial nerve, dorsally the posterior antebrachial cutaneous nerve and the posterior antebrachial interosseous nerve.

Indications. Redness of the eye, tinnitus, epistaxis, sore throat, aching of the hand and arm, and oedema.

Method. Puncture perpendicularly or obliquely 0.5–0.8 cun.

LI 7, WENLIU

The Xi-Cleft point.

Location. On the line joining Yangxi (LI 5) and Quchi (LI 11), 5 cun above Yangxi (LI 5) (see Fig. 16).

Regional anatomy. Between the belly of the m. extensor carpi radialis and the m. abductor pollicis longus; a branch of the radial artery and the cephalic vein; the posterior antebrachial

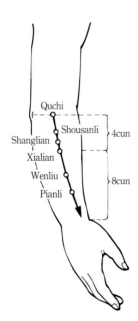

Fig. 16

cutaneous nerve and the deep ramus of the radial nerve.

Indications. Headache, puffiness in the face, congested and sore throat, carbuncles and ulcers, aching of the shoulder and back, borborygmus and abdominal pain.

Method. Puncture perpendicularly 0.5–1.0 cun.

LI 8, XIALIAN

Location. On the line joining Yangxi (LI 5) and Quchi (LI 11), 4 cun below Quchi (LI 11) (see Fig. 16).

Regional anatomy. On the radial side of the radius, the m. extensor carpi radialis brevis and longus, deeply the m. supinator; a branch of the radial artery, the cephalic vein; the posterior antebrachial cutaneous nerve and the deep ramus of the radial nerve.

Indications. Headache, vertigo, pain in the eye, pain in the elbow and arm, abdominal distension and pain.

Method. Puncture perpendicularly 0.5–1.0 cun.

LI 9, SHANGLIAN

Location. On the line joining Yangxi (LI 5) and Quchi (LI 11), 3 cun below Quchi (LI 11) (see Fig. 16).

Regional anatomy. See Xialian (LI 8).

Indications. Headache, aching of the shoulder and arm, hemiplegia, numbness of the arm, borborygmus and abdominal pain.

Method. Puncture perpendicularly 0.5–1.0 cun.

LI 10, SHOUSANLI*

Location. On the line joining Yangxi (LI 5) and Quchi (LI 11), 2 cun below Quchi (LI 11) (see Fig. 16).

Regional anatomy. For musculature and innervation, see Xialian (LI 8); the branches of the radial recurrent artery.

Indications. Toothache, swelling of cheek, motor impairment of the upper limbs, abdominal pain and diarrhoea.

Method. Puncture perpendicularly 0.8–1.2 cun.

LI 11, QUCHI*

The He-sea point.

Location. When the elbow is flexed at a right angle, the point is in the depression at the lateral end of the transverse cubital crease, midway between Chize (Lu 5) and the lateral epicondyle of the humerus (see Fig. 16).

Regional anatomy. The beginning of the m. extensor carpi radialis longus, radial aspect of the m. brachioradialis; the branches of the radial recurrent artery; the posterior antebrachial cutaneous nerve, deeply and on the medial side the radial nerve trunk.

Indications. Congested and sore throat, toothache, redness and pain in the eye, scrofula, faint skin eruptions and febrile diseases, motor impairment of the upper limbs, swelling and pain of the upper limbs, abdominal pain, vomiting and diarrhoea, hypertension, depressive and manic psychosis.

Method. Puncture perpendicularly 1.0–1.5 cun.

Note. According to reports, experimental appendicitis was caused in dogs by injecting directly a mixture of streptococcus and *Staphylococcus aureus* into the appendicular wall. Then needling with a strong stimulation was given to Quchi (LI 11) and Lanweixue (Extra 41) and a definite therapeutic effect was observed.

LI 12, ZHOULIAO

Location. When the elbow is flexed, the point is superior to the lateral epicondyle of the humerus, about 1 cun supero-lateral to Quchi (LI 11), on the medial border of the humerus (see Fig. 17).

Regional anatomy. At the beginning of the m. brachialis of the external epicondyle of the radius, lateral border of the m. triceps brachii; the radial collateral artery; the posterior antebrachial cutaneous nerve and the radial nerve.

Indications. Aching, numbness and spasm of the elbow and arm.

Method. Puncture perpendicularly 0.5–1.0 cun.

LI 13, SHOUWULI

Location. On the line joining Quchi (LI 11),

and Jianyu (LI 15), 3 cun above Quchi (LI 11) (see Fig. 17).

Regional anatomy. At the beginning of the m. brachioradialis, on the radial side of the humerus, laterally the anterior border of the m. triceps brachii; deeply, the radial collateral artery; the posterior antebrachial cutaneous nerve and the radial nerve, deeply on the medial side, the radial nerve.

Indications. Spasmodic pain of the elbow and arm, and scrofula.

Method. Avoid the artery and puncture perpendicularly 0.5–1.0 cun.

LI 14, BINAO*

Location. On the line joining Quchi (LI 11) and Jianyu (LI 15), 7 cun above Quchi (LI 11), at the lower end of the m. deltoideus (see Fig. 17).

Regional anatomy. Radial side of the humerus, lower end of the m. deltoideus, anterior border of the lateral end of the m. triceps brachii; the branches of posterior circumflex humeral artery and the deep brachial artery; the posterior brachial cutaneous nerve, deeply the radial nerve trunk.

Indications. Pain in the shoulder and arm, rigidity of the neck, scrofula and eye disease.

Method. Puncture perpendicularly or obliquely-upwardly 0.8–1.5 cun.

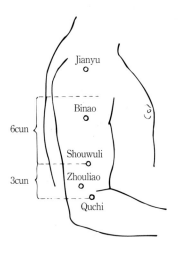

Fig. 17

LI 15, JIANYU*

The Crossing point of the hand Yangming and Yangqiao meridians.

Location. At the lower border of the acromion, between the acromion and the greater tuberosity of humerus, at the centre of the upper portion of the m. deltoideus; when the arm is in full abduction, the point is in the depression appearing at the anterior border of the acromioclavicular joint (see Fig. 17).

Regional anatomy. The posterior circumflex artery and vein; the supraclavicular nerve and axillary nerve.

Indications. Pain and motor impairment of the shoulder and arm, faint skin eruptions and scrofula.

Method. Puncture perpendicularly or downward-obliquely 0.8–1.5 cun.

LI 16, JUGU

The Crossing point of the hand Yangming and Yangqiao meridians.

Location. In the depression between the acromial extremity of the clavicle and the scapular spine (see Fig. 18).

Regional anatomy. On the m. trapezius and m. supraspinatus; deeply the suprascapular artery and vein; a branch of the supraclavicular nerve, a branch of the accessory nerve, deeply the suprascapular nerve.

Indications. Pain and motor impairment of the upper limbs, scrofula and goitre.

Method. Puncture perpendicularly and slightly laterally-downwardly 0.5–1.0 cun.

LI 17, TIANDING

Location. At the posterior border of the m. sternocleidomastoideus, 1 cun directly below Neck-Futu (LI 18) (see Fig. 19).

Regional anatomy. Posterior border of the lower part of the m. sternocleidomastoideus, superficially the m. platysma and deeply the m. scalenus medius (at its beginning); the external jugular vein; the accessory nerve, the cutaneous cervical nerves which emerge at the posterior border of the m. sternocleidomastoideus, deeply the beginning of the phrenic nerve.

Indications. Sudden loss of voice, congested and sore throat, scrofula and goitre.

Method. Puncture perpendicularly 0.5–0.8 cun.

LI 18, NECK-FUTU*

Location. 3 cun lateral to the tip of the Adam's apple, between the sternal head and clavicular head of the m. sternocleidomastoideus (see Fig. 19).

Regional anatomy. At the platysma at the sternal head of the m. sternocleidomastoideus, deeply the beginning of the m. levator scapulae; deeply on the medial side, the ascending cervical artery; the great auricular nerve, cutaneous cervical nerve, lesser occipital nerve and accessory nerve.

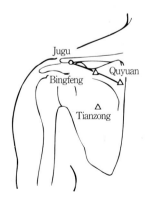

Fig. 18

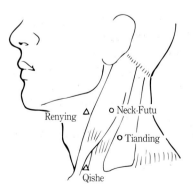

Fig. 19

Indications. Cough, asthmatic breathing, congested and sore throat, sudden loss of voice, scrofula and goitre.

Method. Puncture perpendicularly 0.5–0.8 cun.

LI 19, KOUHELIAO

Location. 0.5 cun lateral to Shuigou (Renzhong, Du 26), right below the lateral margin of the nostril (see Fig. 20).

Regional anatomy. At the canine fossa of the maxilla, end of the m. quadratus labii superioris; the superior labial branches of the facial artery and vein; the facial nerve, anastomotic plexus of the inferior branch of the trigeminal nerve and the infraorbital nerve.

Indications. Nasal obstruction, epistaxis, deviation of the mouth, and trismus.

Method. Puncture perpendicularly or obliquely 0.3–0.5 cun.

LI 20, YINGXIANG*

The Crossing point of the hand and foot Yangming meridians.

Location. In the nasolabial groove, at the level of the midpoint of the lateral border of ala nasi (see Fig. 20).

Regional anatomy. At the m. quadratus labii superioris, deeply the border of the m. piriformis; the facial artery and vein, the branches of

the infraorbital artery and vein; the anastomotic branch of the facial and infraorbital nerves.

Indications. Nasal obstruction, epistaxis, deviation of the mouth, itching of the face and biliary ascariasis.

Method. Puncture obliquely or transversely 0.3–0.5 cun.

Note. The *Medical Secrets of An Official* states that this point is contraindicated in moxibustion.

THE STOMACH MERIDIAN OF THE FOOT YANGMING (WITH 45 ACUPOINTS)

Course

The stomach meridian of foot Yangming starts from the lateral side of the ala nasi (Yingxiang, LI 20) (1), and ascends to the bridge of the nose where it meets the bladder meridian of the foot Taiyang (Jingming, UB 1) (2); turning downward along the lateral side of the nose (Chengqi, St 1) (3) it enters the upper gum (4); reemerging it curves around the lips (5) and descends to meet the Ren meridian at the mentolabial groove

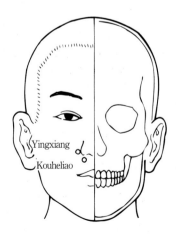

Fig. 20

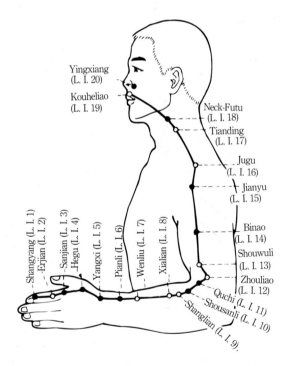

Fig. 21 Points on the large intestine meridian of the hand Yangming.

Table 3.2 An outline of indications of points on the large intestine meridian

Point	Location	Indications	
		primary	secondary
	Hand and elbow: diseases of head, face, eye, ear, nose, mouth and teeth; febrile diseases		
Shangyang* (LI 1)	tip of the index finger	deafness, toothache, swelling of maxillary region, congested and sore throat	loss of consciousness and febrile disease
Erjian (LI 2)	finger	blurred vision, epistaxis, toothache, deviation of mouth	
Sanjian* (LI 3)	finger	ache of lower teeth, congested and sore throat	
Hegu* (LI 4)	dorsum of hand	headache, epistaxis, deafness, toothache, deviation of mouth, congested and sore throat	febrile disease, profuse sweating
Yangxi* (LI 5)	wrist joint	headache, redness of eyes, deafness, toothache	
Pianli (LI 6)*	forearm	epistaxis	oedema
Wenliu (LI 7)	forearm	headache, puffiness in face, congested and sore throat	borborygmus, abdominal pain
Xialian (LI 8)	forearm	pain in elbow and arm	abdominal pain
Shanglian (LI 9)	forearm	motor impairment of upper limbs	abdominal pain, borborygmus
Shousanli* (LI 10)	forearm	toothache, swelling of cheek, motor impairment of upper limbs	abdominal pain and diarrhoea
Quchi* (LI 11)	elbow	congested and sore throat, motor impairment of upper limbs	febrile disease, skin eruptions, abdominal pain, diarrhoea
	Upper arm and shoulder: local diseases mainly		
Zhouliao (LI 12)	upper arm	pain in elbow and arm	
Shouwuli (LI 13)	upper arm	pain in elbow and arm	
Binao* (LI 14)	upper arm	pain in the arm	eye disorders
Jianyu* (LI 15)	scapular joint	pain in shoulder and arm, motor impairment of upper limbs	
Jugu (LI 16)	shoulder	pain in shoulder and arm	
	Neck: diseases of the throat		
Tianding (LI 17)	neck	sudden loss of voice, congested and sore throat	
Neck-Futu* (LI 18)	neck	sudden loss of voice, congested and sore throat	
	Face: diseases of the nose		
Kouheliao (LI 19)	face	nasal obstruction, epistaxis, deviation of mouth	
Yingxiang* (LI 20)	face	nasal obstruction, rhinorrhoea, epistaxis, deviation of mouth	

(Chengjiang, Ren 24) (6); then it runs postero-laterally across the lower portion of the cheek at Daying (St 5) (7); winding along the angle of the mandible (Jiache, St 6) (8), it ascends in front of the ear and traverses Shangguan (GB 3) (9); then it follows the anterior hairline (10) and reaches the forehead (Shenting, Du 24) (11).

A facial branch emerging in front of Daying (St 5) runs downward to Renying (St 9) (12); from there it runs along the throat and enters the supraclavicular fossa (13); descending, it passes through the diaphragm (14), enters the stomach, the organ it pertains to, and connects with the spleen (15).

A straight portion of the meridian arising from the supraclavicular fossa runs downward passing through the nipple (16); then it descends by the umbilicus and enters Qichong (St 30) on the lateral side of the lower abdomen (17).

A branch from the lower orifice of the stomach descends inside the abdomen and joins the previous portion of the meridian at Qichong (St 30) (18); running downward and traversing Biguan (St 31) (19) and further through Futu (St 32) (20) it reaches the knee (21); from there it continues downward along the anterior border of the lateral aspect of the tibia (22), passes through the dorsum of the foot (23) and reaches the lateral side of the tip of the 2nd toe (Lidui, St 45) (24).

The tibial branch emerges from Zusanli (St 36) which is 3 cun below the knee (25), and enters the lateral side of the middle toe (26).

A branch from the dorsum of the foot arises from Chongyang (St 42) and terminates at the medial side of the tip of the great toe (Yinbai, Sp 1) where it links with the spleen meridian of the foot Taiyin (27).

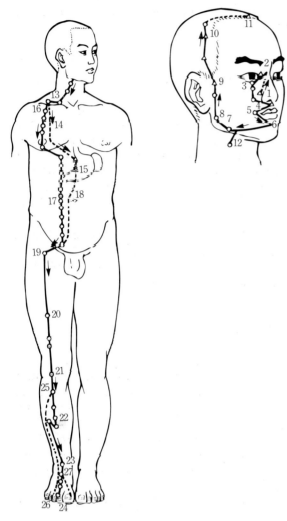

Fig. 22   The course of the stomach meridian of the foot Yangming.

Chief pathological manifestations

Borborygmus, abdominal distension, oedema, stomach-ache, vomiting or polyphagia, thirst, congested and sore throat, epistaxis, pain in the chest and patella and the areas it supplies, febrile diseases and mania.

Outline of therapeutic indications

Points on this meridian are indicated for gastrointestinal diseases, disorders of the head, face, eye, nose, mouth and tooth, mental disorders and other diseases in areas the meridian supplies.

ST 1, CHENGQI*

The Crossing point of the foot Yangming, the Yangqiao and Ren meridians.

Location.   With the eyes looking straight forward, the point is directly below the pupil, between the eyeball and the infraorbital ridge (see Fig. 23).

Regional anatomy.   Above the infraorbital margin, at the m. orbicularis oculi, deeply intraorbitally the m. rectus inferior bulbi and m. obliquus inferior bulbi; the branches of the infraorbital and ophthalmic arteries and veins; a branch of the infraorbital nerve, a muscular branch of the inferior branch of the oculomotor nerve and a branch of the facial nerve.

Indications.   Redness, swelling and pain of the eye, lacrimation, night blindness, twitching of the eyelids and deviation of the mouth and eye.

Method.   Push the eyeball upward with the left thumb and puncture perpendicularly and slowly 0.5–1.0 cun along the infraorbital ridge; to avoid injuring blood vessels and causing haematoma, it is not advisable to lift and thrust the needle.

ST 2, SIBAI*

Location.   With the eyes looking straight for-

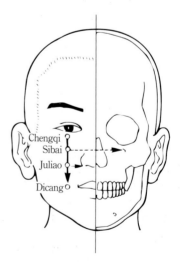

Fig. 23

ward, the point is directly below the pupil, in the depression at the infraorbital foramen (see Fig. 23).

Regional anatomy. At the infraorbital foramen, between the m. orbicularis oculi and m. quadratus labii superioris; the branches of the facial artery and vein, the infraorbital artery and vein; the branches of the facial nerve. The point is just on the course of the infraorbital nerve.

Indications. Redness, pain and itching of the eye, nebula, twitching of eyelids, deviation of the mouth and eye, headache and vertigo.

Method. Puncture perpendicularly or obliquely 0.3–0.5 cun; deep needling is contraindicated.

ST 3, JULIAO

The Crossing point of the foot Yangming and the Yangqiao meridians.

Location. With the eyes looking straight forward, the point is directly below the pupil, level with the lower border of the ala nasi. (see Fig. 23)

Regional anatomy. Superficially the m. quadratus labii superioris, deeply the m. levator anguli oris; the branches of the facial and infraorbital arteries and veins; the branches of the facial and infraorbital nerves.

Indications. Deviation of the mouth and eye, twitching of eyelids, epistaxis, toothache and swelling of the lips and cheek.

Method. Puncture obliquely or transversely 0.3–0.5 cun.

ST 4, DICANG*

The Crossing point of the hand Yangming and the Yangqiao meridians.

Location. 0.4 cun lateral to the corner of the mouth, directly below Juliao (St 3) (see Fig. 23).

Regional anatomy. At the m. orbicularis oris and deeply the m. buccinator; the facial artery and vein; the branches of the facial and infraorbital nerves, deeply the terminal branch of the buccal nerve.

Indications. Deviation of the mouth, salivation, and twitching of eyelids.

Method. Puncture obliquely or transversely 0.5–0.8 cun.

ST 5, DAYING

Location. Anterior to the angle of mandible, on the anterior border of the attached portion of the m. masseter, in the groove-like depression appearing when the cheek is bulged (see Fig. 24).

Regional anatomy. On the anterior border of the attached portion of the m. masseter; anteriorly the facial artery and vein; the facial and buccal nerves.

Indications. Deviation of the mouth, trismus, swelling of cheek and toothache.

Method. Avoid the artery, puncture obliquely or transversely 0.3– 0.5 cun.

ST 6, JIACHE*

Location. One finger-breadth anterior and superior to the lower angle of the mandible where the m. masseter attaches at the prominence of the muscle when the teeth are clenched (see Fig. 24).

Regional anatomy. Anterior to the mandible, the m. masseter; the masseter artery and vein; the great auricular nerve, facial nerve and masseteric nerve.

Indications. Deviation of the mouth, toothache, swelling of cheek and trismus.

Method. Puncture 0.3–0.5 cun perpendicularly or 0.5–1.0 cun transversely.

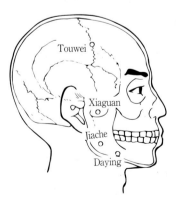

Fig. 24

ST 7, XIAGUAN*

The Crossing point of the foot Yangming and foot Shaoyang meridians.

Location. At the lower border of the zygomatic arch, in the depression anterior to the condyloid process of the mandible and between the notches; the point is located with the mouth closed. (see Fig. 24)

Regional anatomy. At lower border of the arch, with the parotid gland underneath, the beginning of the m. masseter; the transverse facial artery and vein, in the deepest layer the maxillary artery and vein; the zygomatic branch of the facial nerve and the branches of the auriculotemporal nerve, in the deepest layer the mandibular nerve.

Indications. Deafness, tinnitus, otorrhoea, toothache, trismus and deviation of the mouth and eye.

Method. Puncture perpendicularly 0.5–1.0 cun.

ST 8, TOUWEI*

The Crossing point of the foot Yangming, foot Shaoyang and the Yangwei meridians.

Location. Directly above the temporal hairline and 0.5 cun within the anterior hairline at the corner of the forehead (see Fig. 24).

Regional anatomy. Upper border of the m. temporalis, galea aponeurotica; the frontal branches of the superficial temporal artery and vein; a branch of the auriculotemporal nerve and the temporal branch of the facial nerve.

Indications. Headache, blurred vision, pain in the mouth, lacrimation and twitching of eyelids.

Method. Puncture transversely 0.5–1.0 cun.

Note. The *Systematic Classic on Acupuncture and Moxibustion* says this point is contraindicated for moxibustion.

ST 9, RENYING

The Crossing point of the foot Yangming and foot Shaoyang meridians.

Location. Level with and 1.5 cun lateral to the tip of the Adam's apple, just on the course of the common carotid artery, on the anterior border of the m. sternocleidomastoideus (see Fig. 25).

Regional anatomy. The platysma, at the junction of the anterior border of the m. sternocleidomastoideus and the thyroid cartilage; the superior thyroid artery at the bifurcation of the internal and the external carotid artery, the anterior jugular vein and laterally the internal jugular vein; the cutaneous cervical nerve, the cervical branch of the facial nerve, deeply the bulbus arteriosus, in the deepest layer the sympathetic trunk, laterally the descending branch of the hypoglossal nerve and the vagus nerve.

Indications. Congested and sore throat, asthmatic breathing, scrofula, goitre and hypertension.

Method. Avoid the common carotid artery, puncture perpendicularly 0.3–0.8 cun.

Note. In the *Systematic Classic on Acupuncture and Moxibustion* this point is contraindicated for moxibustion.

ST 10, SHUITU

Location. At the midpoint of the line joining Renying (St 9) and Qishe (St 11), on the anterior border of the m. sternocleidomastoideus. (see Fig. 25).

Regional anatomy. The platysma, lateral to the thyroid cartilage, at the crossing point of the m. sternocleidomastoideus and the uppermost belly of the omohyoid muscle; laterally the common carotid artery; the cutaneous cervical nerve, deeply the superior cardiac nerve issuing from the sympathetic nerves.

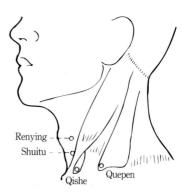

Fig. 25

Indications. Congested and sore throat, cough and asthmatic breathing.

Method. Puncture perpendicularly 0.3–0.8 cun.

ST 11, QISHE

Location. Directly below Renying (St 9), at the superior border of the sternal extremity of the clavicle, between the sternal head and clavicular head of the m. sternocleidomastoideus (see Fig. 25)

Regional anatomy. The platysma, at the beginning of the m. sternocleidomastoideus; superficially the anterior jugular vein, deeply the common carotid artery; the medial supraclavicular nerve and the muscular branch of the ansa hypoglossi.

Indications. Congested and sore throat, asthmatic breathing, hiccup, goitre, scrofula and rigidity of the neck.

Method. Puncture perpendicularly 0.3–0.5 cun.

Note. Deep underneath these points, from Qishe (St 11) to Rugen (St 28), are large arteries and important viscera such as the lung and liver, so deep puncture is contraindicated.

ST 12, QUEPEN

Location. In the centre of the supraclavicular fossa, 4 cun lateral to the Ren meridian (see Fig. 25).

Regional anatomy. At the centre of the supraclavicular fossa, the platysma, the m. omohyoideus; superiorly the transverse cervical artery; the intermediate supraclavicular nerve, deeply the supraclavicular portion of brachial plexus.

Indications. Cough, asthmatic breathing, congested and sore throat, pain in supraclavicular fossa and scrofula.

Method. Puncture perpendicularly or obliquely 0.3–0.5 cun.

Note. Needling is contraindicated at this point for pregnant women.

ST 13, QIHU

Location. At the lower border of the clavicle, 4 cun lateral to the Ren meridian (see Fig. 26).

Regional anatomy. At lower border of the clavicle, the beginning of the m. pectoralis major, deeply the m. subclavius; the branches of the thoracoacromial artery and vein, superiorly the subclavicular vein; the branches of the supraclavicular nerve and the anterior thoracic nerve.

Indications. Cough, asthmatic breathing, hiccup, fullness in the chest and hypochondrium, and pain in the chest.

Method. Puncture obliquely or transversely 0.5–0.8 cun.

ST 14, KUFANG

Location. In the first intercostal space, 4 cun lateral to the Ren meridian (see Fig. 26).

Regional anatomy. The m. pectoralis major and m. pectoralis minor in the first intercostal space, deeply the m. intercostales interni and externi; the thoracoacromial artery and vein and the branches of the lateral thoracic artery and vein; a branch of the anterior thoracic nerve.

Indications. Cough, asthmatic breathing, expectoration of purulent blood and distension and pain in the chest and hypochondrium.

Method. Puncture obliquely or transversely 0.5–0.8 cun.

ST 15, WUYI

Location. In the second intercostal space, 4 cun lateral to the Ren meridian (see Fig. 26).

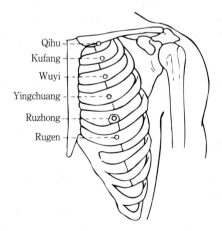

Qihu
Kufang
Wuyi
Yingchuang
Ruzhong
Rugen

Fig. 26

Regional anatomy. The m. pectoralis major and m. pectoralis minor in the 2nd intercostal space, deeply the m. intercostales interni and externi; the thoracoacromial artery and vein and a branch of the anterior thoracic nerve.

Indications. Cough, asthmatic breathing, expectoration of purulent blood, distension and pain in the chest and hypochondrium, and mastitis.

Method. Puncture obliquely or transversely 0.5–0.8 cun.

ST 16, YINGCHUANG

Location. In the third intercostal space, 4 cun lateral to the Ren meridian (see Fig. 26).

Regional anatomy. 3rd intercostal space, the m. pectoralis major, deeply the m. intercostales interni and externi; the lateral thoracic artery and vein and a branch of the anterior thoracic nerve.

Indications. Cough, asthmatic breathing, distension and pain in the chest and hypochondrium, and mastitis.

Method. Puncture obliquely or transversely 0.5–0.8 cun.

ST 17, RUZHONG

Location. In the centre of the nipple (see Fig. 26).

Note. This point is used only as a landmark for locating points on the chest and abdomen, without the application of needling or moxibustion.

ST 18, RUGEN

Location. In the 5th intercostal space, directly below the nipple (see Fig. 26).

Regional anatomy. Lower part of the m. pectoralis major, deeply the m. intercostales interni and externi; the intercostal artery, the superficial epigastric vein, latterly the cutaneous branch of the 5th intercostal nerve, deeply the intercostal nerve trunk.

Indications. Cough, asthmatic breathing, hiccup, pain in the chest, mastitis and insufficient lactation.

Method. Puncture obliquely or transversely 0.5–0.8 cun.

ST 19, BURONG

Location. 6 cun above the umbilicus and 2 cun lateral to the Ren meridian (see Fig. 27).

Regional anatomy. At the m. rectus abdominis and its sheath, deeply the m. transversus abdominis; the branches of the 7th intercostal artery and vein, the branches of the superior epigastric artery and vein; a branch of the 7th intercostal nerve.

Indications. Vomiting, epigastric pain, poor appetite and abdominal distension.

Method. Puncture perpendicularly 0.5–0.8 cun.

ST 20, CHENGMAN

Location. 5 cun above the umbilicus and 2 cun lateral to the Ren meridian (see Fig. 27).

Regional anatomy. At the m. rectus abdominis

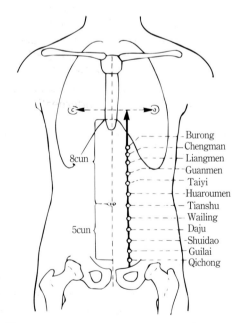

8cun

5cun

Burong
Chengman
Liangmen
Guanmen
Taiyi
Huaroumen
Tianshu
Wailing
Daju
Shuidao
Guilai
Qichong

Fig. 27

and its sheath, deeply the m. transversus abdominis; the branches of the 7th intercostal artery and vein, the branches of the superior epigastric artery and vein, and a branch of the 7th intercostal nerve.

Indications. Epigastric pain, haematemesis, poor appetite and abdominal distension.

Method. Puncture perpendicularly 0.8–1.0 cun.

ST 21, LIANGMEN*

Location. 4 cun above the umbilicus and 2 cun lateral to the Ren meridian (see Fig. 27).

Regional anatomy. At the m. rectus abdominis and its sheath, deeply the m. transversus abdominis; the branches of the 7th intercostal artery and vein, the branches of the superior epigastric artery and vein; a branch of the 8th intercostal nerve (deep underneath on the right side are the lower border of the liver and the pylorus).

Indications. Epigastric pain, vomiting, poor appetite, abdominal distension and diarrhoea.

Method. Puncture perpendicularly 0.8–1.2 cun.

ST 22, GUANMEN

Location. 3 cun above the umbilicus and 2 cun lateral to the Ren meridian (see Fig. 27).

Regional anatomy. At the m. rectus abdominis and its sheath; the branches of the 8th intercostal artery and vein, the branches of the superior epigastric artery and vein; a branch of the 8th intercostal nerve (underneath is the transverse colon).

Indications. Abdominal distension and pain, borborygmus, diarrhoea and oedema.

Method. Puncture perpendicularly 0.8–1.2 cun.

ST 23, TAIYI

Location. 2 cun above the umbilicus and 2 cun lateral to the Ren meridian (see Fig. 27).

Regional anatomy. At the m. rectus abdominis and its sheath; the branches of the 8th intercostal artery and vein and the branches of the inferior epigastric artery and vein; a branch of

the 8th intercostal nerve (underneath is the transverse colon).

Indications. Epigastric pain, restlessness of mind, depressive and manic psychosis.

Method. Puncture perpendicularly 0.8–1.2 cun.

ST 24, HUAROUMEN

Location. 1 cun above the umbilicus and 2 cun lateral to the Ren meridian (see Fig. 27).

Regional anatomy. At the rectus abdominis and its sheath; the branches of the 9th intercostal artery and vein and the branches of the inferior epigastric artery and vein; a branch of the inferior epigastric artery and vein; a branch of the 9th intercostal nerve (underneath is the small intestine).

Indications. Gastric pain, vomiting and depressive and manic psychosis.

Method. Puncture perpendicularly 0.8–1.2 cun.

ST 25, TIANSHU*

The Front-Mu point of the large intestine.

Location. 2 cun lateral to the umbilicus (see Fig. 27).

Regional anatomy. At the m. rectus abdominis and its sheath; the branches of the 9th intercostal artery and vein and the branches of the inferior epigastric artery and vein; a branch of the 10th intercostal nerve (underneath is the small intestine).

Indications. Abdominal distension, borborygmus, pain around the umbilicus, constipation, diarrhoea, dysentery, irregular menstruation and abdominal lumps.

Method. Puncture perpendicularly 1–1.5 cun.

Note. The *Prescriptions Worth A Thousand Gold Coin* says that moxibustion is contraindicated on this point for pregnant women.

ST 26, WAILING

Location. 1 cun below the umbilicus and 2 cun lateral to the Ren meridian (see Fig. 27).

Regional anatomy. At the m. rectus abdominis and its sheath; the branches of the 10th intercostal artery and vein and branches of the inferior epigastric artery and vein; a branch of the 10th intercostal nerve (underneath is the small intestine).

Indications. Abdominal pain, hernia and dysmenorrhoea.

Method. Puncture perpendicularly 1–1.5 cun.

ST 27, DAJU

Location. At the m. rectus abdominis and its sheath; the branches of the 11th intercostal artery and vein, laterally the branches of the inferior epigastric artery and vein; a branch of the 11th intercostal nerve (underneath is the small intestine).

Indications. Distension and fullness in the lower abdomen, dysuria, hernia, seminal emission and premature ejaculation.

Method. Puncture perpendicularly 1–1.5 cun.

ST 28, SHUIDAO

Location. 3 cun below the umbilicus and 2 cun lateral to the Ren meridian, (see Fig. 27).

Regional anatomy. At the m. rectus abdominis and its sheath; the branches of the 12th intercostal artery and vein, laterally the inferior epigastric artery and vein; a branch of the 12th intercostal nerve (underneath is the small intestine).

Indications. Distension and fullness in the lower abdomen, dysuria, dysmenorrhoea, infertility and hernia.

Method. Puncture perpendicularly 1–1.5 cun.

ST 29, GUILAI*

Location. 4 cun below the umbilicus and 2 cun lateral to the Ren meridian (see Fig. 27).

Regional anatomy. At the lateral border of the m. rectus abdominis, the m. obliquus internus abdominis and aponeurosis of the m. transversus abdominis; laterally the branches of the inferior epigastric artery and vein; the iliohypogastric nerve.

Indications. Abdominal pain, hernia, irregular menstruation, morbid leucorrhoea and prolapse of the uterus.

Method. Puncture perpendicularly 1–1.5 cun.

ST 30, QICHONG

Location. 5 cun below the umbilicus and 2 cun lateral to the Ren meridian (see Fig. 27).

Regional anatomy. Lateral and superior to the pubic tubercle, the aponeurosis of the m. obliquus externus abdominis; the lower part of the m. obliquus internus abdominis and m. peritonealis; the branches of the superficial epigastric artery and vein, laterally the inferior epigastric artery and vein; the pathway of the ilioinguinal nerve.

Indications. Borborygmus, abdominal pain, hernia, irregular menstruation, infertility, impotence and swelling of the external genitalia.

Method. Puncture perpendicularly 0.5–1.0 cun.

Note. This is the place where the Chong meridian originates.

ST 31, BIGUAN

Location. At the crossing point of the line drawn directly down from the anterior superior iliac spine and the line level with the lower border of the symphysis pubis, and level with the gluteal groove (see Fig. 28).

Regional anatomy. Between the m. sartorius and m. tensor fasciae latae; deeply the branches of the lateral circumflex femoral artery and vein; the lateral femoral cutaneous nerve.

Indications. Lumbar pain and coldness of knee joints, muscular atrophy and motor impairment, and abdominal pain.

Method. Puncture 1–2 cun perpendicularly.

ST 32, FUTU*

Location. On the line joining the anterior superior iliac spine and the lateral border of

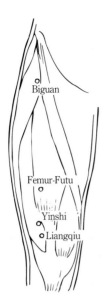

Fig. 28

the patella, 6 cun above the laterosuperior border of the patella (see Fig. 28).

Regional anatomy. In the belly of the m. rectus femoris; the branches of the lateral circumflex femoral artery and vein; the anterior and lateral femoral cutaneous nerves.

Indications. Lumbar pain, coldness in knee joints, paralysis of the lower limbs, hernia and beriberi.

Method. Puncture perpendicularly 1–2 cun.

ST 33, YINSHI

Location. On the line joining the latero-superior border of the patella and the anterior superior iliac spine, 3 cun above the latero-superior border of the patella (see Fig. 28).

Regional anatomy. Between the m. rectus femoris and m. vastus lateralis; the descending branch of the lateral circumflex femoral artery; the anterior and lateral femoral cutaneous nerves.

Indications. Paralysis or motor impairment of the leg and knee, hernia and abdominal distension and pain.

Method. Puncture perpendicularly 1–1.5 cun.

ST 34, LIANGQIU*

The Xi-Cleft point.

Location. On the line joining the latero-superior border of the patella and the anterior superior iliac spine, 2 cun above the latero-superior border of the patella (see Fig. 28).

Regional anatomy. See Yinshi (St 33).

Indications. Swelling and pain of the knee, motor impairment of the lower limbs, gastric pain, mastitis and haematuria.

Method. Puncture 1–1.2 cun.

ST 35, DUBI*

Location. At the lower border of the patella, in the depression lateral to the patellar ligament (see Fig. 29).

Regional anatomy. Lateral border of the patellar ligament; the arterial and venous network around the knee joint; the lateral sural cutaneous nerve and the articular branch of the common peroneal nerve.

Indications. Pain of the knee, motor impairment of the lower limbs and beriberi.

Method. Puncture posteriorly-medially (obliquely) 0.5–1.0 cun.

ST 36, ZUSANLI*

The He-sea point.

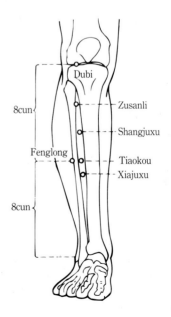

Fig. 29

Location. 3 cun below Dubi (St 35), one finger-breadth from the anterior crest of the tibia (see Fig. 29).

Regional anatomy. Between the m. tibialis anterior and m. extensor digitorum; the anterior tibial artery and vein; the lateral sural cutaneous nerve and the cutaneous branch of the saphenous nerve, deeply the deep peroneal nerve.

Indications. Gastric pain, vomiting, hiccup, abdominal distension, diarrhoea, dysentery, constipation, mastitis, intestinal abscess, pain and motor impairment of the lower limbs, oedema, depressive and manic psychosis, beriberi and emaciation due to general deficiency.

Method. Puncture perpendicularly 1–2 cun.

Note. This is an important tonic point. According to reports, needling Zusanli (St 36) and Shousanli (LI 10) in normal subjects, or patients, makes the contraction of the flaccid stomach strengthen and tension in the stomach relax; it can relieve pyloric spasm. Needling Zusanli (St 36), Hegu (LI 4) and Sanyinjiao (Sp 6) in infants with simple or toxic indigestion, makes the free acid, total acidity, peptase and gastric lipase activity rise rapidly.

Needling Zusanli and Dazhui (St 36 and Du 14) in rabbits makes opsonin increase remarkably, so as to raise the phagocytic index of the white cells and strengthen immunity.

ST 37, SHANGJUXU*

The Lower He-Sea point of the large intestine.

Location. 3 cun below Zusanli (St 36) (see Fig. 29).

Regional anatomy. At the m. tibialis anterior; the anterior tibial artery and vein; the lateral sural cutaneous nerve and the cutaneous branch of the saphenous nerve, deeply the deep peroneal nerve.

Indications. Borborygmus, abdominal pain, diarrhoea, constipation, intestinal abscess, paralysis or motor impairment of the lower limbs and beriberi.

Method. Puncture perpendicularly 1–2 cun.

ST 38, TIAOKOU

Location. 2 cun below Shangjuxu (St 37) (see Fig. 29).

Regional anatomy. See Shangjuxu (St 37).

Indications. Epigastric and abdominal pain, paralysis or motor impairment of the lower limbs, cramp of the gastrocnemius muscle in cholera morbus, swelling of the tarsal region and pain in the shoulder and arm.

Method. Puncture perpendicularly 1–1.5 cun.

ST 39, XIAJUXU*

The Lower He-Sea point of the small intestine.

Location. 3 cun below Shangjuxu (St 37) (see Fig. 29).

Regional anatomy. Between the m. tibialis anterior and m. extensor digitorum longus, deeply the m. extensor hallucis longus; the anterior tibial artery and vein; the branches of the superficial peroneal nerve and the deep peroneal nerve.

Indications. Lower abdominal pain, diarrhoea, dysentery, mastitis, paralysis or motor impairment of the lower limbs, lumbar pain referring to the testis.

Method. Puncture perpendicularly 1–1.5 cun.

ST 40, FENGLONG*

The *luo* point.

Location. 8 cun above the tip of the external malleolus, about one finger-breadth lateral to Tiaokou (St 38) (see Fig. 29).

Regional anatomy. Between the m. extensor digitorum longus and m. peroneus brevis; the branches of the anterior tibial artery; the superficial peroneal nerve.

Indications. Headache, vertigo, profuse sputum and cough, vomiting, constipation, oedema, depressive and manic psychosis and epilepsy, and paralysis or motor impairment of the lower limbs.

Method. Puncture perpendicularly 1–1.5 cun.

ST 41, JIEXI*

The Jing-river point.

Location. At the midpoint of the transverse

crease of the ankle joint, in the depression between the tendons of the m. extensor digitorum longus and hallucis longus (see Fig. 30).

Regional anatomy. Between the tendons of the m. extensor digitorum longus and hallucis longus; the anterior tibial artery and vein; the superficial and deep peroneal nerves.

Indications. Headache, vertigo, depressive-manic psychosis, abdominal distension, constipation, paralysis or motor impairment of the lower limbs.

Method. Puncture perpendicularly 0.5–1.0 cun.

ST 42, CHONGYANG

The *yuan* point.

Location. Distal to Jiexi (St 41), between the tendons of the m. extensor digitorum longus and hallucis longus, between the second and third metatarsal bones and the cuneiform bone, where the dorsal artery of the foot throbs (see Fig. 30).

Regional anatomy. Lateral to the tendon of the m. extensor hallucis longus; the dorsal artery and vein of the foot, the dorsal venous network of the foot; the medial dorsal cutaneous nerve of the foot derived from the superficial peroneal nerve, deeply the deep peroneal nerve.

Indications. Deviation of the mouth and eye, puffiness of face, toothache, depressive-manic psychosis, gastric pain and paralysis or weakness of the foot.

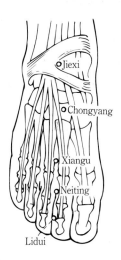

Fig. 30

Method. Avoid the artery, puncture perpendicularly 0.3–0.5 cun.

ST 43, XIANGU

The Shu-stream point.

Location. In the depression distal to the junction of the second and third metatarsal bones (see Fig. 30).

Regional anatomy. In the space of the 2nd metatarsal bone, the m. interossei; the dorsal venous network, deeply the dorsal digital artery of the second toe; the dorsal branch of the superficial peroneal nerve.

Indications. Oedema of the face and body, redness, swelling and pain in the eye, borborygmus, febrile diseases, swelling and pain in the dorsum of the foot.

Method. Puncture perpendicularly or obliquely 0.5–1.0 cun.

ST 44, NEITING*

The Ying-spring point.

Location. Proximal to the web margin between the second and third toes (see Fig. 30).

Regional anatomy. The dorsal venous network and the dorsal branch of the superficial peroneal nerve.

Indications. Toothache, congested and sore throat, deviation of the mouth, epistaxis, gastric pain with sour regurgitation, abdominal distension, diarrhoea, dysentery, constipation, febrile disease, swelling and pain in the dorsum of the foot.

Method. Puncture perpendicularly or obliquely 0.5–0.8 cun.

ST 45, LIDUI*

The Jing-well point.

Location. On the lateral side of the 2nd toe, 0.1. cun posterior to the corner of the nail (see Fig. 30).

Regional anatomy. The arterial and venous network formed by the dorsal digital artery and

Table 3.3   An outline of indications of points on the stomach meridian

Point	Location	Indications	
		primary	secondary
		Head and face: diseases in head, face, eye, nose, mouth and teeth	
Chengqi (St 1)*	face	redness, swelling and pain in the eye	
Sibai (St 2)*	face	redness, swelling and pain in the eye deviation of mouth and eye,	
Juliao (St 3)	face	deviation of mouth and eye, epistaxis, toothache	
Dicang (St 4)*	face	deviation of mouth	
Daying (St 5)	face	deviation of mouth, puffiness of the cheek, toothache	
Jiache (St 6)*	face	deviation of mouth, puffiness of the cheek, toothache, locked jaws	
Xiaguan (St 7)*	face	deviation of mouth, toothache, deafness, lockjaw	
Touwei (St 8)*	lateral head	headache, eye disease	
		Neck and chest: diseases of throat, chest and lung	
Renying (St 9)	neck	congested and sore throat, asthma	
Shuitu (St 10)	neck	congested and sore throat, asthma	
Qishe (St 11)	neck	congested and sore throat	
Quepen (St 12)	chest	cough, asthma, sore throat	
Qihu (St 13)	chest	cough, asthma	
Kufang (St 14)	chest	cough, distension and pain in the chest and hypochondrium	
Wuyi (St 15)	chest	cough, mastitis	
Yingchuan (St 16)	chest	cough, mastitis, distension and pain in the chest and hypochondrium	
Ruzhong (St 17)	chest	contraindicated for needling and moxibustion	
Rugen (St 18)	chest	cough, pain in the chest, insufficient lactation	
		Upper abdomen: gastrointestinal diseases, mental disorders	
Burong (St 19)	upper abdomen	gastric pain, vomiting, abdominal distension	
Chengman (St 20)	"	borborygmus, abdominal distension, gastric pain	
Liangmen (St 21)*	"	poor appetite, gastric pain	
Guanmen (St 22)	"	borborygmus, diarrhoea, abdominal pain	
Taiyi (St 23)	"	gastric pain	depressive-manic psychosis
Huaroumen (St 24)	"	vomiting	"
Tianshu (St 25)*	"	dysentery, borborygmus, abdominal distension, pain around the umbilicus	
		Lower abdomen: diseases of the urinary-genital system, gynaecological problems	
Wailing (St 26)	lower abdomen	abdominal pain	hernia
Daju (St 27)	lower abdomen	distending pain in the lower abdomen, dysuria	hernia
Shuidao (St 28)	"	dysuria	hernia
Guilai (St 29)*	"	irregular menstruation	hernia
Qichong (St 30)	"	irregular menstruation, impotence	hernia
		Above the knee: local disorders of the lower limbs	
Biguan (St 31)	thigh	motor impairment of lower limbs	
Futu (St 32)*	thigh	motor impairment of lower limbs	
Yinshi (St 33)	thigh	motor impairment of lower limbs	
Liangqiu (St 34)*	thigh	gastric pain, pain in the knee joint	
Dubi (St 35)*	knee	pain and numbness in the knee	
		Shank: gastrointestinal diseases and mental disorders	
Zusanli (St 36)*	shank	gastric pain, abdominal distension, diarrhoea, constipation, aching of knee and shank	important point for general tonification
Shangjuxu (St 37)*	"	borborygmus, diarrhoea, abdominal distension	intestinal abscess
Tiaokou (St 38)	"	motor impairment of the lower limbs	
Xiajuxu (St 39)*	"	lower abdominal pain, motor impairment of lower limbs	mastitis
Fenglong (St 40)*	"	vomiting, constipation	profuse sputum, cough, vertigo, mental disorders

Table 3.3 *Contd.*

Foot: diseases of head, face, eye, nose, mouth, teeth, throat; gastrointestinal diseases, mental disorders, febrile diseases			
Jiexi (St 41)*	ankle	headache	mental disorders
Chongyang (St 42)	dorsum of foot	deviation of mouth and eye	
Xiangu (St 43)	dorsum of foot	redness, swelling and pain in the eye, borborygmus, abdominal pain	febrile diseases
Neiting (St 44)*	dorsum of foot	deviation of mouth, toothache, congested and sore throat, abdominal distentsion	febrile diseases
Lldul (St 45)*	tip of toe	toothache, congested and sore throat, abdominal distension	febrile diseases, dream-disturbed sleep, mental disorders

vein of the foot; the dorsal digital nerve derived from the superficial peroneal nerve.

Indications. Epistaxis, toothache, congested and sore throat, abdominal distension, febrile disease, dream-disturbed sleep and depressive-manic psychosis.

Method. Puncture superficially 0.1 cun.

THE SPLEEN MERIDIAN OF THE FOOT TAIYIN (WITH 21 ACUPOINTS)

Course

The spleen meridian of the foot Taiyin starts from the tip of the big toe (Yinbai, Sp 1) (1),

runs along the medial aspect of the foot at the junction of the red and white skin (2), ascends in front of the medial malleolus (3) up to the medial aspect of the leg (4); it follows the posterior aspect of the tibia (5), crosses and goes in front of the liver meridian of the foot Jueyin (6); passing through the anterior medial aspect of the knee and thigh (7), it enters the abdomen (8), and then the spleen, to which it pertains, and connects with the stomach (9); from there it ascends, passing through the diaphragm (10) and running alongside the throat (11); then it reaches the root of the tongue and spreads over its lower surface (12).

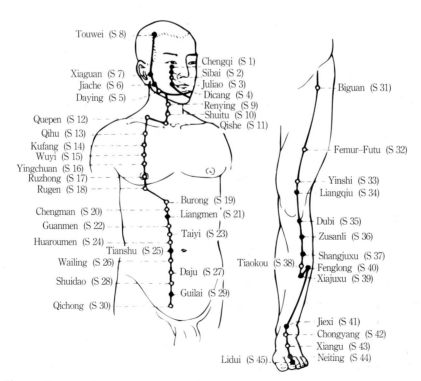

Fig. 31 Points on the stomach meridian of the foot Yangming.

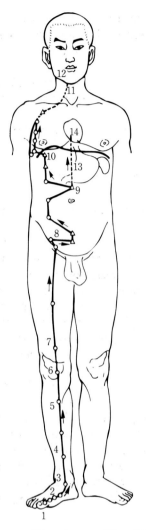

Fig. 32   The course of the spleen meridian of the foot Taiyin.

The branch from the stomach goes upward through the diaphragm (13) and flows into the heart to link with the heart meridian of the hand Shaoyin (14).

Chief pathological manifestations

Epigastric pain, vomiting on eating, belching, abdominal distension, loose stools, jaundice, general heaviness and lassitude, rigidity and pain at the root of the tongue, swelling and distension in the medial aspect of the lower limbs and cold limbs.

Outline of therapeutic indications

Points of this meridian are indicated for spleen and stomach diseases, gynaecological, urinary and genital problems, and other diseases of areas this meridian supplies.

SP 1, YINBAI*

The Jing-well point.
   Location.   On the medial side of the great toe, 0.1 cun posterior to the corner of the nail (see Fig. 33).
   Regional anatomy.   The dorsal digital artery; the dorsal branch derived from the superficial peroneal nerve and the medial plantar nerve at the sole.
   Indications.   Abdominal distension, haematochezia, haematuria, menorrhagia; massive uterine bleeding; depressive-manic psychosis, dream-disturbed sleep, and convulsions.
   Method.   Puncture superficially 0.1 cun.

SP 2, DADU

The Ying-spring point.
   Location.   On the medial side of the great toe, at the anterior border of the first metatarso-digital joint, at the junction of the red and white skin (see Fig. 33).
   Regional anatomy.   At the ending point of the m. abductor hallucis; the branches of the medial plantar artery and vein; the plantar digital proprial nerve derived from the medial plantar nerve.
   Indications.   Abdominal distension, gastric pain, vomiting, diarrhoea, constipation and febrile diseases.
   Method.   Puncture perpendicularly 0.3–0.5 cun.

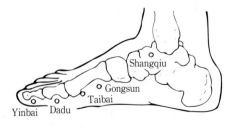

Fig. 33

SP 3, TAIBAI*

The Shu-stream and *yuan* point.

Location. At the posterior border of the head of the first metatarsal bone, at the junction of the red and white skin (see Fig. 33).

Regional anatomy. At the m. abductor hallucis; the dorsal venous network of the foot, the medial plantar artery and the branches of the medial tarsal artery; the branches of the saphenous nerve and superficial peroneal nerve.

Indications. Gastric pain, abdominal distension, borborygmus, diarrhoea, constipation, haemorrhoids, beriberi, general heaviness and joint pain.

Method. Puncture perpendicularly 0.5–0.8 cun.

SP 4, GONGSUN*

The *luo* point, one of the 8 Confluent points of the 8 extra meridians communicating with the Chong meridian.

Location. Anterior and inferior to the base of the first metatarsal bone, at the junction of the red and white skin (see Fig. 33).

Regional anatomy. At the m. abductor hallucis; the medial tarsal artery and the dorsal venous network of the foot; the saphenous nerve and the branch of the superficial peroneal nerve.

Indications. Gastric pain, vomiting, abdominal pain, diarrhoea and dysentery.

Method. Puncture perpendicularly 0.6–1.2 cun.

Note. According to reports, needling Neiguan (P 6) and Zusanli (St 36) in patients with a peptic ulcer, under gastrointestinal X-ray examination, has the effect of increasing the movement of the stomach (especially Zusanli), while the movement of the stomach is weakened by needling Gongsun (Sp 4); needling Gongsun (Sp 4), Neiguan (P 6) and Liangqiu (St 34) can inhibit the secretion of gastric acid.

SP 5, SHANGQIU

The Jing-river point.

Location. In the depression anterior and inferior to the medial malleolus (see Fig. 33).

Regional anatomy. The medial tarsal artery and the great saphenous vein; the saphenous nerve and the branch of the superficial peroneal nerve.

Indications. Abdominal distension, diarrhoea, constipation, jaundice and pain in the foot and ankle.

Method. Puncture perpendicularly 0.5–0.8 cun.

SP 6, SANYINJIAO*

The Crossing point of the three yin meridians of the foot.

Location. 3 cun directly above the tip of the medial malleolus, on the posterior border of the medial aspect of the tibia (see Fig. 34).

Regional anatomy. Between the tibia and m. soleus, deeply the m. flexor digitorum longus; the great saphenous vein, the posterior tibial artery and vein; the medial crural cutaneous nerve, deeply and in the posterior aspect, the tibial nerve.

Indications. Borborygmus, abdominal distension, diarrhoea, irregular menstruation, morbid leucorrhoea, prolapse of the uterus, infertility, delayed labour, seminal emission, impotence, nocturnal enuresis, hernia, insomnia, paralysis or motor impairment of the lower limbs and beriberi.

Method. Puncture perpendicularly 1–1.5 cun.

Note. Contraindicated for pregnant women.

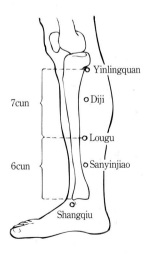

Fig. 34

SP 7, LOUGU

Location.   3 cun above Sanyinjiao (Sp 6) (see Fig. 34).

Regional anatomy.   Between the posterior aspect of the tibia and the m. soleus, deeply the m. flexor digitorum longus; the great saphenous vein, the posterior tibial artery and vein; the medial crural cutaneous nerve and deeply the tibial nerve, in the posterior aspect.

Indications.   Abdominal distension, borborygmus, dysuria, seminal emission, paralysis or motor impairment of the lower limbs.

Method.   Puncture perpendicularly 1–1.5 cun.

SP 8, DIJI*

The Xi-Cleft point.

Location.   3 cun below Yinlingquan (Sp 9) (see Fig. 34).

Regional anatomy.   Between the tibia and m. soleus; anteriorly, the great saphenous vein and the branch of the genu superior artery, deeply the posterior tibial artery and vein; the medial crural cutaneous nerve and deeply the tibial nerve.

Indications.   Abdominal pain, diarrhoea, dysuria, oedema, irregular menstruation, dysmenorrhoea and seminal emission.

Method.   Puncture perpendicularly 1–1.5 cun.

SP 9, YINLINGQUAN*

The He-sea point.

Location.   On the lower border of the medial condyle of the tibia, in the depression on the medial border of the tibia (see Fig. 34).

Regional anatomy.   Between the tibia and m. gastrocnemius, the beginning of the m. soleus; anteriorly, the great saphenous vein, the genu superior artery, deeply, the posterior tibial artery and vein; the medial crural cutaneous nerve, deeply the tibial nerve.

Indications.   Abdominal distension, diarrhoea, oedema, jaundice, dysuria or incontinence of urine, pain in the knee.

Method.   Puncture perpendicularly 1–2 cun.

SP 10, XUEHAI*

Location.   2 cun above the mediosuperior border of the patella (see Fig. 35).

A simple way of locating this point is to cup your right palm to the patient's left knee when the patient's knee is flexed. Have the thumb on the medial side and the other four fingers directed proximally, with the thumb forming an angle of 45 degrees with the index finger. The point is where the tip of your thumb rests.

Regional anatomy.   At the superior border of the epicondylus medialis femoris, medial intermuscular septum of the thigh; the muscular branches of the femoral artery and vein; the anterior femoral cutaneous nerve and the muscular branch of the femoral nerve.

Indications.   Irregular menstruation, massive uterine bleeding, amenorrhoea, skin eruptions, eczema and erysipelas.

Method.   Puncture perpendicularly 1–1.5 cun.

SP 11, JIMEN

Location.   6 cun above Xuehai (Sp 10), on the line joining Xuehai (Sp 10) and Chongmen (Sp 12) (see Fig. 35).

Regional anatomy.   Medial border of the m. sartorius, deeply the m. adductor magnus; the great saphenous vein, deeply and on the lateral side, the femoral artery and vein; the anterior femoral cutaneous nerve and deeply the saphenous nerve.

Indications.   Dysuria, nocturnal enuresis, swelling and pain in the inguinal region.

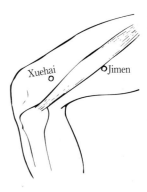

Fig. 35

Method. Avoid the artery, puncture perpendicularly 0.5–1.0 cun.

SP 12, CHONGMEN

The Crossing point of the meridians of the foot Taiyin and foot Jueyin.

Location. 3.5 cun lateral to the midpoint of the upper border of the symphysis pubis (see Fig. 36).

Regional anatomy. Above the lateral aspect of the centre of the ligamentum inguinale, the lower part of the m. obliquus internus abdominis, aponeurosis of the m. obliquus externus abdominis; on the medial aspect, the femoral artery and vein, the femoral nerve.

Indications. Abdominal pain, hernia, massive uterine bleeding and morbid leucorrhoea.

Method. Avoid the artery, puncture perpendicularly 0.5–1.0 cun.

SP 13, FUSHE

The Crossing point of the meridians of the foot Taiyin and foot Jueyin and the Yinwei.

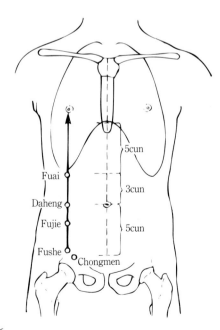

Fig. 36

Location. 0.7 cun laterosuperior to Chongmen (Sp 12), 4 cun lateral to the Ren meridian (see Fig. 36).

Regional anatomy. The ligamentum inguinale, aponeurosis of the m. obliquus externus abdominis, m. obliquus intercostalesminis, deeply the m. transversus abdominis; superficial epigastric artery, intercostal artery and vein; the ilioinguinal nerve (underneath is the caecum on the right side and the colon sigmoideum on the left).

Indications. Abdominal pain, hernia and abdominal masses.

Method. Puncture perpendicularly 1–1.5 cun.

SP 14, FUJIE

Location. 3 cun above Fushe (Sp 13) and 1.3 cun below Daheng (Sp 15) (see Fig. 36).

Regional anatomy. The m. obliquus internus abdominis and m. obliquus externus abdominis; the 11th intercostal artery and vein; the 11th intercostal nerve.

Indications. Abdominal pain, diarrhoea and hernia.

Method. Puncture perpendicularly 1–2 cun.

SP 15, DAHENG

The Crossing point of the meridians of the foot Taiyin and the Yinwei.

Location. 4 cun lateral to the centre of the umbilicus (see Fig. 36).

Regional anatomy. The m. obliquus externus abdominis and m. transversus abdominis; the 11th intercostal artery and vein; the 12th intercostal nerve.

Indications. Diarrhoea, constipation and abdominal pain.

Method. Puncture perpendicularly 1–2 cun.

SP 16, FUAI

The Crossing point of the meridians of the foot Taiyin and the Yinwei.

Location. 3 cun above Daheng (Sp 15), 4 cun lateral to the Ren meridian (see Fig. 36).

Regional anatomy. The m. obliquus externus abdominis and m. obliquus internus abdominis, m. transversus abdominis; the 8th intercostal artery and vein; the 8th intercostal nerve.

Indications. Indigestion, abdominal pain, constipation and dysentery.

Method. Puncture perpendicularly 1–1.5 cun.

SP 17, SHIDOU

Location. In the 5th intercostal space, 6 cun lateral to the Ren meridian (see Fig. 37).

Regional anatomy. In the 5th intercostal space, the m. serratus anterior, deeply the m. intercostales interni and externi; the lateral thoracic artery and vein, thoracoepigastric artery and vein; the lateral cutaneous branch of the 5th intercostal nerve.

Indications. Distension and pain in the chest and hypochondrium, belching, food regurgitation, abdominal distension and oedema.

Method. Puncture obliquely or latero-transversely 0.5–0.8 cun.

Note. Underneath the points from Shidou (Sp 17) to Dabao (Sp 21) of this meridian lies the lung; deep needling is contraindicated.

SP 18, TIANXI

Location. In the 4th intercostal space, 6 cun lateral to the Ren meridian (see Fig. 37)

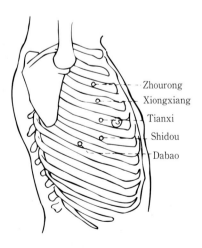

Zhourong
Xiongxiang
Tianxi
Shidou
Dabao

Fig. 37

Regional anatomy. In the 4th intercostal space, the lateral-inferior border of the m. pectoralis major, deeply the m. serratus anterior, more deeply the m. intercostales interni and externi; the branches of the lateral thoracic artery and vein, the thoracoepigastric artery and vein, the 4th intercostal artery and vein; the lateral cutaneous branch of the 4th intercostal nerve.

Indications. Pain in the chest and hypochondrium, cough, mastitis and insufficient lactation.

Method. Puncture obliquely or latero-transversely 0.5–0.8 cun.

SP 19, XIONGXIANG

Location. In the 3rd intercostal space, 6 cun lateral to the Ren meridian (see Fig. 37).

Regional anatomy. In the 3rd intercostal space, the lateral border of the m. pectoralis major and minor, in the m. serratus anterior, deeply the m. intercostales interni and externi; the lateral thoracic artery and vein, the 3rd intercostal artery and vein; the lateral cutaneous branch of the 3rd intercostal nerve.

Indications. Distending pain of the chest and hypochondrium.

Method. Puncture obliquely or latero-transversely 0.5–0.8 cun.

SP 20, ZHOURONG

Location. In the 2nd intercostal space, 6 cun lateral to the Ren meridian (see Fig. 37).

Regional anatomy. In the 2nd intercostal space, the m. pectoralis major, deeply the m. pectoralis minor and m. intercostales interni and externi; the lateral thoracic artery and vein; the 2nd intercostal artery and vein; the lateral cutaneous branch of the 2nd intercostal nerve.

Indications. Cough, upward rebellion of qi, distension and fullness in the chest and hypochondrium.

Method. Puncture obliquely or latero-transversely 0.5–0.8 cun.

SP 21, DABAO*

The major luo (collateral) of the spleen.

Location.   On the mid-axillary line, in the 6th intercostal space (see Fig. 37).

Regional anatomy.   In the 6th intercostal space, the m. serratus anterior; the thoracodorsal artery and vein, the 6th intercostal artery and vein; the 6th intercostal nerve and the terminal branch of the long thoracic nerve.

Indications.   Asthmatic breathing, pain in the chest and hypochondrium, general aching and weakness of the limbs.

Method.   Puncture obliquely or posteriorly-transversely 0.5–0.8 cun.

THE HEART MERIDIAN OF THE HAND SHAOYIN (WITH 9 ACUPOINTS)

Course

The heart meridian of the hand Shaoyin starts from the heart; emerging, it spreads over the "heart system" (i.e. the tissues connecting the heart with the other zangfu organs) (1), passing through the diaphragm to connect with the small intestine (2).

The ascending portion of the meridian derived from the "heart system" (3) runs alongside the throat (4) to connect with the "eye system" (i.e. the tissues connecting the eyes with the brain) (5).

The straight portion of the meridian derived from the "heart system" (3) runs upward to the lung; then it turns downward and emerges from the axilla (Jiquan, H 1) (6); from there it runs along the posterior border of the medial aspect of the upper arm behind the lung meridian of the hand Taiyin and the pericardium meridian of the hand Jueyin (7) down to the cubital fossa from where it descends along the posterior

Table 3.4   An outline of indications of points on the spleen meridian

Point	Location	Indications	
		primary	secondary
Lower limbs: mainly spleen and stomach diseases; then gynaecological diseases and urinary-genital disorders			
Yinbai (Sp 1)*	tip of toe	abdominal distension, menorrhagia	mental disorders
Dadu (Sp 2)	toe	abdominal distension, gastric pain	febrile diseases
Taibai (Sp 3)*	foot	abdominal distension, diarrhoea gastric pain	
Gongsun (Sp 4)*	foot	gastric pain, vomiting, diarrhoea, abdominal pain	dysentery
Shangqiu (Sp 5)	ankle	abdominal distension, diarrhoea, pain of foot and ankle, constipation	
Sanyinjiao (Sp 6)*	shank	borborygmus, abdominal distension, irregular menstruation, seminal emission, dysuria, nocturnal enuresis	insomnia
Lougu (Sp 7)	shank	abdominal distension, borborygmus, motor impairment of the lower limbs	
Diji (Sp 8)*	shank	abdominal pain, diarrhoea, dysuria, irregular menstruation, dysmenorrhea, seminal emission	
Yinlingquan (Sp 9)*	shank	abdominal distension, diarrhoea, dysuria, pain of the knee	oedema
Xuehai (Sp 10)*	shank	irregular menstruation	skin eruptions, eczema
Jimen (Sp 11)	shank	dysuria, nocturnal enuresis	
Abdomen: mainly diseases of the stomach and intestines			
Chongmen (Sp 12)	abdomen	abdominal pain	hernia
Fushe (Sp 13)	abdomen	abdominal pain	hernia
Fujie (Sp 14)	abdomen	abdominal pain	hernia
Daheng (15)	abdomen	constipation, diarrhoea, abdominal pain	
Fuai (Sp 16)	abdomen	abdominal pain, indigestion, constipation, dysentery	
Chest: diseases of the chest and lung			
Shidou (Sp 17)	chest	distending pain in chest and hypochondrium	
Tianxi (Sp 18)	chest	cough, pain in the chest, mastitis	
Xiongxiang (Sp 19)	chest	distending pain in chest and hypochondrium	
Zhourong (Sp 20)	chest	cough, distension and fullness in chest and hypochondrium	
Dabao (Sp 21)*	chest	asthma, pain in chest and hypochondrium	general aching, weakness of limb

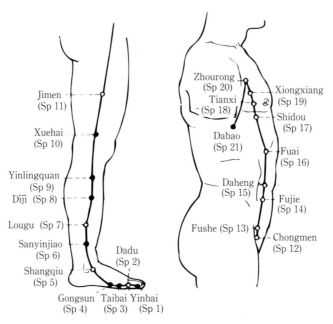

Fig. 38   Points on the spleen meridian of the foot Taiyin.

border of the medial aspect of the forearm (8) to the pisiform region proximal to the palm (9) and enters the palm (10); then it follows the medial aspect of the little finger to its tip (Shaochong, H 9) and links with the small intestine meridian of the hand Taiyang (11).

Chief pathological manifestations

Cardiac pain, dry throat, thirst, yellow sclera, hypochondriacal pain, pain of the medial aspect of the upper arm and feverish sensation in the palms.

Outline of therapeutic indications

Points of this meridian are indicated for diseases of the heart, chest and mental disorders, and other diseases of areas this meridian supplies.

H 1, JIQUAN*

Location.   In the centre of the axilla, on the medial side of the axillary artery (see Fig. 40).

Regional anatomy.   Lateroinferior to the m.

pectoralis major, deeply the m. coracobrachialis, laterally the axillary artery; the ulnar nerve, the median nerve, the medial antebrachial cutaneous nerve and medial brachial nerve.

Indications.   Cardiac pain, dry throat and polydipsia, hypochondriacal pain, scrofula and pain of the shoulder and arm.

Method.   Avoid the axillary artery, puncture perpendicularly or obliquely 0.3–0.5 cun.

H 2, QINGLING

Location.   On the line linking Shaohai (H 3) and Jiquan (H 1), 3 cun above Shaohai (H 3), in the groove medial to the m. biceps brachii (see Fig. 40).

Regional anatomy.   In the groove medial to the m. biceps brachii, the m. triceps brachii; the basilic vein, the superior ulnar collateral artery; the medial antebrachial cutaneous nerve, the medial brachial cutaneous nerve and the ulnar nerve.

Indications.   Headache and coldness, yellow sclera, hypochondriacal pain, pain of the shoulder and arm.

Method.   Puncture perpendicularly 0.5–1.0 cun.

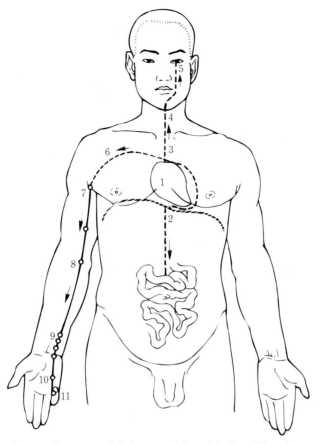

Fig. 39   The course of the heart meridian of the hand Shaoyin.

H 3, SHAOHAI*

The He-sea point.

Location.   When the elbow is flexed, the point is at the midpoint of the line joining the medial end of the transverse cubital crease and the medial epicondyle of the humerus (see Fig. 40).

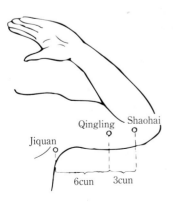

Fig. 40

Regional anatomy.   The round pronator muscle and m. brachii; the basilic vein, the superior and inferior ulnar arteries, the ulnar recurrent artery; the medial antebrachial cutaneous nerve, laterally and anteriorly the median nerve.

Indications.   Cardiac pain, spasmodic pain of the elbow and arm, scrofula, pain in the head and nape, pain in the axilla and hypochondrium.

Method.   Puncture perpendicularly 0.5–1.0 cun.

H 4, LINGDAO

The Jing-river point.

Location.   1.5 cun above the transverse crease of the wrist, on the radial side of the tendon of the m. flexor carpi ulnaris (see Fig. 41).

Regional anatomy.   Between m. flexor carpi ulnaris and m. flexor digitorum superficialis, deeply the m. flexor digitorum profundus; the ulnar artery; the medial antebrachial cutaneous nerve, on the ulnar side, the ulnar nerve.

Indications. Cardiac pain, spasmodic pain of the elbow and arm, sudden loss of voice and alternate spasms of the limbs.

Method. Puncture perpendicularly 0.3–0.5 cun.

H 5, TONGLI*

The *luo* point.

Location. 1 cun above the transverse crease of the wrist, on the radial side of the tendon of the m. flexor carpi ulnaris (see Fig. 41).

Regional anatomy. See Lingdao (H 4).

Indications. Palpitations, sudden loss of voice, aphasia with stiffness of the tongue and pain of the wrist and arm.

Method. Puncture perpendicularly 0.3–0.5 cun.

H 6, YINXI*

The Xi-Cleft point.

Location. 0.5 cun above the transverse crease of the wrist, on the radial side of the tendon m. flexor carpi ulnaris (see Fig. 41).

Regional anatomy. See Lingdao (H 4).

Indications. Cardiac pain, palpitations, hectic tidal fever, haematemesis, epistaxis and sudden loss of voice.

Method. Puncture perpendicularly 0.3–0.5 cun.

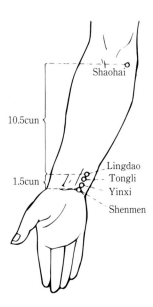

Fig. 41

H 7, SHENMEN*

The Shu-stream and *yuan* point.

Location. At the ulnar end of the transverse crease of the wrist, in the depression on the radial side of the tendon of the m. flexor carpi ulnaris (see Fig. 41).

Regional anatomy. See Lingdao (H 4).

Indications. Cardiac pain, irritability, palpitations, amnesia, insomnia; depressive-manic psychosis, and pain in the chest and hypochondrium.

Method. Puncture perpendicularly 0.3–0.5 cun.

Note. According to reports, needling Shenmen (H 7) in dogs with artificially induced pituitary hypertension, due to injection of pituitary gland, has an obvious antihypertensive effect; needling the points Shenmen (H 7), Yinxi (H 6), Tongli (H 5), Baihui (Du 20) and Daling (P 7) in patients with epilepsy can regularize the EEG, or lower the potential of the pathological brain waves during the epileptic attack.

H 8, SHAOFU

The Ying-spring point.

Location. Between the 4th and 5th metacarpal bones. When a fist is made the point is where the tip of the little finger rests (see Fig. 42).

Regional anatomy. Between the 4th and 5th metacarpal bones; m. lumbricalis, tendons of the m. flexor digitorum superficialis and profundus, deeply the m. interossei; the common palmar digital artery and vein; the 4th common palmar digital nerve derived from the ulnar nerve.

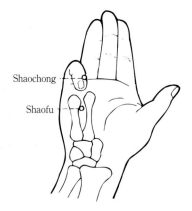

Fig. 42

Table 3.5   An outline of indications of points on the heart meridian

Point	Location	Indications	
		primary	secondary
		Upper limbs: cardiac and chest and mental disorders	
Jiquan (H 1)*	axilla	cardiac and hypochondriacal pain	scrofula
Qingling (H 2)	upper arm	pain in hypochondrium, shoulder and arm	
Shaohai (H 3)*	elbow	cardiac pain, spasmodic pain of elbow and arm	scrofula
Lingdao (H 4)	forearm	cardiac pain, spasmodic pain of elbow and arm	alternate spasm of limbs
Tongli (H 5)*	forearm	palpitation	aphasia with stiffness of tongue, sudden loss of voice
Yinxi (H 6)*	forearm	cardiac pain, palpitation	night sweating
Shenmen (H 7)*	wrist joint	cardiac pain, irritability, palpitation, amnesia, insomnia, mental disorders, pain in the chest and hypochondrium	
Shaofu (H 8)	palm	palpitation, pain in the chest	dysuria, pruritus of external genitalia
Shaochong (H 9)*	tip of finger	palpitation, cardiac pain, pain in chest and hypochondrium, depressive-manic pyschosis	loss of consciousness and febrile disease

Indications. Palpitations, pain in the chest, dysuria, nocturnal enuresis, pruritus and pain of the external genitalia, spasmodic pain of the little finger.

Method. Puncture perpendicularly 0.3–0.5 cun.

H 9, SHAOCHONG*

The Jing-well point.

Location. On the radial side of the little finger, about 0.1 cun posterior to the corner of the nail (see Fig. 42).

Regional anatomy. The arterial and venous network formed by the palmar digital proprial artery and vein; the palmar digital proprial nerve derived from the ulnar nerve.

Indications. Palpitations, cardiac pain, pain in the chest and hypochondrium; depressive-

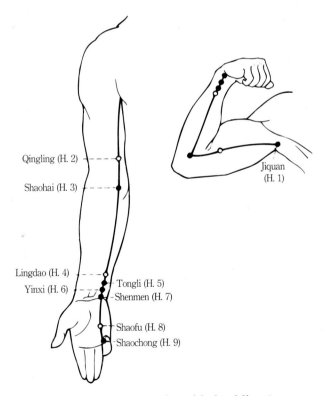

Qingling (H. 2)
Shaohai (H. 3)
Jiquan (H. 1)
Lingdao (H. 4)
Yinxi (H. 6)
Tongli (H. 5)
Shenmen (H. 7)
Shaofu (H. 8)
Shaochong (H. 9)

Fig. 43   Points on the heart meridian of the hand Shaoyin.

manic psychosis, febrile diseases and loss of consciousness.

Method. Puncture superficially 0.1 cun, or prick to cause bleeding.

THE SMALL INTESTINE MERIDIAN OF THE HAND TAIYANG (WITH 19 POINTS)

Course

The small intestine meridian of the hand Taiyang originates from the ulnar side of the tip of the little finger (Shaoze, SI 1) (1), following the ulnar side of the dorsum of the hand it reaches the wrist where it emerges from the styloid process of the ulna (2); from there it ascends along the posterior aspect of the forearm (3), passes between the olecranon of the ulna and the

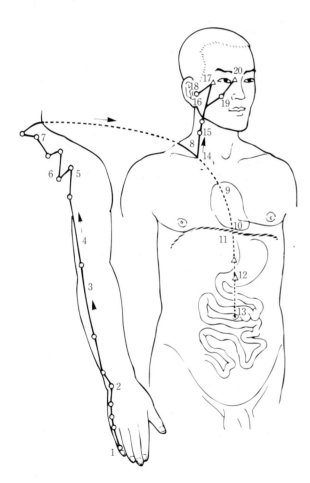

Fig. 44   The course of the small instestine meridian of the hand Taiyang.

medial epicondyle of the humerus, and runs along the posterior border of the lateral aspect of the upper arm (4) to the shoulder joint (5); circling around the scapular region (6), it meets Dazhui (Du 14) on the superior aspect of the shoulder (7); then turning downward to the supraclavicular fossa (8), it connects with the heart (9); from there it descends along the oesophagus (10), passes through the diaphragm (11), reaches the stomach (12), and finally enters the small intestine to which it pertains (13).

The branch from the supraclavicular fossa (14) ascends to the neck (15), and further to the cheek (16), via the outer canthus (17), it enters the ear (Tinggong SI 19) (18).

The branch from the neck (19) runs upward to the infraorbital region (Quanliao, SI 18) and further to the lateral side of the nose; then it reaches the inner canthus (Jingming, UB 1) to link with the urinary bladder meridian of the foot Taiyang (20) and obliquely to link with the zygoma.

Chief pathological manifestations

Lower abdominal pain, lumbar pain referring to the testes, deafness, yellow sclera, swelling of the cheek, congested and sore throat, pain in the lateroposterior border of the shoulder and arm.

Outline of therapeutic indications

Points of this meridian are indicated for diseases of the head, neck, ear, eye, and throat; febrile diseases, mental disorders and other diseases of areas this meridian supplies.

SI 1, SHAOZE*

The Jing-well point.

Location. On the ulnar side of the little finger about 0.1 cun posterior to the corner of the nail (see Fig. 45).

Regional anatomy. The dorsal digital proprial artery and vein, the arterial and venous network formed by the palmar digital artery and vein; the dorsal digital nerve derived from the ulnar nerve.

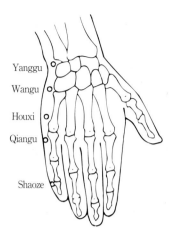

Yanggu
Wangu
Houxi
Qiangu
Shaoze

Fig. 45

Indications. Headache, nebula, congested and sore throat, mastitis, insufficient lactation, loss of consciousness and febrile diseases.

Method. Puncture superficially 0.1 cun, or prick to cause bleeding.

SI 2, QIANGU

The Ying-spring point.

Location. When a loose fist is made, the point is on the ulnar side, distal to the 5th metacarpophalangeal joint, at the junction of the red and white skin (see Fig. 45).

Regional anatomy. The dorsal digital artery and vein; the dorsal digital nerve derived from the ulnar nerve.

Indications. Headache, pain in the eye, tinnitus, congested and sore throat, insufficient lactation and febrile diseases.

Method. Puncture perpendicularly 0.3–0.5 cun.

SI 3, HOUXI*

The Shu-stream point, and one of the 8 Confluent points of the 8 extra meridians communicating with the Du meridian.

Location. When a loose fist is made, the point is on the ulnar side proximal to the metacarpophalangeal joint, at the junction of the red and white skin (see Fig. 45).

Regional anatomy. Ulnar side of the little finger, posterior to the small head of the 5th

metacarpal bone, lateral to the beginning of the m. abductor digiti minimi manus; the dorsal digital artery and vein, the dorsal venous network of the hand; the dorsal branch derived from the ulnar nerve.

Indications. Pain and rigidity of the head and neck, redness of the eye, deafness, congested and sore throat, pain in the back and low back, depressive-manic psychosis, malaria, spasmodic pain of the fingers, elbow and arm.

Method. Puncture perpendicularly 0.5–1.0 cun.

SI 4, WANGU*

The *yuan* point.

Location. Directly above Houxi (SI 3), between the base of the 5th metacarpophalangeal and the triquetral bone, at the junction of the red and white skin (see Fig. 45).

Regional anatomy. On the ulnar side of the dorsum of the hand, lateral border of the m. abductor digiti minimi manus; the posterior carpal artery (the branch of the ulnar artery), the dorsal venous network of the hand; the dorsal branch of the ulnar nerve.

Indications. Rigidity and pain in the head and neck, tinnitus, nebula, jaundice, febrile diseases, malaria, spasm of fingers and pain in the wrist.

Method. Puncture perpendicularly 0.3–0.5 cun.

SI 5, YANGGU

The Jing-river point.

Location. At the ulnar end of the transverse crease on the dorsal aspect of the wrist, in the depression between the styloid process of the ulna and the triquetral bone (see Fig. 45).

Regional anatomy. On the ulnar side of the tendon of the m. extensor carpi ulnaris; the posterior carpal artery; the dorsal branch of the ulnar nerve.

Indications. Headache, blurred vision, tinnitus, deafness, febrile diseases, depressive-manic psychosis and pain of the wrist.

Method. Puncture perpendicularly 0.3–0.5 cun.

SI 6, YANGLAO

The Xi-Cleft point.

Location.   When the palm faces the chest, the point is in the bony cleft on the radial side of the styloid process of the ulna. (see Fig. 46).

Regional anatomy.   Dorsal to the head of the ulna, above the styloid process of the ulna, between the tendon of the m. extensor carpi ulnaris and the tendon of the m. extensor digiti quinti proprius; the terminal branches of the posterior interosseous artery and vein, the dorsal venous network of the wrist; the anastomotic branches of the posterior antebrachial cutaneous nerve and the dorsal branch of the ulnar nerve.

Indications.   Blurred or impaired vision, aching of the shoulder, back, elbow and arm.

Method.   Puncture perpendicularly or obliquely 0.5–0.8 cun.

SI 7, ZHIZHENG*

The *luo* point.

Location.   On the line joining Yanggu (SI 5) and Xiaohai (SI 8), 5 cun above Yanggu (SI 5) (see Fig. 46).

Regional anatomy.   Dorsal to the ulna, ulnar side of the tendon of the m. extensor carpi ulnaris; the terminal branches of the posterior interosseous artery and vein; the branch of the medial antebrachial cutaneous nerve.

Indications.   Headache, blurred vision, febrile

diseases, depressive-manic psychosis, rigidity of the neck, aching of the elbow and arm.

Method.   Puncture perpendicularly 0.5–0.8 cun.

SI 8, XIAOHAI*

The He-sea point.

Location.   When the elbow is flexed, the point is in the depression between the olecranon of the ulna and the medial epicondyle of the humerus (see Fig. 46).

Regional anatomy.   In the groove of ulnar nerve, head of the m. flexor carpi ulnaris; the superior and inferior ulnar collateral arteries and veins, the ulnar recurrent artery and vein; the branches of the medial antebrachial cutaneous nerve, the ulnar nerve.

Indications.   Pain in the elbow and arm, and epilepsy.

Method.   Puncture perpendicularly 0.3–0.5 cun.

SI 9, JIANZHEN

Location.   1 cun above the posterior end of the axillary fold when the arm is adducted (see Fig. 47).

Regional anatomy.   Posterior and inferior to the shoulder joint, lateral border of the scapula, posterior border of the m. deltoideus, deeply the m. teres major; the circumflex scapular artery and vein; the branch of the axillary nerve, deeply the radial nerve, on the superior aspect.

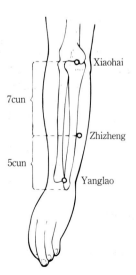

Fig. 46

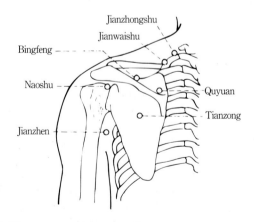

Fig. 47

Indications. Pain in the shoulder and arm, scrofula and tinnitus.

Method. Puncture perpendicularly 1–1.5 cun.

SI 10, NAOSHU

The Crossing point of the hand and foot Taiyang meridians, the Yangwei and Yangqiao.

Location. Directly above the posterior end of the axillary fold, in the depression inferior to the scapular spine (see Fig. 47).

Regional anatomy. In the m. deltoideus, posterior to the scapular articular fossa, deeply the m. infraspinatus; the posterior circumflex humeral artery and vein, deeply the suprascapular artery and vein; the posterior cutaneous nerve of the arm, the axillary nerve, deeply the suprascapular nerve.

Indications. Pain in the shoulder and arm, and scrofula.

Method. Puncture perpendicularly or obliquely 0.5–1.5 cun.

SI 11, TIANZONG*

Location. In the centre of the infrascapular fossa (see Fig. 47).

Regional anatomy. In the m. infraspinatus; the muscular branches of the circumflex humeral artery and vein; the suprascapular nerve.

Indications. Pain in the scapular region, asthmatic breathing and mastitis.

Method. Puncture perpendicularly or obliquely 0.5–1.0 cun.

SI 12, BINGFENG

The Crossing point of the three yang meridians of the hand and the meridian of the foot Shaoyang.

Location. In the centre of the suprascapular fossa, directly above Tianzong (SI 11) (see Fig. 7).

Regional anatomy. Midpoint of upper border of the supraclavicular spine, superficially the m. trapezius and deeply the m. supraspinatus; the suprascapular artery and vein; the supra-

scapular nerve and accessory nerve, deeply the suprascapular nerve.

Indications. Pain in the scapular region, soreness and numbness of the upper limbs.

Method. Puncture perpendicularly or obliquely 0.5–1.0 cun.

SI 13, QUYUAN

Location. On the medial end of the suprascapular fossa, about midway between Naoshu (SI 10) and the spinous process of the 2nd thoracic vertebra (see Fig. 47).

Regional anatomy. At the upper border of the scapular spine, in the m. trapezius and m. supraspinatus; the descending branches of the transverse cervical artery and vein, deeply the muscular branch of the suprascapular artery and vein; the lateral branch of the posterior ramus of the 2nd thoracic nerve, the accessory nerve, deeply the muscular branch of the suprascapular nerve.

Indications. Pain in the scapular region.

Method. Puncture perpendicularly or obliquely 0.5–1.0 cun.

SI 14, JIANWAISHU*

Location. 3 cun lateral to the lower border of the spinous process of the 1st thoracic vertebra (see Fig. 47).

Regional anatomy. At the border of the vertebral angle of the scapula, superficially the m. trapezius and deeply the m. levator scapulae and m. rhomboideus; the transverse cervical artery and vein; the medial cutaneous branches of the posterior ramus of the 1st thoracic nerve, the dorsal scapular nerve and the accessory nerve.

Indications. Pain of the shoulder and back, rigidity of the neck and nape.

Method. Puncture obliquely 0.5–0.8 cun.

SI 15, JIANZHONGSHU

Location. 2 cun lateral to the lower border of the spinous process of the 7th cervical vertebra (see Fig. 47).

Regional anatomy. At the end of the transverse process of the 1st thoracic vertebra; as for the musculature and innervation, see Jianwaishu (SI 14).

Indications. Cough, asthmatic breathing, pain in the shoulder and back and blurred vision.

Method. Puncture obliquely 0.5–0.8 cun.

SI 16, TIANCHUANG

Location. 3.5 cun lateral to the tip of the Adam's apple, at the posterior border of the m. sternocleidomastoideus (see Fig. 48).

Regional anatomy. At the anterior border of the m. trapezius and posterior border of the m. levator scapulae, deeply the m. splenius capitis; the posterior auricular artery and vein and occipital artery and vein; the cutaneous cervical nerve, the emerging portion of the great auricular nerve and the lesser occipital nerve.

Indications. Tinnitus, deafness, congested and sore throat, rigidity and pain of the neck and nape, and sudden loss of voice.

Method. Puncture perpendicularly 0.5–1.0 cun.

SI 17, TIANRONG

Location. Posterior to the angle of the mandible and on the anterior border of the m. sternocleidomastoideus (see Fig. 48).

Regional anatomy. Posterior to the angle of the mandible, the end of the anterior border of the m. sternocleidomastoideus, the lower border of the posterior belly of the digastric muscles; anteriorly the external jugular vein, deeply the internal carotid artery and internal jugular vein; the anterior branch of the great auricular nerve, the cervical branch of the facial nerve, the accessory nerve, the superior cervical ganglion of the sympathetic trunk.

Indications. Tinnitus, deafness, congested and sore throat, swelling and pain of the neck and nape.

Method. Puncture perpendicularly 0.5–1.0 cun.

SI 18, QUANLIAO*

The Crossing point of the meridians of the hand Shaoyang and hand Taiyang.

Location. Directly below the outer canthus, in the depression on the lower border of the zygoma (see Fig. 49).

Regional anatomy. The posterior border of the mandibular process of the zygoma, beginning of the m. masseter, in the m. zygomaticus major; the branches of the transverse facial artery and vein; the facial and infraorbital nerves.

Indications. Deviation of the mouth and eye, twitching of the eyelids, toothache, and swelling of the cheek.

Method. Puncture perpendicularly 0.3–0.5 cun, or obliquely 0.5–1.0 cun.

Note. Contraindicated for moxibustion.

SI 19, TINGGONG*

The Crossing point of the hand and foot Shaoyang and hand Taiyang meridians.

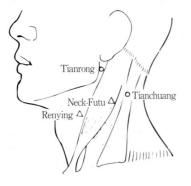

Fig. 48

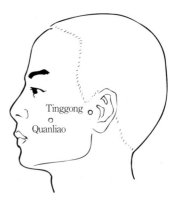

Fig. 49

Table 3.6 An outline of indications of points on the small intestine meridian

Point	Location	Indications primary	secondary
		Hand and elbow: disorders of head, neck, ear, eye, and throat; febrile diseases, mental disorders	
Shaoze (SI 1)*	tip of finger	headache, nebula, sore throat	insufficient lactation, unconsciousness, febrile disease
Qiangu (SI 2)	finger	headache, ache of eye, sore throat	febrile diseases
Houxi (SI 3)*	ulnar side of palm	rigidity of head and neck, redness of eye, deafness, spasmodic pain of finger, elbow and arm	depressive-manic psychosis
Wangu (SI 4)*	wrist	rigidity and pain of head and neck, deafness, nebula, spasm of finger and pain of wrist	jaundice, febrile diseases
Yanggu (SI 5)	wrist	headache, blurred vision, tinnitus, deafness, pain of wrist	mental disorders
Yanglao (SI 6)	forearm	blurred and impaired vision	
Zhizheng (SI 7)*	forearm	rigidity of neck, elbow spasm	mental disorders, febrile diseases
Xiaohai (SI 8)*	elbow	pain of elbow and arm	mental disorders
		Scapular region: disorders in the scapular region	
Jianzhen (SI 9)	scapula	pain of shoulder and arm	
Naoshu (SI 10)	scapula	pain of shoulder and arm	
Tianzong (SI 11)*	scapula	pain in scapular region	mastitis
Bingfeng (SI 12)	scapula	pain in scapular region	
Quyuan (SI 13)	scapula	pain in scapular region	
Jianwaishu (SI 14)*	scapula	pain in shoulder and back, rigidity of neck and nape	
Jianzhongshu (SI 15)	back	pain of elbow and back	
		Neck: disorders of the throat and ear	
Tianchuang (SI 16)	neck	tinnitus, deafness, congested and sore throat	
Tianrong (SI 17)	neck	tinnitus, deafness, congested and sore throat	
		Face: disorders of the face, teeth and ear	
Quanliao (SI 18)*	face	deviation of mouth and eye, twitching of eyelids, toothache	
Tinggong (SI 19)*	ear	tinnitus and deafness	

Location. Anterior to the tragus and posterior to the condyle of the mandible, in the depression formed when the mouth is open (see Fig. 49).

Regional anatomy. The auricular branches of the superficial temporal artery and vein; the branch of the facial nerve and the auriculo-temporal nerve of the trigeminal nerve.

Indications. Tinnitus, deafness, otorrhoea, toothache and depressive-manic psychosis.

Method. Puncture perpendicularly 1.0–1.5 cun when the mouth is open.

THE URINARY BLADDER MERIDIAN OF THE FOOT TAIYANG (WITH 67 POINTS)

Course

The urinary bladder meridian of the foot Taiyang starts from the inner canthus (Jingming, UB 1) (1); ascending to the forehead (2), it joins the Du meridian at the vertex (Baihui, Du 20)

(3), where a branch arises running to the temple (4).

The straight portion of the meridian enters and communicates with the brain from the vertex (5); then it emerges and bifurcates to descend along the posterior aspect of the neck (6); running downward alongside the medial aspect of the scapular region and parallel to the vertebral column (7) it reaches the lumbar region (8), where it enters the body cavity via the paravertebral muscle (9) to connect with the kidney (10) and joins the organ to which it pertains, the bladder (11).

The branch of the lumbar region descends through the gluteal region (2) and ends in the popliteal fossa (13).

The branch from the posterior aspect of the neck goes straight downward along the medial border of the scapula (14); passing through the gluteal region (Huantiao, GB 30) (15) downward along the lateral aspect of the thigh (16) it meets

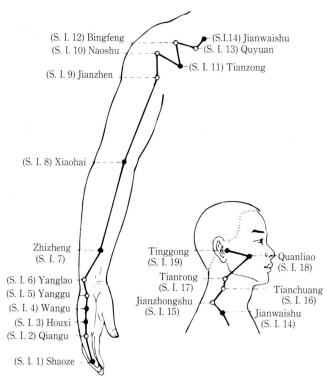

(S. I. 12) Bingfeng
(S. I. 10) Naoshu
(S.I.14) Jianwaishu
(S. I. 13) Quyuan
(S. I. 11) Tianzong
(S. I. 9) Jianzhen
(S. I. 8) Xiaohai
Zhizheng
(S. I. 7)
(S. I. 6) Yanglao
(S. I. 5) Yanggu
(S. I. 4) Wangu
(S. I. 3) Houxi
(S. I. 2) Qiangu
(S. I. 1) Shaoze
Tinggong
(S. I. 19)
Tianrong
(S. I. 17)
Jianzhongshu
(S. I. 15)
Quanliao
(S. I. 18)
Tianchuang
(S. I. 16)
Jianwaishu
(S. I. 14)

Fig. 50   Points on the small intestine meridian of the hand Taiyang.

the preceding branch descending from the lumbar region in the popliteal fossa (17); from there it descends to the leg (18) and further to the posterior aspect of the external malleolus (19); then running along the tuberosity of the 5th metatarsal bone (20), it reaches the lateral side of the tip of the little toe (Zhiyin, UB 67), where it links with the kidney meridian of the foot Shaoyin (21).

Chief pathological manifestations

Retention of urine, nocturnal enuresis, depressive-manic psychosis, malaria, aching of the eye, lacrimation on facing wind, nasal obstruction and discharge, epistaxis, headache, pain of the nape (neck), back, low back and gluteal region and posterior aspect of the lower limbs which this meridian supplies.

Outline of therapeutic indications

Points of this meridian are indicated for diseases of the head, nape (neck), eye, back, low back, lower limbs, and mental disorders. The Back-Shu points on the 1st lateral line, and points on the 2nd lateral line which are level with those Back-Shu points on the 1st lateral line, are indicated for diseases of their related zangfu organs and related tissues and organs.

UB 1, JINGMING*

The Crossing point of the hand and foot Taiyang meridians, the foot Yangming meridian, the Yinqiao and Yangqiao.

Location.   0.1 cun beside the inner canthus (see Fig. 52).

Regional anatomy.   In the intraorbital medial palpebral ligament, deeply the internus; the angular artery and vein, the supratrochlear and infratrochlear arteries and veins, deeply and superiorly the oculomotor artery and vein; the supratrochlear and infratrochlear nerves, deeply the ophthalmic nerve, superiorly the nasociliary nerve.

Indications.   Congested and swollen eyes, lacrimation, blurred vision and impaired vision, myopia, night blindness and colour blindness.

Method.   Ask the patient to close his eyes when gently pushing the eyeball to the lateral

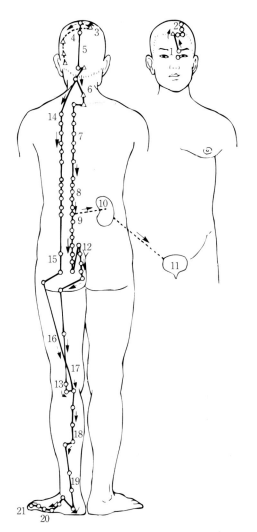

Fig. 51   The course of the urinary bladder of the foot Taiyang.

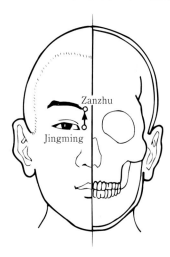

Fig. 52

side; then puncture slowly and perpendicularly 0.5–1.0 cun close against the orbital wall. It is not advisable to rotate or lift and thrust the needle (or only to do so very gently). To avoid bleeding, press the puncture for a while; moxibustion is contraindicated on this point.

UB 2, ZANZHU*

Location.   In the depression on the medial end of the eyebrow (see Fig. 52).

Regional anatomy.   The m. frontalis and m. corrugator supercilii; the frontal artery and vein; the medial branch of the frontal nerve.

Indications.   Headache, deviation of the mouth and eye, impaired vision, lacrimation, congested, swollen and painful eyes, twitching of the eyelids, pain in the supraorbital region, ptosis of the eyelid.

Method.   Puncture transversely 0.5–0.8 cun; moxibustion is contraindicated.

UB 3, MEICHONG

Location.   Directly above Zanzhu (UB 2), 0.5 cun within the anterior hairline (see Fig. 53).

Regional anatomy.   The m. frontalis; the frontal artery and vein; the medial branch of the frontal nerve.

Indications.   Headache, vertigo, nasal obstruction, epilepsy.

Method.   Puncture transversely 0.3–0.5 cun.

UB 4, QUCHAI

Location.   1.5 cun lateral to Shenting (Du 24), at the point one-third medially and two-thirds laterally of the distance from Shenting (Du 24) to Touwei (St 8) (see Fig. 53).

Regional anatomy.   See Meichong (UB 3).

Indications.   Headache, nasal obstruction, epistaxis and impaired vision.

Method.   Puncture transversely 0.5–0.8 cun.

UB 5, WUCHU

Location.   0.5 cun above Quchai (UB 4),

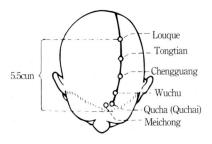

Fig. 53

1.5 cun lateral to the median line on the head (see Fig. 53).

Regional anatomy. See Meichong (UB 3).

Indications. Headache, blurred vision and epilepsy.

Method. Puncture transversely 0.5–0.8 cun.

UB 6, CHENGGUANG

Location. 1.5 cun posterior to Wuchu (UB 5) (see Fig. 53).

Regional anatomy. The galea aponeurotica; the anastomotic network of the frontal artery and vein, the superficial temporal artery and vein, the occipital artery and vein; the anastomotic branch of the lateral branch of the frontal nerve and the great occipital nerve.

Indications. Headache, blurred vision, nasal obstruction and febrile diseases.

Method. Puncture transversely 0.3–0.5 cun.

UB 7, TONGTIAN*

Location. 1.5 cun posterior to Chengguang (UB 6) (see Fig. 53).

Regional anatomy. The galea aponeurotica; the anastomotic network of the superficial temporal artery and vein, the occipital artery and vein; the branch of the great occipital nerve.

Indications. Headache, vertigo, nasal obstruction, epistaxis and rhinorrhoea.

Method. Puncture transversely 0.3–0.5 cun.

UB 8, LUOQUE

Location. 1.5 cun posterior to Tongtian (UB 7) (see Fig. 53).

Regional anatomy. The ending point of the m. occipitalis; the branches of the occipital artery and vein; the branch of the great occipital nerve.

Indications. Vertigo, impaired vision, tinnitus and mental disorders.

Method. Puncture transversely 0.3–0.5 cun.

UB 9, YUZHEN

Location. 2.5 cun directly above the midpoint of the posterior hairline, then 1.3 cun lateral (see Fig. 54).

Regional anatomy. The m. occipitalis; the occipital artery and vein; the branch of the great occipital nerve.

Indications. Ache in the head and nape, ache of the eye, nasal obstruction.

Method. Puncture transversely 0.3–0.5 cun.

UB 10, TIANZHU*

Location. 0.5 cun directly above the midpoint of the posterior hairline, then 1.3 cun lateral, in the depression on the lateral border of the m. trapezius (see Fig. 54).

Regional anatomy. At the beginning of the m. trapezius, deeply the m. semispinalis capitis; the occipital artery and vein; the great occipital nerve.

Indications. Headache, stiffness of neck (nape), nasal obstruction, depressive-manic psychosis and epilepsy, pain of the shoulder and back, febrile diseases.

Method. Puncture perpendicularly or obliquely 0.5–0.8 cun; puncture in a medial or upward direction is forbidden, to avoid injuring the medulla.

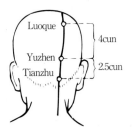

Fig. 54

UB 11, DAZHU*

The influential point of bone, the Crossing point of the Taiyang meridians of the hand and foot.

Location. Level with the lower border of the spinous process of the 1st thoracic vertebra, 1.5 cun lateral (see Fig. 55).

Regional anatomy. The m. trapezium, m. rhomboideus, m. serratus posterior superior, deeply the m. longissimus; the posterior branches of the 1st intercostal artery and vein; the cutaneous branches of the posterior rami of the 1st thoracic nerve, deeply their lateral cutaneous branches.

Indications. Cough, fever, stiffness of the neck, pain of the shoulder and back.

Method. Puncture obliquely 0.5–0.8 cun.

Note. Deep puncture is contraindicated for the points on the back along this meridian, to avoid injuring important viscera beneath.

UB 12, FENGMEN*

The Crossing point of the foot Taiyang and Du meridians.

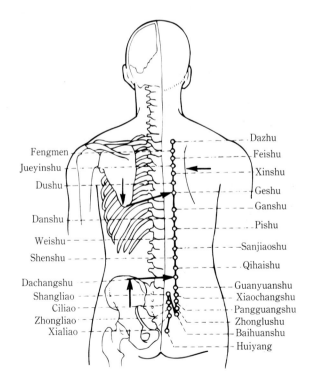

Fengmen
Jueyinshu
Dushu

Danshu

Weishu
Shenshu

Dachangshu
Shangliao
Ciliao
Zhongliao
Xialiao

Dazhu
Feishu
Xinshu
Geshu
Ganshu
Pishu
Sanjiaoshu
Qihaishu
Guanyuanshu
Xiaochangshu
Pangguangshu
Zhonglushu
Baihuanshu
Huiyang

Fig. 55

Location. Level with the lower border of the 2nd thoracic vertebral process, 1.5 cun lateral (see Fig. 55).

Regional anatomy. The m. trapezius, m. rhomboideus, m. serratus posterior superior, deeply the m. longissimus; the posterior branches of the 2nd intercostal artery and vein; the cutaneous branches of the posterior rami of the 2nd and 3rd thoracic nerves, deeply the lateral branch of the 3rd thoracic nerve (posterior rami).

Indications. Common cold, cough, fever, headache, stiffness of the neck, pain in the chest and back.

Method. Puncture obliquely 0.5–0.8 cun.

UB 13, FEISHU*

The Back-Shu point of the lung.

Location. Below the spinous process of the 3rd thoracic vertebra, 1.5 cun lateral (see Fig. 55).

Regional anatomy. The m. trapezius, m. rhomboideus, m. serratus posterior superior, deeply the m. longissimus; the posterior branches of the 3rd intercostal artery and vein; the cutaneous branches of the posterior rami of the 3rd or 4th thoracic nerve, deeply the lateral branch of the posterior rami of the 3rd thoracic nerve.

Indications. Cough, asthma, haematemesis, hectic fever, night sweating and nasal obstruction.

Method. Puncture obliquely 0.5–0.8 cun.

UB 14, JUEYINSHU

The Back-Shu point of the pericardium.

Location. Level with the lower border of the spinous process of the 4th thoracic vertebra, 1.5 cun lateral (see Fig. 55).

Regional anatomy. The m. trapezius, m. rhomboideus, m. serratus posterior superior, deeply the m. longissimus; the posterior branches of the 4th intercostal artery and vein; the cutaneous branches of the posterior rami of the 4th or 5th thoracic nerve, deeply the lateral branch of the posterior rami of the 4th thoracic nerve.

Indications. Cough, cardiac pain, stuffiness in the chest; vomiting.

Method. Puncture obliquely 0.5–0.8 cun.

UB 15, XINSHU*

The Back-Shu point of the heart.

Location. Level with the lower border of the spinous process of the 5th thoracic vertebra, 1.5 cun lateral (see Fig. 55).

Regional anatomy. M. trapezius, m. rhomboideus, m. longissimus; the posterior branches of the 5th intercostal artery and vein; the cutaneous branches of the posterior rami of the 5th or 6th thoracic nerve, deeply the lateral branch of the posterior rami of the 5th thoracic nerve.

Indications. Cardiac pain, palpitations, cough, haematemesis, insomnia, amnesia, night sweating, nocturnal emission, epilepsy.

Method. Puncture obliquely 0.5–0.8 cun.

UB 16, DUSHU

Location. Level with the lower border of the spinous process of the 6th thoracic vertebra, 1.5 cun lateral (see Fig. 55).

Regional anatomy. The m. trapezius, m. latissimus, m. longissimus; the posterior branches of the 6th intercostal artery and vein; the cutaneous branches of the posterior rami of the 6th or 7th thoracic nerve, deeply the lateral branch of the posterior rami of the 6th thoracic nerve.

Indications. Cardiac pain, stuffiness in the chest, abdominal pain, chilliness and fever, asthmatic breathing.

Method. Puncture obliquely 0.5–0.8 cun.

UB 17, GESHU*

One of the 8 Influential points, the Influential point of blood.

Location. Level with the lower border of the spinous process of the 7th thoracic vertebra, 1.5 cun lateral (see Fig. 55).

Regional anatomy. The m. trapezius, m. longissimus; the posterior branches of the 7th intercostal artery and vein; the cutaneous branches of the posterior rami of the 7th or 8th thoracic nerve, deeply the lateral branch of the posterior rami of the 7th thoracic nerve.

Indications. Vomiting, hiccup, asthma, cough, haematemesis, hectic fever and night sweating.

Method. Puncture obliquely 0.5–0.8 cun.

Note. According to reports, needling Geshu (UB 17) and Gaohuang (UB 43) in rabbits with artificially caused anaemia has the effect of rapidly correcting the anaemic state. The effect in the needling group was much faster than that of the control group.

UB 18, GANSHU*

The Back-Shu point of the liver.

Location. Level with the lower border of the spinous process of the 9th thoracic vertebra, 1.5 cun lateral (see Fig. 55).

Regional anatomy. The m. latissimus, m. longissimus, m. iliocostalis; the posterior branches of the 9th intercostal artery and vein; the cutaneous branches of the posterior rami of the 9th or 10th thoracic nerve, deeply the lateral branch of the posterior rami of the 9th thoracic nerve.

Indications. Jaundice, hypochondriacal pain, haematemesis, congested eye, blurred vision, night blindness, depressive-manic psychosis and epilepsy and back pain.

Method. Puncture obliquely 0.5–0.8 cun.

UB 19, DANSHU*

The Back-Shu point of the gallbladder.

Location. Level with the lower border of the spinous process of the 10th thoracic vertebra, 1.5 cun lateral (see Fig. 55).

Regional anatomy. The m. latissimus, m. longissimus, m. iliocostalis, the posterior branches of the 10th intercostal artery and vein; the cutaneous branches of the posterior rami of the 10th thoracic nerve, deeply the lateral branch of the posterior rami of the 10th thoracic nerve.

Indications. Jaundice, bitter taste in the mouth, hypochondriacal pain, pulmonary tuberculosis and hectic fever.

Method. Puncture obliquely 0.5–0.8 cun.

UB 20, PISHU*

The Back-Shu point of the spleen.

Location. Level with the lower border of the spinous process of the 11th thoracic vertebra, 1.5 cun lateral (see Fig. 55).

Regional anatomy. The m. latissimus, m. longissimus, m. iliocostalis; the posterior branches of the 11th intercostal artery and vein; the cutaneous branches of the posterior rami of the 11th thoracic nerve, deeply the lateral branch of the posterior rami of the 11th thoracic nerve.

Indications. Abdominal distension, jaundice, vomiting, diarrhoea, dysentery, haematochezia, oedema, back pain.

Method. Puncture obliquely 0.5–0.8 cun.

UB 21, WEISHU*

The Back-Shu point of the stomach.

Location. Level with the lower border of the spinous process of the 12th thoracic vertebra, 1.5 cun lateral (see Fig. 55).

Regional anatomy. Between the lumbodorsal fascia, m. longissimus and m. iliocostalis; the posterior branches of the 12th intercostal artery and vein; the cutaneous branches of the posterior rami of the 12th thoracic nerve, deeply the lateral branch of the posterior rami of the 12th thoracic nerve.

Indications. Pain in the chest and hypochondrium, epigastric pain, vomiting, abdominal distension and borborygmus.

Method. Puncture obliquely 0.5–0.8 cun.

UB 22, SANJIAOSHU

The Back-Shu point of the Sanjiao.

Location. Level with the lower border of the spinous process of the 1st lumbar vertebra, 1.5 cun lateral (see Fig. 55).

Regional anatomy. Between the lumbodorsal fascia, m. longissimus, m. iliocostalis; the posterior branches of the 1st lumbar artery and vein; the cutaneous branch of the posterior ramus of the 1st lumbar nerve, deeply the lateral branch of the posterior ramus of the 1st lumbar nerve.

Indications. Borborygmus, abdominal distension, vomiting, diarrhoea, dysentery, oedema, rigidity and pain in the low back and back.

Method. Puncture perpendicularly 0.5–1.0 cun.

UB 23, SHENSHU*

The Back-Shu point of the kidney.

Location. Level with the lower border of the spinous process of the 2nd lumbar vertebra, 1.5 cun lateral (see Fig. 55).

Regional anatomy. Between the lumbodorsal fascia, m. longissimus, m. iliocostalis; the posterior branches of the 2nd lumbar artery and vein; the cutaneous branch of the posterior ramus of the 2nd lumbar nerve. Deeply the lateral branch of the posterior ramus of the 2nd lumbar nerve, deeply the 1st lumbar plexus.

Indications. Nocturnal enuresis, nocturnal emission, impotence, irregular menstruation, morbid leucorrhoea, oedema, tinnitus, deafness, and lumbar pain.

Method. Puncture perpendicularly 0.5–1.0 cun.

UB 24, QIHAISHU

Location. Level with the lower border of the spinous process of the 3rd lumbar vertebra, 1.5 cun lateral (see Fig. 55).

Regional anatomy. Between the lumbodorsal fascia, m. longissimus, m. iliocostalis; the posterior branches of the 2nd lumbar artery and vein; the lateral branch of the posterior ramus of the 2nd lumbar nerves, deeply the 1st lumbar plexus.

Indications. Borborygmus, abdominal distension, haemorrhoids, dysmenorrhoea, lumbar pain.

Method. Puncture perpendicularly 0.5–1.0 cun.

UB 25, DACHANGSHU*

The Back-Shu point of the large intestine.

Location. Level with the lower border of the spinous process of the 4th lumbar vertebra, 1.5 cun lateral (see Fig. 55).

Regional anatomy. Between the lumbodorsal fascia, m. longissimus, m. iliocostalis; the posterior branches of the 4th lumbar artery and vein; the cutaneous branch of the posterior ramus of the 3rd lumbar nerve, deeply the lumbar plexus.

Indications. Abdominal distension, diarrhoea, constipation, and lumbar pain.

Method. Puncture perpendicularly 0.8–1.2 cun.

UB 26, GUANYUANSHU

Location. Level with the lower border of the spinous process of the 5th lumbar vertebra, 1.5 cun lateral (see Fig. 55).

Regional anatomy. The m. sacrospinalis; the medial rami of the posterior branches of the lowest lumbar artery and vein; the posterior ramus of the 5th lumbar nerve.

Indications. Abdominal distension, diarrhoea, frequent urination or dysuria, nocturnal enuresis and lumbar pain.

Method. Puncture perpendicularly 0.8–1.2 cun.

UB 27, XIAOCHANGSHU

The Back-Shu point of the small intestine.

Location. Level with the lower border of the spinous process of the 1st sacral vertebra, 1.5 cun lateral (see Fig. 55).

Regional anatomy. Between m. sacrospinalis and m. gluteus maximus; the posterior branches of the lateral sacral artery and vein; the posterior branches of the 5th lumbar nerve.

Indications. Abdominal pain, diarrhoea, dysentery, nocturnal enuresis, haematuria, haemorrhoids, seminal emission, morbid leucorrhoea and lumbar pain.

Method. Puncture perpendicularly or obliquely 0.8–1.2 cun.

UB 28, PANGGUANGSHU

The Back-Shu point of the urinary bladder.

Location. Level with the lower border of the spinous process of the 2nd sacral vertebra, 1.5 cun lateral (see Fig. 55).

Regional anatomy. Between m. sacrospinalis and m. gluteus maximus; the posterior branches of the lateral sacral artery and vein; the branch of the middle clunial nerves.

Indications. Dysuria, nocturnal enuresis, diarrhoea, constipation, and rigidity and pain of the back and low back.

Method. Puncture perpendicularly or obliquely 0.8–1.2 cun.

UB 29, ZHONGLUSHU

Location. Level with the lower border of the spinous process of the 3rd sacral vertebra, 1.5 cun lateral (see Fig. 55).

Regional anatomy. The m. gluteus maximus, sacrotuberous ligament; the branches of the inferior clunial artery and vein; the inferior clunial nerves.

Indications. Diarrhoea, hernia, and rigidity and pain in the low back.

Method. Puncture perpendicularly 1–1.5 cun.

UB 30, BAIHUANSHU

Location. Level with the lower border of the spinous process of the 4th sacral vertebra, 1.5 cun lateral (see Fig. 55).

Regional anatomy. The m. gluteus maximus, sacrotuberous ligament; the inferior clunial artery and vein, deeply the pudendal artery and vein; the inferior clunial nerves, deeply the pudendal nerve.

Indications. Nocturnal enuresis, nocturnal emission, irregular menstruation, morbid leucorrhoea and lumbar and sacral pain.

Method. Puncture perpendicularly 1.0–1.5 cun.

UB 31, SHANGLIAO

Location. In the 1st posterior sacral foramen, about the midpoint of the posterior superior iliac spine and the Du meridian (see Fig. 55).

Regional anatomy. The m. sacrospinalis and m. gluteus maximus; the posterior branches of the lateral sacral artery and vein; the posterior ramus of the 1st sacral nerve.

Indications. Constipation and dysuria, irregular menstruation, morbid leucorrhoea, prolapse of the uterus, seminal emission, impotence and lumbar pain.

Method. Puncture perpendicularly 1–1.5 cun.

UB 32, CILIAO*

Location. In the 2nd posterior sacral foramen,

about the midpoint of the posterior superior iliac spine and the Du meridian (see Fig. 55).

Regional anatomy. The m. gluteus maximus; the posterior branches of the lateral sacral artery and vein; the posterior ramus of the 2nd sacral nerve.

Indications. Hernia, irregular menstruation, dysmenorrhoea, morbid leucorrhoea, dysuria, seminal emission, lumbar pain, paralysis of the lower limbs.

Method. Puncture perpendicularly 1–1.5 cun.

UB 33, ZHONGLIAO

Location. In the 3rd posterior sacral foramen, about the midpoint between Zhonglushu (UB 29) and the Du meridian (see Fig. 55).

Regional anatomy. The m. gluteus maximus; the posterior branches of the lateral sacral artery and vein; the site where the posterior ramus of the 3rd sacral nerve passes.

Indications. Constipation, diarrhoea, dysuria, irregular menstruation, morbid leucorrhoea and lumbar pain.

Method. Puncture perpendicularly 1–1.5 cun.

UB 34, XIALIAO

Location. In the 4th posterior sacral foramen, about the midpoint between Baihuanshu (UB 30) and the Du meridian (see Fig. 55).

Regional anatomy. The m. gluteus maximus; the branches of the inferior gluteal artery and vein; at the site where the posterior ramus of the 4th sacral nerve passes.

Indications. Abdominal pain, constipation, dysuria, morbid leucorrhoea and lumbar pain.

Method. Puncture perpendicularly 1–1.5 cun.

UB 35, HUIYANG

Location. 0.5 cun lateral to the tip of the coccyx (see Fig. 55).

Regional anatomy. The m. gluteus maximus; the branches of the inferior gluteal artery and vein; the coccygeal nerve, deeply the pudendal nerve.

Indications. Diarrhoea, haematochezia, haemorrhoids, impotence and morbid leucorrhoea.

Method. Puncture perpendicularly 1–1.5 cun.

UB 36, CHENGFU

Location. In the middle of the transverse gluteal fold (see Fig. 56).

Regional anatomy. At the lower border of the m. gluteus maximus; the artery and vein running alongside the sciatic nerve; the posterior femoral cutaneous nerve, deeply the sciatic nerve.

Indications. Pain in the lumbar, sacral and gluteal regions, and haemorrhoids.

Method. Puncture perpendicularly 1–2 cun.

UB 37, YINMEN

Location. On the line linking Chengfu (UB 36) and Weizhong (UB 40), 6 cun below Chengfu (UB 36) (see Fig. 56).

Regional anatomy. Between the m. semitendinosus and m. biceps femoris, deeply the m. adductor magnus; the third perforating branch of the deep femoral artery and vein; the posterior femoral cutaneous nerve, the sciatic nerve.

Indications. Lumbar pain, paralysis or motor impairment of the lower limbs.

Method. Puncture perpendicularly 1–2 cun.

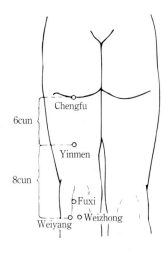

Fig. 56

UB 38, FUXI

Location. 1 cun above Weiyang (UB 39), on the medial aspect of the m. biceps femoris (see Fig. 56).

Regional anatomy. On the medial aspect of the m. biceps femoris; the superolateral genicular artery and vein; the posterior femoral cutaneous nerve and the common peroneal nerve.

Indications. Constipation, femoropopliteal pain and numbness.

Method. Puncture perpendicularly 1–1.5 cun.

UB 39, WEIYANG*

The Lower He-Sea point of the Sanjiao.

Location. At the lateral end of the transverse crease of the popliteal fossa, on the medial border of the tendon of the m. biceps femoris (see Fig. 56).

Regional anatomy. See Fuxi (UB 38).

Indications. Abdominal fullness; dysuria, lumbar rigidity and pain, and spasmodic pain of the leg and foot.

Method. Puncture perpendicularly 1–1.5 cun.

UB 40, WEIZHONG*

The Lower He-sea point.

Location. In the middle of the transverse crease of the popliteal fossa (see Fig. 56).

Regional anatomy. In the middle of the popliteal fossa, the popliteal fascia; the femoropopliteal vein, deeply and medially the popliteal vein and further deeply the popliteal artery; the posterior femoral cutaneous nerve, the tibial nerve.

Indications. Lumbar pain, paralysis of lower limbs, abdominal pain, vomiting and diarrhoea, dysuria, nocturnal enuresis and erysipelas.

Method. Puncture perpendicularly 1–1.5 cun, or prick the popliteal vein with a three-edged needle to cause bleeding.

UB 41, FUFEN

The Crossing point of the hand Taiyang and foot Taiyang meridians.

Location. Level with the lower border of the spinous process of the 2nd thoracic vertebra, 3 cun lateral, on the spinal border of the scapula (see Fig. 57).

Regional anatomy. The medial border of spina scapulae; m. trapezius, m. rhomboideus, deeply the m. iliocostalis; the descending branch of the transverse cervical artery, the posterior branches of the 2nd intercostal artery and vein; the lateral branches of the posterior rami of the 2nd thoracic nerve.

Indications. Rigidity and pain in the nape; spasm of the shoulder and back, numbness of the elbow and arm.

Method. Puncture obliquely 0.5–0.8 cun.

UB 42, POHU

Location. Level with the lower border of the spinous process of the 3rd thoracic vertebra, 3 cun lateral (see Fig. 57).

Regional anatomy. On the spinal border of the scapula, the m. trapezius, m. rhomboideus,

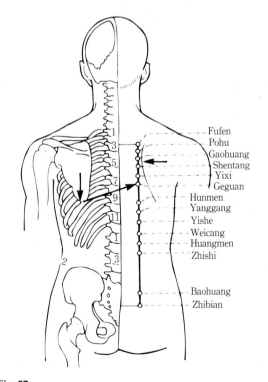

Fufen
Pohu
Gaohuang
Shentang
Yixi
Geguan
Hunmen
Yanggang
Yishe
Weicang
Huangmen
Zhishi

Baohuang
Zhibian

Fig. 57

m. iliocostalis; the dorsal lateral branches of the 3rd intercostal artery and vein, the descending branch of the transverse cervical artery; the posterior branches of the 2nd and 3rd thoracic nerve.

Indications. Cough, asthma, pulmonary tuberculosis, rigidity of the nape and pain in the shoulder and back.

Method. Puncture obliquely 0.5–0.8 cun.

UB 43, GAOHUANG*

Location. Level with the lower border of the spinous process of the 4th thoracic vertebra, 3 cun lateral (see Fig. 57).

Regional anatomy. On the spinal border of the scapula, m. trapezius, m. rhomboideus, m. iliocostalis; the posterior branch of the 4th intercostal artery and vein and the descending branch of the transverse cervical artery; the posterior branches of the 3rd and 4th thoracic nerves.

Indications. Cough, asthma, pulmonary tuberculosis, amnesia, seminal emission and diarrhoea with undigested food in it.

Method. Puncture obliquely 0.5–0.8 cun.

UB 44, SHENTANG

Location. Level with the lower border of the spinous process of the 5th thoracic vertebra, 3 cun lateral (see Fig. 57).

Regional anatomy. On the spinal border of the scapula; the m. trapezius, m. rhomboideus, m. iliocostalis; the posterior branch of the 5th intercostal artery and vein and the descending branch of the transverse cervical artery; the posterior branches of the 4th and 5th thoracic nerves.

Indications. Cough, asthma, stuffiness in the chest, rigidity and pain in the back.

Method. Puncture obliquely 0.5–0.8 cun.

UB 45, YIXI

Location. Level with the lower border of the spinous process of the 6th thoracic vertebra, 3 cun lateral (see Fig. 57).

Regional anatomy. On the lateral border of the m. trapezius, the m. iliocostalis; the posterior branches of the 6th intercostal artery and vein; the posterior branches of the 5th and 6th thoracic nerves.

Indications. Cough, asthma, malaria, febrile diseases, pain in the shoulder and back.

Method. Puncture obliquely 0.5–0.8 cun.

UB 46, GEGUAN

Location. Level with the lower border of the spinous process of the 7th thoracic vertebra, 3 cun lateral (see Fig. 57).

Regional anatomy. The m. latissimus dorsi, m. iliocostalis; the posterior branches of the 7th intercostal artery and vein; the posterior branch of the 6th thoracic nerve.

Indications. Stuffiness in the chest; belching, vomiting, rigidity and pain in the back.

Method. Puncture obliquely 0.5–0.8 cun.

UB 47, HUNMEN

Location. Level with the lower border of the spinous process of the 9th thoracic vertebra, 3 cun lateral (see Fig. 57).

Regional anatomy. The m. latissimus dorsi, m. iliocostalis; the posterior branches of the 9th intercostal artery and vein; the posterior branches of the 8th and 9th thoracic nerves.

Indications. Pain in the chest and hypochondrium, vomiting, diarrhoea and pain in the back.

Method. Puncture obliquely 0.5–0.8 cun.

UB 48, YANGGANG

Location. Level with the lower border of the spinous process of the 10th thoracic vertebra, 3 cun lateral (see Fig. 57).

Regional anatomy. The m. latissimus dorsi, m. iliocostalis; the posterior branches of the 10th intercostal artery and vein; the posterior branches of the 9th and 10th thoracic nerves.

Indications. Borborygmus, abdominal pain, diarrhoea, jaundice and diabetes.

Method. Puncture obliquely 0.5–0.8 cun.

UB 49, YISHE

Location. Level with the lower border of the spinous process of the 11th thoracic vertebra, 3 cun lateral (see Fig. 57).

Regional anatomy. The m. latissimus dorsi, m. iliocostalis; the posterior branches of the 11th intercostal artery and vein; the posterior branches of the 10th and 11th thoracic nerves.

Indications. Abdominal distension, borborygmus, vomiting and diarrhoea.

Method. Puncture obliquely 0.5–0.8 cun.

UB 50, WEICANG

Location. Level with the lower border of the spinous process of the 12th thoracic vertebra, 3 cun lateral (see Fig. 57).

Regional anatomy. The m. latissimus dorsi, m. iliocostalis; the posterior branches of the subcostal artery and vein; the posterior branches of the 12th and 13th thoracic nerves.

Indications. Epigastric pain, abdominal distension, infantile retention of food, oedema and pain in the back.

Method. Puncture obliquely 0.5–0.8 cun.

UB 51, HUANGMEN

Location. Level with the lower border of the spinous process of the 1st lumbar vertebra, 3 cun lateral (see Fig. 57).

Regional anatomy. The m. latissimus dorsi, m. iliocostalis; the posterior branches of the 1st lumbar artery and vein; the posterior branch of the 12th thoracic nerve.

Indications. Abdominal pain, constipation, abdominal masses and disease of the breast.

Method. Puncture obliquely 0.5–0.8 cun.

UB 52, ZHISHI*

Location. Level with the lower border of the spinous process of the 2nd lumbar vertebra, 3 cun lateral (see Fig. 57).

Regional anatomy. The m. latissimus dorsi,

m. iliocostalis; the posterior branches of the 2nd lumbar artery and vein; the lateral branch of the posterior ramus of the 12th thoracic nerve and the lateral branch of the 1st lumbar nerve.

Indications. Seminal emission, impotence, dysuria, oedema, rigidity and pain in the low back.

Method. Puncture obliquely 0.5–0.8 cun.

UB 53, BAOHUANG

Location. Level with the lower border of the spinous process of the 2nd sacral vertebra, 3 cun lateral (see Fig. 57).

Regional anatomy. The m. gluteus maximus, m. gluteus medius and minimus; the superior gluteal artery and vein; the superior clunial nerves, deeply the superior gluteal nerve.

Indications. Borborygmus, abdominal distension, constipation, retention of urine, rigidity and pain in the low back.

Method. Puncture perpendicularly 1–1.5 cun.

UB 54, ZHIBIAN*

Location. Level with the lower border of the spinous process of the 4th sacral vertebra, 3 cun lateral (see Fig. 57).

Regional anatomy. The m. gluteus maximus, lower border of the m. piriformis; the inferior gluteal artery and vein; the inferior gluteal nerve, the posterior femoral cutaneous nerve and the sciatic nerve laterally.

Indications. Dysuria, constipation, haemorrhoids, lumbar and sacral pain, motor impairment of the lower limbs.

Method. Puncture perpendicularly 1.5–2 cun.

UB 55, HEYANG

Location. 2 cun directly below Weizhong (UB 40) (see Fig. 58).

Regional anatomy. Between the medial and lateral heads of the m. gastrocnemius; the small saphenous vein, deeply the popliteal artery and vein; the medial sural cutaneous nerve, deeply the tibial nerve.

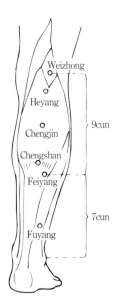

Fig. 58

Indications. Stiffness and pain of the low back, motor impairment of the lower limbs, hernia and massive uterine bleeding.

Method. Puncture perpendicularly 1–2 cun.

UB 56, CHENGJIN

Location. At the midpoint of the line joining Heyang (UB 55) and Chengshan (UB 57) (see Fig. 58).

Regional anatomy. In the centre of the belly of the m. gastrocnemius; the small saphenous vein, deeply the posterior tibial artery and vein; the medial sural cutaneous nerve, deeply the tibial nerve.

Indications. Haemorrhoids, spasm and pain in the low back and leg.

Method. Puncture perpendicularly 1–1.5 cun.

UB 57, CHENGSHAN*

Location. At the top of the depression formed in the belly of the m. gastrocnemius (see Fig. 58).

Regional anatomy. Below the junction of the two halves of the belly of the m. gastrocnemius; the small saphenous vein, deeply the posterior tibial artery and vein; the medial sural cutaneous nerve, deeply the tibial nerve.

Indications. Haemorrhoids, beriberi, constipation, spasm and pain in the low back and leg.

Method. Puncture perpendicularly 1–3 cun.

UB 58, FEIYANG*

The *luo* point.

Location. 7 cun directly above Kunlun (UB 60), lateral and inferior to Chengshan (UB 57) (see Fig. 58).

Regional anatomy. The m. gastrocnemius, m. soleus; the lateral sural cutaneous nerve.

Indications. Headache, blurred vision, epistaxis, pain in the low back and leg, and haemorrhoids.

Method. Puncture perpendicularly 1–1.5 cun.

UB 59, FUYANG

The Xi-Cleft point of the Yangqiao meridian.

Location. 3 cun directly above Kunlun (UB 60) (see Fig. 58).

Regional anatomy. At the posterior aspect of the fibula, lateroanterior border of tendo calcaneus, deeply the m. flexor hallucis longus; the small saphenous vein, deeply the terminal branch of the peroneal artery; the sural nerve.

Indications. Headache, lumbar sacral pain, motor impairment of the lower limbs, swelling and pain of the external malleolus.

Method. Puncture perpendicularly 0.8–1.2 cun.

UB 60, KUNLUN*

The Jing-river point.

Location. In the depression between the tip of the external malleolus and the tendo calcaneus (see Fig. 59).

Regional anatomy. The m. peroneus brevis; the small saphenous vein, the posterior external malleolar artery and vein; the sural nerve.

Indications. Headache, rigidity of the neck, blurred vision, epistaxis, epilepsy, difficult labour, lumbar-sacral pain, swelling and pain of the heel.

Method. Puncture perpendicularly 0.5–0.8 cun.

Note. The *Compendium of Acupuncture*

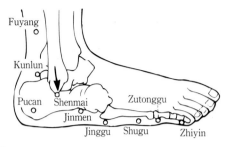

Fig. 59

and Moxibustion states that abortion may be induced by needling this point in pregnant women.

UB 61, PUCAN (ALSO CALLED PUSHEN)

Location. Directly below Kunlun (UB 60) at the junction of the red and white skin (see Fig. 59).

Regional anatomy. The external calcaneal branches of the peroneal artery and vein; the external calcaneal branch of the sural nerve.

Indications. Motor impairment of the lower limbs, pain in the heel, and epilepsy.

Method. Puncture perpendicularly 0.3–0.5 cun.

UB 62, SHENMAI*

One of the 8 Confluent points of the 8 extra meridians, communicating with the Yangqiao.

Location. In the depression directly below the external malleolus (see Fig. 59).

Regional anatomy. At the upper border of the tendon of the m. peroneus longus and brevis; network of artery at external malleolus and the small saphenous vein; the lateral dorsal cutaneous nerve of the foot.

Indications. Headache, vertigo, depressive-manic psychosis and epilepsy, aching of the low back and leg, redness and pain in the eye, and insomnia.

Method. Puncture perpendicularly 0.3–0.5 cun.

UB 63, JINMEN

The Xi-Cleft point.

Location. Midpoint of the line joining Shenmai (UB 62) and Jinggu (UB 64) in the depression lateral to the cuboid bone (see Fig. 59).

Regional anatomy. Between the tendon of the m. peroneus longus and m. abductor digiti minimi pedis; the lateral plantar artery and vein; the lateral dorsal cutaneous nerve of the foot, deeply the lateral plantar nerve.

Indications. Headache, epilepsy, infantile convulsions, lumbar pain, motor impairment of the lower limbs and pain of the external malleolus.

Method. Puncture perpendicularly 0.3–0.5 cun.

UB 64, JINGGU

The *yuan* point.

Location. Below the tuberosity of the 5th metatarsal bone, at the junction of the red and white skin (see Fig. 59).

Regional anatomy. Inferior to the m. abductor digiti minimi pedis; the lateral plantar artery and vein; the lateral dorsal cutaneous nerve of the foot, deeply the lateral plantar nerve.

Indications. Headache, rigidity in the neck, nebula, epilepsy and lumbar pain.

Method. Puncture perpendicularly 0.3–0.5 cun.

UB 65, SHUGU*

The Shu-stream point.

Location. Posterior to the head of the 5th metatarsal bone, at the junction of the red and white skin (see Fig. 59).

Regional anatomy. Inferior to the m. abductor digiti minimi pedis; the 4th common plantar digital artery and vein; the 4th common plantar digital nerve and the lateral dorsal cutaneous nerve of the foot.

Indications. Headache, rigidity in the neck, blurred vision, depressive-manic psychosis, pain in the low back and leg.

Method. Puncture perpendicularly 0.3–0.5 cun.

UB 66, ZUTONGGU

The Ying-spring point.

Table 3.7   Indications of points on the bladder meridian

Point	Location	Indications	
		primary	secondary
Head and nape: diseases of head, nape, eye and nose; mental disorders			
Jingming (UB 1)*	inner canthus	eye diseases	
Zanzhu (UB 2)*	medial end of the eyebrow	headache, congested, swollen and aching eye	
Meichong (UB 3)	anterior head	headache, vertigo, nasal obstruction	epilepsy
Quchai (UB 4)	anterior head	headache, nasal obstruction, epistaxis	
Wuchu (UB 5)	anterior head	headache, vertigo	epilepsy
Chengguang (UB 6)	anterior head	headache, nasal obstruction	
Tongtian (UB 7)*	anterior head	headache, vertigo, nasal obstruction, epistaxis	
Luoque (UB 8)	posterior head	vertigo, tinnitus	mental disorders
Yuzhen (UB 9)	posterior head	pain in the head and nape, pain in eye, nasal obstruction	
Tianzhu (UB 10)*	nape	headache, rigidity of nape, nasal obstruction	
Vertebrae 1–7 on the 1st lateral line: mainly diseases of the heart and lung			
Dazhu (UB 11)*	back	cough, fever, rigidity of nape, pain of shoulder and back	
Fengmen (UB 12)*	back	common cold, cough, rigidity of nape, pain of chest and back	
Feishu (UB 13)*	back	cough, asthma, haematemesis, hectic fever	nasal obstruction
Jueyinshu (UB 14)	back	cough, cardiac pain	
Xinshu (UB 15)*	back	cough, haematemesis, cardiac pain	palpitation, amnesia, epilepsy
Dushu (UB 16)	back	cardiac pain	
Geshu (UB 17)*	back	cough, haematemesis, vomiting	
Vertebrae 9–13 on the 1st lateral line: gastrointestinal diseases mainly; chest and lung diseases as well			
Ganshu (UB 18)*	back	hypochondriacal pain, haematemesis, blurred vision	jaundice, mental disorders
Danshu (UB 19)*	back	hypochondriacal pain	jaundice
Pishu (UB 20)*	back	abdominal distension, diarrhoea, dysentery	oedema, back pain
Weishu (UB 21)*	back	epigastric pain, vomiting, borborygmus	
Sanjiaoshu (UB 22)	low back	borborygmus, abdominal distension, stiffness and pain of the low back	
The 14th vertebra – buttock, on 1st lateral line: diseases of intestines, gynaecology, external genitalia			
Shenshu (UB 23)*	low back	nocturnal enuresis, nocturnal emission, impotence, irregular menstruation, lumbar pain	oedema, tinnitus, deafness
Qihaishu (UB 24)	low back	borborygmus, abdominal distension, dysmenorrhoea, lumbar pain	
Dachangshu (UB 25)*	low back	abdominal distension, diarrhoea, constipation, lumbar pain	
Guanyuanshu (UB 26)	buttock	diarrhoea, lumbar pain	
Xiaochangshu (UB 27)	buttock	abdominal pain, diarrhoea, nocturnal enuresis	
Pangguangshu (UB 28)	buttock	nocturnal enuresis, rigidity and pain of the lower back	
Zhonglushu (UB 29)	buttock	diarrhoea, rigidity and pain of the low back	
Baihuanshu (UB 30)	buttock	nocturnal emission, irregular menstruation, leucorrhoea, lumbar and sacral pain	
Shangliao (UB 31)	sacrum	dysuria, leucorrhoea, prolapse of uterus, lumbar pain	
Ciliao (UB 32)*	sacrum	irregular menstruation, leucorrhoea, dysuria, lumbar pain	
Zhongliao (UB 33)	sacrum	irregular menstruation, leucorrhoea, dysuria, lumbar pain	
Xialiao (UB 34)	sacrum	dysuria, leucorrhoea, constipation	
Huiyang (UB 35)	buttock	diarrhoea, haemorrhoids, leucorrhoea	
Above popliteal fossa: local disorders, intestinal disorders			
Chengfu (UB 36)	thigh	pain of low back, sacrum, buttock and thigh	
Yinmen (UB 37)	thigh	lumbar pain, motor impairment of the lower limbs	
Fuxi (UB 38)	thigh	pain and numbness of the thigh and popliteal fossa	
Weiyang (UB 39)*	popliteal fossa	abdominal fullness, dysuria, spasmodic pain of leg and foot	

Table 3.7 *Contd.*

Point	Location	Indications		secondary
		primary		
Weizhong (UB 40)*	popliteal fossa	dysuria, nocturnal enuresis, lumbar pain, lower-limb paralysis		abdominal pain, vomiting, diarrhoea
Vertebrae 1–7 on the 2nd lateral line: chest and lung diseases				
Fufen (UB 41)	back	rigidity of nape, shoulder and back		
Pohu (UB 42)	back	cough, pulmonary tuberculosis, rigidity of nape, pain of shoulder and back		
Gaohuang (UB 43)*	back	cough, asthma, pulmonary tuberculosis cough,		amnesia, nocturnal emission
Shentang (UB 44)	back	asthma, stuffiness in chest		
Yixi (UB 45)	back	cough, pain in shoulder and back		malaria, febrile diseases
Geguan (UB 46)	back	stuffiness in chest, belching, vomiting		
Vertebrae 9–13, on the 2nd lateral line: gastrointestinal diseases				
Hunmen (UB 47)	back	vomiting, pain in chest, hypochondrium and back		
Yanggang (UB 48)	back	borborygmus, abdominal pain, diarrhoea		jaundice
Yishe (UB 49)	back	abdominal distension, vomiting, diarrhoea		
Weicang (UB 50)	low back	epigastric pain, abdominal distension		
Huangmen (UB 51)	low back	abdominal pain, constipation		
Vertebrae 14–21, on the 2nd lateral line: diseases of intestines, gynaecology, external genitalia				
Zhishi (UB 52)*	low back	nocturnal emission, dysuria, lumbar rigidity and pain		
Baohuang (UB 53)	buttock	constipation, retention of urine, lumbar sacral pain		
Zhibian (UB 54)*	buttock	dysuria, haemorrhoids, pain of lower back		
Shank and foot: diseases of the head, nape, eye, nose, back and low back; mental disorders, and disorders of the posterior aspect of the lower limbs				
Heyang (UB 55)	shank	lumbar rigidity and pain		
Chengjin (UB 56)	shank	haemorrhoids, spasm and pain of low back and leg		
Chengshan (UB 57)*	shank	constipation, haemorrhoids, pain of low back and leg		
Feiyang (UB 58)*	shank	headache, blurred vision, pain of low back and leg		
Fuyang (UB 59)	shank	headache, lumbar sacral pain, paralysis of lower limbs		
Kunlun (UB 60)*	ankle	headache, nape rigidity, blurred, vision, lumbar pain		difficult labour, epilepsy
Pucan (UB 61)	foot	pain in the heel		mental disorders
Shenmai (UB 62)*	foot	congested eye, insomnia, headache, vertigo, soreness and pain of low back and leg		mental disorders
Jinmen (UB 63)	foot	headache		epilepsy
Jinggu (UB 64)	foot	headache, nape rigidity, pain in lower back and leg		epilepsy
Shugu (UB 65)*	foot	headache, nape rigidity, blurred vision, pain in low back and leg		epilepsy
Zutonggu (UB 66)	foot	headache, nape rigidity, blurred vision, epistaxis		mental disorders
Zhiyin (UB 67)*	tip of toe	headache, eye pain, nasal obstruction, epistaxis		difficult labour, malposition of fetus

Location. In the depression anterior to the 5th metatarsophalangeal joint, at the junction of the red and white skin (see Fig. 59).

Regional anatomy. The plantar digital artery and vein; the plantar digital proprial nerve and the lateral dorsal cutaneous nerve of the foot.

Indications. Headache, rigidity of the neck, blurred vision, epistaxis, depressive-manic psychosis.

Method. Puncture perpendicularly 0.2–0.3 cun.

UB 67, ZHIYIN*

The Jing-well point.

Location. On the lateral side of the small toe, about 0.1 cun posterior to the corner of the nail (see Fig. 59).

Regional anatomy. The network formed by the dorsal digital artery and plantar digital proprial artery; the plantar digital proprial nerve and the lateral dorsal cutaneous nerve of the foot.

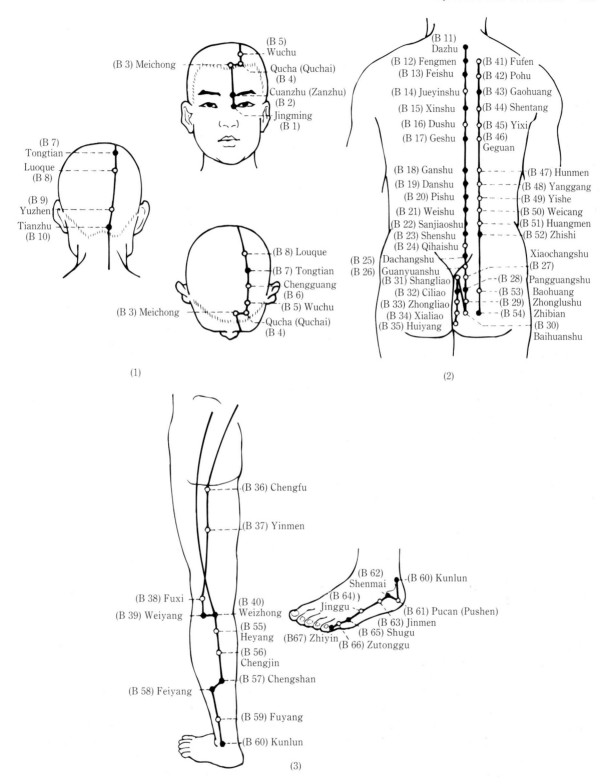

Fig. 60 Points on the urinary bladder of the foot Taiyang.

Indications. Headache, pain in the eye, nasal obstruction, epistaxis, malposition of the fetus and difficult labour.

Method. Puncture superficially 0.1 cun; moxibustion is applied onto this point to correct malposition of the fetus.

THE KIDNEY MERIDIAN OF THE FOOT SHAOYIN (WITH 27 POINTS)

Course

The kidney meridian of the foot Shaoyin originates from the inferior aspect of the small toe (1)

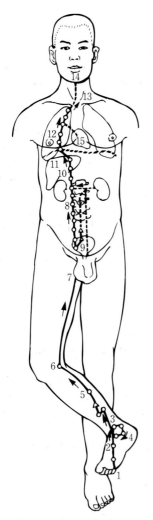

Fig. 61 The course of the kidney meridian of the foot Shaoyin.

and goes obliquely towards the sole (Yongquan, K 1); emerging from the lower aspect of the tuberosity of the navicular bone (2) and running behind the medial malleolus (3), it enters the heel (4); then it ascends along the medial side of the leg (5) to the medial side of the popliteal fossa, (6) and goes further upward and along the posterior and medial aspect of the thigh (7) towards the vertebral column (Changqiang, Du 1), where it enters the kidney which is the organ it pertains to (8), and connects with the bladder (9).

The straight portion of the meridian re-emerges from the kidney ascending and passing through the liver and diaphragm (11); it enters the lung (12), runs along the throat (13) and terminates at the root of the tongue (14).

A branch emerges from the lung, joins the heart and runs into the chest to link with the pericardium meridian of the hand Jueyin (15).

Chief pathological manifestations

Haemoptysis, asthma, dryness of the tongue, congested and sore throat, oedema, constipation, diarrhoea, lumbar pain, pain in the medial aspect of the thigh, motor impairment and weakness, feverishness in the sole, etc.

Outline of therapeutic indications

Points of this meridian are indicated for diseases of gynaecology, external genitalia, kidney, lung and throat, and other diseases at areas it supplies.

K 1, YONGQUAN*

The Jing-well point.

Location. On the sole, in the depression when the foot is in plantar flexion, approximately at the junction of the anterior one-third and posterior two-thirds of the sole (see Fig. 62).

Regional anatomy. Between the 2nd and 3rd plantar metatarsal bones, the plantar aponeurosis, the tendon of the m. flexor digitorum brevis, tendon of the m. flexor digitorum longus, the 2nd m. lumbricalis, deeply the m. interossei; deeply the plantar arterial arch derived from the

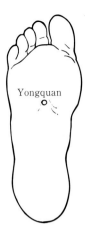

Fig. 62

anterior tibial artery; the branches of the medial plantar nerve.

Indications. Headache, dizziness, insomnia, blurred vision, congested and sore throat, sudden loss of voice, constipation, dysuria, infantile convulsions, depressive-manic psychosis, and loss of consciousness.

Method. Puncture perpendicularly 0.5–1.0 cun.

K 2, RANGU*

The Ying-spring point.

Location. In the depression on the lower border of the tuberosity of the navicular bone (see Fig. 63).

Regional anatomy. In the m. abductor hallucis; the medial tarsal artery; the medial plantar nerve.

Indications. Irregular menstruation, morbid leucorrhoea, seminal emission, diabetes, diarrhoea, haemoptysis, congested and sore throat, dysuria, acute infantile omphalitis, and trismus.

Method. Puncture perpendicularly 0.5–1 cun.

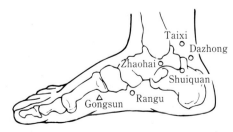

Fig. 63

K 3, TAIXI*

The Shu-stream and *yuan* point.

Location. In the depression between the tip of the medial malleolus and the tendo calcaneus (see Fig. 63).

Regional anatomy. Anteriorly the posterior tibial artery and vein; the medial crural cutaneous nerve, on the course of the tibial nerve.

Indications. Irregular menstruation, seminal emission, impotence, frequent urination, constipation, diabetes, haemoptysis, asthma, sore throat, insomnia, lumbar pain, deafness and tinnitus.

Method. Puncture perpendicularly 0.5–1 cun.

K 4, DAZHONG*

The *luo* point.

Location. 0.5 cun below Taixi (K 3) and slightly posterior, at the medial border of the tendo calcaneus (see Fig. 63).

Regional anatomy. At the medial anterior border of the attachment of tendo calcaneus; the medial calcaneal branch of the posterior tibial artery; the medial crural cutaneous nerve, on the course of the medial calcaneal ramus derived from the tibial nerve.

Indications. Retention of urine, nocturnal enuresis, constipation, haemoptysis, asthma, dementia and pain in the heel.

Method. Puncture perpendicularly 0.3–0.5 cun.

K 5, SHUIQUAN

The Xi-Cleft point.

Location. 1 cun directly below Taixi (K 3) (see Fig. 63).

Regional anatomy. See Dazhong (K 4).

Indications. Irregular menstruation, dysmenorrhoea, amenorrhoea, prolapse of the uterus, and dysuria.

Method. Puncture perpendicularly 0.3–0.5 cun.

K 6, ZHAOHAI*

One of the 8 Confluent points of the 8 extra meridians, communicating with the Yinqiao.

Location. In the depression at the lower border of the medial malleolus (see Fig. 63).

Regional anatomy. Inferior to the medial malleolus, the ending point of the m. abductor hallucis; posteriorly and inferiorly, the posterior tibial artery and vein; the medial crural cutaneous nerve, deeply the tibial nerve.

Indications. Irregular menstruation, morbid leucorrhoea, prolapse of the uterus, frequent urination, retention of urine, constipation, dryness and pain of the throat, epilepsy and insomnia.

Method. Puncture perpendicularly 0.3–0.5 cun.

Note. According to reports, needling Zhaohai (K 6) in normal subjects has an obvious effect in promoting diuresis.

K 7, FULIU*

The Jing-river point.

Location. 2 cun above Taixi (K 3) (see Fig. 64).

Regional anatomy. Posterior to the tibia, inferior to the m. soleus and medial to the tendo calcaneus; deeply and anteriorly the posterior tibial artery and vein; the medial sural and medial crural cutaneous nerves, deeply the tibial nerve.

Indications. Oedema, abdominal distension, diarrhoea, night sweating, anhidrosis in febrile diseases, motor impairment of the lower limbs.

Method. Puncture perpendicularly 0.6–1 cun.

K 8, JIAOXIN

The Xi-Cleft point of the Yinqiao meridian.

Location. About 0.5 cun anterior to Fuliu (K 7) (see Fig. 64).

Regional anatomy. Posterior to the medial border of tibia, in the m. flexor digitorum longus; deeply the posterior tibial artery and vein; the medial crural cutaneous nerve, deeply the tibial nerve.

Indications. Irregular menstruation, massive uterine bleeding, prolapse of the uterus, hernia, diarrhoea and constipation.

Method. Puncture perpendicularly 0.6–1.2 cun.

K 9, ZHUBIN

The Xi-Cleft point of the Yinwei meridian.

Location. 5 cun above Taixi (K 3), on the line linking Taixi (K 3) and Yingu (K 10) (see Fig. 64).

Regional anatomy. At the lower end of the belly of the m. gastrocnemius, tendo calcaneus, m. soleus; deeply, the posterior tibial artery and vein; the medial sural and medial crural cutaneous nerves, deeply the tibial nerve.

Indications. Depressive-manic psychosis, hernia, vomiting, pain in the shank.

Method. Puncture perpendicularly 1–1.5 cun.

K 10, YINGU*

The He-sea point.

Location. When the knee is flexed, the point is on the medial side of the popliteal fossa, between the tendons of the m. semitendinosus and semimembranosus (see Fig. 65).

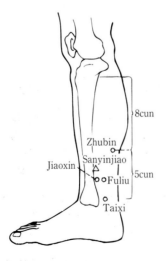

Fig. 64

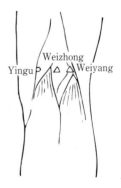

Fig. 65

Regional anatomy. Posterior to the tibia and medial malleolus, between the tendons of the m. semitendinosus and semimembranosus; the medial superior genicular artery and vein; the medial femoral cutaneous nerve.

Indications. Impotence, hernia, massive uterine bleeding, dysuria, and soreness and pain in the popliteal fossa.

Method. Puncture perpendicularly 1–1.5 cun.

K 11, HENGGU

The Crossing point of the kidney and Chong meridians.

Location. 5 cun below the umbilicus, on the superior border of the symphysis pubis, 0.5 cun lateral to the Ren meridian (see Fig. 66).

Regional anatomy. Aponeurosis of the m. obliquus internus and externus abdominis, aponeurosis of m. transversus abdominis and lateral border of the m. pyramidalis; the inferior epigastric artery and vein; the branch of the iliohypogastric nerve (underneath are the small intestine and the fundus of the bladder).

Indications. Distending pain in the lower abdomen, dysuria, nocturnal enuresis, seminal emission, impotence and hernia.

Method. Puncture perpendicularly 1–1.5 cun.

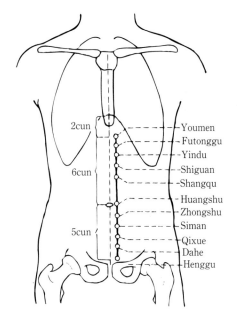

Fig. 66

K 12, DAHE

The Crossing point of the kidney and Chong meridians.

Location. 4 cun below the umbilicus, 0.5 cun lateral to the Ren meridian (see Fig. 66).

Regional anatomy. The aponeurosis of the m. obliquus internus and externus abdominis, aponeurosis of the m. transversus abdominis, lateral border of pyramidalis; the inferior epigastric artery and vein; the branches of the iliohypogastric nerve and the 12th intercostal nerve (underneath are the fundus of the small intestine and fundus of the bladder when it is full).

Indications. Seminal emission, impotence, prolapse of the uterus and morbid leucorrhoea.

Method. Puncture perpendicularly 1–1.5 cun.

K 13, QIXUE

The Crossing point of the kidney and Chong meridians.

Location. 3 cun below the umbilicus, 0.5 cun lateral to the Ren meridian (see Fig. 66)

Regional anatomy. Musculature and vasculature are the same as that of Dahe (K 12); the 12th intercostal nerve (underneath is the small intestine).

Indications. Irregular menstruation, morbid leucorrhoea, dysuria and diarrhoea.

Method. Puncture perpendicularly 1–1.5 cun.

K 14, SIMAN

The Crossing point of the kidney and Chong meridians.

Location. 2 cun below the umbilicus, 0.5 cun lateral to the Ren meridian (see Fig. 66).

Regional anatomy. See Dahe (K 12) for musculature and vasculature; the 11th intercostal nerve (underneath is the small intestine).

Indications. Irregular menstruation, leucorrhoea, nocturnal enuresis, seminal emission, hernia, constipation, abdominal pain and oedema.

Method. Puncture perpendicularly 1–1.5 cun.

K 15, ZHONGZHU

The Crossing point of the kidney and Chong meridians.

Location. 1 cun below the umbilicus, 0.5 cun lateral to the Ren meridian (see Fig. 66).

Regional anatomy. See Dahe (K 12) for musculature and vasculature; the 10th intercostal nerve (underneath is the small intestine).

Indications. Irregular menstruation, abdominal pain, constipation, and diarrhoea.

Method. Puncture perpendicularly 1–1.5 cun.

K 16, HUANGSHU

The Crossing point of the kidney and Chong meridians.

Location. 0.5 cun lateral to the umbilicus (see Fig. 66).

Regional anatomy. See Dahe (K 12) for musculature and vasculature; the 10th intercostal nerve (underneath is the small intestine).

Indications. Abdominal pain and distension, vomiting, constipation and diarrhoea.

Method. Puncture perpendicularly 1–1.5 cun.

K 17, SHANGQU

The Crossing point of the kidney and Chong meridians.

Location. 2 cun above the umbilicus, 0.5 cun lateral to the Ren meridian (see Fig. 66).

Regional anatomy. At the medial border of the m. rectus abdominis; the branches of the superior and inferior epigastric arteries and veins; the 9th intercostal nerve (at the pylorus).

Indications. Abdominal pain, diarrhoea and constipation.

Method. Puncture perpendicularly 1–1.5 cun.

K 18, SHIGUAN

The Crossing point of the kidney and Chong meridians.

Location. 3 cun above the umbilicus, 0.5 cun lateral to the Ren meridian (see Fig. 66).

Regional anatomy. See Shangqu (K 17).

Indications. Vomiting, abdominal pain, constipation and infertility.

Method. Puncture perpendicularly 1–1.5 cun.

K 19, YINDU

The Crossing point of the kidney and Chong meridians.

Location. 4 cun above the umbilicus, 0.5 cun lateral to the Ren meridian (see Fig. 66).

Regional anatomy. At the medial border of the m. rectus abdominis; the branches of the superior epigastric artery and vein; the 8th intercostal nerve.

Indications. Abdominal distension and pain, constipation and infertility.

Method. Puncture perpendicularly 1–1.5 cun.

K 20, FUTONGGU

The Crossing point of the kidney and Chong meridians.

Location. 5 cun above the umbilicus, 0.5 cun lateral to the Ren meridian (see Fig. 66).

Regional anatomy. See Yindu (K 19).

Indications. Abdominal distension and pain, vomiting.

Method. Puncture perpendicularly 0.5–1 cun.

K 21, YOUMEN

The Crossing point of the kidney and Chong meridians.

Location. 6 cun above the umbilicus, 0.5 cun lateral to the Ren meridian (see Fig. 66).

Regional anatomy. See Futonggu (K 20) for musculature and vasculature; the 7th intercostal nerve.

Indications. Abdominal pain and distension, vomiting and diarrhoea.

Method. Puncture perpendicularly 0.5–1 cun.

Note. Deep needling is forbidden, to avoid injuring the liver.

K 22, BULANG

Location. At the 5th intercostal space, 2 cun lateral to the Ren meridian (see Fig. 67).

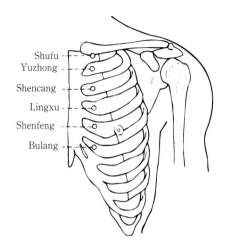

Fig. 67

Regional anatomy. The m. pectoralis major, m. intercostales interni and the external intercostal ligaments; the branches of the 5th intercostal artery and vein; the cutaneous branch of the 5th intercostal nerve, deeply the 5th intercostal nerve.

Indications. Cough, asthma, distension and fullness in the chest and hypochondrium, and vomiting.

Method. Puncture obliquely or transversely 0.5–0.8 cun.

Note. For points along this meridian on the chest, deep needling is contraindicated so as not to injure the heart and lung.

K 23, SHENFENG

Location. At the 4th intercostal space, 2 cun lateral to the Ren meridian (see Fig. 67).

Regional anatomy. The m. pectoralis, m. intercostales interni and the external intercostal ligaments; the branches of the 4th intercostal artery and vein; the cutaneous branch of the 4th intercostal nerve, deeply the 4th intercostal nerve.

Indications. Cough, asthma, abdominal and hypochondriacal fullness, vomiting and mastitis.

Method. Puncture obliquely or transversely 0.5–0.8 cun.

K 24, LINGXU

Location. At the 3rd intercostal space, 2 cun lateral to the Ren meridian (see Fig. 67).

Regional anatomy. See Bulang (K 22) for musculature; the 3rd intercostal artery and vein; the cutaneous branch of the 3rd intercostal nerve, deeply the 3rd intercostal nerve.

Indications. See Shenfeng (K 23).

Method. Puncture obliquely or transversely 0.5–0.8 cun.

K 25, SHENCANG

Location. At the 2nd intercostal space, 2 cun lateral to the Ren meridian (see Fig. 67).

Regional anatomy. See Bulang (K 22) for musculature; the 2nd intercostal artery and vein; the cutaneous branch of the 2nd intercostal nerve, deeply it is on the course of the 2nd intercostal nerve.

Indications. Cough, asthma, pain in the chest and vomiting.

Method. Puncture obliquely or transversely 0.5–0.8 cun.

K 26, YUZHONG

Location. At the 1st intercostal space, 2 cun lateral to the Ren meridian (see Fig. 67).

Regional anatomy. See Bulang (K 22) for musculature; the 1st intercostal artery and vein; the cutaneous branch of the 1st intercostal nerve, deeply the 1st intercostal nerve.

Indications. Cough, asthma, fullness in the chest and hypochondrium.

Method. Puncture obliquely or transversely 0.5–0.8 cun.

K 27, SHUFU*

Location. At the lower border of the clavicle, 2 cun lateral to the Ren meridian (see Fig. 67).

Regional anatomy. In the m. pectoralis major between the clavicle, sternum and the 1st rib; the anterior perforating branches of the internal mammary artery and vein; the medial supraclavicular nerve.

Indications. Cough, asthma, pain in the chest, and vomiting.

Method. Puncture obliquely or transversely 0.5–0.8 cun.

Table 3.8   Indications of points on the kidney meridian

Point	Location	Indications	
		primary	secondary
Foot: gynaecological, external genitalia, intestinal, lung and throat diseases			
Yongquan (K 1)*	sole	sore throat, dysuria, constipation, unconsciousness	headache, blurred vision, infantile convulsion, mental disorders
Rangu (K 2)*	foot	irregular menstruation, seminal emission, haemoptysis	diabetes
Taixi (K 3)*	foot	sore throat, haemoptysis, irregular menstruation	toothache, insomnia, tinnitus
Dazhong (K 4)*	foot	retention of urine, nocturnal enuresis, constipation, pain in the heel	dementia
Shuiquan (K 5)	foot	irregular menstruation, dysmenorrhoea, dysuria	
Zhaohai (K 6)*	foot	dryness and pain of throat, irregular menstruation, constipation	mental disorders, insomnia
Shank: gynaecological, external genitalia, and intestinal diseases			
Fuliu (K 7)*	shank	abdominal distension, diarrhoea, oedema	night sweating, antihidrosis in febrile cases
Jiaoxin (K 8)	shank	irregular menstruation, prolapse of uterus	
Zhubin (K 9)	shank	hernia, vomiting, pain in the shank	mental disorders
Yingu (K 10)*	popliteal fossa	impotence, massive uterine bleeding, dysuria	
Lower abdomen: gynaecological, external genitalia and intestinal diseases			
Henggu (K 11)	lower abdomen	seminal emission, dysuria	
Dahe (K 12)	lower abdomen	seminal emission, leucorrhoea	
Qixue (K 13)	lower abdomen	irregular menstruation, diarrhoea	
Siman (K 14)	lower abdomen	irregular menstruation, hernia, abdominal pain	
Zhongzhu (K 15)	lower abdomen	irregular menstruation, constipation	
Upper abdomen: gastrointestinal diseases			
Huangshu (K 16)	upper abdomen	abdominal pain, constipation	
Shangqu (K 17)	upper abdomen	abdominal pain, constipation, diarrhoea	
Shiguan (K 18)	upper abdomen	vomiting, abdominal pain	
Yindu (K 19)	upper abdomen	abdominal distension and pain	
Futonggu (K 20)	upper abdomen	vomiting, abdominal pain	
Youmen (K 21)	upper abdomen	abdominal pain, vomiting, diarrhoea	
Chest: diseases of the chest and lung			
Bulang (K 22)	chest	cough, asthma, fullness in chest and hypochondrium	
Shenfeng (K 23)	chest	″ ″	
Lingxu (K 24)	chest	″ ″	
Shencang (K 25)	chest	cough, asthma, pain in the chest	
Yuzhong (K 26)	chest	cough, asthma, fullness in chest and hypochondrium	
Shufu (K 27)*	chest	cough, asthma, pain in the chest	

THE PERICARDIUM MERIDIAN OF THE HAND JUEYIN (WITH 9 POINTS)

Course

The pericardium meridian of the hand Jueyin originates from the chest (1); emerging, it enters the pericardium, the organ it pertains to and then descends through the diaphragm (2) to the abdomen, connecting successively with the upper-jiao, middle-jiao and the lower-jiao (the Sanjiao) (3).

A branch arising from the chest goes inside the chest, emerging from the costal region at a point 3 cun below the anterior axillary fold (Tianchi P 1) (5) and ascends to the axilla (6); following the medial aspect of the upper arm, it goes downward between the lung meridian of the hand Taiyin and the heart meridian of the hand Shaoyin (7) to the cubital fossa (8), further downward to the forearm between the two tendons (i.e. the tendons of the m. palmaris longus and m. flexor carpi radialis) (9), ending in the palm (10); from there it passes along the middle finger right down to its tip (Zhongchong P 9) (11).

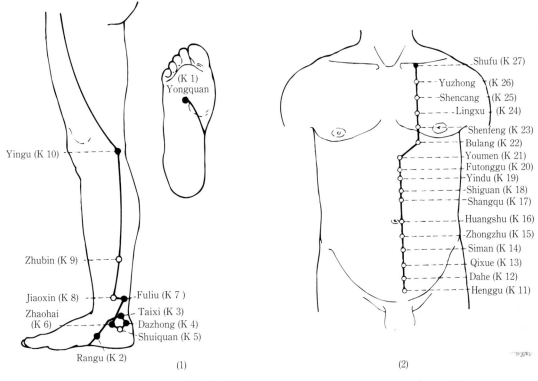

Fig. 68   Points in the kidney meridian of the foot Shaoyin.

Another branch arises from the palm at Laogong (P 8), goes along the ring finger to its tip (Guanchong SJ 1), and links with the Sanjiao meridian of the hand Shaoyang (12).

Chief pathological manifestations

Cardiac pain, stuffiness in the chest, palpitations, irritability, depressive-manic psychosis, swelling in the axilla, spasm in the elbow and arm, feverish sensation in the palm, etc.

Outline of therapeutic indications

Points of this meridian are indicated for diseases of the heart, chest and stomach, and mental disorders, and other diseases of areas this meridian supplies.

P 1, TIANCHI*

The Crossing point of the meridians of the hand Jueyin and foot Shaoyang.

Location. At the 4th intercostal space, 1 cun lateral to the nipple (see Fig. 70).

Regional anatomy. The m. pectoralis major, m. pectoralis minor, m. intercostales interni and externi (the 4th); the thoracoepigastric vein, the branches of the lateral thoracic artery and vein; the muscular branch of the anterior thoracic nerve, the 4th intercostal nerve.

Indications. Cough, asthma, stuffiness in the chest, hypochondriacal and costal pain, scrofula and mastitis.

Method. Puncture obliquely or transversely 0.3–0.5 cun.

Note. Deep needling is contraindicated so as not to injure the lung.

P 2, TIANQUAN

Location. On the palmar side of the upper arm, 2 cun below the level of the anterior axillary fold, between the two heads of the m. biceps brachii (see Fig. 71).

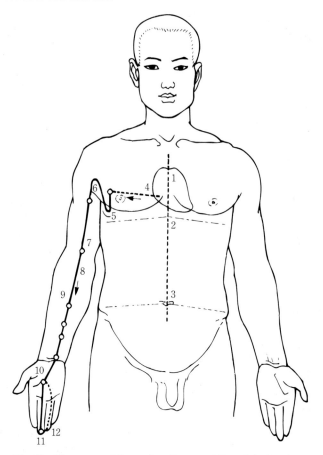

Fig. 69   The course of the pericardium meridian of the hand
Jueyin.

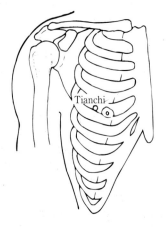

Fig. 70

Regional anatomy.   Between the two heads of
the m. biceps brachii; the muscular branches of
the brachial artery and vein; the medial brachial
cutaneous nerve and the musculocutaneous
nerve.

Indications.   Cardiac pain, cough, distending
pain in the chest and hypochondrium, and pain
in the arm.

Method.   Puncture perpendicularly 1–1.5 cun.

P 3, QUZE*

The He-sea point.

Location.   On the transverse cubital crease, at
the ulnar side of the tendon of the m. biceps
brachii (see Fig. 71).

Regional anatomy.   On the ulnar side of the
tendon of the m. biceps brachii; on the pathway

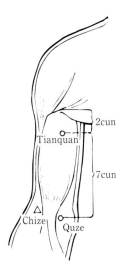

Fig. 71

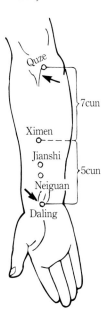

Fig. 72

of the brachial artery and vein; the median nerve.

Indications. Cardiac pain, palpitations, gastric pain, vomiting, diarrhoea, febrile diseases, spasmodic pain of the elbow and arm.

Method. Puncture perpendicularly 1–1.5 cun, or prick to cause bleeding.

P 4, XIMEN

The Xi-Cleft point.

Location. 5 cun above the transverse crease of the wrist, between the tendons of the m. palmaris longus and m. flexor carpi radialis (see Fig. 72).

Regional anatomy. The m. flexor digitorum superficialis, m. flexor digitorum profundus; the median artery and vein, deeply the anterior interosseous artery and vein; the medial antebrachial cutaneous nerve, deeply the median nerve, more deeply the anterior interosseous nerve.

Indications. Cardiac pain, palpitations, vomiting, bloody haemoptysis, carbuncles and boils, epilepsy.

Method. Puncture perpendicularly 0.8–1.2 cun.

P 5, JIANSHI*

The Jing-river point.

Location. 3 cun above the transverse crease of the wrist, between the tendons of the m. palmaris longus and m. flexor carpi radialis (see Fig. 72)

Regional anatomy. See Ximen (P 4).

Indications. Cardiac pain, palpitations, gastric pain, vomiting, febrile diseases, depressive-manic psychosis.

Method. Puncture perpendicularly 0.5–1 cun.

P 6, NEIGUAN*

The *luo* point of the meridian of the hand Jueyin, one of the 8 Confluent points of the 8 extra meridians communicating with the Yinwei.

Location. 2 cun above the transverse crease of the wrist, between the tendons of the m. palmaris longus and flexor carpi radialis (see Fig. 72).

Regional anatomy. See Ximen (p 4).

Indications. Cardiac pain, palpitations, stuffiness in the chest, gastric pain, vomiting, epilepsy, febrile diseases, motor impairment of the upper limbs, hemiplegia, insomnia, vertigo, unilateral headache (migraine).

Method. Puncture perpendicularly 0.5–1 cun.

Note. According to reports, electroneedling Neiguan (P 6), Hegu (LI 4) and Zusanli (St 36) in normal subjects caused no obvious change in serum amylase, but in patients with pancreatitis it caused a rapid lowering in serum amylase.

P 7, DALING*

The Shu-stream and *yuan* point.

Location. In the middle of the transverse crease of the wrist, between the tendons of the m. palmaris longus and m. flexor carpi radialis (see Fig. 72).

Regional anatomy. Between the tendons of the m. palmaris longus and m. flexor carpi radialis, m. flexor pollicis longus and tendon of the m. flexor digitorum profundus; the palmar arterial and venous network of the wrist; deeply the median nerve, the medial antebrachial cutaneous nerve.

Indications. Cardiac pain, palpitations, gastric pain, vomiting, depressive-manic psychosis, boils and ulcers, pain in the chest and hypochondrium.

Method. Puncture perpendicularly 0.5–0.8 cun.

P 8, LAOGONG*

The Ying-spring point.

Location. Between the 2nd and 3rd metacarpal bones. When the fist is clenched, the point is just below the tip of the middle finger (see Fig. 73).

Regional anatomy. Between the 2nd and 3rd metacarpal bones; the palmar aponeurosis, the 2nd m. lumbricales, the tendons of the m. flexor digitorum superficialis and profundus, deeply the transverse head of the m. abductor of the thumb, the interossei muscle; the common palmar digital artery; the median nerve.

Indications. Cardiac pain, vomiting, depressive-manic psychosis, oral ulcers and foul breath.

Method. Puncture perpendicularly 0.3–0.5 cun.

P 9, ZHONGCHONG*

The Jing-well point.

Location. In the centre of the tip of the middle finger (see Fig. 73). (According to records in the

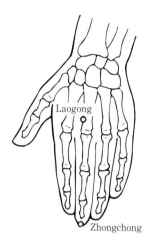

Fig. 73

Systematic Classic of Acupuncture and Moxibustion (the *Jia Yi Jing*), some hold that it should be located at the corner of the nail on the radial side of the middle finger.)

Regional anatomy. The arterial and venous network formed by the palmar digital proprial artery and vein; the palmar digital proprial nerve of the median nerve.

Indications. Cardiac pain, unconsciousness, stiffness, swelling and pain in the tongue, febrile diseases, infantile crying during the night, heat stroke and syncope.

Method. Puncture superficially 0.1 cun or prick to cause bleeding.

THE SANJIAO MERIDIAN OF THE HAND SHAOYANG (WITH 23 POINTS)

Course

The Sanjiao meridian of the hand Shaoyang starts from the tip of the ring finger (Guanchong, SJ 1) (1), running upward between the 4th and 5th metacarpal bones (2), along the dorsal aspect of the wrist (3) to the lateral aspect of the forearm between the radius and ulna (4); passing through the olecranon (5) and along the lateral aspect of the upper arm (6), it reaches the shoulder region (7), where it runs across and passes behind the gallbladder meridian of the foot Shaoyang (8); winding over to the supraclavicular fossa (9), it spreads in the chest to connect with the pericardium (10); then it descends

Table 3.9   Indications of points on the pericardium meridian

Point	Location	Indications primary	secondary
		Chest and forearm: diseases in the heart and chest	
Tianchi (P 1)*	chest	stuffiness in chest, scrofula	
Tianquan (P 2)	forearm	cardiac pain, distending pain in the chest and hypochondrium	
		Hand and arm: diseases of heart, chest, stomach, mental disorders, febrile diseases	
Quze (P 3)*	elbow	cardiac pain, gastric pain	febrile diseases
Ximen (P 4)	forearm	cardiac pain, palpitation, haematemesis	
Jianshi (P 5)*	forearm	cardiac pain, vomiting, mental disorders	malaria
Neiguan (P 6)*	forearm	cardiac pain, palpitation, stuffiness in the chest, vomiting, epilepsy	febrile diseases
Daling (P 7)*	wrist joint	cardiac pain, vomiting, depressive-manic psychosis	boils and ulcers
Laogong (P 8)*	palm	cardiac, depressive-manic psychosis, epilepsy	oral ulcer
Zhongchong (P 9)*	tip of finger	cardiac pain, loss of consciousness	febrile diseases

through the diaphragm down to the abdomen, and joins the Sanjiao, i.e. the upper, middle and lower-jiao, the organ it pertains to (11).

A branch starts from the chest (12); running upward it emerges from the supraclavicular fossa (13); from there it ascends to the neck (14), running along the posterior border of the ear (15), and further to the corner of the anterior hairline (16); then it turns downward to the cheek and terminates in the infraorbital region (17).

The auricular branch arises from the retroauricular region and enters the ear, then it emerges in front of the ear, crosses the previous branch at the cheek and reaches the outer canthus (Sizhukong, SJ 23) to link with the gallbladder meridian of the foot Shaoyang (19).

Chief pathological manifestations

Abdominal distension, oedema, nocturnal enuresis, dysuria, deafness, tinnitus, sore throat, congested eye, swelling of the cheek, retroauricular pain and pain on the lateral aspect of the shoulder, elbow and arm.

Outline of therapeutic indications

Points of this meridian are indicated for diseases of the lateral aspect of the head, of the ear, eye, chest, hypochondrium and throat; febrile diseases and other diseases of areas this meridian supplies.

SJ 1, GUANCHONG*

The Jing-well point.

Location.   On the ulnar side of the ring finger, about 0.1 cun posterior to the corner of the nail (see Fig. 76).

Regional anatomy.   The arterial and venous network formed by the palmar digital proprial artery and vein; the palmar digital proprial nerve derived from the ulnar nerve.

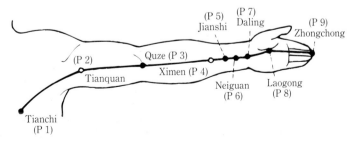

Fig. 74   Points on the pericardium meridian of the hand Jueyin.

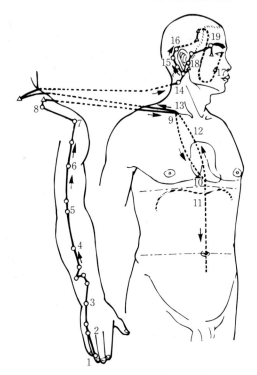

Fig. 75 The course of the Sanjiao meridian of the hand Shaoyang.

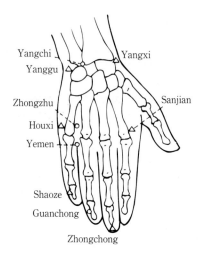

Fig. 76

Indications. Headache, congested eye, deafness, sore throat, febrile diseases, loss of consciousness.

Method. Puncture superficially 0.1 cun or prick to cause bleeding.

SJ 2, YEMEN*

The Ying-spring point.

Location. When the fist is clenched, the point is between the ring and small fingers, in the depression proximal to the margin of the web.

Regional anatomy. The dorsal digital artery and the dorsal digital nerve.

Indications. Headache, congested eye, deafness, sore throat and malaria.

Method. Puncture perpendicularly 0.3–0.5 cun.

SJ 3, ZHONGZHU*

The Shu-stream point.

Location. When the fist is clenched, the point

is on the dorsum of the hand between the 4th and 5th metacarpal bones, in the depression proximal to the metacarpophalangeal joint, 1 cun posterior to Yemen (SJ 2) (see Fig. 76).

Regional anatomy. The m. interossei; the dorsal venous network of the wrist and the posterior carpal artery; the dorsal metacarpal branch derived from the ulnar nerve.

Indications. Headache, congested eye, tinnitus, deafness, sore throat, febrile diseases, motor impairment of the fingers.

Method. Puncture perpendicularly 0.3–0.5 cun.

SJ 4, YANGCHI*

The *yuan* point.

Location. On the transverse crease of the dorsum of wrist, in the depression on the ulnar side of the tendon of the m. extensor digitorum communis.

Regional anatomy. At the articulation of the ulna and carpal bone; between the tendon of the m. extensor digitorum communis and the tendon of the m. extensor digiti minimi; the dorsal venous network of the wrist and the posterior carpal artery; the dorsal branch of the ulnar nerve and the terminal branch of the posterior antebrachial cutaneous nerve.

Indications. Congested eye, deafness, sore throat, malaria, pain in the wrist and diabetes.

Method. Puncture perpendicularly 0.3–0.5 cun.

SJ 5, WAIGUAN*

The *luo* point, one of the 8 Confluent points of the 8 extra meridians communicating with the Yangwei meridian.
Location.   2 cun above the transverse crease on the dorsum of the wrist, between the radius and ulna (see Fig. 77).
Regional anatomy.   Between the m. extensor digitorum and m. extensor pollicis longus; deeply, the posterior and anterior antebrachial interosseous arteries and veins; the posterior antebrachial cutaneous nerve, deeply the posterior interosseous nerve.
Indications.   Febrile diseases, headache, congested eye, tinnitus, deafness, scrofula, costal and hypochondriacal disorders, and pain of the upper limbs.
Method.   Puncture perpendicularly 0.5–1 cun.

SJ 6, ZHIGOU*

The Jing-river point.
Location.   3 cun above the transverse crease on the dorsum of the wrist. between the radius and ulna (see Fig. 77).
Regional anatomy.   See Waiguan (SJ 5).

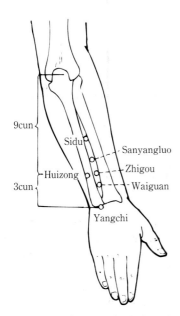

Fig. 77

Indications.   Tinnitus, deafness, sudden hoarseness of voice, scrofula, costal and hypochondriacal pain, constipation and febrile diseases.
Method.   Puncture perpendicularly 0.8–1.2 cun.

SJ 7, HUIZONG

Xi-Cleft point.
Location.   About 1 cun lateral to Zhigou (SJ 6), on the radial side of the ulna (see Fig. 77).
Regional anatomy.   Between m. extensor carpi ulnaris and m. extensor digiti minimi, deeply m. extensor indicis; deeply the posterior antebrachial interosseous arteries and veins; the posterior antebrachial cutaneous nerve, deeply the posterior interosseous nerve and the anterior interosseous nerve.
Indications.   Deafness, epilepsy and pain of the upper limbs.
Method.   Puncture perpendicularly 0.5–1 cun.

SJ 8, SANYANGLUO

Location.   1 cun above Zhigou (SJ 6), between the radius and ulna (see Fig. 77).
Regional anatomy.   Between m. extensor digitorum communis and m. abductor pollicis longus; the posterior antebrachial interosseous artery and vein; the posterior antebrachial cutaneous nerve, deeply the posterior and anterior interosseous nerves.
Indications.   Deafness, sudden hoarseness of voice, toothache, and pain in the upper limbs.
Method.   Puncture perpendicularly 0.5–1 cun.

SJ 9, SIDU

Location.   5 cun below the olecranon of the ulna, between the radius and the ulna (see Fig. 77).
Regional anatomy.   Between m. extensor digitorum communis and m. extensor carpi ulnaris; for vasculature and innervation see Sanyangluo (SJ 8).
Indications.   Deafness, sore throat, sudden hoarseness of voice, toothache, and pain in the upper limbs.
Method.   Puncture perpendicularly 0.5–1 cun.

SJ 10, TIANJING*

The He-sea point.

Location. When the elbow is flexed, the point is in the depression about 1 cun above the olecranon of the ulna (see Fig. 78).

Regional anatomy. In the olecranon fossa, posterior to the lower end of the humerus, upper border of the olecranon, the tendon of the m. triceps brachii; the arterial and venous network of the elbow; the posterior brachial cutaneous nerve and the muscular branch of the radial nerve.

Indications. Migraine, deafness, scrofula and epilepsy.

Method. Puncture perpendicularly 0.5–1 cun.

SJ 11, QINGLENGYUAN

Location. When the elbow is flexed, the point is 1 cun above Tianjing (SJ 10) (see Fig. 78).

Regional anatomy. At the posterior aspect of the humerus, above the tip of the olecranon, in the centre of the lower part of the m. triceps brachii; the median collateral artery and vein; the posterior brachial cutaneous nerve and muscular branch of the radial nerve.

Indications. Headache, pain in the upper limbs, and yellow sclera.

Method. Puncture perpendicularly 0.8–1.2 cun.

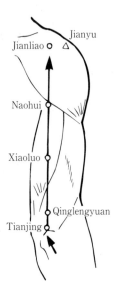

Fig. 78

SJ 12, XIAOLUO

Location. On the line linking the olecranon of the ulna and Jianliao (SJ 14), 3 cun above Qinglengyuan (SJ 11) (see Fig. 78).

Regional anatomy. Posterior to the humerus, in the centre of the belly of the m. triceps brachii; the median collateral artery and vein; the posterior brachial cutaneous nerve and the muscular branch of the radial nerve.

Indications. Headache, toothache, rigidity of the neck, and pain in the shoulder and back.

Method. Puncture perpendicularly 1–1.5 cun.

SJ 13, NAOHUI

Location. On the line linking the olecranon and Jianliao (SJ 14), 3 cun below Jianliao (SJ 14), on the posterior border of the m. deltoideus (see Fig. 78).

Regional anatomy. At the posterior aspect of the upper part of the humerus, in the m. triceps brachii; the median collateral artery and vein; the posterior brachial cutaneous nerve, the muscular branch of the radial nerve, and the radial nerve deeply.

Indications. Goitre, scrofula and pain in the upper limbs.

Method. Puncture perpendicularly 1–1.5 cun.

SJ 14, JIANLIAO*

Location. Posterior and inferior to the acromion, in the depression about 1 cun posterior to Jianyu (LI 15) when the arm is abducted (see Fig. 78).

Regional anatomy. Posterior and inferior to the acromion, In the m. deltoideus; the muscular branch of the posterior circumflex humeral artery; the muscular branch of the axillary nerve.

Indications. Spasmodic pain and motor impairment in the shoulder and arm.

Method. Puncture perpendicularly 1–1.5 cun towards the shoulder joint.

SJ 15, TIANLIAO

The crossing point of the hand Shaoyang meridian and the Yangwei.

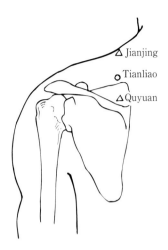

Fig. 79

Location. On the superior angle of the scapula, 1 cun above Quyuan (SI 13) (see Fig. 79).

Regional anatomy. In the supraspinous fossa at the upper part of the scapula, superficially the m. trapezius and deeply m. supraspinatus; the descending branch of the transverse cervical artery, deeply the muscular branch of the suprascapular artery; the accessory nerve and the branch of the suprascapular nerve.

Indications. Pain in the shoulder and arm, stiffness in the neck.

Method. Puncture perpendicularly 0.5–0.8 cun.

SJ 16, TIANYOU

Location. Posterior and inferior to the mastoid process, on the posterior border of the m. sternocleidomastoideus, almost level with the angle of the mandible (see Fig. 80).

Regional anatomy. Posterior to the ending point of the m. sternocleidomastoideus; the posterior auricular artery and vein and external jugular vein; the lesser occipital nerve.

Indications. Headache, pain in the eye, deafness, scrofula, and stiffness of the neck.

Method. Puncture perpendicularly 0.5–1 cun.

SJ 17, YIFENG*

The Crossing point of the hand and foot Shaoyang meridians.

Location. Anterior and inferior to the mastoid process, in the depression level with the posterior lower border of the ear lobe (see Fig. 81).

Regional anatomy. The posterior auricular artery and vein, the external jugular vein; the great auricular nerve, deeply at the site where the facial nerve emerges from the stylomastoid foramen.

Indications. Tinnitus, deafness, deviation of the mouth and eye, trismus, toothache, swelling of the cheek, and scrofula.

Method. Puncture perpendicularly 0.8–1.2 cun.

SJ 18, QIMAI

Location. In the centre of the mastoid process, at the junction of the lower one-third and the upper two-thirds of the curved line joining Yifeng (SJ 17) and Jiaosun (SJ 20) behind the helix (see Fig. 81).

Regional anatomy. Posterior to the root of the

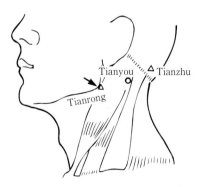

Fig. 80

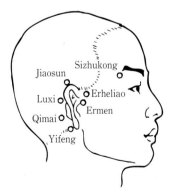

Fig. 81

auricle, in the m. auricularis posterior; the posterior auricular artery and vein; the posterior auricular branch of the great auricular nerve.

Indications. Headache, tinnitus, deafness, and infantile convulsions.

Method. Puncture transversely 0.3–0.5 cun, or prick to cause bleeding.

SJ 19, LUXI

Location. Posterior to the ear, at the junction of the upper one-third and the lower two-thirds of the curved line joining Yifeng (SJ 17) and Jiaosun (SJ 20) behind the helix (see Fig. 81).

Regional anatomy. Posterior to the root of the auricle, in the m. auricularis posterior; the posterior auricular artery and vein; the posterior auricular branch of the great auricular nerve and the lesser occipital nerve.

Indications. Headache, tinnitus, deafness, and infantile convulsions.

Method. Puncture transversely 0.3–0.5 cun.

SJ 20, JIAOSUN

The Crossing point of the hand and foot Shaoyang meridians and the meridian of the hand Yangming.

Location. Within the hairline directly above the ear apex (see Fig. 81).

Regional anatomy. At the upper border of the root of the auricle, in the m. auricularis superior; the branches of the superficial temporal artery and vein; the branches of the auriculotemporal nerve.

Indications. Swelling of the cheek, nebula, toothache, stiffness in the neck.

Method. Puncture transversely 0.3–0.5 cun.

SJ 21, ERMEN*

Location. Anterior to the supratragic notch, in the depression at the posterior border of the condylar process of the mandible (see Fig. 81).

Regional anatomy. The superficial temporal artery and vein; the branches of the auriculotemporal nerve and facial nerve.

Indications. Tinnitus, deafness, otorrhoea and toothache.

Method. Puncture, perpendicularly 0.5–1 cun, with mouth open.

SJ 22, ERHELIAO

The Crossing point of the hand and foot Shaoyang meridians and the hand Taiyang.

Location. On the posterior border of the hairline where the superficial temporal artery passes, at the level with the root of the auricle (see Fig. 81).

Regional anatomy. The m. temporalis; posteriorly, the superficial temporal artery and vein; the branch of the auriculotemporal nerve, the temporal branch of the facial nerve.

Indications. Headache, tinnitus, trismus, and deviation of the mouth and eye.

Method. Avoid the artery, puncture obliquely or transversely 0.3–0.5 cun.

SJ 23, SIZHUKONG*

Location. In the depression at the lateral end of the eyebrow (see Fig. 81).

Regional anatomy. Subcutaneously the m. orbicularis oculi; the frontal branches of the superficial temporal artery and vein; the zygomatic branch of the facial nerve and the branch of the auriculotemporal nerve.

Indications. Headache, congested eye, twitching of the eyelids, toothache, and depressive-manic psychosis.

Method. Puncture transversely 0.5–1 cun.

THE GALLBLADDER MERIDIAN OF THE FOOT SHAOYANG (WITH 44 POINTS)

Course

The gallbladder meridian of the foot Shaoyang starts from the outer canthus (Tongziliao, GB 1) (1), ascends to the corner of the forehead (Hanyan, GB 4) (2), then curves downward to the retroauricular region (Fengchi, GB 20) (3) and goes along the side of the neck in front of

Table 3.10 Indications of points on the Sanjiao meridian

Point	Location	Indications primary	secondary
		Hand and elbow: diseases of lateral head, ear, eye, chest, hypochondrium, throat; febrile diseases	
Guanchong (SJ 1)*	tip of finger	headache, redness of eye, deafness, congested and sore throat	febrile diseases
Yemen (SJ 2)*	between the fingers	headache, redness of eye, deafness, congested and sore throat	malaria
Zhongzhu (SJ 3)*	dorsum of hand	headache, redness of eye, tinnitus, deafness, sore throat	febrile diseases
Yangchi (SJ 4)*	forearm	headache, congested eye, deafness, congested and sore throat	diabetes, malaria
Waiguan (SJ 5)*	forearm	headache, congested eye, tinnitus, deafness, hypochondriacal pain, pain in upper limbs	febrile diseases
Zhigou (SJ 6)*	forearm	sudden hoarseness of voice, hypochondriacal pain, constipation	febrile diseases
Huizong (SJ 7)	forearm	deafness	epilepsy
Sanyangluo (SJ 8)	forearm	deafness, hoarseness of voice, pain in upper limbs	
Sidu (SJ 9)	forearm	deafness, hoarseness of voice, hypochondriacal pain, pain in upper limb	
Tianjing (SJ 10)*	elbow	migraine, scrofula	epilepsy
		Neck and lateral head: diseases of the lateral aspect of head, the ear and eye	
Qinglengyuan (SJ 11)	upper	arm pain in upper limbs	yellow sclera
Xiaoluo (SJ 12)	upper arm	stiffness in the neck	
Naohui (SJ 13)	upper arm	pain in upper limbs	
Jianliao (SJ 14)*	shoulder	spasmodic pain or motor impairment of upper limbs	
Tianliao (SJ 15)	shoulder	pain in shoulder and back, stiffness in neck	
Tianyou (SJ 16)	neck	headache, deafness, scrofula, stiffness in neck	
Yifeng (SJ 17)*	ear	tinnitus, deafness, deviation of mouth and eye, swelling of cheek	
Qimai (SJ 18)	ear	headache, tinnitus, deafness, infantile convulsion	
Luxi (SJ 19)	ear	headache, tinnitus, deafness	
Jiaosun (SJ 20)	ear	swelling of cheek, toothache, nebula	
Ermen (SJ 21)*	anterior to ear	headache, tinnitus, toothache	
Erheliao (SJ 22)	anterior to ear	headache, tinnitus, trismus	
Sizhukong (SJ 23)*	end of eyebrow	headache, eye disease	

the Sanjiao meridian of the hand Shaoyang to the shoulder (4); turning back it traverses and passes behind the Sanjiao meridian of the hand Shaoyang down to the supraclavicular fossa (5).

The retroauricular branch arises from the retroauricular region (6) and enters the ear, then it comes out and passes the preauricular region (7) to the posterior aspect of the outer canthus (8).

The branch arising from the outer canthus (9) runs downward to Daying (St 5) (10) and meets the Sanjiao meridian of the hand Shaoyang in the infraorbital region (11); then passing through Jiache (St 6) (12), it descends to the neck and enters the supraclavicular fossa where it meets the main meridian (13); from there it further descends into the chest (14); passes through the diaphragm to link with the liver (15) and enters the gallbladder, the organ it pertains to (16); then it runs inside the hypochondriacal region (17),

comes out from the lateral side of the lower abdomen near the femoral artery at the inguinal region (18); from there it goes superficially along the margin of the pubic hair (19) and goes transversely into the hip region (Huantiao, GB 30) (20).

The straight portion of the meridian goes downward from the supraclavicular fossa (21), passes in front of the axilla (22) along the lateral aspect of the chest (23) and through the free ends of the floating ribs to the hip region where it meets the previous branch (25); then it descends along the lateral aspect of the thigh (26) to the lateral side of the knee (27); going further downward along the anterior aspect of the fibula (28) all the way to its lower end (Xuanzhong, GB 39) (29), it reaches the anterior aspect of the external malleolus (30); it then follows the dorsum of the foot to the lateral side of the tip of the 4th toe (foot Qiaoyin, GB 44) (31).

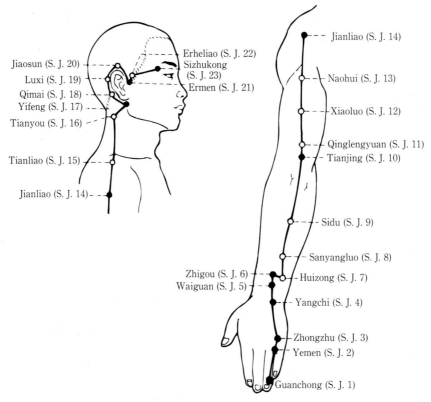

Jiaosun (S. J. 20)
Luxi (S. J. 19)
Qimai (S. J. 18)
Yifeng (S. J. 17)
Tianyou (S. J. 16)

Erheliao (S. J. 22)
Sizhukong (S. J. 23)
Ermen (S. J. 21)

Tianliao (S. J. 15)

Jianliao (S. J. 14)

Zhigou (S. J. 6)
Waiguan (S. J. 5)

Jianliao (S. J. 14)
Naohui (S. J. 13)
Xiaoluo (S. J. 12)
Qinglengyuan (S. J. 11)
Tianjing (S. J. 10)

Sidu (S. J. 9)
Sanyangluo (S. J. 8)
Huizong (S. J. 7)
Yangchi (S. J. 4)
Zhongzhu (S. J. 3)
Yemen (S. J. 2)
Guanchong (S. J. 1)

Fig. 82   Points on the Sanjiao meridian of the hand Shaoyang.

The branch of the dorsum of the foot starts from Foot Linqi (GB 41), goes between the 1st and 2nd metatarsal bones to the distal portion of the great toe and terminates at its hairy region (Dadun, Liv 1), where it links with the liver meridian of the foot Jueyin (32).

Chief pathological manifestations

Bitter taste in the mouth, blurred vision, malaria, headache, neck pain above the Adam's apple, pain in the outer canthus, swelling and pain in the supraclavicular region, axillary swelling, pain in the chest, hypochondrium, buttock and lateral aspect of the lower limbs, pain in the lateral aspect of the foot, feverish sensation in the lateral aspect of the foot.

Outline of therapeutic indications

Points of this meridian are indicated for diseases of lateral head, eye, ear and throat; mental disorders, febrile diseases, and other diseases of areas the meridian supplies.

GB 1, TONGZILIAO*

The Crossing point of the hand Taiyang and hand and foot Shaoyang meridians.

Location.   0.5 cun lateral to the outer canthus, in the depression on the lateral side of the orbit (see Fig. 84).

Regional anatomy.   The m. orbicularis oculi, deeply m. temporalis; the zygomaticoorbital artery and vein; the zygomaticofacial and zygomaticotemporal nerves, the temporal branch of the facial nerve.

Indications.   Headache, congested eye with swelling and pain, nebula and optic atrophy.

Method.   Puncture transversely 0.3–0.5 cun.

GB 2, TINGHUI*

Location.   Anterior to the intertragic notch, at the posterior border of the condylar process of the mandible. The point is needled with the mouth open (see Fig. 84).

Regional anatomy.   The rami auricularis an-

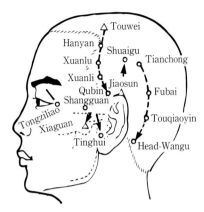

Fig. 84

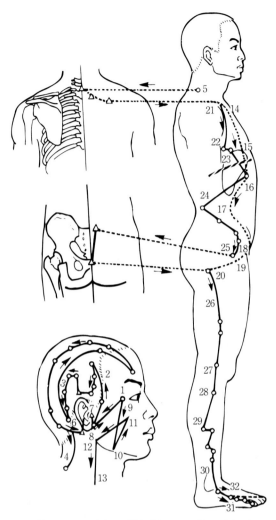

Fig. 83 The course of the gallbladder meridian of the foot Shaoyang.

teriores, deeply the external carotid artery and posterior facial vein; the great auricular nerve and subcutaneously the facial nerve.

Indications. Tinnitus, deafness, toothache and deviation of the mouth.

Method. Puncture perpendicularly 0.5–1 cun, with the mouth open.

GB 3, SHANGGUAN (ALSO CALLED KEZHUREN)

The Crossing point of the hand and foot Shaoyang and foot Yangming meridians.

Location. Directly above Xiaguan (St 7), on

the upper border of the zygomatic arch (see Fig. 84).

Regional anatomy. In the m. temporalis; the zygomaticoorbital artery and vein; the zygomatic branch of the facial nerve and the small branch of the trigeminal nerve.

Indications. Migraine, tinnitus, deafness, deviation of the mouth and eye, toothache, and trismus.

Method. Puncture perpendicularly 0.5–1 cun.

GB 4, HANYAN

The Crossing point of the hand and foot Shaoyang and the foot Yangming meridians.

Location. At the junction of the upper one-quarter and the lower three-quarters of the curved line linking Touwei (St 8) and Qubin (GB 7) (see Fig. 84).

Regional anatomy. In the m. temporalis; the parietal branches of the superficial temporal artery and vein; the temporal branch of the auriculotemporal nerve.

Indications. Migraine, blurred vision, tinnitus, toothache, and epilepsy.

Method. Puncture transversely 0.5–0.8 cun.

GB 5, XUANLU

Location. Midpoint of the curved line linking Touwei (St 8) and Qubin (GB 7) (see Fig. 84).

Regional anatomy. See Hanyan (GB 4).

Indications. Migraine, congested eye with swelling and pain, and toothache.

Method. Puncture transversely 0.5–0.8 cun.

GB 6, XUANLI

The Crossing point of the hand and foot Shaoyang and the foot Yangming meridians.

Location. At the junction of the lower one-quarter and the upper three-quarters of the curved line linking Touwei (St 8) and Qubin (GB 7) (see Fig. 84).

Regional anatomy. See Hanyan (GB 4).

Indications. Migraine, congested eye with swelling and pain, and tinnitus.

Method. Puncture transversely 0.5–0.8 cun.

GB 7, QUBIN

The Crossing point of the foot Shaoyang and foot Taiyang meridians.

Location. Directly above the posterior border of the pre-auricular hairline, about the level of Jiaosun (SJ 20) (see Fig. 84).

Regional anatomy. See Hanyan (GB 4).

Indications. Headache, toothache, trismus and sudden hoarseness of the voice.

Method. Puncture transversely 0.5–0.8 cun.

GB 8, SHUAIGU*

The Crossing point of the foot Shaoyang and foot Taiyang meridians.

Location. Directly above the ear apex, 1.5 cun within the hairline. (see Fig. 84).

Regional anatomy. In the m. temporalis; the parietal branches of the superficial temporal artery and vein; the anastomotic branch of the auriculotemporal nerve and the great occipital nerve.

Indications. Migraine, vertigo, acute and chronic infantile convulsions.

Method. Puncture transversely 0.5–0.8 cun.

GB 9, TIANCHONG

The Crossing point of the foot Shaoyang and foot Taiyang meridians.

Location. Directly above the posterior border of the root of the auricle, 2 cun within the hairline (see Fig. 84).

Regional anatomy. The posterior auricular artery and vein; the branch of the great occipital nerve.

Indications. Headache, depressive psychosis or epilepsy, swelling and pain of the gums.

Method. Puncture transversely 0.5–0.8 cun.

GB 10, FUBAI

The Crossing point of the foot Shaoyang and foot Taiyang meridians.

Location. Posterior to the upper border of the root of the auricle, 1 cun transversely within the hairline (see Fig. 84).

Regional anatomy. See Tianchong (GB 9).

Indications. Headache, tinnitus, deafness, pain in the eye and goitre.

Method. Puncture transversely 0.5–0.8 cun.

GB 11, TOUQIAOYIN

The Crossing point of the foot Shaoyang and foot Taiyang meridians.

Location. Directly below Fubai (GB 10), at the root of the mastoid process (see Fig. 84).

Regional anatomy. The branches of the posterior auricular artery and vein; the anastomotic branch of the great and lesser occipital nerves.

Indications. Headache, tinnitus and deafness.

Method. Puncture transversely 0.5–0.8 cun.

GB 12, WANGU

The Crossing point of the foot Shaoyang and foot Taiyang meridians.

Location. In the depression posterior and inferior to the mastoid process (see Fig. 84).

Regional anatomy. Superior to the site where m. sternocleidomastoideus attaches; the posterior auricular artery and vein; the lesser occipital nerve.

Indications. Headache, stiffness and pain in the neck, toothache, deviation of the mouth and epilepsy.

Method. Puncture obliquely 0.5–0.8 cun.

GB 13, BENSHEN

The Crossing point of the meridians of the foot Shaoyang and Yangwei.

Location. 3 cun lateral to Shenting (Du 24), at the junction of the medial two-thirds and the lateral one-third of the line joining Shenting (Du 24) and Touwei (St 8) (see Fig. 85).

Regional anatomy. In the m. frontalis; the frontal branches of the superficial temporal artery and vein, and the lateral branches of the frontal artery and vein; the lateral branch of the frontal nerve.

Indications. Headache, blurred vision, epilepsy and infantile convulsions.

Method. Puncture transversely 0.5–0.8 cun.

GB 14, YANGBAI*

The Crossing point of the foot Shaoyang and Yangwei meridians.

Location. With the eyes looking straight forward, the point is directly above the pupil, 1 cun above the eyebrow (see Fig. 85).

Regional anatomy. In the m. frontalis; the lateral branches of the frontal artery and vein; the lateral branch of the frontal nerve.

Indications. Headache, pain in the eye, blurred vision, twitching of the eyelids.

Method. Puncture transversely 0.3–0.5 cun.

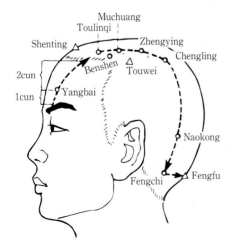

Fig. 85

GB 15, TOULINQI*

The Crossing point of the meridians of the foot Shaoyang and foot Taiyang and Yangwei.

Location. Directly above Yangbai (GB 14), 0.5 cun within the hairline (see Fig. 85).

Regional anatomy. In the m. frontalis; the frontal artery and vein; the anastomotic branch of the medial and lateral branches of the frontal nerve.

Indications. Headache, blurred vision, lacrimation, nasal obstruction, infantile convulsions and epilepsy.

Method. Puncture transversely 0.3–0.5 cun.

GB 16, MUCHUANG

The Crossing point of the meridians of the foot Shaoyang, foot Taiyang and Yangwei.

Location. 1 cun posterior to Toulinqi (GB 15) (see Fig. 85).

Regional anatomy. In the galea aponeurotica; the frontal branches of the superficial temporal artery and vein; the anastomotic branch of the medial and lateral branches of the frontal nerve.

Indications. Headache, congested eye with swelling and pain, optic atrophy, nasal obstruction, epilepsy and puffiness in the face.

Method. Puncture transversely 0.3–0.5 cun.

GB 17, ZHENGYING

The Crossing point of the meridians of the foot Shaoyang and Yangwei.

Location. 1 cun posterior to Muchuang (GB 16) (see Fig. 85).

Regional anatomy. In the galea aponeurotica; the anastomotic plexus formed by the parietal branches of the superficial temporal artery and vein and the occipital artery and vein; the anastomotic branch of the frontal and great occipital nerve.

Indications. Headache, blurred vision, rigidity of the lips and toothache.

Method. Puncture transversely 0.3–0.5 cun.

GB 18, CHENGLING

The Crossing point of the foot Shaoyang and Yangwei meridians.

Location. 1.5 cun posterior to Zhengying (GB 17) (see Fig. 85).

Regional anatomy. In the galea aponeurotica; the branches of the occipital artery and vein; the branch of the great occipital nerve.

Indications. Headache, vertigo, pain in the eye, nasal obstruction and epistaxis.

Method. Puncture transversely 0.3–0.5 cun.

GB 19, NAOKONG

The Crossing point of the foot Shaoyang and Yangwei meridians.

Location. 1.5 cun directly above Fengchi (GB 20) (see Fig. 85).

Regional anatomy. In the m. occipitalis; the branches of the occipital artery and vein; the branch of the great occipital nerve.

Indications. Headache, blurred vision, depressive-manic psychosis, epilepsy, and stiffness and pain in the neck.

Method. Puncture transversely 0.3–0.5 cun.

GB 20, FENGCHI*

The Crossing point of the foot Shaoyang and Yangwei meridians.

Location. In the depression between the m. sternocleidomastoideus and m. trapezius, on the same level with Fengfu (Du 16) (see Fig. 85).

Regional anatomy. In the depression between m. sternocleidomastoideus and m. trapezius, deeply m. splenius capitis; the branches of the occipital artery and vein; the branch of the lesser occipital nerve.

Indications. Headache, vertigo, congested eye with swelling and pain, rhinorrhoea, epistaxis, tinnitus, stiffness and pain in the neck, common cold, epilepsy, windstroke, febrile diseases, malaria and goitre.

Method. With the needle tip slightly downwards, puncture obliquely 0.8–1.2 cun towards the tip of the nose; or puncture transversely towards Fengfu (Du 16).

Note. In the centre of the deep portion is the medulla; correct angle and depth of needling are strictly demanded.

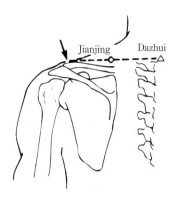

Fig. 86

GB 21, JIANJING*

The Crossing point of the hand and foot Shaoyang, and Yangwei meridians.

Location. Midpoint of the line linking Dazhui (Du 14) and the acromion (see Fig. 86).

Regional anatomy. The m. trapezius, deeply m. levator scapulae and m. supraspinatus; the transverse cervical artery and vein; the branches of the axillary nerve, deeply the radial nerve.

Indications. Stiffness and pain in the head and neck, pain in the shoulder and back, motor impairment of the upper limbs, difficult labour, mastitis, insufficient lactation and scrofula.

Method. Puncture perpendicularly 0.5–0.8 cun.

Note. Underneath is the apex of the lung and deep needling is contraindicated; contraindicated for pregnant women.

GB 22, YUANYE

Location. On the mid-axillary line when the arm is raised, at the 4th intercostal space (see Fig. 87).

Regional anatomy. The m. serratus anterior, m. intercostales interni and externi; the thoraco-epigastric vein, the lateral thoracic artery and vein, the 4th intercostal artery and vein; the lateral cutaneous branch of the 4th intercostal nerve, the branch of the long thoracic nerve.

Indications. Fullness in the chest, hypochondriacal pain and pain in the upper limbs.

Method. Puncture obliquely or transversely 0.5–0.8 cun.

Note. For points of this meridian from Yuanye

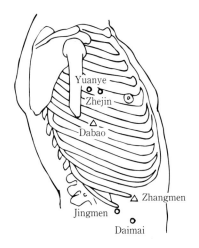

Fig. 87

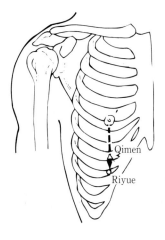

Fig. 88

(GB 22) to Jingmen (GB 25), deep needling is contraindicated so as not to injure the important viscera underneath.

GB 23, ZHEJIN

Location. 1 cun anterior to Yuanye (GB 22), at the 4th intercostal space (see Fig. 87).

Regional anatomy. The m. pectoralis major, m. serratus anterior, m. intercostales interni and externi; the lateral thoracic artery and vein, the 4th intercostal artery and vein; the lateral cutaneous branch of the 4th intercostal nerve.

Indications. Fullness in the chest, hypochondriacal pain, asthma, vomiting and sour regurgitation.

Method. Puncture obliquely or transversely 0.5–0.8 cun.

GB 24, RIYUE*

The Front-Mu point of the gallbladder, the Crossing point of the foot Shaoyang and foot Taiyin meridians.

Location. Directly below the nipple, at the 7th intercostal space (see Fig. 88).

Regional anatomy. In the aponeurosis of the m. obliquus externus abdominis, m. transversus abdominis; the 7th intercostal artery and vein; the 7th intercostal nerve.

Indications. Vomiting, sour regurgitation, cos-

tal and hypochondriacal pain, hiccup and jaundice.

Method. Puncture obliquely or transversely 0.5–0.8 cun.

GB 25, JINGMEN

The Front-Mu point of the kidney.

Location. On the free end of the 12th rib (see Fig. 87).

Regional anatomy. The m. obliquus externus abdominis, m. obliquus internus abdominis and m. transversus abdominis; the 11th intercostal artery and vein; the 11th intercostal nerve.

Indications. Dysuria, oedema, lumbar pain, hypochondriacal pain, abdominal distension and diarrhoea.

Methods. Puncture perpendicularly 0.5–1 cun.

GB 26, DAIMAI*

The Crossing point of the foot Shaoyang and Dai meridians.

Location. Directly below the free end of the 11th rib, level with the umbilicus (see Fig. 87).

Regional anatomy. The m. obliquus internus and externus abdominis, m. transversus abdominis; the 12th intercostal artery and vein; the 12th intercostal nerve (underneath is the ascending colon on the right and the descending colon on the left).

Indications. Abdominal pain, amenorrhoea, irregular menstruation, morbid leucorrhoea, hernia, and lumbar and hypochondriacal pain.

Method. Puncture perpendicularly 1–1.5 cun.

GB 27, WUSHU

The Crossing point of the foot Shaoyang and Dai meridians.

Location. On the lateral side of the abdomen, 0.5 cun anterior to the superior iliac spine, 3 cun below the level of the umbilicus (see Fig. 89).

Regional anatomy. Anterior and inferior to the iliac spine; m. obliquus internus and externus abdominis, m. transversus abdominis; the superficial and deep circumflex iliac arteries and veins; the iliohypogastric nerve.

Indications. Abdominal pain, hernia, morbid leucorrhoea, constipation and prolapse of uterus.

Method. Puncture perpendicularly 1–1.5 cun.

GB 28, WEIDAO

The Crossing point of the foot Shaoyang and Dai meridians.

Location. 0.5 cun anterior and inferior to Wushu (GB 27) (see Fig. 89).

Regional anatomy. The m. obliquus internus and externus abdominis, m. transversus abdominis; the superficial and deep circumflex iliac arteries and veins; the ilioinguinal nerve.

Indications. Abdominal pain, hernia, leucorrhoea and prolapse of the uterus.

Method. Puncture perpendicularly or anteriorly-inferiorly 1–1.5 cun.

GB 29, JULIAO

The Crossing point of the foot Shaoyang and Yangqiao meridians.

Location. At the midpoint of the line linking the anterio-superior iliac spine and the highest point of the great trochanter (see Fig. 89).

Regional anatomy. Superficially the m. tensor fasciae latae, deeply the m. vastus lateralis; the branches of the superficial circumflex iliac artery and vein, the ascending branches of the lateral circumflex femoral artery and vein; the lateral femoral cutaneous nerve.

Indications. Lumbar pain, motor impairment of the lower limbs and hernia.

Method. Puncture perpendicularly 1–1.5 cun.

GB 30, HUANTIAO*

The Crossing point of the foot Shaoyang and Taiyang meridians.

Location. At the junction of the lateral one-third and the medial two-thirds of the line linking the highest point of the great trochanter and the hiatus of the sacrum (see Fig. 90).

Regional anatomy. At the inferior border of the m. gluteus maximus and m. piriformis; medially the inferior gluteal artery and vein; the inferior gluteal cutaneous nerve, the inferior gluteal nerve and deeply the sciatic nerve.

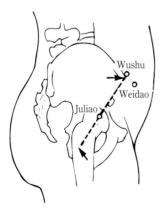

Fig. 89

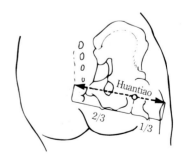

Fig. 90

Indications.   Motor impairment or paralysis of the lower limbs, and lumbar pain.
Method.   Puncture perpendicularly 2–3 cun.

GB 31, FENGSHI*

Location.   On the midline of the lateral aspect of the thigh, 7 cun above the transverse popliteal crease (see Fig. 91) or, more simply, when the patient is standing erect with the hands close to the sides, the point is where the tip of the middle finger touches.
Regional anatomy.   Below the m. tensor fasciae latae, in the m. vastus lateralis; the muscular branches of the lateral circumflex femoral artery and vein; the lateral femoral cutaneous nerve, the muscular branch of the femoral nerve.
Indications.   Motor impairment or paralysis of the lower limbs, general pruritus, and beriberi.
Method.   Puncture perpendicularly 1–2 cun.

GB 32, ZHONGDU

Location.   2 cun below Fengshi (GB 31) (see Fig. 91).
Regional anatomy.   See Fengshi (GB 31).
Indications.   Motor impairment or paralysis of the lower limbs.
Method.   Puncture perpendicularly 1–2 cun.

GB 33, XIYANGGUAN*

Location.   3 cun above Yanglingquan (GB 34), in the depression superior to the epicondylus lateralis femoris (see Fig. 91).
Regional anatomy.   Posterior to the iliotibial tract, anterior to the tendon of the m. biceps femoris; the superior lateral genicular artery and vein; the terminal branch of the lateral femoral cutaneous nerve.
Indications.   Popliteal swelling, pain and swelling, numbness of the shank.
Method.   Puncture perpendicularly 1–1.5 cun.

GB 34, YANGLINGQUAN*

The He-sea point, the Influential point of the tendons.
Location.   In the depression anterior-inferior to the small head of the fibula (see Fig. 92).
Regional anatomy.   In the m. peroneus longus and brevis; the inferior lateral genicular artery and vein; just at the site where the common peroneal nerve bifurcates into the superficial and deep peroneal nerves.
Indications. Hypochondriacal pain, bitter taste in the mouth, vomiting, motor impairment of the lower limbs, beriberi, jaundice and infantile convulsions.
Method.   Puncture perpendicularly 1–1.5 cun.

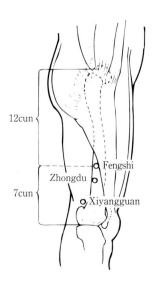

Fig. 91

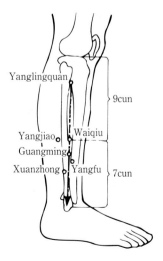

Fig. 92

Note. According to reports, observation of cholecystography under X-ray showed that needling Yanglingquan (GB 34) in normal subjects (without disorders of the gallbladder) reduced markedly the concentration of the contrast medium. This indicates that needling can increase the movement and evacuation of the gallbladder which started as soon as the needling sensation appeared. The effect was especially obvious 10 minutes after the withdrawal of the needle.

GB 35, YANGJIAO

The Xi-Cleft point of the Yangwei meridian.
Location.   7 cun above the tip of the external malleolus, at the posterior border of the fibula (see Fig. 92).
Regional anatomy.   At the site where the m. peroneus longus attaches; the branches of the peroneal artery and vein; the lateral sural cutaneous nerve.
Indications.   Distension and fullness in the chest and hypochondrium, motor impairment of the lower limbs, and depressive-manic psychosis.
Method.   Puncture perpendicularly 1–1.5 cun.

GB 36, WAIQIU

The Xi-Cleft point of the gallbladder meridian.
Location.   7 cun above the tip of the external malleolus, at the anterior border of the fibula (see Fig. 92).
Regional anatomy.   Between the m. peroneus longus and the m. extensor digitorum communis, deeply the m. peroneus brevis; the branches of the anterior tibial artery and vein; the superficial peroneal nerve.
Indications.   Distension and fullness in the chest and hypochondrium, motor impairment of the lower limbs, depressive-manic psychosis.
Method.   Puncture perpendicularly 1–1.5 cun.

GB 37, GUANGMING*

The *luo* point.
Location.   5 cun above the tip of the external malleolus, at the anterior border of the fibula (see Fig. 92).
Regional anatomy.   Between the m. extensor digitorum longus and the m. peroneus brevis; the branches of the anterior tibial artery and vein; the superior peroneal nerve.
Indications.   Pain in the eye, night blindness, motor impairment of the lower limbs, distending pain in the breasts.
Method.   Puncture perpendicularly 1–1.5 cun.

GB 38, YANGFU

The Jing-river point.
Location.   4 cun above the tip of the external malleolus, slightly anterior to the anterior border of the fibula (see Fig. 92).
Regional anatomy.   See Guangming (GB 37).
Indications.   Migraine, pain of the outer canthus, scrofula, beriberi, axillary swelling and pain, sore throat, distending pain in the chest and hypochondrium and motor impairment of the lower limbs.
Method.   Puncture perpendicularly 1–1.5 cun.

GB 39, XUANZHONG* (ALSO CALLED JUEGU)

The Influential point of marrow.
Location.   3 cun above the tip of the external malleolus, at the posterior border of the fibula (see Fig. 92).
Regional anatomy.   At the site where the m. peroneus brevis and the m. extensor digitorum longus part from each other; the branches of the anterior tibial artery and vein; the superficial peroneal nerve.
Indications.   Stiffness of the neck, distending pain in the chest and hypochondrium, motor impairment of the lower limbs, sore throat, beriberi and haemorrhoids.
Method.   Puncture perpendicularly 1–1.5 cun.

GB 40, QIUXU*

The *yuan* point.

Location. Anterior and inferior to the external malleolus, in the depression on the lateral side of the tendon of the m. extensor digitorum longus (see Fig. 93).

Regional anatomy. The m. extensor digitorum brevis; the branch of the anterior-lateral malleolar artery and vein; the branches of the lateral dorsal cutaneous nerve and superficial peroneal nerve.

Indications. Distending pain in the chest and hypochondrium, motor impairment of the lower limbs, and malaria.

Method. Puncture perpendicularly 0.5–0.8 cun.

Note. According to reports, when doing a cholangiography (after an injection of morphine) in cases of the drainage from the common bile duct, needling Qiuxu (GB 40), Yanglingquan (GB 34) and Riyue (GB 24) produced obvious regular contractions which increased.

GB 41, ZULINQI*

The Shu-stream point, one of the 8 Confluent points of the 8 extra meridians communicating with the Dai meridian.

Location. In the depression distal to the junction of the 4th and 5th metatarsal bones, on the lateral side of the tendon of the m. extensor digiti minimi of the foot (see Fig. 93).

Regional anatomy. The dorsal arterial and venous network of the foot, the 4th dorsal metatarsal artery and vein; the branch of the intermediate dorsal cutaneous nerve of the foot.

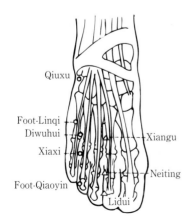

Fig. 93

Indications. Congested eye with swelling and pain, hypochondriacal and costal pain, irregular menstruation, nocturnal enuresis, mastitis, malaria and pain in the tarsal region.

Method. Puncture perpendicularly 0.3–0.5 cun.

GB 42, DIWUHUI

Location. Between the 4th and 5th metatarsal bones, on the medial side of the tendon of the m. extensor digiti minimi of the foot (see Fig. 93).

Regional anatomy. See Zulinqi (GB 41).

Indications. Headache, congested eye, tinnitus, hypochondriacal pain, mastitis, haematemesis due to internal injuries, and swelling and pain on the dorsum of the foot.

Method. Puncture perpendicularly 0.3–0.5 cun.

GB 43, XIAXI*

The Ying-spring point.

Location. On the dorsum of the foot, between the 4th and 5th toes, proximal to the margin of the web (see Fig. 93).

Regional anatomy. The dorsal digital artery and vein; the dorsal digital nerve.

Indications. Headache, blurred vision, tinnitus, deafness, congested eye with swelling and pain, costal and hypochondriacal pain, febrile diseases and mastitis.

Method. Puncture perpendicularly 0.3–0.5 cun.

GB 44, ZUQIAOYIN

The Jing-well point.

Location. On the lateral side of the 4th toe, about 0.1 cun posterior to the corner of the nail.

Regional anatomy. The arterial and venous network formed by the dorsal digital artery and vein and plantar digital artery and vein; the dorsal digital nerve.

Indications. Headache, congested eye with swelling and pain, deafness, congested and sore throat, febrile diseases, insomnia, hypochondriacal pain, hiccup, and irregular menstruation.

Method. Puncture superficially 0.1 cun, or prick to cause bleeding.

Table 3.11 Indications of points on the gallbladder meridian

Point	Location	Indications primary	secondary
Head: diseases of the head, neck and five sense organs			
Tongziliao (GB 1)*	outer canthus	headache, eye diseases	
Tinghui (GB 2)*	pre-auricle	tinnitus, deafness, toothache	
Shangguan (GB 3)	pre-auricle	migraine, tinnitus, deafness, toothache, deviation of mouth	
Hanyan (GB 4)	lateral head	migraine, blurred vision, tinnitus	
Xuanlu (GB 5)	lateral head	migraine, congested eye with swelling and pain	
Xuanli (GB 6)	lateral head	headache, trismus	
Qubin (GB 7)	lateral head	migraine, congested eye with swelling and pain	
Shuaigu (GB 8)*	lateral head	migraine, vertigo	
Tianchong (GB 9)	lateral head	headache, swelling and pain of gums	
Fubai (GB 10)	posterior head	headache, ear disease	
Head-Qiaoyin (GB 11)	posterior head	headache, ear diseases	
Head-Wangu(GB 12)	posterior head	headache, stiffness and pain in neck	
Benshen (GB 13)	front head	headache, blurred vision	epilepsy
Yangbai (GB 14)*	front head	frontal headache, eye diseases	
Head-Linqi (GB 15)*	front head	headache, eye diseases, nasal obstruction	
Muchuang (GB 16)	front head	headache, eye diseases, nasal obstruction	
Zhengying (GB 17)	front head	migraine, blurred vision	
Chengling (GB 18)	posterior head	headache, rhinorrhoea	
Naokong (GB 19)	posterior head	headache, stiffness and pain in the neck	mental disorders, epilepsy
Shoulder and neck: diseases of head, neck and shoulder			
Fengchi (GB 20)*	neck	headache, eye disease, rhinorrhoea, pain in the neck	common cold, epilepsy
Jianjing (GB 21)*	shoulder	stiffness and pain in head and shoulder and back	mastitis, delayed labour
Chest and hypochondrium: diseases of chest and hypochondrium			
Yuanye (GB 22)	hypochondrium	fullness in chest, hypochondriacal pain	
Zhejin (GB 23)	hypochondrium	fullness in chest, asthma	
Riyue (GB 24)*	costal region	hypochondriacal and costal pain, vomiting, hiccup	jaundice
Costal region: diseases of gynaecology, external genitalia, intestines			
Jingmen (GB 25)	lumbar	dysuria, oedema, lumbar and hypochondriacal pain	
Daimai (GB 26)*	lateral abdomen	abdominal pain, irregular menstruation, leucorrhoea	
Wushu (GB 27)	lateral abdomen	abdominal pain, leucorrhoea	
Weidao (GB 28)	lateral abdomen	abdominal pain, leucorrhoea, hernia prolapse of uterus	
Hip to knee: lumbar and leg diseases			
Femur-Juliao (GB 29)	hip	lumbar pain, motor impairment of lower limbs	
Huantiao (GB 30)*	hip	lumbar pain, motor impairment of lower limbs	
Fengshi (GB 31)*	thigh	motor impairment of lower limbs	general pruritus
Femur-Zhongdu (GB 32)	thigh	motor impairment of lower limbs	
Xiyangguan (GB 33)*	knee	swelling and pain in the knee	
Shank and foot: diseases of head, eye, ear, throat, hypochondrium; mental disorders, febrile diseases			
Yanglingquan (GB 34)*	shank	hypochondriacal pain, motor impairment of lower limbs	jaundice, infantile convulsion
Yangjiao (GB 35)	shank	distending pain in chest and hypochondrium, motor impairment of limbs	mental disorders
Waiqiu (GB 36)	shank	distending pain in chest and hypochondrium, motor impairment of lower limbs	mental disorders
Guangming (GB 37)*	shank	eye diseases, motor impairment of lower limbs	
Yangfu (GB 38)	shank	migraine, motor impairment of lower limbs	
Xuanzhong (GB 39)*	shank	pain of knee, motor impairment of lower limbs	stiffness of neck and nape
Qiuxu (GB 40)*	foot, tarsal region	distending pain of chest and hypochondrium, motor impairment of lower limbs	
Foot-Linqi (GB 41)*	foot, tarsal region	eye diseases, hypochondriacal pain, mastitis, irregular menstruation	
Diwuhui (GB 42)	foot, tarsal region	headache, mastitis, swelling and pain of dorsum of foot	
Xiaxi (GB 43)*	between toes	headache, eye diseases, tinnitus, deafness, hypochondriacal pain	febrile diseases
Foot-Qiaoyin (GB 44)	tip of toe	headache, congested eye with swelling and pain, and pain, congested and sore throat	febrile disease, insomnia

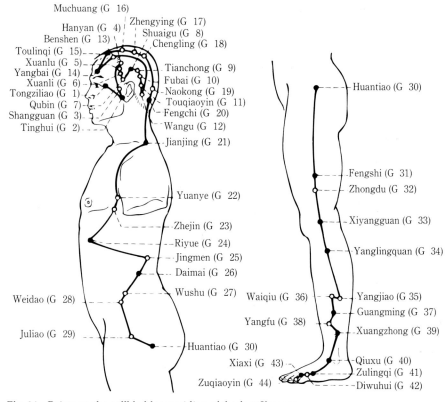

Muchuang (G 16)
Hanyan (G 4)
Zhengying (G 17)
Shuaigu (G 8)
Benshen (G 13)
Chengling (G 18)
Toulinqi (G 15)
Xuanlu (G 5)
Yangbai (G 14)
Tianchong (G 9)
Xuanli (G 6)
Fubai (G 10)
Tongziliao (G 1)
Naokong (G 19)
Qubin (G 7)
Touqiaoyin (G 11)
Shangguan (G 3)
Fengchi (G 20)
Tinghui (G 2)
Wangu (G 12)
Jianjing (G 21)

Huantiao (G 30)

Yuanye (G 22)

Zhejin (G 23)
Riyue (G 24)
Jingmen (G 25)
Daimai (G 26)
Weidao (G 28)
Wushu (G 27)
Waiqiu (G 36)
Juliao (G 29)
Huantiao (G 30)
Xiaxi (G 43)
Zuqiaoyin (G 44)
Yangfu (G 38)

Fengshi (G 31)
Zhongdu (G 32)
Xiyangguan (G 33)
Yanglingquan (G 34)
Yangjiao (G 35)
Guangming (G 37)
Xuangzhong (G 39)
Qiuxu (G 40)
Zulingqi (G 41)
Diwuhui (G 42)

Fig. 94   Points on the gallbladder meridian of the foot Shaoyang.

THE LIVER MERIDIAN OF THE FOOT JUEYIN (WITH 14 POINTS)

Course

The liver meridian of the foot Jueyin originates from the dorsal hairy region of the great toe (Dadun, Liv 1) (1); running upward along the dorsum of the foot (2), passing through Zhongfeng (Liv 4), 1 cun in front of the medial malleolus (3), it ascends to an area 8 cun above the medial malleolus, where it goes across and behind the spleen meridian of the foot Taiyin (4); then it goes further upward to the medial side of the knee (5) and along the medial aspect of the thigh (6) to the pubic region (7), where it curves around the external genitalia (8) and goes up to the lower abdomen (9); then it goes upward and curves around the stomach to enter the liver, the organ it pertains to, and connects with the gallbladder (10); from there it continues to ascend, passing through the diaphragm (11), and branching out in the costal and hypochondriacal region (12); then it ascends along the posterior aspect of the throat (13) to the nasopharynx (14) and connects with the "eye system" (15); running further upward, it emerges from the forehead (16) and meets the Du meridian at the vertex (17).

The branch arising from the "eye system" goes downward into the cheek (18) and curves around the inner surface of the lips (19).

The branch arising from the liver (20) passes through the diaphragm and flows upward into the lung and links with the lung meridian of the hand Taiyin (22).

Chief pathological manifestations

Lumbar pain, fullness in the chest, hiccup, nocturnal enuresis, dysuria, hernia, and swelling in the lower abdomen.

Outline of therapeutic indications

Points of this meridian are indicated for liver

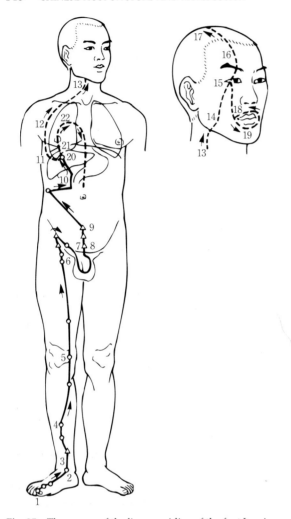

Fig. 95 The course of the liver meridian of the foot Jueyin.

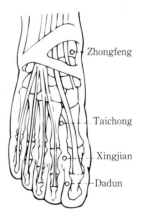

Fig. 96

diseases, gynaecological diseases, diseases of the external genitalia and other diseases of areas the meridian supplies.

LIV 1, DADUN*

The Jing-well point.

Location. On the lateral side of the great toe, about 0.1 cun posterior to the corner of the nail (see Fig. 96).

Regional anatomy. The dorsal digital artery and vein; the dorsal digital nerve.

Indications. Hernia, nocturnal enuresis, amenorrhoea, massive uterine bleeding, prolapse of the uterus and epilepsy.

Method. Puncture obliquely 0.1–0.2 cun, or prick to cause bleeding.

Note. Contraindicated for pregnant women (before and after the labour) when treated with moxibustion. This is mentioned in the *Supplement with Diagnosis to the Systematic Compilation of the Internal Classic.*

LIV 2, XINGJIAN*

The Ying-spring point.

Location. On the dorsum of the foot between the 1st and 2nd toes, proximal to the margin of the web (see Fig. 96).

Regional anatomy. The dorsal venous network of the foot, the 1st dorsal digital artery; the site where the dorsal digital nerves split from the lateral dorsal metatarsal nerve of the deep peroneal nerve.

Indications. Headache, blurred vision, congested eye with swelling and pain, optic atrophy, deviation of the mouth, hypochondriacal pain, hernia, dysuria, massive uterine bleeding, epilepsy, irregular menstruation, dysmenorrhoea, morbid leucorrhoea and windstroke.

Method. Puncture obliquely 0.5–0.8 cun.

LIV 3, TAICHONG*

The Shu-stream and *yuan* point.

Location. On the dorsum of the foot, in the depression distal to the junction of the 1st and 2nd metatarsal bones (see Fig. 96).

Regional anatomy. Lateral border of the tendon of the m. extensor hallucis longus; the dorsal venous network of the foot, the 1st dorsal metatarsal artery; the dorsal digital nerve.

Indications. Headache, vertigo, congested eye with swelling and pain, deviation of the mouth, hypochondriacal pain, nocturnal enuresis, hernia, massive uterine bleeding, irregular menstruation, epilepsy, nausea, infantile convulsions and motor impairment of the lower limbs.

Method. Puncture 0.5–0.8 cun perpendicularly.

Note. According to reports, needling Zusanli (St 36), Yanglingquan (GB 34) or unilaterally Taichong (Liv 3) in patients with an acute disease of the biliary tract undergoing a cholecystectomy operation or exploratory choledochostomy, made the biliary pressure (after an injection of morphine) not only cease to rise but also rapidly lower. The effect of relieving the spasm of Oddi's sphincter at the orifice of the biliary tract whilst needling Taichong (Liv 3) is stronger and more powerful than that whilst needling Zusanli (St 36) and Yanglingquan (GB 34).

LIV 4, ZHONGFENG*

The Jing-river point.

Location. 1 cun anterior to the medial malleolus, on the medial side of the tendon of the m. tibialis anterior (see Fig. 96).

Regional anatomy. The dorsal venous network of the foot and the anterior medial malleolar artery; the branch of the medial dorsal cutaneous nerve of the foot and the saphenous nerve.

Indications. Hernia, seminal emission, dysuria and abdominal pain.

Method. Puncture perpendicularly 0.5–0.8 cun.

LIV 5, LIGOU

The *luo* point.

Location. 5 cun above the tip of the medial malleolus, at the middle of the medial aspect of the tibia (see Fig. 97).

Regional anatomy. Posteriorly the great saphenous vein; the anterior branch of the saphenous nerve.

Indications. Dysuria, nocturnal enuresis, irre-

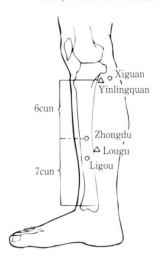

Fig. 97

gular menstruation, leucorrhoea and motor impairment of the lower limbs.

Method. Puncture transversely 0.5–0.8 cun.

LIV 6, ZHONGDU

The Xi-Cleft point.

Location. 7 cun above the tip of the medial malleolus, at the middle of the medial aspect of the tibia (see Fig. 97).

Regional anatomy. The great saphenous vein; the branch of the saphenous nerve.

Indications. Hernia, massive uterine bleeding.

Method. Puncture transversely 0.5–0.8 cun.

LIV 7, XIGUAN

Location. 1 cun posterior to Yinlingquan (Sp 9) (see Fig. 97).

Regional anatomy. Posterior and inferior to the medial condyle of the tibia, in the upper portion of the medial head of the m. gastrocnemius; deeply the posterior tibial artery; the branch of the medial sural cutaneous nerve, deeply the tibial nerve.

Indications. Swelling and pain in the knee region.

Method. Puncture perpendicularly 1–1.5 cun.

LIV 8, QUQUAN*

The He-sea point.

Location. When the knee is flexed, the point is in the depression above the medial end of the transverse popliteal crease (see Fig. 98).

Regional anatomy. Posterior to the medial epicondyle of the femur, on the anterior part of the insertion of the m. semimembranosus and m. semitendinosus, posterior border of the m. sartorius; superficially the great saphenous vein and deeply the popliteal artery and vein; superficially the saphenous nerve and deeply the tibial nerve.

Indications. Abdominal pain, dysuria, seminal emission, pruritus vulvae, pain in the knee, irregular menstruation, dysmenorrhoea and leucorrhoea.

Method. Puncture perpendicularly 1–1.5 cun.

LIV 9, YINBAO

Location. 4 cun above the medial epicondyle of the femur, at the posterior border of the m. sartorius (see Fig. 98)

Regional anatomy. Between the m. vastus medialis and the m. sartorius, the m. abductor longus; deeply the m. abductor brevis; deeply the femoral artery and vein on the lateral side, the superficial branch of the medial circumflex femoral artery; the anterior femoral cutaneous nerve, on the course of the superficial and deep branches of the obturator nerve.

Indications. Abdominal pain, nocturnal enuresis, dysuria and irregular menstruation.

Method. Puncture perpendicularly 1–2 cun.

LIV 10, ZUWULI

Location. 2 cun lateral to Qugu (Ren 2) and then 3 cun below (see Fig. 99).

Regional anatomy. Inferior to the pubic spine; m. abductor longus and brevis; the superficial branches of the medial femoral artery; the superficial and deep branches of the obturator nerve.

Indications. Lower abdominal pain, retention of urine, prolapse of the uterus, swelling and pain of the testes, preference for lying in bed, and scrofula.

Method. Puncture perpendicularly 1–2 cun.

LIV 11, YINLIAN

Location. 2 cun lateral to Qugu (Ren 2) and then 2 cun below (see Fig. 99).

Regional anatomy. Inferior to the pubic spine; the m. abductor longus and brevis; the branches of the medial circumflex femoral artery and vein; the branch of the medial femoral cutaneous nerve, the superficial and deep branches of the obturator nerve.

Indications. Irregular menstruation, leucorrhoea and lower abdominal pain.

Method. Puncture perpendicularly 1–2 cun.

LIV 12, JIMAI

Location. 2.5 cun lateral to the lower border of the pubic spine, in the inguinal groove lateral and inferior to Qichong (St 30) (see Fig. 99).

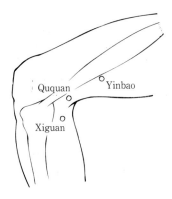

Fig. 98

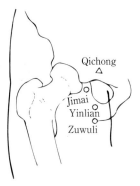

Fig. 99

Regional anatomy. The branches of the external pudendal artery and vein, the pubic branches of the inferior epigastric artery and vein, laterally the femoral vein; the ilioinguinal nerve, deeply the branch of the obturator nerve.

Indications. Lower abdominal pain, hernia and prolapse of the uterus.

Method. Avoid the artery first, puncture perpendicularly 0.5–0.8 cun.

Note. The *Plain Questions* states that moxibustion is applicable but needling contraindicated at this point.

LIV 13, ZHANGMEN*

Front-Mu point of the spleen, one of the 8 Influential points—the Influential point of the zang organs, the Crossing point of the liver and gallbladder meridians.

Location. At the free end of the 11th floating rib (see Fig. 100).

Regional anatomy. In the m. obliquus internus and externus abdominis and m. transversus abdominis; the terminal branch of the 10th intercostal artery; the 10th and 11th intercostal nerves (underneath is the lower border of the liver on the right and the lower border of the spleen on the left).

Indications. Abdominal distension, diarrhoea, hypochondriacal pain and abdominal masses.

Method. Puncture perpendicularly 0.8–1 cun.

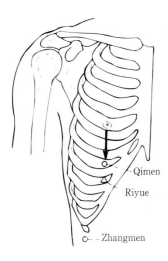

Qimen
Riyue
Zhangmen

Fig. 100

LIV 14, QIMEN*

The Front-Mu point of the liver, the Crossing point of the foot Jueyin, foot Taiyin and Yinwei meridians.

Location. Directly below the nipple, at the 6th intercostal space (see Fig. 100).

Regional anatomy. In the aponeurosis of the m. obliquus internus and externus abdominis, m. intercostalis; the 6th intercostal artery and vein; the 6th intercostal nerve.

Indications. Distending pain in the chest and hypochondrium, abdominal distension, vomiting and mastitis.

Method. Puncture obliquely or transversely 0.5–0.8 cun.

The 8 extra meridians

THE DU MERIDIAN (WITH 28 ACUPOINTS)

Course

The Du meridian arises from the lower abdomen and emerges from the perineum (1); then it goes posteriorly along the interior of the spinal column (2) to Fengfu (Du 16) at the nape, where it enters the brain (3); it further ascends to the vertex (4) and winds along the forehead to the columnella of the nose (5).

Chief pathological manifestations

Spinal stiffness and pain, opisthotonos, etc.

Outline of therapeutic indications

Points of this meridian are indicated for mental disorders, febrile diseases, local disorders of the lumbar-sacral regions, back, head and nape, and diseases of related internal organs.

DU 1, CHANGQIANG*

The Crossing point of the Du, foot Shaoyang and foot Shaoyin meridians, the *luo* point of the Du meridian.

Location. 0.5 cun below the tip of the coccyx,

Table 3.12   Indications of points on the liver meridian

Point	Location	Indications primary	secondary
Lower limbs: gynaecological diseases and external genitalia diseases mainly; intestinal diseases as well			
Dadun (Liv 1)*	tip of big toe	hernia, nocturnal enuresis, uterine bleeding, prolapse of uterus	epilepsy
Xingjian (Liv 2)*	between the toes	uterine bleeding, dysuria	headache, congested eye, deviation of mouth, hypochondriacal pain, epilepsy
Taichong (Liv 3)*	metatarsal region	uterine bleeding, nocturnal enuresis, hernia	headache, vertigo, deviation of mouth, hypochondriacal pain, epilepsy
Zhongfeng (Liv 4)*	ankle	hernia, seminal emission, dysuria	
Ligou (Liv 5)	shank	irregular menstruation, leucorrhoea, dysuria	
Zhongdu (Liv 6)	shank	hernia, uterine bleeding, abdominal pain	
Xiguan (Liv 7)	shank	pain in the knee	
Ququan (Liv 8)*	knee	abdominal pain, dysuria, hernia, seminal emission	
Yinbao (Liv 9)	thigh	nocturnal enuresis, dysuria, irregular menstruation	
Zuwuli (Liv 10)	thigh	retention of urine	
Yinlian (Liv 11)	thigh	irregular menstruation	
Hypochondriacal and abdominal regions: gastrointestinal diseases mainly; and gynaecological diseases as well			
Jimai (Liv 12)	abdomen	hernia, lower abdominal pain	
Zhangmen (Liv 13)*	hypochondrium	abdominal distension, diarrhoea, hypochondriacal pain	
Qimen (Liv 14)*	costal region	distending pain in chest and hypochondrium, vomiting	

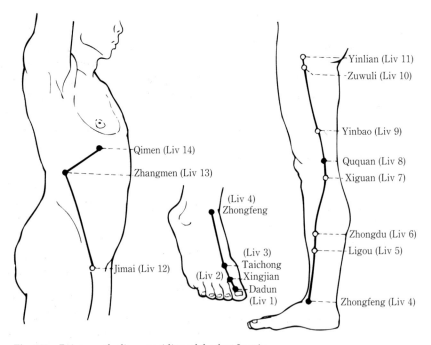

Fig. 101   Points on the liver meridian of the foot Jueyin.

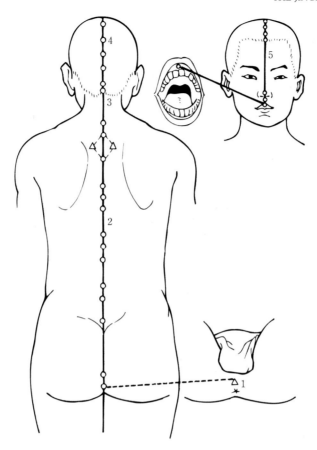

Fig. 102   The course of the Du meridian.

midway between the tip of the coccyx and the anus (see Fig. 103).

Regional anatomy. In the anococcygeal diaphragm; the branches of the inferior haemorrhoid artery and vein, the extending part of the interspinal venous plexus; the posterior ramus of the coccygeal nerve.

Indications. Diarrhoea, haematochezia, constipation, haemorrhoids, prolapse of the anus, depressive-manic psychosis and epilepsy.

Method. Puncture in obliquely close to the front of the coccyx 0.8–1 cun. Perpendicular puncture easily injures the rectum.

DU 2, YAOSHU

Location. In the hiatus of the sacrum (see Fig. 103).

Regional anatomy. The sacrococcygeal liga-

ment; the posterior branches of the median sacral artery and vein and interspinal venous plexus; the coccygeal nerve.

Indications. Irregular menstruation, haemorrhoids, lumbar and spinal stiffness and pain, motor impairment of the lower limbs, and epilepsy.

Method. Puncture upwardly and obliquely 0.5–1 cun.

DU 3, YAOYANGGUAN*

Location. Below the spinous process of the 4th lumbar vertebra (see Fig. 103).

Regional anatomy. The lumbodorsal fascia, supraspinal ligament and interspinal ligament; the posterior branch of the lumbar artery, the interspinal venous plexus; the medial branch of the posterior ramus of the lumbar nerve.

Indications. Irregular menstruation, nocturnal

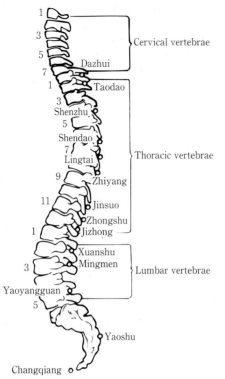
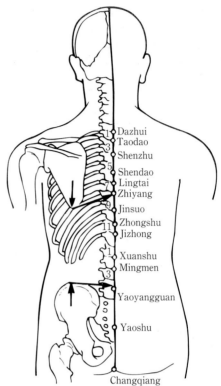

Fig. 103

emission, impotence, lumbosacral pain and motor impairment of the lower limbs.

Method. Puncture upwardly and obliquely 0.5–1 cun.

DU 4, MINGMEN*

Location. Below the spinous process of the 2nd lumbar vertebra (see Fig. 103).

Regional anatomy. See Yaoyangguan (Du 3).

Indications. Impotence, nocturnal emission, leucorrhoea, irregular menstruation, diarrhoea, lumbar spinous stiffness and pain.

Method. Puncture upwardly obliquely 0.5–1 cun.

DU 5, XUANSHU

Location. Below the spinous process of the 1st lumbar vertebra (see Fig. 103).

Regional anatomy. See Yaoyangguan (Du 3).

Indications. Diarrhoea, abdominal pain, lumbo-spinous stiffness and pain.

Method. Puncture upwardly obliquely 0.5–1 cun.

DU 6, JIZHONG

Location. Below the spinous process of the 11th thoracic vertebra (see Fig. 103).

Regional anatomy. The lumbodorsal fascia, supraspinal ligament and interspinal venous plexus; the posterior branch of the 11th intercostal artery and the interspinal venous plexus; the medial branch of the posterior ramus of the 11th thoracic nerve.

Indications. Diarrhoea, jaundice, haemorrhoids, epilepsy, infantile malnutrition, and prolapse of the anus.

Method. Puncture upwardly obliquely 0.5–1 cun.

DU 7, ZHONGSHU

Location. Below the spinous process of the 10th thoracic vertebra (see Fig. 103).

Regional anatomy. See Jizhong (Du 6) for musculature and ligament; the posterior branch of the 10th intercostal artery and the interspinal venous plexus; the medial branch of the posterior ramus of the 10th intercostal nerve.

Indications. Jaundice, vomiting, abdominal fullness and lumbar stiffness and pain.

Method. Puncture upwardly obliquely 0.5–1 cun.

DU 8, JINSUO

Location. Below the spinous process of the 9th thoracic vertebra (see Fig. 103).

Regional anatomy. See Jizhong (Du 6) for musculature and ligament; the posterior branch of the 9th intercostal artery and the interspinal venous plexus; the medial branch of the posterior ramus of the 9th intercostal nerve.

Indications. Epilepsy, stiffness of the back and gastric pain.

Method. Puncture upwardly obliquely 0.5–1 cun.

DU 9, ZHIYANG*

Location. Below the spinous process of the 7th thoracic vertebra (see Fig. 103).

Regional anatomy. See Jizhong (Du 6) for musculature and ligament; the posterior branch of the 7th intercostal artery and interspinal venous plexus; the medial branch of the posterior ramus of the 7th intercostal nerve.

Indications. Jaundice, distension and fullness in chest and hypochondrium, cough and asthmatic breathing, stiffness in the back and pain in the back.

Method. Puncture upwardly obliquely 0.5–1 cun.

DU 10, LINGTAI

Location. Below the spinous process of the 6th thoracic vertebra (see Fig. 103).

Regional anatomy. See Jizhong (Du 6) for musculature and ligament; the posterior branch of the 6th intercostal artery and interspinal venous plexus; the branch of the posterior ramus of the 6th intercostal nerve.

Indications. Cough, asthma, carbuncle and boils, stiffness and pain in the back.

Method. Puncture upwardly obliquely 0.5–1 cun.

DU 11, SHENDAO

Location. Below the spinous process of the 5th thoracic vertebra (see Fig. 103).

Regional anatomy. See Jizhong (Du 6) for musculature and ligament; the posterior branch of the 5th intercostal artery and interspinal venous plexus; the medial branch of the posterior ramus of the 5th thoracic nerve.

Indications. Palpitations, amnesia, cough, and stiffness and pain in the back.

Method. Puncture upwardly and obliquely 0.5–1 cun.

DU 12, SHENZHU

Location. Below the spinous process of the 3rd thoracic vertebra (see Fig. 103).

Regional anatomy. See Jizhong (Du 6) for musculature and ligament; the posterior branch of the 3rd intercostal artery and the interspinal venous plexus; the medial branch of the posterior ramus of the 3rd intercostal nerve.

Indications. Cough, asthma, scrofula, stiffness and pain in the back.

Method. Puncture upwardly obliquely 0.5–1 cun.

DU 13, TAODAO

The Crossing point of the Du and foot Taiyang meridians.

Location. Below the spinous process of the 1st thoracic vertebra (see Fig. 103).

Regional anatomy. See Jizhong (Du 6) for musculature and ligament; the posterior branch of the 1st intercostal artery and the interspinal venous plexus; the medial branch of the posterior ramus of the 1st intercostal nerve.

Indications. Headache, malaria, febrile diseases and stiffness of the back.

Method. Puncture upwardly and obliquely 0.5–1 cun.

DU 14, DAZHUI*

Location. Below the spinous process of the 7th cervical vertebra (see Fig. 103).

Regional anatomy. See Jizhong (Du 6) for musculature and ligament; the interspinal venous plexus; the posterior branch of the 8th cervical nerve.

Indications. Febrile diseases, malaria, cough, asthma, hectic fever and night sweating, epilepsy, stiffness and pain in the head and neck, and rubella.

Method. Puncture upwardly obliquely 0.5–1 cun.

Note. According to reports, on needling Dazhui (Du 14), Hegu (LI 4) and Zusanli (St 36) in patients with leucorrhoea due to radiotherapy or chemotherapy, a marked effect was observed. In treating trophic eosinophilia by needling Dazhui (Du 14), Feishu (UB 13) and Zusanli (St 36), a gradual decrease in eosinophils was observed.

DU 15, YAMEN*

The Crossing point of the Du and Yangwei meridians.

Location. 0.5 cun directly above the midpoint of the posterior hairline (see Fig. 104).

Regional anatomy. Between the 1st and 2nd cervical vertebrae; the branches of the occipital artery and vein and interspinal venous plexus; the 3rd occipital nerve and the great occipital nerve.

Indications. Sudden loss of voice, aphasia with tongue stiffness, depressive-manic psychosis and epilepsy, and stiffness and pain in the head and back.

Method. Puncture perpendicularly or downward obliquely 0.5–1 cun; upward oblique or deep puncture is forbidden.

Note. The point is near the medulla in its

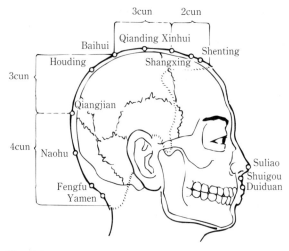

Fig. 104

deep portion, and the correct angle and depth of needling should be strictly enforced.

DU 16, FENGFU*

The Crossing point of the Du and Yangwei meridians.

Location. 1 cun directly above the midpoint of the posterior hairline (see Fig. 104).

Regional anatomy. Between the occipital bone and the 1st cervical vertebra; the branch of the occipital artery and interspinal venous plexus; the branches of the 3rd cervical nerve and the great occipital nerve.

Indications. Headache, stiffness in the nape, vertigo, sore throat, loss of voice, depressive-manic psychosis and windstroke.

Method. Puncture perpendicularly or downward obliquely 0.5–1 cun; deep puncture is forbidden.

Note. Deep underneath is the medulla, and caution is needed while needling this point.

DU 17, NAOHU

The Crossing point of the Du and foot Taiyang meridians.

Location. 1.5 cun directly above Fengfu (Du 16) (see Fig. 104).

Regional anatomy. At the upper border of the

external occipital protuberance and between the m. occipitalis; the branches of the occipital arteries and veins of both sides; the branch of the great occipital nerve.

Indications. Dizziness and vertigo, stiffness in the nape, loss of voice and epilepsy.

Method. Puncture transversely 0.5–0.8 cun.

DU 18, QIANGJIAN

Location. 1.5 cun directly above Naohu (Du 17) (see Fig. 104).

Regional anatomy. At the junction of the sagittal suture and lambdoid suture, in the galea aponeurotica; the anastomotic network formed by branches of the occipital arteries and veins of both sides; the branch of the great occipital nerve.

Indications. Headache, blurred vision, stiffness in the nape, and depressive-manic psychosis.

Method. Puncture transversely 0.5–0.8 cun.

DU 19, HOUDING

Location. 1.5 cun directly above Qiangjian (Du 18) (see Fig. 104).

Regional anatomy. In the galea aponeurotica; the anastomotic network formed by the branches of the occipital arteries and veins on both sides; the branch of the great occipital nerve.

Indications. Headache, vertigo and depressive-manic psychosis.

Method. Puncture transversely 0.5–0.8 cun.

DU 20, BAIHUI*

The Crossing point of the Du and foot Taiyang meridians.

Location. 7 cun directly above the midpoint of the posterior hairline (see Fig. 104). A simple way to locate this point is to look directly above the ear apex, at the middle of the vertex.

Regional anatomy. In the galea aponeurotica; the anastomotic network formed by the superficial temporal arteries and veins and the occipital arteries and veins on both sides; the branch of

the great occipital nerve and branch of the frontal nerve.

Indications. Headache, vertigo, windstroke and aphasia, depressive-manic psychosis, prolapse of anus, prolapse of uterus, and insomnia.

Method. Puncture transversely 0.5–0.8 cun.

DU 21, QIANDING

Location. 1.5 cun anterior to Baihui (Du 20) (see Fig. 104).

Regional anatomy. In the galea aponeurotica; the anastomotic network formed by the superficial temporal arteries and veins and the occipital arteries and veins on both sides; the branch of the frontal nerve and the branch of the great occipital nerve.

Indications. Headache, vertigo, rhinorrhoea and epilepsy.

Method. Puncture transversely 0.5–0.8 cun.

DU 22, XINHUI

Location. 2 cun directly above the midpoint of the anterior hairline (see Fig. 104).

Regional anatomy. At the junction of the coronal suture and sagittal suture, in the galea aponeurotica; the anastomotic network formed by the branches of the superficial temporal arteries and veins and branch of the frontal nerve.

Indications. Headache, vertigo, rhinorrhoea, epilepsy.

Method. Puncture transversely 0.5–0.8 cun.

Note. This point is prohibited in infants with a patent frontal suture.

DU 23, SHANGXING*

Location. 1 cun directly above the midpoint of the anterior hairline (see Fig. 104).

Regional anatomy. At the junction of the m. frontalis on both sides; the branches of the frontal artery and vein, and the branches of the superficial temporal artery and vein; the branch of the frontal nerve.

Indications. Headache, pain in the eye, rhinorrhoea, epistaxis, depressive-manic psychosis, malaria and febrile diseases.

Method. Puncture transversely 0.5–1 cun.

DU 24, SHENTING

The crossing point of the Du, foot Taiyang and foot Yangming meridians.

Location. 0.5 cun directly above the midpoint of the anterior hairline (see Fig. 104).

Regional anatomy. At the junction of the m. frontalis on both sides; the branches of the frontal artery and vein; the branch of the frontal nerve.

Indications. Headache, vertigo, insomnia, rhinorrhoea, and epilepsy.

Method. Puncture transversely 0.5–0.8 cun.

Note. In the *Systematic Classic of Acupuncture and Moxibustion*, it says that needling this point is contraindicated, otherwise it may cause mental disorders.

DU 25, SULIAO*

Location. On the tip of the nose (see Fig. 104).

Regional anatomy. In the cartilage of the apex nasi; the nasal dorsal branches of the facial artery and vein; the buccal branch of the facial nerve (the branch of the infraorbital nerve).

Indications. Rhinorrhoea, epistaxis, asthmatic breathing, coma, convulsions, suffocation in the newborn.

Method. Puncture upwardly obliquely 0.3–0.5 cun.

Note. According to reports, on needling Suliao (Du 25), Shuigou (Du 26) and Huiyin (Ren 1) in animals (rabbits, cats and dogs), an immediate increase in respiration was observed. Furthermore, the degree and the positive rate of increase of respiration in needling Suliao and Shuigou was higher than that in needling Huiyin.

DU 26, SHUIGOU* (RENZHONG)

The Crossing point of the Du, hand and foot Yangming meridians.

Location. At the junction of the upper one-third and the lower two-thirds of the philtrum (see Fig. 104).

Regional anatomy. In the m. orbicularis oris; the superior labial artery and vein; the buccal branch of the facial nerve, and the branch of the infraorbital nerve.

Indications. Depressive-manic psychosis and epilepsy, infantile convulsions, coma, deviation of the mouth and eye, and lumbar stiffness and pain.

Method. Puncture upwardly obliquely 0.3–0.5 cun.

DU 27, DUIDUAN

Location. On the medial tubercle of the upper lip, at the junction of the skin and the lip (see Fig. 104).

Regional anatomy. In the m. orbicularis oris; the superior labial artery and vein; the buccal branch of the facial nerve and the branch of the infraorbital nerve.

Indications. Depressive-manic psychosis, swelling and pain of the gums, deviation of the mouth, and epistaxis.

Method. Puncture upwardly obliquely 0.2–0.3 cun.

DU 28, YINJIAO

Location. At the junction of the gum and the frenulum of the upper lip (see Fig. 105).

Regional anatomy. The superior labial artery and vein; the branch of the superior alveolar nerve.

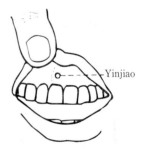

Fig. 105

Table 3.13   Indications of points on the Du meridian

Point	Location	Indications primary	secondary
Coccygeal end to 14th vertebra: mental disorders, diseases of gynaecology, external genitalia and intestines			
Changqiang (Du 1)*	coccygeal end	haematochezia, haemorrhoids	mental disorders
Yaoshu (Du 2)	iliac bone	irregular menstruation, lumbar stiffness and pain	
Yaoyangguan (Du 3)*	lumbar vertebra	irregular menstruation, nocturnal emission, lumbosacral pain, motor impairment of lower limbs	
Mingmen (Du 4)*	lumbar vertebra	impotence, nocturnal emission, leucorrhoea, lumbar pain	diarrhoea, irregular menstruation
Vertebrae 13–9: mental disorders, gastrointestinal diseases			
Xuanshu (Du 5)	lumbar	diarrhoea, lumbar stiffness and vertebral pain	
Jizhong (Du 6)	thoracic vertebra	diarrhoea, jaundice	epilepsy
Zhongshu (Du 7)	thoracic vertebra	jaundice, vomiting, lumbar stiffness and pain	
Jinsuo (Du 8)	thoracic vertebra	gastric pain, lumbar stiffness	epilepsy
Vertebrae 7–1: mental disorders, heart and lung diseases, febrile diseases			
Zhiyang (Du 9)*	thoracic vertebra	jaundice, cough and asthma	back stiffness, back pain
Lingtai (Du 10)	thoracic vertebra	cough, asthma	boils and ulcers
Shendao (Du 11)	thoracic vertebra	cough	palpitation, amnesia
Shenzhu (Du 12)	thoracic vertebra	cough, asthma	epilepsy, back stiffness and pain
Taodao (Du 13)	thoracic vertebra	headache	malaria, febrile diseases
Dazhui (Du 14)*	cervico-thoracic	cough, asthma, headache, neck stiffness	febrile disease, malaria, epilepsy
Nape: mental disorders, diseases of head and nape			
Yamen (Du 15)*	cervical vertebra	sudden hoarseness of voice, aphasia with tongue stiffness	mental disorders
Fengfu (Du 16)*	posterior head	headache, neck stiffness, vertigo, sore throat	mental disorders
Head: mental disorders, diseases of head, face, five sense organs			
Naohu (Du 17)	posterior head	dizziness, neck stiffness	epilepsy
Qiangjian (Du 18)	posterior head	headache, blurred vision	epilepsy
Houding (Du 19)	posterior head	headache, vertigo	mental disorders, epilepsy
Baihui (Du 20)*	vertex	headache, vertigo, windstroke	mental disorders, prolapse of anus, prolapse of uterus
Qianding (Du 21)	anterior head	headache, rhinorrhoea	epilepsy
Xinhui (Du 22)	anterior head	headache, vertigo, rhinorrhoea	epilepsy
Shangxing (Du 23)*	anterior head	headache, rhinorrhoea, epistaxis	mental disorders
Shenting (Du 24)	anterior head	headache, vertigo	epilepsy
Mouth and nose: mental disorders, pain of nose, mouth and teeth			
Suliao (Du 25)*	nose tip	nose diseases	convulsions, coma
Shuigou (Du 26)*	philtrum	deviation of mouth and eye	mental disorders, infantile convulsions, coma, lumbar stiffness and pain
Duiduan (Du 27)	upper lip	deviation of mouth, swelling and pain of gums	mental disorders
Yinjiao (Du 28)	gum	swelling and pain in gums	mental disorders

Indications. Depressive-manic psychosis, swelling and pain of the gums, and rhinorrhoea.

THE REN MERIDIAN (WITH 24 ACUPOINTS)

Course

The Ren meridian originates from inside the lower abdomen and emerges from the perineum (1); it goes anteriorly to the pubic region (2) and ascends along the interior of the abdomen, passing through Guanyuan (Ren 4) and some other points along the front midline (3) to the throat (6); ascending further, it curves around the lips (5), passes through the cheek and enters the infraorbital region (Chengqi, St 1) (7).

Chief pathological manifestations

Hernia, morbid leucorrhoea, abdominal masses, etc.

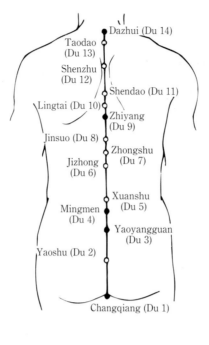

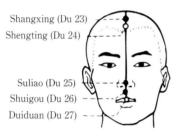

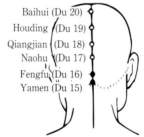

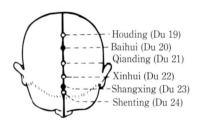

Fig. 106   Points on the Du meridian.

Outline of therapeutic indications

Points of this meridian are indicated for local diseases of the abdomen, chest, neck, head and face and their related internal organs; a few points have tonic functions or can be used in treating mental disorders.

REN 1, HUIYIN

The Crossing point of the Ren, Du and Chong meridians.

Location.   Between the anus and the root of the scrotum in males and between the anus and the posterior labial commissure in females (see Fig. 107).

Regional anatomy.   In the centre of the m. bulbospongiosus; m. transversus perineal superficialis and profundus; the branches of the perineal artery and vein; the branch of the perineal nerve.

Indications.   Dysuria, haemorrhoids, nocturnal emission, irregular menstruation, depressive-manic psychosis and coma.

Method.   Puncture perpendicularly 0.5–1 cun.

REN 2, QUGU

The Crossing point of the Ren and foot Jueyin meridians.

Location.   On the midpoint of the upper border of the symphysis pubis (see Fig. 108).

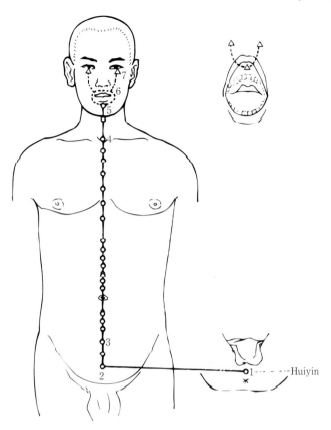

Fig. 107   The course of the Ren meridian.

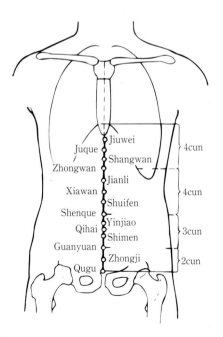

Fig. 108

Regional anatomy. With the m. pyramidalis on both sides; the branches of the inferior epigastric artery and the obturator artery; the branch of the iliohypogastric nerve.

Indications. Dysuria, nocturnal enuresis, nocturnal emission, impotence, irregular menstruation, and morbid leucorrhoea.

Method. Puncture perpendicularly 1–1.5 cun.

Note. Points of this meridian from Qugu (Ren 2) to Shangwan (Ren 13) can only be used with special caution for acupuncture or moxibustion treatment in pregnant women.

REN 3, ZHONGJI*

The Crossing point of the Ren and the 3 foot yin meridians, the Front-Mu point of the bladder.

Location. 4 cun below the umbilicus (see Fig. 108).

Regional anatomy. On the linea alba; the

branches of the superficial epigastric artery and vein, and the branches of the inferior epigastric artery and vein; the branch of the iliohypogastric nerve. (Underneath is the sigmoid colon.)

Indications. Nocturnal enuresis, dysuria, hernia, nocturnal emission, impotence, irregular menstruation, uterine bleeding and leucorrhoea, prolapse of the uterus and infertility.

Method. Puncture perpendicularly 1–1.5 cun.

REN 4, GUANYUAN

The Crossing point of the Ren and the 3 foot yin meridians, the Front-Mu point of the small intestine.

Location. 3 cun below the umbilicus (see Fig. 108).

Regional anatomy. See Zhongji (Ren 3) for vasculature; the medial cutaneous branches of the anterior ramus of the 12th intercostal nerve. (Underneath is the small intestine.)

Indications. Nocturnal enuresis, frequent urination, retention of urine, diarrhoea, abdominal pain, nocturnal emission, impotence, hernia, irregular menstruation, leucorrhoea, infertility, and emaciation due to consumption or other causes.

Method. Puncture perpendicularly 1–2 cun.

Note. This point has tonic functions; it is an important point for nurturing health.

REN 5, SHIMEN

The Front-Mu point of the Sanjiao.

Location. 2 cun below the umbilicus (see Fig. 108).

Regional anatomy. See Zhongji (Ren 3) for vasculature; the medial cutaneous branches of the anterior ramus of the 11th intercostal nerve. (Underneath is the small intestine.)

Indications. Abdominal pain, oedema, hernia, dysuria, diarrhoea, amenorrhoea, leucorrhoea and massive uterine bleeding.

Method. Puncture perpendicularly 1–2 cun.

REN 6, QIHAI*

Location. 1.5 cun below the umbilicus (see Fig. 108).

Regional anatomy. See Shimen (Ren 5).

Indications. Abdominal pain, diarrhoea, constipation, nocturnal enuresis, hernia, nocturnal emission, irregular menstruation, amenorrhoea and prostration or shock.

Method. Puncture perpendicularly 1–2 cun.

Note. This point has tonic functions and is an important point for nurturing health.

REN 7, YINJIAO

The Crossing point of the Ren and Chong meridians.

Location. 1 cun below the umbilicus (see Fig. 108).

Regional anatomy. See Zhongji (Ren 3) for vasculature; the medial cutaneous branches of the anterior ramus of the 10th intercostal nerve. (Underneath is the small intestine.)

Indications. Abdominal pain, oedema, hernia, irregular menstruation and leucorrhoea.

Method. Puncture perpendicularly 1–2 cun.

REN 8, SHENQUE*

Location. In the centre of the umbilicus (see Fig. 108).

Regional anatomy. The inferior epigastric artery and vein; the anterior cutaneous branch of the 10th intercostal nerve.

Indications. Abdominal pain, diarrhoea, prolapse of the rectum, oedema, prostration or shock.

Method. Generally needling is not applied in this point owing to the inconvenience of sterilization; moxibustion with moxa stick or cones, over a layer of salt, is applicable.

Note. The *Systematic Classic of Acupuncture and Moxibustion* states that needling is contraindicated.

REN 9, SHUIFEN

Location. 1 cun above the umbilicus (see Fig. 108).

Regional anatomy. The inferior epigastric artery and vein; the anterior cutaneous branch of the 8th and 9th intercostal nerves. (Underneath is the small intestine.)

Indications. Oedema, retention of urine, abdominal pain, diarrhoea, food regurgitation.

Method. Puncture perpendicularly 1–2 cun.

Note. The *Illustrated Manual on the Points for Acupuncture and Moxibustion on a Bronze Figure* states that moxibustion applied on this point is very effective for oedema while needling is contraindicated.

REN 10, XIAWAN*

The Crossing point of the Ren and foot Taiyin meridians.

Location. 2 cun above the umbilicus (see Fig. 108).

Regional anatomy. The inferior epigastric artery and vein; the anterior cutaneous branches of the 8th intercostal nerve. (Underneath is the transverse colon.)

Indications. Abdominal pain, abdominal distension, diarrhoea, vomiting, indigestion, abdominal masses.

Method. Puncture perpendicularly 1–2 cun.

REN 11, JIANLI

Location. 3 cun above the umbilicus (see Fig. 108).

Regional anatomy. See Xiawan (Ren 10).

Indications. Gastric pain, vomiting, anorexia, abdominal distension and oedema.

Method. Puncture perpendicularly 1–2 cun.

REN 12, ZHONGWAN

Front-Mu point of the stomach, Influential point of the fu organs, the Crossing point of the Ren, hand Taiyang and hand Shaoyang, and foot Yangming meridians.

Location. 4 cun above the umbilicus (see Fig. 108).

Regional anatomy. The superficial epigastric artery and vein; the anterior cutaneous branch of the 7th intercostal nerve. (Underneath is the pylorus.)

Indications. Gastric pain, vomiting, sour regurgitation, abdominal distension, diarrhoea, jaundice and depressive-manic psychosis.

Method. Puncture perpendicularly 1–1.5 cun.

REN 13, SHANGWAN

The Crossing point of the Ren, foot Yangming, hand Taiyang meridians.

Location. 5 cun above the umbilicus (see Fig.108).

Regional anatomy. See Zhongwan (Ren 12) for vasculature and innervation. (Underneath is the lower border of the liver and the pylorus.)

Indications. Gastric pain, vomiting, abdominal distension and epilepsy.

Method. Puncture perpendicularly 1–1.5 cun.

REN 14, JUQUE

Front-Mu point of the heart.

Location. 6 cun above the umbilicus (see Fig. 108).

Regional anatomy. See Shangwan (Ren 13).

Indications. Pain in the chest, palpitations, vomiting, sour regurgitation, and depressive-manic psychosis.

Method. Puncture downward obliquely 0.5–1 cun.

REN 15, JIUWEI

The *luo* point.

Location. Below the xiphoid process, 7 cun above the umbilicus (see Fig. 108).

Regional anatomy. The superior epigastric artery and vein; the anterior cutaneous branch of the 6th intercostal nerve.

Indications. Pain in the chest, abdominal distension, and depressive-manic psychosis.

Method. Puncture downward obliquely 0.4–0.6 cun.

REN 16, ZHONGTING

Location. At the midpoint of the junction of sternum and xiphoid (see Fig. 109).

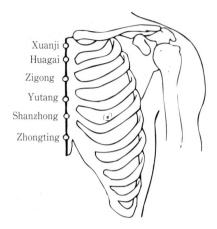

Xuanji
Huagai
Zigong
Yutang
Shanzhong
Zhongting

Fig. 109

Regional anatomy. The anterior perforating branches of the internal mammary artery and vein; the medial branch of the anterior cutaneous ramus of the 5th intercostal nerve.

Indications. Distension and fullness in the chest and hypochondrium, cardiac pain, vomiting, infantile milk regurgitation.

Method. Puncture transversely 0.3–0.5 cun.

REN 17, SHANZHONG* (ALSO PRONOUNCED AS TANZHONG)

Front-Mu point of the pericardium, Influential point of the qi.

Location. On the interior midline, at the level of the 4th intercostal space (see Fig. 109).

Regional anatomy. On the sternum; the anterior perforating branches of the internal mammary artery and vein; the medial branch of the anterior cutaneous ramus of the 4th intercostal nerve.

Indications. Cough, asthma, pain in the chest, palpitations, insufficient lactation, vomiting, and dysphagia.

Method. Puncture transversely 0.3–0.5 cun.

REN 18, YUTANG

Location. On the anterior midline, at the level of the 3rd intercostal space (see Fig. 109).

Regional anatomy. The anterior perforating branches of the internal mammary artery and vein; the medial branch of the anterior ramus of the 3rd intercostal nerve.

Indications. Cough, asthma, pain in the chest and vomiting.

Method. Puncture transversely 0.3–0.5 cun.

REN 19, ZIGONG

Location. On the anterior midline, at the level of the 2nd intercostal space (see Fig. 109).

Regional anatomy. The anterior perforating branches of the internal mammary artery and vein; the medial branch of the anterior cutaneous ramus of the 2nd intercostal nerve.

Indications. Cough, asthma, and pain in the chest.

Method. Puncture transversely 0.3–0.5 cun.

REN 20, HUAGAI

Location. On the anterior midline, at the midpoint of the sternal angle (see Fig. 109).

Regional anatomy. Between the sternal manubrium and the sternum; the anterior perforating branches of the internal mammary artery and vein; the medial branch of the anterior cutaneous ramus of the 1st intercostal nerve.

Indications. Cough, asthma, distension and pain in the chest and hypochondrium.

Method. Puncture transversely 0.3–0.5 cun.

REN 21, XUANJI

Location. On the anterior midline, in the middle of the sternal manubrium (see Fig. 109).

Regional anatomy. On the sternum; the anterior perforating branches of the internal mammary artery and vein; the anterior branch of the supraclavicular nerve and the anterior cutaneous branch of the 1st intercostal nerve.

Indications. Cough, asthma, pain in the chest, and congested and sore throat.

Method. Puncture transversely 0.3–0.5 cun.

REN 22, TIANTU*

The Crossing point of the Ren and Yinwei meridians.

Location. In the centre of the suprasternal fossa (see Fig. 110).

Regional anatomy. In the middle of the sternal notch; between the m. sternocleidomastoideus, deeply the m. sternohyoideus and m. sternothyroideus; subcutaneously the jugular arch, and the branch of the inferior thyroid artery, deeply the trachea, inferiorly the innominate vein and aortic arch at the posterior aspect of the sternum; the anterior branch of the supraclavicular nerve.

Indications. Cough, asthma, pain in the chest, sore throat, sudden hoarseness of voice, goitre, globus hystericus, and dysphagia.

Method. Puncture perpendicularly 0.2 cun first, then tip the needle downward and puncture along the posterior aspect of the sternum, 1–1.5 cun.

Note. Correct angle and depth of needling should be stressed so as not to injure the lung and related arteries and veins. According to reports, when needling Tiantu (Ren 22), Feishu (UB 13), Dashu (UB 19), Taiyuan (LI 9) and Zusanli (St 36), the resistance of the passage of the breath during either inhalation and exhalation (especially during the exhalation), obviously decreased. Also, when needling Tiantu (Ren 22), Shanzhong (Ren 17) and Hegu (Li 4), the movement of the oesophagus was strengthened, the oesophageal lumen was enlarged and a barium meal made faster downward progress. When needling Tiantu (Ren 22), Hegu (LI 4), Taiyang (K 1) and Lianquan (Ren 23) in patients

with hyperthyroidism, the symptoms disappeared, the enlarged gland reduced and the basal metabolism was markedly decreased.

REN 23, LIANQUAN*

The Crossing point of the Ren and Yinwei meridians.

Location. At the midpoint of the upper border of the hyoid bone (see Fig. 110)

Regional anatomy. Above the hyoid bone, between m. geniohyoideus on both sides; the anterior superficial jugular vein, the branch of the cutaneous cervical nerve, deeply the root of the tongue, the hypoglossal nerve and the branch of the glossopharyngeal nerve.

Indications. Swelling and pain of the subglossal region, salivation with glossoplegia, aphasia with stiffness of the tongue as seen in apoplexy, sudden hoarseness of voice and dysphagia.

Method. Puncture obliquely towards the root of the tongue 0.5–0.8 cun.

REN 24, CHENGJIANG*

The Crossing point of the Ren and foot Yangming meridians.

Location. In the centre of the mentolabial groove (see Fig. 110).

Regional anatomy. At the lower border of the m. orbicularis oris, between m. quadratus labii inferioris and m. mentalis; the branches of the inferior labial artery and vein; the branch of the facial nerve, i.e. the ramus of mandible and the mental ramus.

Indications. Deviation of the mouth, swelling and pain of gums, salivation, sudden hoarseness of voice and depressive-manic psychosis.

Method. Puncture obliquely 0.3–0.5 cun.

THE CHONG MERIDIAN

Course

The Chong meridian originates from the inside of the lower abdomen and emerges at the perineum (1); ascending, it goes inside the spinal

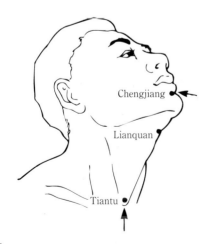

Fig. 110

Table 3.14 Indications of points on the Ren meridian

Point	Location	Indications primary	secondary
Lower abdomen: gynaecological diseases, diseases of external genitalia and intestinal diseases; (Guanyuan and Qihai have tonic functions)			
Huiyin (R 1)	perineum	dysuria, nocturnal emission, irregular menstruation	coma
Qugu (R 2)	lower abdomen	dysuria, nocturnal emission, impotence, leucorrhoea	
Zhongji (R 3)*	lower abdomen	nocturnal enuresis, dysuria, nocturnal emission, irregular menstruation	prolapse of uterus
Guanyuan (R 4)	lower abdomen	nocturnal enuresis, retention of urine, diarrhoea, impotence, irregular menstruation	consumption and impairment
Shimen (R 5)	lower abdomen	abdominal pain, oedema, diarrhoea, amenorrhoea	
Qihai (R 6)*	lower abdomen	abdominal pain, diarrhoea, nocturnal enuresis and uterine bleeding	prostration or shock
Yinjiao (R 7)	lower abdomen	abdominal pain, oedema and irregular menstruation	
Upper abdomen: mainly gastrointestinal diseases; also mental disorders			
Shenque (R 8)*	umbilicus	abdominal pain, diarrhoea	shock
Shuifen (R 9)	upper abdomen	retention of urine, oedema, diarrhoea	
Xiawan (R 10)*	upper abdomen	abdominal pain, diarrhoea, vomiting	
Jianli (R 11)	upper abdomen	gastric pain, vomiting, anorexia	oedema
Zhongwan (R 12)	upper abdomen	gastric pain, vomiting, abdominal distension, diarrhoea	mental disorders
Shangwan (R 13)	upper abdomen	gastric pain, vomiting	epilepsy
Juque (R 14)	upper abdomen	pain in the chest, palpitation, vomiting	mental disorders and epilepsy
Jiuwei (R 15)	upper abdomen	abdominal pain and abdominal distension	mental disorders and epilepsy
Chest: mainly diseases of heart, chest and lung; also disorders of oesophagus			
Zhongting (R 16)	chest	distension and fullness in the chest and hypochondrium, cardiac pain	
Shanzhong (R 17)*	chest	asthma, pain in the chest, palpitation, vomiting	insufficient lactation
Yutang (R 18)	chest	cough, asthma, pain in the chest	
Zigong (R 19)	chest	cough, asthma, pain in the chest	
Huagai (R 20)	chest	cough, asthma, pain in the chest	
Xuanji (R 21)	chest	cough, asthma, pain in the chest	
Neck: disorders of the tongue and throat			
Tiantu (R 22)*	neck	cough, asthma, sudden hoarseness of voice, congested and sore throat	dysphagia
Lianquan (R 23)*	neck	aphasia with stiffness of tongue, subglossal swelling and pain,	dysphagia
Lips: disorders of the mouth and tooth			
Chengjiang (R 24)*	chin	deviation of mouth, toothache	

column (2) where its superficial branch passes through the region of Qichong (St 30)(3) and communicates with the kidney meridian of the foot Shaoyin; running along both sides of the abdomen, it goes up to the throat (4) and curves around the lips (5) (see Fig. 112).

Chief pathological manifestations

Abdominal spasm and rebellion of qi.

Coalescent points

The coalescent points of the Chong meridian are: Huiyin (Ren 1), Yinjiao (Ren 7), Qichong (St 30), Henggu (K 11), Dahe (K 12), Qixue (K 13), Siman (K 14), Zhongshu (K 15), Huangshu (K 16), Shangqu (K 17), Shiguan (K 18), Yindu (K 19), Zutonggu (K 20) and Youmen (K 21).

THE DAI MERIDIAN

Course

The Dai meridian originates below the hypochondriacal region and goes obliquely downward through Daimai (GB 26), Wushu (GB 27) and Weidao (GB 28) (1); it goes transversely around the waist like a belt or girdle (2) (see Fig. 113).

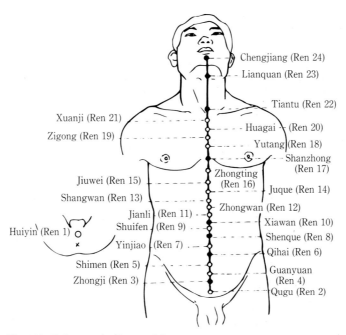

Fig. 111   Points on the Ren meridian.

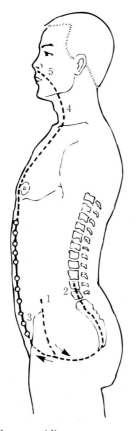

Fig. 112   The Chong meridian.

Chief pathological manifestations

Abdominal fullness, cold sensation in the waist as if soaked in cold water.

Coalescent points

The coalescent points of the Dai meridian are: Daimai (GB 26), Wushu (GB 27) and Weidao (GB 28).

THE YINWEI MERIDIAN

Course

The Yinwei meridian originates from the medial aspect of the shank (1), and goes up along the medial aspect of the thigh to the abdomen (2) to communicate with the spleen meridian of the foot Taiyin (3); then it goes along the chest (4) and communicates with the Ren meridian at the neck (5) (see Fig. 114).

Chief pathological manifestations

Cardiac pain and mental depression.

Coalescent points

The coalescent points of the Yinwei meridian

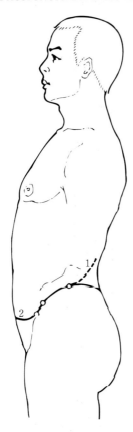

Fig. 113   The Dai meridian.

are: Zhubin (K 9), Fushe (Sp 13), Daheng (Sp 15),
Fuai (Sp 16), Qimen (Liv 14), Tiantu (Ren 22)
and Lianquan (Ren 23).

THE YANGWEI MERIDIAN

Course

The Yangwei meridian originates from the lateral aspect of the heel (1) and emerges from the
external malleolus (2); ascending along the gall-bladder meridian of the foot Shaoyang it passes
through the hip region (3); then it goes further
upward along the posterior aspect of the hypo-chondriacal and costal regions (4) and the poste-rior aspect of the axilla to the shoulder (5) and to
the forehead (6); then it turns backward to the
posterior aspect of the neck where it communi-cates with the Du meridian (7) (see Fig. 115).

Chief pathological manifestations

Chilliness and fever, and lumbar pain.

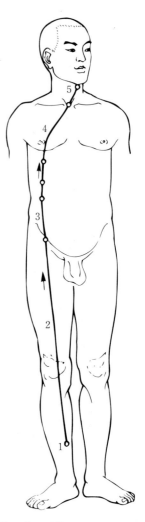

Fig. 114   The Yinwei meridian.

Coalescent points

The coalescent points of the Yangwei meridian
are: Jinmen (UB 63), Yangjiao (GB 35), Naoshu
(SI 10), Tianliao (SJ 15), Jianjing (GB 21), Touwei
(St 8), Benshen (GB 13), Yangbai (GB 14),
Toulinqi (GB 15), Muchuang (GB 16), Zhengying
(GB 17), Chengling (GB 18), Naokong (GB 19),
Fengchi (GB 20), Fengfu (Du 16) and Yamen
(Du 15).

THE YINQIAO MERIDIAN

Course

The Yinqiao meridian originates from the pos-terior aspect of the navicular bone (1); ascending

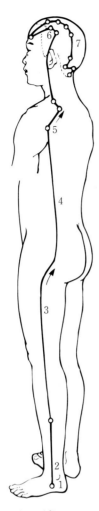

Fig. 115 The Yangwei meridian.

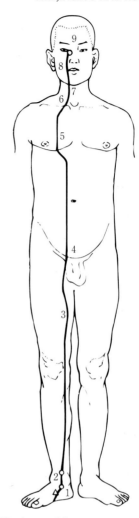

Fig. 116 The Yinqiao meridian.

to the upper portion of the medial malleolus (2), it goes straight upward along the posterior border of the medial aspect of the thigh (3) to the external genitalia (4); then it goes upward along the chest (5) to the supraclavicular fossa (6) and runs further upward and passes anteriorly by Renying (St 9) (7) and passes the zygoma (8); then it reaches the inner canthus and communicates with the foot Taiyang and the Yangqiao meridians (9) (see Fig. 116).

Chief pathological manifestations

Somnolence and retention of urine.

Coalescent points

The coalescent points of the Yinqiao meridian

are: Zhaohai (K 6), Jiaoxin (K 8) and Jingming (UB 1).

THE YANGQIAO MERIDIAN

Course

The Yangqiao meridian originates from the lateral aspect of the heel (1); it runs upward along the external malleolus and passes the posterior border of the fibula (2); then it goes onwards along the lateral side of the thigh and the posterior side of the hypochondrium to the shoulder; from there it passes up the neck to the corner of the mouth and enters the inner canthus to communicate with the Yinqiao meridian; running further upward along the bladder meridian of the foot Taiyang to the forehead, it meets the meridian of the foot Shaoyang at Fengchi (GB 20) (3) (see Fig. 117).

Chief pathological manifestations

Eye pain initiated from the inner canthus, and insomnia.

Coalescent points

The coalescent points of the Yangqiao meridian are: Shenmai (UB 62), Pucan (UB 61), Fuyang (UB 55), Femur-Juliao (GB 29), Naoshu (SI 10),

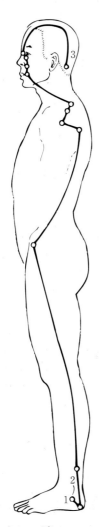

Fig. 117   The Yangqiao meridian.

Jianyu (LI 15), Jugu (LI 16), Tianliao (SJ 15), Dicang (St 4), Nose-Juliao (St 3), Chengqi (St 1), and Jingming (UB 1).

The fifteen collateral luo-connecting points

THE HAND TAIYIN—LIEQUE (LU 7)

For the luo (collateral) of the lung meridian of the hand Taiyin, the *luo* point is Lieque (Lu 7). It arises from the cleft of the tendons and bone on the radial side of the wrist and proximal to the wrist, follows the lung meridian of the hand Taiyin into the palm of the hand and spreads through the thenar eminence.

Its pathological manifestations are a feverish sensation at the wrist and palm in excess cases, and frequent yawning, incontinence of urine and frequent urination in deficiency cases. Then this point can be selected for treatment.

The point is 1.5 cun above the transverse crease of the wrist; from there a branch runs to the large intestine meridian of the hand Yangming.

THE HAND SHAOYIN—TONGLI (H 5)

The luo of the heart meridian of the hand Shaoyin has as its *luo* point Tongli (H 5), which is one cun above the transverse crease of the wrist. The luo branches out at Tongli (H 5) and ascends along the heart meridian of the hand Shaoyin and enters the heart, then goes to the root of the tongue and connects with the system of the eye.

Its pathological manifestations are a stuffiness and fullness in the chest, as seen in excess cases, and aphasia in deficiency cases. Then this point can be selected for treatment.

From this point a branch runs to the small intestine meridian of hand Taiyang.

THE HAND JUEYIN—NEIGUAN (P 6)

For the luo of the pericardium meridian of the

hand Jueyin, the *luo* point is Neiguan (P 6), which is 2 cun above the transverse crease on the palmar aspect of the wrist and between the two tendons. It disperses and runs to the Sanjiao meridian of the hand Shaoyang, runs along the pericardium meridian of the hand Jueyin upwardly to the pericardium, and finally connects with the system of the heart.

Its pathological manifestations are cardiac pain in excess cases, and stiffness of the neck in deficiency cases. Then this point can be selected for treatment.

THE HAND TAIYANG—ZHIZHENG (SI 7)

The luo of the small intestine meridian of the hand Taiyang has as its *luo* point Zhizheng (SI 7), which is 5 cun above the wrist. The luo runs inward to connect with the heart meridian of the hand Shaoyin, and its branch runs upward to the elbow to connect with Jianyu (LI 15).

Its pathological manifestations are a motor impairment of the elbow joint in excess cases, and skin warts and scabs on fingers in deficiency cases. Then this point can be selected for treatment.

THE HAND YANGMING—PIANLI (LI 6)

The luo of the large intestine meridian of the hand Yangming has as its *luo* point Pianli (LI 6), which is 3 cun above the wrist. The luo starts from Pianli (LI 6) and joins the lung meridian of the hand Taiyin. Its branch goes upward along the arm to Jianyu (LI 15), to the jaw and further spreads into the area of the teeth; still another branch ascends and enters the ear to join the chief meridians supplying this area.

Its pathological manifestations are dental caries and deafness in excess cases; cold, sore and aching teeth, and blockage in the interior of the body in deficiency cases. Then this point can be selected for treatment.

THE HAND SHAOYANG—WAIGUAN (SI 5)

The luo of the Sanjiao meridian of the hand

Shaoyang has as its *luo* point Waiguan (SJ 5), which is 2 cun above the dorsal transverse crease of the wrist. The luo travels laterally winding to the buttock, ascending up and flowing into the chest, then it runs to join the pericardium meridian of the hand Jueyin.

Its pathological manifestations are a spasm of the elbow in excess cases, and flaccidity of the elbow in deficiency cases. Then this point can be selected for treatment.

THE FOOT TAIYANG—FEIYANG (UB 58)

The luo of the bladder meridian of the foot Taiyang has as its *luo* point Feiyang (UB 56), which is 7 cun above the external malleolus. The luo runs to the kidney meridian of the foot Shaoyin.

Its pathological manifestations are a nasal obstruction or discharge, pain in the head and back, in excess cases; nasal discharge or bleeding in deficiency cases. Then this point can be selected for treatment.

THE FOOT SHAOYANG—GUANGMING (GB 37)

The luo of the gallbladder meridian of the foot Shaoyang has its *luo* point in Guangming (GB 37), which is 5 cun above the external malleolus. The luo runs to the liver meridian of the foot Jueyin, then goes downward to connect with the dorsum of the foot.

Its pathological manifestations are cold lower limbs in excess cases, and weakness and motor impairment of the lower limbs, with difficulty in standing up from a sitting position, in deficiency cases. Then this point can be selected for treatment.

THE FOOT YANGMING—FENGLONG (ST 40)

The luo of the stomach meridian of the foot Yangming has its *luo* point in Fenglong (St 40), which is 8 cun above the external malleolus. The luo runs to the spleen meridian of the foot

Taiyin; a branch runs along the lateral aspect of the tibia upward to the neck and head, and converges with the other meridians to run downward to connect with the throat.

Its pathological manifestations are an upward rebellion of the qi leading to Bi syndrome of the throat with sudden loss of voice. In excess, mental disorders occur; in deficiency cases, motor impairment of the lower limbs, and muscular atrophy in the leg. Then this point can be selected for treatment.

THE FOOT TAIYIN—GONGSUN (SP 4)

The luo of the spleen meridian of the foot Taiyin has its *luo* point in Gongsun (Sp 4), which is one cun posterior to the base of the 1st metatarsal bone. The luo runs to the stomach meridian of the foot Yangming. A branch runs upward to the abdomen and connects with the stomach and intestines.

The upward rebellion of its qi leads to morbid cholera, in excess cases with severe pain in the intestines, and in deficiency cases with abdominal distension and fullness. Then this point can be selected for treatment.

THE FOOT SHAOYIN—DAZHONG (K 4)

The luo of the kidney meridian of the foot Shaoyin has its *luo* point in Dazhong (K 4), which is posterior to the medial malleolus. The luo crosses the heel and joins the bladder meridian of the foot Taiyang; a branch follows the kidney meridian of the foot Shaoyin upward to a point below the pericardium, then goes laterally to pierce through the lumbar vertebrae.

Its pathological manifestations are dysuria in excess cases, lumbar pain in deficiency cases. Then this point can be used for treatment.

THE FOOT JUEYIN—LIGOU (LIV 5)

The luo of the liver meridian of the foot Jueyin has its *luo* point in Ligou (Liv 5), which is 5 cun above the medial malleolus. The luo runs to the

gallbladder meridian of the foot Shaoyang; a branch runs up the leg to the testis and terminates at the penis.

Its pathological manifestations are rebellion of its qi leading to swelling of the testes and hernia; in excess cases priapism, and in deficiency cases sudden pudendal pruritus. Then this point can be selected for treatment.

THE REN MERIDIAN—JIUWEI (REN 15)

The luo of the Ren meridian has its *luo* point in Jiuwei (Ren 15), which is below the xiphoid process. The luo runs and spreads over the abdomen.

Its pathological manifestations are a cutaneous pain of the abdomen in excess cases, and pruritus in deficiency cases. Then this point can be selected for treatment.

THE DU MERIDIAN—CHANGQIANG (DU 1)

The luo of the Du meridian has its *luo* point in Changqiang (Du 1). The luo runs upward along both sides of the spine to the nape, and spreads over the top of the head; then it goes to the scapular regions on both sides and connects with the bladder meridian to pierce through the spine.

Its pathological manifestations are a stiffness of the spine and back with motor impairment in excess cases; heaviness in the head and shaking of the upper part of the body in deficiency cases. For such disorders along the spine, this point can be selected.

THE MAJOR COLLATERAL OF THE SPLEEN—DABAO (SP 21)

The major luo of the spleen has its *luo* point in Dabao (Sp 21), which is 3 cun below Yuanye (GB 22). The luo runs and spreads through the chest and the hypochondriacal region.

Its pathological manifestations are a general aching in excess cases, and general flaccidity and weakness in the body and joints in deficiency cases. This collateral spreads over the whole body like a network—if haematomas are seen in the network, this point can be selected for treatment.

The extraordinary points

HEAD AND NECK

EXTRA 1, SISHENCONG

Location. 1 cun respectively posterior, anterior and lateral to Baihui (Du 20). Four points in all (see Fig. 118).

Regional anatomy. In the galea aponeurotica; the occipital artery and vein, the parietal branches of the superficial temporal artery and vein and the anastomotic network of the supraorbital artery and vein; the greater occipital nerve, the auriculotemporal nerve and the branch of the supraorbital nerve.

Indications. Headache, vertigo, insomnia, amnesia, and epilepsy.

Method. Puncture transversely 0.5–0.8 cun.

EXTRA 2, YINTANG

Location. Midway between the medial ends of the two eyebrows (see Fig. 119).

Regional anatomy. In the m. procerus; on both sides there are branches of the medial frontal artery and vein; the supratrochlear ramus of the trigeminal nerve.

Indications. Headache, vertigo, epistaxis, rhinorrhoea, infantile convulsions and insomnia.

Method. Puncture transversely 0.3–0.5 cun.

EXTRA 3, YUYAO

Location. At the midpoint of the eyebrow (see Fig. 119).

Regional anatomy. In the m. orbicularis oculi; the lateral branches of the frontal artery and vein; the branches of the supraorbital nerve and facial nerve.

Indications. Pain in the supraorbital region, twitching of eyelids, ptosis of eyelids, congested eye with swelling and pain, and nebula.

Method. Puncture transversely 0.3–0.5 cun.

EXTRA 4, SHANGMING

Location. At the midpoint of the superciliary arch, below the supraorbital margin (see Fig. 119).

Regional anatomy. In the m. orbicularis oculi; the frontal artery and vein, the supraorbital artery; the branches of the supraorbital nerve and the facial nerve.

Indications. Eye disease.

Method. Push the eyeball slightly downward, puncture perpendicularly and slowly 0.5–1.5 cun towards the orbital border; lifting and thrusting manipulation of the needle is not allowed.

EXTRA 5, TAIYANG

Location. In the depression about 1 cun posterior to the midpoint between the lateral end of the eyebrow and the outer canthus (see Fig. 120).

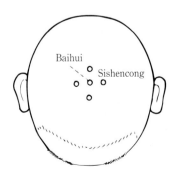

Fig. 118

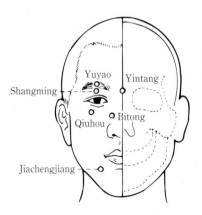

Fig. 119

Regional anatomy.   In the temporal fascia and m. temporalis; the superficial temporal artery and vein; the 2nd and 3rd branches of the trigeminal nerve, the temporal branch of the facial nerve.

Indications.   Headache, and eye diseases.

Method.   Puncture perpendicularly 0.3–0.5 cun, or prick to cause bleeding.

EXTRA 6, QIUHOU

Location.   At the junction of the lateral one-quarter and the medial three-quarters of the infraorbital margin (see Fig. 119).

Regional anatomy.   In the m. orbicularis oculi, deeply m. oculi; superficially the facial artery and vein; the zygomatic branch of the facial nerve and the infraorbital nerve; the optic nerve, deeply the ophthalmic nerve.

Indications.   Eye diseases.

Method.   Push the eyeball slightly upward, puncture perpendicularly and slowly 0.5–1.5 cun towards the orbital margin, without lifting and thrusting manipulation.

EXTRA 7, BITONG

Location.   At the upper end of the nasolabial groove (see Fig. 119).

Regional anatomy.   In the m. quadratus labii superioris; the branches of the facial artery and vein; the anterior ethmoidal nerve, the branch of the infraorbital nerve and the infratrochlear nerve.

Indications.   Rhinorrhoea, and nasal scabs.

Method.   Puncture transversely internally and upwardly 0.3–0.5 cun.

EXTRA 8, YUYE, JINJIN

Location.   On the veins on both sides of the frenulum of the tongue; Jinjin is on the left, while Yuye is on the right (see Fig. 121).

Regional anatomy.   The sublingual vein, hypoglossal nerve and lingual nerve.

Indications.   Oral ulcers, glossal swelling, vomiting, and diabetes.

Method.   Prick to cause bleeding.

EXTRA 9, JIACHENGJIANG

Location.   1 cun lateral to Chengjiang (Ren 24) (see Fig. 119).

Regional anatomy.   In the m. orbicularis oris; the branch of the facial artery; the 3rd branch of the trigeminal nerve (the mental nerve).

Indications.   Swelling and pain of the gums, and deviation of the mouth.

Method.   Puncture obliquely or transversely 0.5–1 cun.

EXTRA 10, QIANZHENG

Location.   0.5–1 cun anterior to the auricular lobe (see Fig. 120).

Regional anatomy.   In the m. masseter; subcutaneously the parotid gland; the branches of

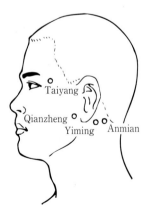

Fig. 120

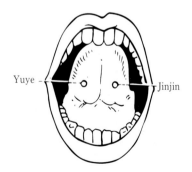

Fig. 121

the masseteric artery and vein; the branch of the facial nerve.

Indications. Deviation of the mouth, and oral and glossal ulcers.

Method. Puncture obliquely or transversely 0.5–1 cun.

EXTRA 11, YIMING

Location. 1 cun posterior to Yifeng (SJ 17) (see Fig. 120).

Regional anatomy. Above the m. sternocleidomastoideus; the posterior auricular artery and vein; the greater auricular nerve and the lesser occipital nerve.

Indications. Eye diseases, tinnitus, and insomnia.

Method. Puncture perpendicularly 0.5–1 cun.

EXTRA 12, ANMIAN

Location. Midway between Yifeng (SJ 17) and Fengchi (GB 20) (see Fig. 120).

Regional anatomy. In the m. sternocleidomastoideus and m. splenicus; the occipital artery and vein; the greater auricular nerve and lesser occipital nerve.

Indications. Insomnia, vertigo, headache, palpitations and depressive-manic psychosis.

Method. Puncture perpendicularly 0.8–1.2 cun.

THE TRUNK

EXTRA 13, JINGBI

Location. At the junction of the medial one-third and lateral two-thirds of the clavicle, 1 cun directly above (see Fig. 122).

Regional anatomy. The m. sternocleidomastoideus; the branches of the external carotid artery and vein; the brachial plexus.

Indications. Numbness of the arms and paralysis of the upper limbs.

Method. Puncture perpendicularly 0.5–0.8 cun.

EXTRA 14, SANJIAOJIU

Location. Take the length between the angles formed at either corner of the mouth as one side of an equilateral triangle. Lay the triangle so formed below the umbilicus with its top situated at the centre of the umbilicus; the point is located at the two other angles at either end of the lower side, on the same level (see Fig. 123).

Regional anatomy. In the m. rectus abdominis; the muscular branches of the inferior epigastric artery and vein; the 10th intercostal nerve.

Indications. Hernia and abdominal pain.

Method. 5–7 cones with moxibustion.

EXTRA 15, TITUO

Location. 4 cun lateral to Guanyuan (Ren 4) (see Fig. 123).

Regional anatomy. At the m. obliquus internus and externus abdominis and m. transversus abdominis; the superficial iliac circumflex artery and vein; the iliohypogastric nerve.

Indications. Prolapse of the uterus, hernia, abdominal pain.

Method. Puncture perpendicularly 0.8–1.2 cun.

EXTRA 16, ZIGONGXUE

Location. 3 cun lateral to Zhongji (Ren 3) (see Fig. 123).

Regional anatomy. At the m. obliquus internus

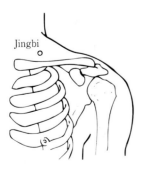

Fig. 122

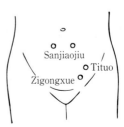

Fig. 123

and externus abdominis; the superficial epigastric artery and vein; the iliohypogastric nerve.

Indications.   Prolapse of the uterus, irregular menstruation and infertility.

Method.   Puncture perpendicularly 0.8–1.2 cun.

EXTRA 17, DINGCHUAN

Location.   0.5 cun lateral to Dazhui (Du 14) (see Fig. 124).

Regional anatomy.   The m. trapezius, m. rhomboideus, m. splenius capitis, m. longissimus; the branches of the transverse cervical artery and deep cervical artery; the posterior branch of the 8th cervical nerve.

Indications.   Asthma and cough.

Method.   Puncture perpendicularly 0.5–0.8 cun.

EXTRA 18, JIEHEXUE

Location.   3.5 cun lateral to Dazhui (Du 14) (see Fig. 124).

Regional anatomy.   The m. trapezius, m. splenius capitis, deeply the m. levator scapulae; the transverse cervical artery and vein; the medial cutaneous branch of the posterior rami of the 1st thoracic nerve, the dorsal nerve of scapula and the accessory nerve.

Indications.   Pulmonary tuberculosis and other tubercular diseases.

Method.   Puncture perpendicularly 0.5–0.8 cun.

EXTRA 19, JIAJI (ALSO KNOWN AS THE HUATUOJIAJI POINTS)

Location.   0.5 cun lateral to the lower border of the spinous process of the vertebrae from the first thoracic to the fifth lumbar (see Fig. 124).

Regional anatomy.   The intertransverse ligaments and muscles, which vary in three ways: superficially the m. trapezius, m. latissimus dorsi, m. rhomboideus; at a medium depth the m. serratus superior and inferior; deeply the m. brevis

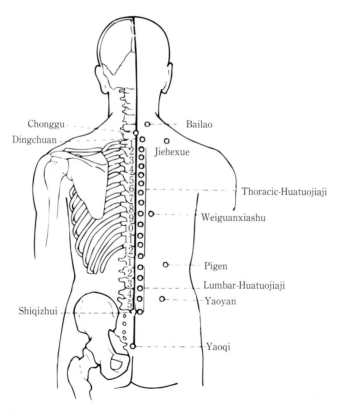

Chonggu
Dingchuan
Bailao
Jiehexue
Thoracic-Huatuojiaji
Weiguanxiashu
Pigen
Lumbar-Huatuojiaji
Yaoyan
Shiqizhui
Yaoqi

Fig. 124

between the m. sacrospinalis and transverse process; the posterior ramus of the spinal nerve derived from each vertebra and their arterial and venous plexuses.

Indications. See Table 3.15.

Method. Puncture obliquely 0.5–1 cun.

EXTRA 20, WEIGUANXIASHU (ALSO KNOWN AS BASHU, CUISHU)

Location. 1.5 cun lateral to the lower border of the 8th thoracic vertebra (see Fig. 124).

Regional anatomy. At the lower border of the m. trapezius, m. latissimus dorsi, m. longissimus; the medial branches of the posterior rami of the 8th intercostal artery and vein; the medial cutaneous branch of the posterior ramus of the 8th thoracic nerve; deeply the lateral branch of the posterior ramus of the 8th thoracic nerve.

Indications. Diabetes, and dryness of the throat.

Method. Puncture obliquely 0.5–0.8 cun.

EXTRA 21, PIGEN

Location. 3.5 cun lateral to the lower border of the spinous process of the 1st thoracic vertebra (see Fig. 124).

Regional anatomy. The m. latissimus, m. iliocostalis; the dorsal branch of the 1st lumbar artery and vein; the lateral branch of the posterior ramus of the 12th thoracic nerve, deeply the posterior branch of the 1st lumbar nerve.

Indications. Abdominal masses, and lumbar pain.

Method. Puncture perpendicularly 0.8–1.2 cun.

EXTRA 22, YAOYAN

Location. In the depression 3–4 cun lateral to the lower border of the spinous process of the 4th lumbar vertebra (see Fig. 124).

Regional anatomy. In the lumbodorsal fascia, m. latissimus, m. iliocostalis; the dorsal branches of the 4th lumbar artery and vein; the posterior branch of the 3rd lumbar nerve, deeply the lumbar plexus.

Indications. Lumbar pain, irregular menstruation, and leucorrhoea.

Method. Puncture perpendicularly 1–1.5 cun.

EXTRA 23, SHIQIZHUI

Location. Below the spinous process of the 5th lumbar vertebra (see Fig. 124).

Regional anatomy. In the lumbar dorsal fascia, supraspinal ligament and interspinal ligament; the posterior branch of the lumbar artery, interspinal cutaneous venous plexus; the medial branch of the posterior ramus of the lumbar nerve.

Indications. Lumbar pain, paralysis of the lower limbs, massive uterine bleeding and irregular menstruation.

Method. Puncture upwardly obliquely 1–1.5 cun.

THE FOUR LIMBS

EXTRA 24, SHIXUAN

Location. On the tips of the ten fingers, about 0.1 cun distal to the nails (see Fig. 125), ten points in all.

Regional anatomy. The network of arteries and veins formed by the proper palmar digital artery and vein; the proper palmar digital nerve and receptors of pain sensation.

Indications. Coma or loss of consciousness, epilepsy, high fever and congested and sore throat.

Table 3.15 Indications of the Huatuojiaji points

Huatuojiaji points		Indications
Thoracic	1 2 3	Diseases in the upper limbs
	4 5 6	Diseases in the chest region
	7 8 9 10 11 12	Diseases in the abdominal region
Lumbar	1 2 3 4 5	Diseases in the lower limbs

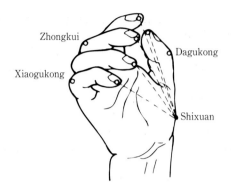

Fig. 125

Method. Puncture superficially 0.1–0.2 cun, or prick to cause bleeding.

EXTRA 25, SIFENG

Location. On the palmar surface, in the midpoint of the transverse crease of the proximal interphalangeal joints of the index, middle, ring and little fingers (see Fig. 126), four points on either hand.

Regional anatomy. The fibrous sheath, digital synovial sheaths, the tendon of the m. flexor digitalis profundus; deeply the cavity of the interphalangeal joints of the hand; the branches of the proper palmar digital artery and vein; the proper palmar digital nerves.

Indications. Infantile malnutrition, whooping cough.

Method. Prick to cause bleeding, or squeeze out a small amount of yellowish viscous fluid locally.

Note. According to reports, after needling Sifeng in children with malnutrition and indigestion accompanied by rickets, the calcium and phosphate level in the blood serum were increased, and the activity of the alkaline phosphatase decreased, which greatly facilitated their skeletal development and growth. Needling Sifeng in children with roundworm increases digestive enzyme activity.

EXTRA 26, ZHONGKUI

Location. On the midpoint of the proximal interphalangeal joint of the middle finger at the dorsal aspect (see Fig. 125).

Regional anatomy. The dorsal digital nerve and artery.

Indications. Vomiting, anorexia, and hiccup.

Method. 5–7 cones with moxibustion, or puncture superficially 0.2–0.3 cun.

EXTRA 27, BAXIE

Location. On the dorsum of the hand, at the junction of the red and white skin of the hand webs, eight points in all (see Fig. 127).

Regional anatomy. At the m. interossei; the dorsal venous network of the hand, dorsal metacarpal arteries; the dorsal branches of the ulnar and radial nerves.

Indications. Polydipsia, eye pain, and poisonous snake-bite with swelling and pain in the hand and arm.

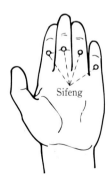

Fig. 126

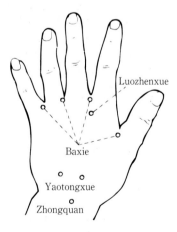

Fig. 127

Method. Puncture obliquely 0.5–0.8 cun, or prick to cause bleeding.

EXTRA 28, LUOZHENXUE

Location. On the dorsum of the hand, between the 2nd and 3rd metacarpal bones (see Fig. 127).

Regional anatomy. At the m. interossei dorsalis; the dorsal metacarpal arteries, dorsal venous network of the hand; the branches of the radial nerve.

Indications. Neck sprain, pain in the hand and arm, and gastric pain.

Method. Puncture perpendicularly or obliquely 0.5–0.8 cun.

EXTRA 29, YAOTONGXUE

Location. On the dorsum of the hand, on both sides of the m. extensor digitorum communis, 1 cun below the transverse crease of the wrist; 2 points on either hand (see Fig. 127).

Regional anatomy. The m. interossei lateral dorsalis; the dorsal venous network of the hand; the dorsal branches of the radial and ulnar nerves.

Indications. Acute lumbar sprain.

Method. Puncture obliquely from both sides towards the centre of the palm.

EXTRA 30, ZHONGQUAN

Location. In the depression between Yangxi (LI 5) and Yangchi (SJ 4) (see Fig. 127).

Regional anatomy. Between the m. extensor pollicis longus and extensor indicis; the dorsal carpal ligament; the dorsal carpal branch of the radial artery, the dorsal carpal venous network; the superficial branch of the radial nerve.

Indications. Stuffiness in the chest, gastric pain, and haematemesis.

Method. Puncture perpendicularly 0.3–0.5 cun.

EXTRA 31, ERBAI

Location. 4 cun above the transverse crease of the wrist, on both sides of the tendon of the m. flexor carpi radialis, two points on each hand (see Fig. 128).

Regional anatomy. The m. flexor digitorum superficialis; the radial artery and vein, interosseous artery and vein; medial cutaneous ramus of the antebrachial nerve, the lateral cutaneous branch of the antebrachial nerve, the median nerve and the radial nerve.

Indications. Haemorrhoids and prolapse of the rectum.

Method. Puncture perpendicularly 0.5–1 cun.

EXTRA 32, BIZHONG

Location. Midway between the transverse carpal crease and the transverse cubital crease, between the radius and ulna (see Fig. 128).

Regional anatomy. Between the m. palmaris longus, m. flexor carpi radialis, the m. flexor digitorum superficialis and profundus; the median antebrachial artery and vein; the medial antebrachial cutaneous nerve, the antebrachial interossei palmar nerve.

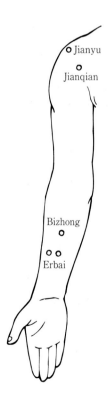

Jianyu

Jianqian

Bizhong

Erbai

Fig. 128

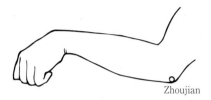

Zhoujian

Fig. 129

Indications. Paralysis and spasm of the upper limbs, neuralgia of the forearm, and hysteria.

Method. Puncture perpendicularly 1–1.5 cun.

EXTRA 33, ZHOUJIAN

Location. On the tip of the ulnar olecranon, when the elbow is flexed (see Fig. 129).

Regional anatomy. The superficial fascia, the cubital articular arterial network; the posterior ramus of the antebrachial cutaneous nerve.

Indications. Scrofula.

Method. 5–7 moxa cones with moxibustion.

EXTRA 34, JIANQIAN (ALSO KNOWN AS JIANNEILING)

Location. Midpoint of the line joining the upper end of the anterior axillary fold and Jianyu (LI 15) (see Fig. 128). It can also be located 1 cun above the upper end of the anterior axillary fold, according to another way of locating this point.

Regional anatomy. In the m. deltoideus; the thoracoacromial artery and vein; the posterior branch of the supraclavicular nerve.

Indications. Pain in the shoulder and arm, and motor impairment of the arm.

Method. Puncture perpendicularly 1–1.5 cun.

EXTRA 35, HUANZHONG

Location. At the midpoint of the line joining Huantiao (GB 30) and Yaoshu (Du 2) (see Fig. 130).

Regional anatomy. In the m. gluteus maximus; the inferior gluteal artery and vein; the inferior clunial nerves, deeply the inferior gluteal nerve and sciatic nerve.

Indications. Sciatica, lumbar and leg pain.

Method. Puncture perpendicularly 2–3 cun.

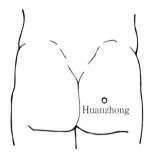

Huanzhong

Fig. 130

EXTRA 36, SIQIANG

Location. 4.5 cun directly above the midpoint of the upper border of the patella (see Fig. 131).

Regional anatomy. The m. rectus femoris, m. vastus intermedius; the muscular branches of the femoral artery; superficially the anterior cutaneous branch of the femoral nerve and deeply the femoral nerve.

Indications. Motor impairment and paralysis of the lower limbs.

Method. Puncture perpendicularly 1.5–2 cun.

EXTRA 37, BAICHONGWO

Location. 1 cun above Xuehai (Sp 10) (see Fig. 131).

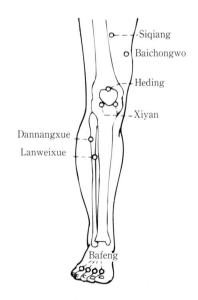

Siqiang
Baichongwo
Heding
Xiyan
Dannangxue
Lanweixue
Bafeng

Fig. 131

Regional anatomy. In the m. vastus medialis; the femoral artery and vein; the anterior cutaneous branch of the femoral nerve, deeply the muscular branch of the femoral nerve.

Indications. Rashes, skin eruptions and pruritus due to *feng* and damp, and boils and ulcers in the lower part of the body.

Method. Puncture perpendicularly 1.5–2 cun.

EXTRA 38, HEDING

Location. In the depression at the midpoint of the upper border of the patella (see Fig. 131).

Regional anatomy. At the upper border of the patella; the tendon of the m. quadriceps femoris; the arterial network of the knee joint; the anterior cutaneous branch and the muscular branch of the femoral nerve.

Indications. Lumbar pain, weakness of the leg, and paralysis.

Method. Puncture perpendicularly 1–1.5 cun.

EXTRA 39, XIYAN

Location. A pair of points, located in the depressions medial and lateral to the patellar ligament (see Fig. 131).

Regional anatomy. Medial and lateral to the patellar ligament; the arterial and venous network of the knee joint; the branch of the saphenous nerve, the femoral lateral cutaneous nerve, and branch of the common tibiofibular nerve.

Indications. Knee-joint pain, heaviness and pain in the leg and feet, and beriberi.

Method. Puncture obliquely 0.5–1 cun towards the centre of the knee, or puncture transversely through Xiyan on one side towards that on the opposite side.

EXTRA 40, DANNANGXUE

Location. 1–2 cun below Yanglingquan (GB 34) (see Fig. 131).

Regional anatomy. The m. peroneus longus and m. flexor digitorum longus; the branches of the anterior tibial artery and vein; the lateral gastrocnemius cutaneous nerve, the deep peroneal nerve.

Indications. Acute and chronic cholecystitis, cholelithiasis, biliary ascariasis, and motor impairment of the lower limbs.

Method. Puncture perpendicularly 1–2 cun.

EXTRA 41, LANWEIXUE

Location. About 2 cun below Zusanli (St 36) (see Fig. 131).

Regional anatomy. In the m. tibialis anterior and m. flexor digitorum longus; the anterior artery and vein of the tibia; the lateral gastrocnemius cutaneous nerve and deep peroneal nerve.

Indications. Acute and chronic appendicitis, indigestion and paralysis of the lower limbs.

Method. Puncture perpendicularly 1.5–2 cun.

Note. According to reports, during operations on patients with acute appendicitis or an acute attack of chronic appendicitis, strong stimulation was applied by needling Lanweixue on both sides for 0.5–3 minutes. Increased movement of the appendix was observed in most cases and even a whirling movement in a few cases. 1–2 minutes after needling, evacuation of the appendix was observed under an X-ray barium meal test, while congestion of different degrees was observed in all cases.

EXTRA 42, BAFENG

Location. On the dorsum of the foot, in the depressions on the webs between toes, proximal to the web margin, eight points in all (see Fig. 131).

Regional anatomy. In the m. metatarsal interossei at the small head of the phalanx; the dorsal digital arteries and veins; the superficial and deep nerves.

Indications. Beriberi, pain of the toes, poisonous snakebites, and swelling and pain of the dorsum of the foot.

Method. Puncture obliquely 0.5–0.8 cun, or prick to cause bleeding.

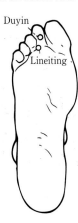

Fig. 132

EXTRA 43, DUYIN

Location.   On the sole, at the midpoint of the transverse crease of the 2nd distal interphalangeal joint (see Fig. 132).

Regional anatomy.   The tendon of the m. flexor digitorum brevis; the medial plantar artery and vein; the medial plantar nerve and the proper plantar digital nerve.

Indications.   Hernia and irregular menstruation.

Method. 3–5 moxa cones applied in moxibustion.

EXTRA 44, LINEITING

Location.   On the sole, between the 2nd and 3rd toes, on the site just opposite to Neiting (St 44) (see Fig. 132).

Regional anatomy.   The plantar aponeurosis; the medial plantar nerve and the branch of the lateral plantar artery.

Indications.   Pain of the toes, infantile convulsions, epilepsy and acute gastric pain.

Method.   Puncture perpendicularly 0.3–0.5 cun.

TECHNIQUES OF ACUPUNCTURE AND MOXIBUSTION

PART
2

The techniques of needling and the techniques of moxibustion are two therapeutic methods which are unalike. Needling, or acupuncture, is a therapy which treats disease by stimulating acupoints on the human body with metal needles, via certain manipulative techniques, while moxibustion treats and prevents disease by applying heat to the skin with ignited moxa wool, mainly made from the leaves of the plant *Artemisia vulgaris*.

However, these two, although differing in the materials and instruments used, and in their manipulative techniques, fall into the same category of *wai zhi* (外治) or "external treatment" which is applied by stimulating acupoints, and consequently the jingluo and zangfu organs, in order to regulate yin and yang, to *fu zheng* (扶正) or "strengthen the antipathogenic qi", *qu xie* (祛邪) or "eliminate the pathogenic qi", remove obstruction from the jingluo, and activate the circulation of qi and blood. This is all with the same aim of preventing and treating disease.

Acupuncture and moxibustion are often applied in combination, within clinical practice, and so often termed together *zhen jiu* or "acupuncture and moxibustion" (针灸).

In the therapy of acupuncture, the needle is the main instrument, and in ancient times reference was made in the *Miraculous Pivot* to the "nine needles" of differing shapes, names and therapeutic purposes (see Fig. 133).[1] Needles used in modern times are developed on the basis of the Nine Needles of ancient times, although made of different materials such as gold, silver, stainless steel, and other alloys. The technology used in making the needles and their shapes also differ from those of the *Miraculous Pivot*.

Clinically the most commonly used needles are the "filiform needle", the "three-edged needle", the "cutaneous needle" and the "intradermal needle". They are all applied with differing methods of manipulation.

The Nine Needles of ancient times were the following, according to Chapter 1 ("On 9 Needles and 12 Yuan-source Points", see Appendix 1) in the *Miraculous Pivot*:

The arrow-head needle. 1.6 inches long, with a round head and sharp tip, often used in superficial puncture of the skin or bloodletting in heat syndromes of the head and body.

The round needle. 1.6 inches long, with an oval rounded tip and a cylindrically

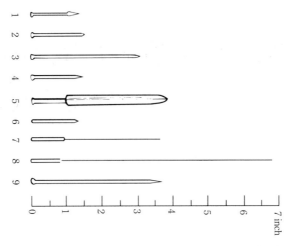

Fig. 133   The nine needles of ancient times: 1 Arrow-head
needle, 2 Round needle, 3 Blunt needle, 4 Sharp-edged
needle, 5 Sword-shaped needle, 6 Round-sharp needle,
7 Filiform needle, 8 Long needle, 9 Large needle.

shaped body, used in massage treatment for qi stagnation in the muscles (without
injuring the muscles during treatment).

The blunt needle.   3.5 inches long, with a round yet slightly sharp tip, the shape of
a millet grain, used in pressing on the jingluo (pressing only, not puncturing).

The sharp-edged needle.   1.6 inches long, with a cylindrically shaped body and a
sharp pyramidal or triangular tip, used for bloodletting in treating carbuncles and
febrile diseases.

The sword-shaped needle.   4 inches long and 0.25 inches wide, shaped like a sword,
used for cutting in external diseases, for instance draining abscesses.

The round-sharp needle.   1.6 inches long, with a slightly larger head but thin body,
used in deep needling for carbuncles and in Bi syndrome.

The filiform needle.   3.6 inches long, as thin as the hair, used in cold, heat or painful conditions, or Bi syndrome.

The long needle.   7 inches long, used in deep needling when treating disorders of
the deep tissues and persistent Bi syndrome.

The large needle.   4 inches long with a thick and round body, used in joint disorders with retention of fluid, and later used for hot needling when treating scrofula
and mastitis.

In the following chapters, the most commonly used therapeutic methods of acupuncture and moxibustion are introduced: filiform needling, moxibustion (and
cupping), other methods of needling (including three-edged needling, cutaneous
needling, intradermal needling, electroneedling, and point injection), scalp acupuncture, ear acupuncture and acupuncture anaesthesia.

Techniques of filiform needling 4

THE STRUCTURE, SPECIFICATION, STORAGE AND REPAIR OF THE FILIFORM NEEDLE

STRUCTURE AND SPECIFICATION

The filiform needle is the main and the most widely used instrument in the treatment of disease in the acupuncture clinic, and almost all the points indicated for acupuncture can be punctured by the filiform needle.

The filiform needle most commonly used in clinics nowadays, although it has its origin in the needles used in ancient times, differs very much from them, both in terms of the material used, gauge or length of the needle body, and the technology used in manufacture. Nowadays most needles are made of stainless steel, whilst others are made from gold, silver, or alloys, etc.

A filiform needle consists of five parts: the handle, tail, tip, body and root.

Handle. The place for holding the needle during manipulation. It is wound around in a filigree, either of copper or aluminium.

Tail. The part at the end of the handle. It is the place for putting moxa-wool in warm needling.

Tip. The sharp point of the needle, also known as the awn. Pointed like a pine needle, it leads the needle into the acupoint when puncturing.

Body. The part between the handle and the tip, which should be smooth, straight and flexible.

Root. The demarcation line between the body and the handle.

"Length" and "gauge" refer to the dimensions of the needle body. The length and gauge of the more commonly used filiform needles are listed below:

The filiform needles listed in the tables vary in length and gauge, yet needles 28 to 31 gauge in diameter, and 1.5 to 3.5 inches in length are commonly in use in the clinic.

Table 4.1 Lenghts of filiform needles

cun	0.5	1.0	1.5	2.0	2.5	3.0	3.5	4.0	4.5
mm	15	25	40	50	65	75	90	100	115

STORAGE AND REPAIR

Storage refers particularly to preventing the tip from being damaged and the body from being bent, rusting or staining. Therefore needles should be well kept in a box or tube.

Line the box with several layers of sterilized gauze. The sterilized needles are fixed in the gauze according to their length and again covered by sterilized gauze, then the box is closed and the needles are ready for use.

If a tube is used, dry cotton balls are placed at both ends to protect the needle-tip. The needles in the tube are sterilized in an autoclave and then are ready for use.

Being therapeutic instruments, needles must be carefully examined before use. A bent body, or dull or bent needle-tip may make it difficult to insert into the patient. As a result the curative effect is hampered. Thus examination and needle repair are at all times an absolute necessity. The following are the basic methods.

During examination, attention should be paid to whether the body of the needle is at all rusty, and slightly or acutely bent. An obtusely bent needle can be straightened by clamping the body with the fingers or pieces of bamboo. A rusty needle with an abrupt bend is often thrown away so as to avoid the breaking of the needle in the patient. Examination also includes examining the connection between handle and body. Badly connected or loosely connected needles are not fit for use.

Also check the tip, to see if it is hooked, blunted, or deviated. If bent, blunted or deviated, the tip can be corrected with fine sand paper or a fine grind stone. The best needle is like a pine needle, straight and smooth. A too

Tip   Body   Root   Handle   Tail

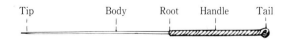

Fig. 134 The structure of the filiform needle.

Table 4.2 Gauges of filiform needles

No.	26	27	28	29	30	31	32	33
Diameter (mm)	0.45	0.42	0.38	0.34	0.32	0.30	0.28	0.26

sharp tip is easily bent, while if it is too blunt it may cause pain on insertion.

NEEDLING PRACTICE

Needling practice refers to practising the finger force and manipulation technique necessary during needling. As the filiform needle is fine and flexible, it is very difficult to insert easily with a minimum of pain, without strength in the fingers, neither can all the varying kinds of manipulation be conducted freely. Thus the results are not as desired. Therefore practice in needling is the basic training for beginners.

PRACTISING WITH SHEETS OF PAPER

Fold some soft tissue paper into a small packet about 8 cm in length, 5 cm in breadth and 2–3 cm in thickness, surround it with gauze and then bind it with thread into the shape of the Chinese character "#". Hold the packet in the left hand, and the handle of the needle about 1 inch along with the right thumb, index and middle fingers, using the fingers as if holding a Chinese brush or pen.

Place the needle-tip on the packet, then rotate the handle with the right thumb, index and middle fingers clockwise and counter-clockwise with gradual pressure. Repeat the same practice, at another place, again and again. This is useful mainly for strengthening the finger force and gaining skill in manipulating and rotating the needle (see Fig. 135).

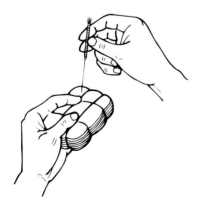

Fig. 135 Practising needling on sheets of paper.

PRACTISING WITH A COTTON CUSHION

Wrap some cotton into a cushion about 6–7 cm in diameter, surround it with gauze and bind the opening with thread. The method is the same as that with sheets of paper, the only difference being that a soft cotton cushion is suitable for practising many manipulative techniques, such as lifting, thrusting, rotating, etc. (see Fig. 136).

In practice, one must try to rotate the needle at a moderate speed and control the angle of rotation; at the same time, practise lifting and thrusting the needle until you can manipulate it freely.

Generally speaking, lifting and thrusting the needle should be performed to an equal extent, rotation of the needle should be to the same amplitude, and all must be done at a moderate speed.

But there is a great difference between practising with a paper packet or cotton cushion, and needling the human body. In order to experience the differing sensations of the manipulations, it is best to practise puncturing points on your own body. Only in this way can you gain experience and, at the same time, improve your needling technique.

PREPARATIONS PRIOR TO TREATMENT

CHOICE OF NEEDLE

Nowadays the most commonly used needles are made of stainless steel, for not only is it rust-proof and heatproof, but also very hard, flexible and tough. Needles made of gold and silver are seldom used in clinic because of their poor flexibility and expense.

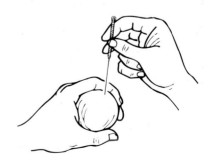

Fig. 136 Practising needling on a cotton cushion.

Needles should be carefully inspected according to the above-mentioned requirements in order to avoid inflicting unnecessary pain on the patient. As well as this, needles of differing lengths and gauges are chosen on the basis of the patient's sex, age, build, constitution, the condition of antipathogenic factors and pathogenic factors, the situation of the affected area and the location of the point.

It is said in the *Miraculous Pivot*[2] that the nine kinds of needles are shaped differently according to their various functions. For example, a relatively thick and long needle is suitable for a man who has a strong constitution, and is well built, with a deep-seated illness; but in a woman who is thin and weak, with a superficially located illness, puncture should be made with a relatively short and thin needle.

As for the location of the acupoint, usually a short, small-gauged needle is chosen for a point on an area where the skin and muscles are thin and which is punctured superficially; while a long and thick needle is chosen for a point located where there is thick muscle and which has to be punctured deeply.

The proper choice of needle in the clinic is to select a needle which is a little longer than the required length—namely, when the needle is inserted to a given depth, some of the needle body should be left exposed above the skin. For example, if the required depth of the point is 0.5 cun, a needle of 1 cun should be selected; if the depth is 1 cun, then a needle of 1.5 cun is the choice.

CHOICE OF POSTURE

An appropriate posture for the patient is significant for the correct location of points, the manipulation or prolonged retention of the needle, and also in preventing fainting, stuck needles, bent needles or even broken needles.

A patient who is nervous or severely ill may find a sitting position tiring, which could lead to fainting. Similarly, in an uncomfortable posture during treatment, the patient may move his body, giving rise to a bent or stuck needle or even breaking it. Thus the selection of a proper posture, according to the location of the points used, is of great importance. Not only can it help to locate the point correctly, but also help in the manipulation of the needle or its prolonged retention.

The more commonly used postures adopted in the clinic are the supine, lateral recumbent, prone, sitting-reclining, sitting in flexion and sitting in flexion with the head resting on the arm:

Supine posture. Suitable for points on the head, face, chest and abdominal regions and some points on the four limbs (see Fig. 137).

Lateral recumbent. Suitable for points on the lateral side of the body, namely points of Shaoyang meridians and some points on the four limbs (see Fig. 138).

Prone posture. Suitable for points on the head, neck, back, lumbar region and buttocks, the posterior regions of the lower limbs and some points on the upper limbs (see Fig. 139).

Sitting-reclining posture. Suitable for points on the front of the head, face and neck (see Fig. 140).

Sitting in flexion. Suitable for points on the back, head and nape (see Fig. 141).

Sitting in flexion with the lateral side of the head resting on one arm. Suitable for points on one side of the head and face and areas around the ear (see Fig. 142).

In addition to the above postures, others may be adopted according to the situation of the point; but it is better to select a posture which is suitable for all prescribed points instead of adopting two or more. If two or more postures have to be adopted for therapeutic purposes, or because of the locations of the points, then the patient's constitution and the condition of the illness should be taken into consideration.

The lying position is usually to be preferred, especially for those patients who have never been treated by acupuncture before, or who are nervous, severely ill, elderly, etc.

STERILIZATION

Before the needles are inserted into the points, sterilization must be applied. This includes the

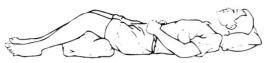

Fig. 137 Supine.

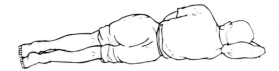

Fig. 138 Lateral recumbent.

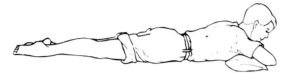

Fig. 139 Prone.

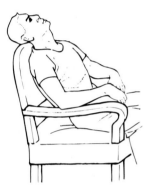

Fig. 140 Sitting-reclining.

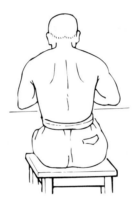

Fig. 141 Sitting in flexion.

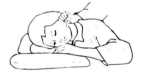

Fig. 142 Sitting in flexion with the lateral side of the head resting on one arm.

sterilization of the needles, the area around the points and the practitioner's fingers.

The following are the methods of sterilization which may be selected according to differing conditions:

Needle sterilization

Wrapped in gauze, the needles and other instruments should be sterilized in an autoclave at 1.5 times atmospheric pressure and 120 °C, for 15 minutes, if at all possible. Otherwise the needles may be boiled in water for 15–30 minutes.

Besides this, alcohol can be used for sterilization. Soak the needles in 75% alcohol for 30 minutes. Then take them out and wipe off the liquid from the needles. At the same time, soak the other instruments, such as the forceps, in a fluid of 2% lysol or 1:1000 mercuric chloride for one or two hours.

The needles used in treating infectious diseases should be put in another place and strictly sterilized before reuse. In this case the rule should be a separate needle for each point.

Sterilization of the area around the point and the practitioner's fingers

The area on the body surface selected for needling may be sterilized by rubbing the skin in a circular manner from the centre of the point to the outside, with a cotton ball of 75% alcohol (at first with 2.5% iodine, and then removed with a 75% alcohol cotton ball). Then the area should be kept clean.

Before inserting the needles the practitioner should wash his hands with soap and rub his hands with 75% alcohol. During the manipulation, the practitioner should try to avoid touching the needle body. If it is necessary, a dry cotton ball should be used to separate the needle from the finger.

NEEDLING METHODS

INSERTION

The needle should be inserted in a coordinated manner with the help of both hands.

In the *Classic on Medical Problems*, it says, "an experienced acupuncturist believes in the important function of the left hand, while one inexperienced believes in the important function of the right hand".[3] It further states in the *Guide to Acupuncture and Moxibustion*, "press heavily with the left hand to disperse the qi, insert the needle gently and slowly with the right hand to avoid pain".[4] Generally the needle should be held with the thumb, index and middle finger of the right hand, as if holding a Chinese brush (see Fig. 143)—this hand is known as the "puncturing hand". The left hand is known as the "pressing hand", it presses firmly on the area close to the point with the finger-nail and helps to support the needle body.

The function of the puncturing hand is to control and manipulate the needle. On insertion, it conducts finger force to the needle-tip to enter it into the skin, and on manipulation it may either rotate, lift, thrust, flick, vibrate, scrape, twist or withdraw the needle.

The function of the pressing hand is to fix the point and hold the needle body during insertion. In this way, the needle can be kept straight and the finger force reach the needle-tip, causing less pain and helping to regulate and control the needle-sensation.

The following are some methods of insertion.

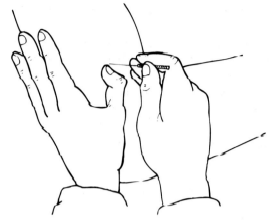

Fig. 144   Inserting the needle aided by pressure from the finger of the pressing hand.

Inserting the needle aided by pressing with the finger-nail of the pressing hand

Press the skin beside the acupoint with the nail of the thumb and index finger of the left hand. Hold the needle with the right hand and keep the needle-tip close against the nail, then insert the needle into the point (see Fig. 144).

This method is suitable for insertion with short needles.

Inserting the needle with the help of the puncturing and pressing hands

Hold and expose slightly the needle-tip with a dry sterilized cotton ball in the thumb and the index finger of the left hand, then insert the needle into the point with the right hand (see Fig. 145).

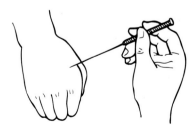

Fig. 143   Holding the needle.

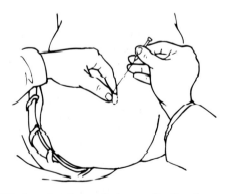

Fig. 145   Inserting the needle by coordinating the puncturing and pressing hands.

This method is suitable for insertion of long needles.

Clinically, there is also the method of inserting the needle with only one hand, i.e. holding the needle-tip with a dry sterilized cotton ball with the thumb and the index finger of the right hand, leaving 0.7–1 cm of its tip exposed. Then insert the needle swiftly into the skin. The pressing hand may also be made use of, according to circumstances.

Inserting the needle with the fingers stretching the skin

Stretch the skin where the point is located, with the thumb and index finger of the left hand, and insert the needle into the space between the two fingers (see Fig. 146).

This method is suitable for inserting the needle into points on areas where the skin is loose.

Inserting the needle by pinching up the skin

Pinch the skin up around the point with the thumb and index finger of the left hand and insert the needle into the upper portion of the skin (see Fig. 147).

This method is suitable for inserting the needle into points on areas where the muscle and skin are thin, such as Yintang (Extra 2).

In order to make the insertion easy and cause no pain, these methods can be adapted according to need, for instance by varying them according to anatomical characteristics, the depth of the point and manipulation needed of the needle.

Additionally, the needle may be inserted with the help of a needling tube, which is made of glass or metal, and 0.7–1 cm shorter than the needle, so as to expose the needle handle. The gauge of the tube is determined on the basis that it must be broad enough to let the needle tail pass through.

Firstly put the needle into the tube, keeping the tip at the same level as the lower end of the tube. Then, holding the tube with the left hand, position the tip directly on the selected point and tap the needle tail with the index finger of the right hand, or flick it with the middle finger, and the needle is inserted into the skin. After removal of the tube, manipulate the needle.

ANGLE AND DEPTH OF INSERTION

In the process of insertion, the angle and depth are of especial importance.

A correct angle and depth of insertion helps to induce the needling sensation, brings about the desired therapeutic results and guarantees the safety of the needling. However, the correct location of the point on the body surface does not necessarily imply the correct insertion of the needle into the point; so, clinically, a differing angle, direction or depth of insertion at the same point may produce varying needling sensations—inducing the meridional qi in differing directions with differing therapeutic effects.

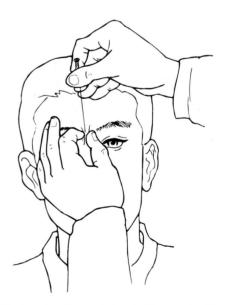

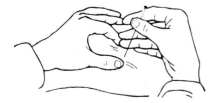

Fig. 146   Inserting the needle by stretching the skin.

Fig. 147   Inserting the needle by pinching up the skin.

Therefore the angle, direction and depth of insertion should be decided according to the location of the point, the patient's condition, the therapeutic requirements and the methods of manipulation chosen for the needle.

The angle formed by the needle and the skin-surface

The angle is decided both by the location of the point and by the therapeutic purpose of needling.

Generally there are three types of angle (see Fig 148):

— perpendicular,
— oblique,
— horizontal.

Perpendicular. The needle is inserted perpendicularly, forming a 90-degree angle with the skin-surface. Most points on the body can be inserted in this way.

Oblique. The needle is inserted obliquely to form an angle of approximately 45 degrees with the skin-surface. This is suitable when inserting the needle into points close to important viscera or where the muscle is thinner, and the points cannot be punctured perpendicularly or deeply.

Horizontal. This is also known as transverse insertion. The needle is inserted horizontally at an angle of 15 degrees with the skin-surface. This method is used to insert the needle into points in areas where the skin and muscle are thin, such as on the head.

Depth of insertion

The depth of insertion at each point has been discussed earlier in the detailed description of each acupoint (Ch. 3). Only a brief summary of the principles deciding the depth of insertion is given here. The following conditions may be borne in mind:

— constitution,
— age,
— condition of the disease,
— location of the points.

Constitution. For thin and weak patients, superficial insertion is advisable; for those who are fleshy and strong, deep insertion is adopted.

Age. For the elderly whose constitution is weak or delicate, or in the case of infants, superficial insertion is applicable; for the young and middle-aged, and those with a strong constitution, deep insertion is advisable.

Condition of the disease. For yang syndromes and recent illnesses, superficial insertion is applied; for yin syndromes and in chronic cases, deep insertion is used.

Location of the points. For points on the head, face, chest, back and areas where the skin and muscles are thin, superficial insertion is employed; for points on the four limbs, buttocks, abdomen, and areas where the skin and muscle are abundant, deep insertion is advisable.

The angle of insertion has a close relationship with the depth of insertion. Generally, deep insertion is usually performed by inserting the needle perpendicularly, superficial insertion by inserting obliquely or horizontally. However special attention should be paid to the angle and depth of such points as Tiantu (Ren 22), Yamen

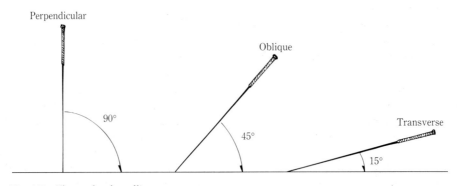

Fig. 148   The angle of needling.

(Du 15), Fengfu (Du 16), etc., and those near the eyes, and viscera such as the liver, lungs, etc.

At the same time, changes in angle and depth of the insertion should be made according to the variation of the seasons.

NEEDLE MANIPULATION AND "DE QI"

Here needle manipulation refers to particular kinds of hand techniques, which are performed after inserting the needle in order to enable the practitioner to *de qi* (得气). This is an important technical term, meaning variously "to gain the qi", "the arrival of the qi", or "needling sensation". These manipulative techniques are used to regulate the needling sensation so as to achieve a reinforcing or reducing action.

The *de qi* in this case refers to the reaction of the meridional qi after the needle is inserted into the point.

When the qi arrives, the practitioner may feel a kind of moderate, sinking or tight sensation under the needle-tip; the patient, too, may have a sensation of soreness, numbness, heaviness or distension around the point, or even a sensation travelling to a certain place or transmitting in a certain direction.

If the qi doesn't arrive, the practitioner may feel a hollow sensation around the needle or else the patient will have no sensation at all.

Dou Hanqing described this vividly in his *Lyric of Standard Profundities* (see Appendix 2) where he states that a "hollow, smooth and loose sensation around the needle suggests the absence of qi, which lets you feel as if you are walking on a wild and empty ground, but a heavy, uneven and tense feeling suggests the *de qi*, which is felt as a fish biting at the hook and pulling the line downward".

The *de qi* and the speed of its arrival are not only closely related to the acupuncture effect, but also to the prognosis. As it says in the *Miraculous Pivot*, "the needling sensation must be achieved no matter how many methods are used or how long it may take".[5] This reveals fully the importance of the *de qi*.

As for the relationship between the acupuncture effect and the speed of qi arrival: generally, a quick *de qi* suggests a quick effect from treatment, while a slow *de qi* means a slow result, while absence of qi may lead to no effect. This is also described in the *Ode to the Golden Needle* (see Appendix 2).

Therefore in the clinic, if there is no needling sensation, the cause must be discovered, such as an inaccurate location of the point, an imperfect manipulation of the needle or a mistaken angle or depth of insertion. Then measures should be taken at once, i.e. to readjust the location of the point and manipulate the needle sufficiently.

If the absence of qi is caused by the patient's weak constitution, or other pathological factors, leading to a dullness in sensation, then other means—such as manipulating, retaining or warming the needle or moxibustion—should be taken to promote the qi. Then, if the qi still refuses to arrive, it shows that the disease can't be cured, because the meridional qi of the zangfu organs is greatly exhausted.

In the *Great Compendium of Acupuncture and Moxibustion* it says, "the *de qi* alone is the measure of the treatment. If the qi does not arrive, there is no treatment".[6] No *de qi* suggests there is no hope in curing the disease with acupuncture, so other therapeutic methods should be considered.

As for needling manipulations there are two main categories: fundamental techniques, and auxiliary techniques.

Fundamental techniques

The two most commonly used in the clinic are lifting-thrusting and rotating.

Lifting-thrusting

After the needle-tip reaches a certain depth, the needle body is perpendicularly lifted and thrusted. The needle penetrating in from the superficial region to the deep region is known as thrusting. Withdrawal of the needle from the deep region to the superficial region is called lifting (see Fig. 149).

The amplitude, frequency and duration of the lifting-thrusting depends on the patient's constitution, the condition of the yin and yang,

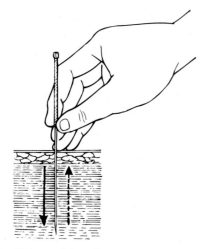

Fig. 149 Lifting and thrusting.

the location of the points and the therapeutic requirements.

Rotating

After the needle reaches its desired depth, twirl and rotate the needle, backward and forward, with the thumb and index finger of the right hand (see Fig. 150).

The amplitude, frequency and duration of the needle rotation depends on the patient's constitution, the conditions of the illness with regard to yin and yang, the characteristics of the points and the therapeutic requirements.

The two methods mentioned above can be used singly or in combination, according to the conditions.

Auxiliary manipulations

Local massaging

Slightly massage the skin around the point, or along the course of the meridian, with the left or right hand.

This promotes the circulation of qi and blood so as to facilitate the needling sensation, and also may help disperse qi and blood when there is a tense sensation around the needle.

Scraping

After the needle reaches the required depth, the belly of the thumb or index finger is put on the tail to hold the needle steady, and then the nail of the thumb, index finger or middle finger scrapes the handle of the needle, from below to above (see Fig. 151).

This is used to stimulate the meridional qi and promote the *de qi*.

Flicking

When the needle arrives at the required depth, flick the needle gently causing it to tremble, to make the meridional qi flow rapidly (see Fig. 152).

It is said in the *Questions and Answers on Acupuncture and Moxibustion*, that "if the qi doesn't flow smoothly, flick the needle gently

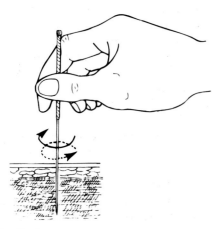

Fig. 150 Rotating.

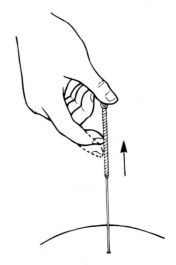

Fig. 151 Scraping.

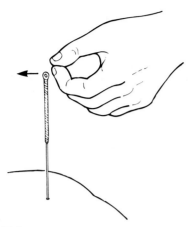

Fig. 152   Flicking.

and accelerate it, this is known as promoting qi by flicking".

Twisting

After inserting the needle to the required depth, rotate the needle in one direction with the thumb, index and middle fingers, as if twisting thread, either 2–3 rotations, or else 3–5 rotations each time; at the same time, lift and thrust the needle to avoid it being entwined in muscle fibre.

It is recorded in the *Great Compendium of Acupuncture and Moxibustion* that "when twisting the needle one should follow the course of the meridional qi without causing tensity, otherwise the muscle may twine about the needle, causing pain".[7]

This method is used to promote the circulation and arrival of qi, to strengthen the body's resistance and expel pathogenic factors.

Shaking

After the needle is inserted to the required depth, shake the handle of the needle as if working a scull or a windlass.

This method may be used to expel the pathogen by shaking the needle during its lifting from the deep region to the superficial region, and then removing it.

The method may also be used to conduct the qi, or needling sensation, in a certain direction. Shake the needle obliquely or horizontally, from left to right, without a change of depth. This is the method sometimes described as *qing long bai wei* (青龙摆尾) or "the green dragon shaking its tail".

In the *Questions and Answers on Acupuncture and Moxibustion* it says, "shaking the needle is the way to promote qi circulation".

Trembling

After inserting the needle to the required depth, hold the handle with the right hand and apply swift lifting and thrusting movements, of a small amplitude, in order to cause a type of vibration.

This is used to promote the *de qi*, or to encourage the function of dispelling the pathogen and strengthening the bodily resistance.

METHODS OF REINFORCING AND REDUCING

The methods of reinforcing and reducing are derived from the *Miraculous Pivot*, where it says that "reducing is used in treating excess syndromes, reinforcing in deficiency syndromes, swift needling in heat syndromes, retaining the needle in cold syndromes and moxibustion in cases with a feeble pulse".[8]

Reinforcing and reducing are two distinct therapeutic techniques based upon the essential principles behind acupuncture and moxibustion.

It says in the *Miraculous Pivot* that "the key to the reinforcing and reducing method lies in manipulating the nine kinds of needles".[9] The *Prescriptions Worth a Thousand Gold Coin* states that, "reinforcing and reducing are the leading methods among all acupuncture manipulative techniques". They play an important role in the treatment of disease by acupuncture, but more especially form the core content of the filiform needling technique.

The method by which one is able to invigorate the bodily resistance, and strengthen weakened physiological functions, is called *bu* (补) or "reinforcing", while the method by which one is able to eliminate pathogenic factors and to check hyperactive physiological functions, restoring them to normal, is called *xie* (泻) or "reducing".

Both reinforcing and reducing with needles are performed by puncturing the points with the proper manipulation.

The production of the reinforcing or reducing effect may be discussed under three main aspects: the functional conditions, the characteristics of the specific point, and the particular manipulation of the needle.

Functional conditions

The internal environment forms a base for various kinds of pathological changes. Therefore, under differing pathological conditions, acupuncture may exert differing regulatory functions, produced through the effects of reinforcing and reducing.

For instance, if someone is weak and manifesting deficiency symptoms, then acupuncture functions to invigorate the bodily resistance. Alternatively, when they are suffering from a syndrome of excessive heat or *feng* stroke, the acupuncture functions to expel the heat outwards, and to restore consciousness. Again acupuncture can not only relieve intestinal spasm, and alleviate pain, but also strengthen intestinal peristalsis and keep the digestion working properly.

So it says in the *Plain Questions* that "reducing is applied to treat excess syndromes, reinforcing is employed for deficiency syndromes . . . no matter how many times it may have to be performed, the purpose is to harmonize yin and yang".[10]

This regulatory function of acupuncture is closely related to the condition of the antipathogenic factors within the human body. If they are vigorous, the meridional qi is easy to activate. If they are weakened, it is difficult to excite or only slightly stimulated after repeated tries. For this reason, the *Miraculous Pivot* says that the flowing of the meridional qi suggests the effect of reinforcing and reducing.[11]

Characteristics of the points

Points are characterized not only by common features but also by a relative specificity. For instance, some points are suitable for treating deficiency syndromes, such as Zusanli (S 36) and Guanyuan (Ren 4), for they have the property of tonifying the body; while some points, such as Shaoshang (LI 11) and Shixuan (Extra), are especially chosen to treat excess syndromes, for they function in expelling pathogens.

Needle manipulation

Acupuncture is a method which can promote the transformation of internal factors within the organism. For this purpose the ancient acupuncturists developed and summarized a great number of reinforcing and reducing methods, which are still commonly used in the clinic.

Reinforcing and reducing by rotating

After the *de qi*, rotate the needle gently and slowly, within a small amplitude and for a short duration; this is called reinforcing. Rotate the needle rapidly and forcefully, within a large amplitude and for a long duration; this is known as reducing.

Reinforcing and reducing methods are also distinguished by the direction of rotation. A forceful leftward rotation within a large amplitude is reinforcing, whilst a forceful rightward rotation within a large amplitude is reducing.

Reinforcing and reducing by lifting and thrusting

After the *de qi*, reinforcing is performed by thrusting the needle heavily and lifting the needle gently and manipulating the needle for a short while, whilst reducing is performed by lifting the needle heavily and swiftly, thrusting the needle gently, and manipulating the needle for a longer period.

Reinforcing and reducing obtained by rapid and slow insertion and withdrawal

Reinforcing is performed by slow insertion with less rotation and rapid withdrawal of the needle, whilst reducing is applied by rapid insertion, more rotation and a slow withdrawal.

Reinforcing and reducing achieved by directing the needle-tip

Reinforcing is applied by directing the needle-tip along the course of the meridian, whilst reducing is applied by directing the tip against the course of the meridian.

Reinforcing and reducing method by means of the patient's respiration

Reinforcing is achieved by inserting the needle when the patient breathes in and withdrawing the needle when the patient breathes out. Reducing is performed contrariwise.

Reinforcing and reducing achieved by keeping the puncture-hole open or closed

Pressing the hole as soon as the needle is withdrawn is known as reinforcing; conversely, shaking the needle to enlarge the hole on withdrawal of the needle is called reducing.

Even reinforcing and reducing

After the *de qi*, lift and thrust, twist and rotate the needle at a moderate speed, then withdraw it.

In clinical practice these methods can be used together. There are also some well-known methods which combine the above, for example, "setting the mountain on fire" and "penetrating the heaven's coolness".

Setting the mountain on fire

First insert the needle to the superficial region, about one-third of the required depth (Heaven). After the *de qi*, rotate the needle with the reinforcing method, then thrust the needle to the medium region, about two-thirds of the required depth (Man). After the needle sensation is felt, rotate the needle with the reinforcing method, then thrust it to the deep region (Earth); rotate it with the reinforcing method after the *de qi*, then lift it slowly back to the superficial region. This is repeated thrice before the needle is thrust to the required depth and retained.

During the operation reinforcing by means of the breathing may be adopted as well.

This method is often used to treat diseases of a deficiency-cold nature, such as Bi syndrome of the cold type (intractable arthralgia) and numbness.

Penetrating the heaven's coolness

Thrust the needle to the deep region (to the given depth), and rotate it with a reducing method after the *de qi*. Then lift the needle rapidly back to the medium region, rotate it with the reducing method after the *de qi*, then lift it rapidly to the superficial region, rotate it with the reducing method after the de qi, and then finally thrust the needle slowly into the deep region. This is repeated thrice before the needle is rapidly lifted to the superficial region and retained.

During the operation, the reducing method by means of the breathing may be employed as well.

This method is often used to treat diseases of an excess heat nature, such as Bi syndrome of the heat type and acute carbuncles.

RETAINING AND WITHDRAWING THE NEEDLE

Retaining the needle means keeping the needle in the point after it has been inserted to the given depth. The purpose is to strengthen the function of the acupuncture and to enable continuous further manipulation. Usually the needle is withdrawn, or retained for 10–20 minutes after the *de qi*, whilst proper manipulation of the reinforcing and reducing methods is employed; but in some special cases, such as acute abdominal pain, tetanus, opisthotonos, intractable pain of cold nature or spastic cases, the time for retaining the needle may be prolonged, sometimes lasting as long as several hours.

During this period, manipulate the needle at intervals to increase and consolidate the effect. If no sensation is felt, then wait quietly until the qi arrives. Clinically, whether the needle is retained or not, and the duration for retaining the needle, is decided by the patient's constitution and the conditions of the illness.

Withdrawing the needle refers to the usual method of removing the needle after the manipulation, or else after it has been retained.

When withdrawing the needle, press the skin around the point with the thumb and index finger of the left hand, rotate the needle gently, and lift it slowly to the subcutaneous level. Then withdraw it quickly and press the hole with a sterilized cotton ball to prevent bleeding.

If the methods of reinforcing and reducing by rapid or slow insertion and withdrawal, or by keeping the hole open or closed, are adopted, then the needle should be withdrawn according to these rules. The number of the needles used should be checked to make sure that none are unremoved, and then the patient should rest for a brief while before leaving.

THE PREVENTION AND MANAGEMENT OF POSSIBLE ACCIDENTS

Although acupuncture is safe, some accidents may take place owing to carelessness, imperfect manipulation, negligence of the contraindications or lack of a comprehensive knowledge of anatomy. The possible accidents are as follows.

LOSS OF CONSCIOUSNESS

Loss of consciousness during acupuncture can be avoided. Care should be taken to prevent it.

Cause

This is often due to a delicate constitution, nervousness or fatigue, hunger, profuse sweating, severe diarrhoea, an improper position or too forceful manipulation.

Manifestation

Sudden spiritlessness, dizziness, vertigo, pale complexion, fidgeting, nausea, profuse sweating, palpitations, cold limbs, drop in blood pressure, deep and thready pulse, fainting, falling to the ground, cyanosis of the lips and nails, faecal and urinary incontinence and an extremely weak pulse.

Management

Withdraw all needles at once. Help the patient to lie down and keep him warm. In mild cases offer the patient some warm water or water with sugar. The symptoms will disappear spontaneously. In severe cases, in addition to the above management, puncture Shuigou (Du 26), Suliao (Du 25), Neiguan (P 6), and Zusanli (St 36), and apply moxibustion to Baihui (Du 20), Guanyuan (Ren 4) and Qihai (Ren 6). Generally the patient will respond.

If the patient still remains unconscious, with feeble respiration and a weak pulse, other treatment or emergency measures should be taken.

Prevention

In the case of loss of consciousness, prevention is of great importance. Firstly an explanation of acupuncture procedure should be given to new patients who have never been needled before, to those who are over-sensitive, or to those with a delicate constitution, in order to remove their nervousness. At the same time, select a good posture, such as lying down. Prescribe fewer points and puncture the patient gently. If they feel hungry, tired or thirsty, they should first eat, rest or drink before the acupuncture. During the procedure, the practitioner should concentrate his attention on watching the mental state of the patient, and inquire as to his or her feelings. Then if the first signs of loss of consciousness appear, the doctor can take steps quickly to prevent it.

STUCK NEEDLES

This takes place during the manipulation or after the retention of the needles. The practitioner may feel a stuck sensation around the needle and find it difficult to rotate, lift, thrust, or withdraw, while the patient may feel pain. This is known as a stuck needle.

Cause

This may arise from nervousness, for when the needle is inserted into the body, the patient may contract the muscles violently; or it may be caused by imperfect manipulation, such as twirling the needle only in one direction, resulting in the needle becoming entwined in muscle fibres, or by a too lengthy retention of the needle.

Manifestation

The needle is found to be impossible or difficult to rotate, lift, thrust or withdraw, and the patient feels severe pain.

Management

If the needle is stuck due to the contraction of the muscle, it can be left where it is for a while; otherwise, massage the skin around the point, pluck the handle of the needle, or insert another needle nearby, to disperse the qi and blood and thus release the tension in the muscle. If it is caused by imperfect manipulation or rotation then twirl the needle in the opposite direction. At the same time, pluck and scrape the handle to release the muscle fibre.

Prevention

Sensitive patients should be encouraged to relax, and care should be taken during manipulation to avoid rotating the needle only in one direction; further, twirling should always be performed along with lifting and thrusting.

BENT NEEDLES

Bent needles means that the needle bends when or after it has been inserted into the point.

Cause

This may result from unskilful manipulation, too forceful or rapid manipulation, or from the needle striking hard tissue, a sudden change of the patient's posture, or from foreign pressure on the needle.

Manifestation

It is difficult to lift, thrust, rotate or withdraw the needle. At the same time, the patient feels pain.

Management

When the needle is bent, then lifting, thrusting or rotating the needle should in no case be applied further. If the needle is slightly bent, withdraw it slowly. If it is acutely bent, withdraw it following the course of the bend. If it is caused by a change in the patient's posture, turn him gently back to his original position, relax the local muscle and remove the needle. Never try to withdraw the needle by force.

Prevention

Perfect insertion and even finger-force are required, and a too rapid or forceful insertion is forbidden. Select a proper position and ask the patient to keep still during the time the needle is retained. At the same time, protect the needle from being impacted or pressed on by external forces.

BROKEN NEEDLE

This means that the needle has broken inside the body. It can be avoided by careful examination of the needle before puncture and proper attention during manipulation.

Cause

This may arise from a poor quality needle or an eroded base of the needle, a complete insertion of the needle body into the point, or from too forceful lifting, thrusting or rotating of the needle which causes the muscle to contract suddenly, a sudden change of the patient's posture, or from improper management of a bent or stuck needle.

Manifestation

The needle body is broken during manipulation or on withdrawal of the needle. The broken part is left in the point below the skin surface, sometimes with part of the needle body exposed.

Management

The practitioner should keep calm and ask the

patient to maintain his original position to prevent the broken part from going deeper into the body. If the broken part protrudes from the skin, remove it with forceps or fingers. If the broken part is at the same level or just below the level of the skin, press the tissue around the point with the thumb and index finger of the left hand until the broken end is exposed, then remove it with forceps. If it is completely under the skin or in the deep muscle, it should be located with an X-ray and removed by operation.

Prevention

To prevent accidents, careful inspection of the needle should be made prior to treatment in order to reject needles which do not conform to the specified requirements, and furthermore also avoid manipulating the needle too violently and forcefully. During the manipulation or retention of the needle the patient should be asked to remain still. The needle body should not be inserted into the body completely and part should always be exposed above the skin in case it needs to be taken out if broken. On needle insertion, if it is bent the needle should be withdrawn immediately. Never try to insert or manipulate a needle with too much force. The correct procedure should always be followed immediately in the case of accidents, such as finding a stuck needle. Never try to withdraw a needle with too much force.

HAEMATOMA

This indicates a swelling around the punctured part due to cutaneous bleeding.

Cause

This may result from injuring the skin and muscle or blood vessels with a hooked needle.

Manifestation

Local swelling, distension and pain after withdrawing the needle. Then the skin turns blue or purplish.

Management

In mild cases the haematoma will disappear by itself. In cases of local swelling, severe pain and a haematoma over a large area of the skin with limitation of functional activities, apply a cold compress to stop the bleeding and then apply a hot compress or light massage to disperse the stagnation of blood.

Prevention

Examine the needles carefully, pay attention to the regional anatomy and avoid injuring blood vessels. Press the point with a sterilized cotton ball as soon as the needle is withdrawn.

PRECAUTIONS IN ACUPUNCTURE

In performing acupuncture, attention should be paid to the following aspects, because each patient's physiological environment and particular condition is different.

1. It is not advisable to give acupuncture to patients who are over-hungry, tired or nervous. Those who are weak or deficient both in qi and blood should be punctured gently in a supine position.
2. It is contraindicated to puncture the abdomen and lumbosacral region within the first three months of pregnancy. For pregnancy over three months, the points on the upper abdomen and lumbosacral region, and those points which activate the blood circulation, such as Sanyinjiao (Sp 6), Hegu (LI 4), Kunlun (UB 60) and Zhiyin (UB 67), are contraindicated. No acupuncture treatment is to be given to women during the period of menstruation except for the purpose of regulating menstruation.
3. Points on the vertex of infants should not be needled when the fontanelle is not yet closed.
4. It is contraindicated to puncture a patient who has a tendency to spontaneous haemorrhage or continuous bleeding after injury.
5. It is not suitable to puncture points on an area where there is an infection, ulcer, scar or tumour.
6. Points in areas where there are important

viscera, as on the chest, ribs, waist, and back, should not be punctured perpendicularly or deeply, especially on those with hepatomegaly, splenomegaly or pulmonary emphysema. Puncturing deeply the points on the chest, back, axilla, costal regions or supraclavicular fossa may injure the lung, causing traumatic pneumothorax. In mild cases such manifestations as chest pain, a full sensation in the chest, palpitations and difficulty in breathing may appear. In severe cases, dyspnoea, purple lips and nails, sweating, and a drop in the blood pressure may be manifest.

On a physical examination, the intercostal spaces of the impacted side may become wider, and there may be over-resonance on percussion. Furthermore, if the trachea is pushed to the healthy side, the sound of respiration is obvi-

ously reduced or disappears. Diagnosis can be made with the help of an X-ray, which shows the amount of air and the condition of the lung. In such a case immediate therapeutic steps should be taken. Therefore the acupuncturist should fully concentrate his mind on the needling, keep the patient in a proper position, and strictly control the depth and angle of insertion.

7. When the points around the eyes and vertex, such as Fengfu (Du 16) and Yamen (Du 15) are needled, attention should be paid to the angle of needling, and no rotation, lifting or thrusting within a large amplitude is allowed.

8. As for those patients suffering retention of urine, it is necessary to control the direction, angle and depth of the needle when puncturing points on the lower abdomen, so as to avoid accidents caused through injuring the bladder.

NOTES

1. See for example the *Miraculous Pivot*, Ch. 1, "On the 9 Needles and 12 Yuan-sources" (Appendix 1).
2. *Miraculous Pivot*, Ch. 7, "A Just Choice in Needling".
3. *Classic on Medical Problems*, Problem 78.
4. This phrase is first contained within Dou Hanqing's poem the *Lyric of Standard Profundities*, see Appendix 2. It was first presented in this book.
5. *Miraculous Pivot*, Ch. 1, "On the 9 Needles and 12 Yuan-sources".
6. The *Great Compendium* was complied by Yang Jizhou, in 1601 AD. This quote is from "Questions and Answers on

the Jingluo, how to Needle with or against the Qi", towards the end of Book Four.
7. This is contained within Book Four of the *Great Compendium*. The section outlines Yang Jizhou's own technique, developing and refining the technique of the *Ode to the Golden Needle*.
8. *Miraculous Pivot*, Ch. 10, "Meridians".
9. *Miraculous Pivot*, Ch. 1, "On the 9 Needles and 12 Yuan-sources".
10. *Plain Questions*, Ch. 20, "Discussion over the 3 Sections and 9 Divisions".
11. *Miraculous Pivot*, Ch. 9, "Looking to Endings and Beginnings".

Moxibustion 5

Moxibustion is a therapeutic method which treats and prevents disease by applying the stimulation of warmth and heat to the acupoints and jingluo. In the *Introduction to Medicine* it says, "When a disease fails to respond to herbal medicine and acupuncture, moxibustion is suggested".

There are many raw materials used in moxibustion, but *Artemisia vulgaris* is the most common in use in the clinic. It is a species of perennial herb belonging to the chrysanthemum family. Its leaf is fragrant and inflammable, and, when burned, its heat penetrates into the jingluo, activates the qi and blood circulation, eliminates cold and damp, disperses swelling and accumulation, restores the primary yang qi after collapse and prevents disease.

In the *Other Records by Famous Physicians*, it says "*Artemisia vulgaris* is nonpoisonous and slightly bitter in taste, it is indicated in the treatment of various kinds of diseases". The material for moxibustion is called *qi* (艾) or "moxa", made of the leaves of the plant, which are pestled after removing any impurities. They are then dried for use later.

MOXIBUSTION METHODS IN COMMON USE

There are many moxibustion methods. Table 5.1 illustrates those in common use in the clinic.

MOXIBUSTION WITH A MOXACONE

Place some moxa wool on a board, knead and shape it by hand into a cone the size of a grain of wheat, a xanthium seed, a lotus seed or about the size of half an olive. In the book *Bianque's Medical Experiences*, it records that a lotus-seed sized moxa cone, about 0.3 cm in diameter, is suitable for moxibustion on an adult, a xanthium-seed sized cone for the four limbs and for infants, and a wheat-grain sized cone for moxibustion on the head or face.

In the clinic, moxibustion with moxa cones may be direct or indirect.

Direct moxibustion

A moxa cone placed directly on the point and ignited is called direct moxibustion. In this, the

moxibustion leads to a local burn, blistering, festering and finally a scar after healing. It is known as scarring moxibustion. If no local scar is formed, it is known as non-scarring moxibustion.

Scarring moxibustion

This is also known as festering moxibustion. Prior to moxibustion, apply a little garlic juice to the point in order to increase the adhesion of the moxa cone to the skin. Then put the cone on the point and ignite it until it completely burns out; repeat the procedure according to the required number of cones.

Because the fire of the moxa cone burns the skin, the patient may feel severe pain, and the practitioner should pat the skin around the point to relieve the pain. In normal conditions, the skin begins to fester and forms post-moxibustion sores one week after the moxibustion. In 5–6 weeks, the sore is healed, the scab has dropped off and a scar is left behind. This method must therefore be chosen only after seeking permission from the patient.

It is indicated in chronic diseases, such as asthma, lung disorders and scrofula.

Non-scarring moxibustion

Apply a small amount of vaseline over the point prior to moxibustion so as to increase the adhesion of the moxa cone to the skin. Then place a cone the size of a xanthium-seed onto the point and ignite it.

When three-fifths or three-quarters of the cone is burnt, and the patient feels discomfort, remove the cone and put on another one. If a wheat-grain sized cone is used, the practitioner may remove it with forceps, then put on another. Generally this procedure is repeated until the local skin reddens, but no blister forms, and there is no scar left.

The indications are all diseases of a cold-deficiency nature.

Indirect moxibustion

Moxibustion with some medicine separating the moxa cone and the skin is known as indirect moxibustion. The medicines used are many—

Table 5.1   Methods of moxibustion

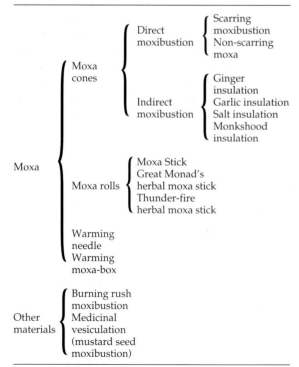

Moxa	Moxa cones	Direct moxibustion	Scarring moxibustion / Non-scarring moxa
		Indirect moxibustion	Ginger insulation / Garlic insulation / Salt insulation / Monkshood insulation
	Moxa rolls		Moxa Stick / Great Monad's herbal moxa stick / Thunder-fire herbal moxa stick
	Warming needle / Warming moxa-box		
Other materials	Burning rush moxibustion / Medicinal vesiculation (mustard seed moxibustion)		

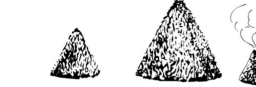

Fig. 153   Moxa cones.

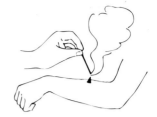

Fig. 154   Direct moxibustion.

ginger, garlic, salt, etc. The following are commonly used in clinics:

— moxibustion with ginger,
— moxibustion with garlic,
— moxibustion with salt,
— moxibustion with monkshood cake.

Moxibustion with ginger

Cut a slice of ginger about 0.2–0.3 cm thick, punch holes in it and place it on the point selected. On top of this piece of ginger, a moxa cone is placed and ignited. When it burns out, remove the cone and put on another. This procedure is repeated until the skin reddens.

This method is indicated in vomiting, abdominal pain, diarrhoea and pain of a cold nature.

Moxibustion with garlic

Cut a slice of fresh garlic about 0.2– 0.3 cm thick, punch holes in it, (or pestle it into a paste), and put it on the point. On top of the garlic, place a moxa cone and ignite it; when it burns out, remove it and put on another. This is repeated up to the given number.

The indications are scrofula, tuberculosis and the early stage of skin ulcers with boils.

Moxibustion with salt

Fill the umbilicus with salt, or put a piece of ginger in place, with a large moxa cone on top of it and ignite it.

This method is often indicated in febrile diseases of the yin type—vomiting and diarrhoea, prostration syndrome arising from apoplexy, etc. It has the function of restoring the yang, or resuscitation in the case of collapse. But it must be used continuously, and many cones applied, until the pulse is restored, the four extremities become warm, and the symptoms partly disappear.

Moxibustion with monkshood cake

A cake about 0.8 cm thick and 3 cm in diameter is made of monkshood powder mixed with alcohol. Then numerous holes are punched in it and it is placed on the site for moxibustion, with an ignited moxa cone placed on top of it.

This method is suitable for treating impotence, ejaculatio praecox caused by decline of the *mingmen* (命门) fire or "fire of the gate of life", and persistent skin ulcers.

MOXIBUSTION WITH A MOXA ROLL

Place 24 g of moxa wool on a piece of paper

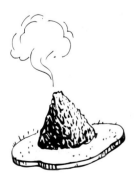

Fig. 155   Indirect moxibustion with ginger.

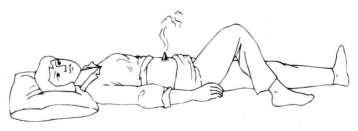

Fig. 156   Indirect moxibustion with salt.

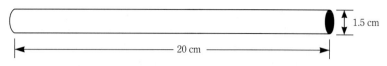

Fig. 157 Moxa stick.

about 26 cm long and 20 cm wide, roll it up tightly into the shape of a stick about 1.5 cm in diameter, then wrap it with paper made of mulberry bark and seal the opening with paste or glue (see Fig 157).

The moxa wool may be mixed with other herbal medicines, such as 6 g each of Rougui (*Cortex Cinnamonis*), Ganjiang (*Rhizoma Zingiberis*), Dingxiang (*Zios caryophylli*), Duhuo (*Radix Angelicas pubescentis*), Xixin (*Herba Asari*), Baizhi (*Radix Angelicas dahuricae*), Xionghuang (realgar), Cangzhu (*Rhizoma Atractylodis*), Moyao (*Myrrh Resina Olibani*), Ruxiang (*Resina Boswelliae carterii*), Chuanjiao (*Pericardium Zanthoxyli*), etc. These herbs are mixed together and ground into a fine powder. A moxa stick mixed with herbal medicines is called a "medicated moxa stick".

Moxibustion with a moxa stick is divided into mild-warm moxibustion and sparrow-pecking moxibustion.

Mild-warm moxibustion

Apply an ignited moxa stick over selected points at a distance of 2–3 cm, causing a mild warmth without a burning sensation. Carry on for 5–7 minutes, until the skin is locally red.

The index and middle fingers of the practitioner should be placed on both sides of the point for those who are unconscious or have dulled sensation in the area. In this way you control the heat produced by the stick, by adjusting the distance between the stick and the skin, and prevent accidents.

Sparrow-pecking moxibustion

When this method is applied, the ignited moxa stick is moved rapidly over the point, just like a pecking sparrow. The distance between the stick and the skin is not fixed. The stick is evenly moved back and forth, vertically or transversely, or in a repeated circular fashion.

The above-mentioned methods are used for most ordinary cases, but mild-warm moxibustion is often used in treating chronic disease, whilst the sparrow-pecking method is appropriate in acute cases. There are also the particular uses of the Great Monad's herbal moxa stick, and the thunder-fire moxa stick:

The Great Monad's herbal moxa stick

Combine together: 125 g of Rensheng (*Radix Ginseng*), 250 g of Chuanshanjiao (*Squama Manitis*), 90 g of Shanyangxue (goat's blood), 500 g of Qiannianjian (*Rhizoma Homalomenae*), 300 g of Gudifeng (*Rubus Ellipticus*), 500 g of Rougui (*Cortex Cinnamomi*), 500 g of Xiaohuixiang (*Fuctus Foenicuii*), 500 g of Cangzhu (*Rhizoma Atractylodis*), 1000 g of Gancao (*Radix Glycyrrhizae*), 2000 g

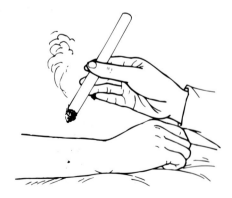

Fig. 158 Mild-warm moxibustion.

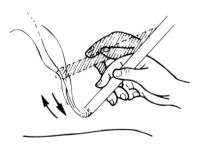

Fig. 159 Sparrow-pecking moxibustion.

of Fangfeng (*Radix Ledebouriellae*) and a little musk. These herbs are mixed and ground together into a fine powder. Then take 24 g of the medicine and mix it with 150 g of moxa wool, put this on a piece of paper about 40 cm square and roll it up into a long stick, the shape of a Chinese fire-cracker. The whole paper stick is glued together with egg-white and dried in a cool place for use.

Ignite one end of the stick and rapidly place it in a piece of dry cloth which has been folded into several layers. Then direct the cloth with the ignited moxa stick in it onto the skin, to function as a hot compress and produce a sensation of heat over the point or affected site. When it cools ignite it again. Repeat this 7–10 times.

It is effective in treating painful joints (Bi syndrome) caused by *feng*, cold or damp, intractable numbness, motor impairment, hemiplegia, etc.

The Thunder-fire moxa stick

The method of production is the same as for the Great Monad's stick except for the medical prescription. Use 125 g of fine moxa wool, 9 g each of Chenxiang (*Lignum Aquilariae Radix Aucklandiae*), Muxiang (*Resina Olibani*), Ruxiang (*Resina Boswelliae carterii*), Qianghuo (*Rhizoma sea Radix Notopterygii*), Ganjiang (dried ginger), and Chuanshanjiao (*Squama Monitis*). Grind them into powder and mix with a little musk.

The method and clinical indications are almost the same as those of the Great Monad's stick. In the *Great Compendium of Acupuncture and Moxibustion* it says it is used "to check the pain caused by injury to the muscles or bones, or pain of a cold damp nature, or else in those who are afraid of being needled".

MOXIBUSTION WITH A WARMING NEEDLE

Moxibustion with a warming needle is a method of combining acupuncture with moxibustion, and is used in conditions where both retention of the needle and moxibustion are needed.

The manipulation is as follows. After the *de qi*, rotate the needle, either reinforcing or reducing, then retain the needle. Wrap the top of the handle with some fine moxa wool, or place a small piece of moxa stick about 2 cm long on it, then ignite it. After it burns out, remove it and withdraw the needle. This method is easy and can be widely used in the clinic.

MOXIBUSTION WITH A MOXA-BOX

The device is a special metal apparatus shaped like a small round box. The bottom may be flat or pointed, with an even smaller box inside it, which is full of small holes. The box carrying the ignited moxa wool, or prescribed medicines, is then covered with a lid. Keep it on the point, or the site, until the local skin becomes red.

Its function is to regulate qi and blood, and warm the middle-jiao to dispel cold. It can be used in all cases in which moxibustion is indicated, especially with children, women and those who are afraid of direct moxibustion.

OTHER MOXIBUSTION METHODS

BURNING RUSH MOXIBUSTION

This is also known as "The Fire of January 13th", a time in the depth of the winter according to the Chinese lunar calendar. It is performed by soaking a rush in oil, then igniting the rush and placing it directly over the point.

It can expel exterior syndromes caused by the *feng*, promote qi circulation and resolve *tan*, clear *feng* and stop convulsions. Indications are tetanus neonatorum and stomach-ache, abdominal pain, and acute diseases such as gastroenteritis, etc.

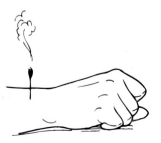

Fig. 160 Moxibustion with a warming needle.

MUSTARD SEED MOXIBUSTION

This is one form of "cold moxibustion" which causes blisters by herbal materials applied externally on acupoints. However it does not use ignited moxa, and so is also known as the "blister-inducing method".

It is performed by grinding mustard seed into a powder, mixing it with water and applying the paste to the point or affected area. With a strong stimulation, it can form blisters so as to treat painful joints (Bi syndrome), facial paralysis, or, together with other medications, asthma.

PRECAUTIONS

In addition to the basic theory and principles of diagnosis and treatment, based upon an overall analysis of symptoms and signs according to TCM, attention should be paid to the following.

THE PROCESS OF MOXIBUSTION

In *Prescriptions Worth a Thousand Gold Coin* it says "Moxibustion is generally applied firstly to the yang, and then to the yin.... first above, then below".

In the clinic, first apply moxibustion to the upper region of the body, then to the lower region, first to the yang areas, then to the yin, first to an area needing fewer cones, then to that needing more cones, first to the point needing a small cone then to the point needing a large cone. But the sequence should be decided according to the particular conditions.

For example, in the case of a rectal prolapse, first apply moxibustion to Changqiang (Du 1) to "draw" the anus back, then to Baihui (Du 20) to elevate the qi in the middle-jiao.

REINFORCING AND REDUCING METHODS OF MOXIBUSTION

In the *Miraculous Pivot* it says, "the reinforcing method of moxibustion is to wait for the fire of the ignited cone to die out by itself, without being extinguished artificially. The reducing method is to blow on the ignited cone, and then put another cone on top to extinguish it."[1] This makes the effect of the moxa more penetrating into the point.

This is the method used by the ancient physicians. Nowadays it may be adopted according to the patient's conditions and the characteristics of the selected points.

CONTRAINDICATIONS

1. It is not advisable to apply moxibustion to a patient suffering from a heat syndrome of the excess type, or high fever due to yin deficiency.
2. Scarring moxibustion should not be applied to the face, near the sense organs or any area near large blood vessels.
3. The abdominal and lumbosacral regions of pregnant women are contraindicated for the use of moxibustion.

MANAGEMENT AFTER MOXIBUSTION

After moxibustion, slight redness and heat may remain in the local region; this is nothing serious and needs no special management.

If small blisters are caused by overstimulation by the moxa, take care not to break them, they will be absorbed and heal by themselves. Large blisters should be punctured and drained by a sterilized needle or a syringe. Put some gentian violet over the lesion, then wrap it with gauze. If pus forms in scarring moxibustion, the patient should have a good rest to strengthen the bodily resistance, and at the same time keep the site clean. The blisters should be dressed to prevent further infection and they will heal naturally.

If the pus is yellow or green, or mixed with blood, apply an anti-inflammatory plaster or a "Yuhong plaster".

Additionally, take care not to let the ignited moxa cone burn the skin or clothes. The used moxa sticks and the Great Monad's herbal moxa stick should be put into a glass bottle with a small opening or a pail made from iron to prevent it from burning.

Appendix: The methods of cupping

Cupping is a therapy in which a jar is attached to the skin surface, causing local congestion through the negative pressure created by introducing heat in the form of an ignited material, with the aim of treating disease.

Cupping was also known as the horn method (using animal horns) in ancient times, when it was recorded in the *Book of the Fifty-two Prescriptions* unearthed from the Mawangdui Tombs of the Han Dynasty (see *Introduction*), and also in many other ancient Chinese medical classics. It was mainly used by surgeons to suck out pus, while treating the skin, and other external conditions.

Along with the development of clinical practice, not only were the materials for making jars and cupping methods greatly improved, but also the range of indications was expanded, and consequently cups were used in both internal medicine and surgery. Cupping is often used together with acupuncture, as it functions similarly to moxibustion.

TYPES OF JARS

There are a great variety of jars, but those most commonly used in the clinic are made of bamboo, pottery or glass.

The bamboo jar

Cut down a section of good bamboo 3–5 cm in diameter, forming a cylinder 6–8 cm or 6–10 cm in length. The jointed end is used as the bottom, and the other end as the opening. Remove the outer skin and internal membrane with a knife, making the rim of the jar smooth with sandpaper. The bamboo jar is available in many places for it is economical, easy to make, light and free from being damaged. But it easily dries out, tending to break here and there, letting in the air, which affects suction.

The pottery jar

This is made of clay and may be large or small in size, with a smooth rim, large belly and small opening at the bottom like a drum. It can exert great suction but is easily damaged.

The glass cup

This is made of glass, its shape being based on the pottery jar, round like a ball. The rim is smooth. It is made in three sizes, large, medium and small, or sometimes can be replaced by a bottle with a large opening. Since it is transparent, local congestion can be observed, thus the duration of cupping can be controlled. But it is also easily damaged.

METHODS

Cupping methods are various. Cupping with fire, and cupping after boiling are commonly used in the clinic.

CUPPING WITH FIRE

Attach the cup to the skin by applying fire inside the cup to cause negative pressure. There are various manipulations as follows:

Fire twiddling method

Ignite a long piece of paper or cotton-wool ball, held by forceps, with alcohol and flame. Let it circle inside the cup, one to three times (taking care not to burn the rim), remove it from the cup

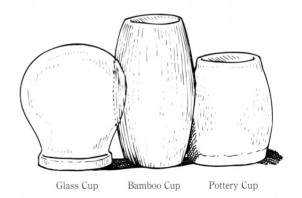

Glass Cup   Bamboo Cup   Pottery Cup

Fig. 161 Types of cup.

and place the cup on the selected position as quickly as possible. Since there is no fire in the cup, this method is safe and commonly used.

Fire throwing method

Throw a piece of ignited paper or cotton ball soaked in alcohol into the cup, then rapidly place the mouth of the cup firmly against the skin at a selected position. This method is applied for the side of the body.

Alcohol method

Drop 1–3 drops of 95% alcohol or strong spirit (not too much, to prevent burning the skin) into the cup, let it spread along the internal surface, ignite the alcohol, then place the cup rapidly onto the required place.

Cotton-wool sticking method

Stick a piece of a cotton-wool ball with alcohol to the lower one-third of the internal surface, ignite the cotton, then rapidly put the cup onto the given site.

Fire burning in the lid method

Fill a lid or a small glass, whose diameter is smaller than that of the cup, with a few drops of 95% alcohol or an alcohol-soaked cotton-wool

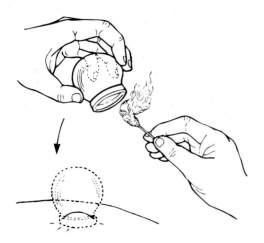

Fig. 162   Fire twiddling method.

ball. Put it on the selected site, ignite and rapidly place the cup over it.

The above-mentioned methods, except the fire twiddling method, are all employed with fire burning inside the cup, so care should be taken to prevent the skin from being burnt.

CUPPING AFTER BOILING

Boil 5–10 bamboo cups in water, take them out with the opening downwards, cover the opening quickly with a cold towel and rapidly place the cup on the affected site. The water may be mixed with herbal medicines which dispel *feng* and activate blood circulation, such as Qianghuo (*Rhizoma seu Radix Notopterygii*), Duhuo (*Radix Angelicas pubescentis*), Danggui (*Radix Angelicas sinensis*), Honghua (*Flos. Carthami*), Mahuang (*Herba Ephedrae*), Aiye (*Folium Artemisiae*), Chuanjiao (*Pericardium Zanthoxyli*), Mugua (*Fructus Chaenomelis*), Chuanniao (*Radix Aconiti*) or Caoniao (*Radix Aconiti kusnezoffii*), etc.

The method is called medicated cupping and is indicated in Bi syndromes due to *feng*, cold or damp.

In the above-mentioned methods, the cup may be retained on the point for 10–15 minutes until local congestion appears; if the cup is large, with a strong suction, the duration may be shortened for fear of causing blisters.

Indications for cupping are Bi syndromes (painful joints) caused by *feng*, cold or damp, common cold, cough, stomach-ache, vomiting, abdominal pain, diarrhoea, etc.

There are also some other cupping methods for application in the clinic according to the particular conditions.

Mobile cupping

This is also known as "pushing cup". Apply some lubricating oil, such as vaseline, onto the rim of the cup or the skin of the affected site. Put the cup on the skin then push the cup with the right hand back and forth, up and down, vertically or horizontally, until the local skin gets red, congested or even until a blood stasis is created.

This method is suitable for treating numbness, pain or Bi syndromes involving *feng* and damp, over large areas where the muscles are thick, such as the back, thighs, buttocks and lumbar region.

Quickly-replaced cupping

Put the cup on the skin then remove it at once. Repeat this procedure until the skin turns red, becomes congested or forms a blood stasis. It is often used to treat numbness of the skin, pain, and declined or weakened functions.

Bloodletting cupping

First sterilize the area for cupping. Then prick a small vein with a three-edged needle or tap the skin with an intradermal needle, and adopt cupping to promote the bloodletting. This is suitable for treating erysipelas, sprain, mastitis, etc.

Cupping while needling

This is also known as cupping on the needle. Place the cup over the needle which is inserted into the point, for 5–10 minutes until the skin becomes congested or a blood stasis forms. This method can combine the functions of both needling and cupping.

WITHDRAWING THE CUP

Don't try to remove the cup when the suction is too forceful. Hold the cup with the left hand, and press the skin around the rim of the cup with the right hand to allow air in.

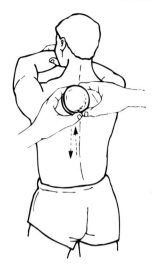

Fig. 163 Mobile cupping.

PRECAUTIONS

1. Cupping should be applied in a comfortable position and in an area with abundant muscle. An improper position, too much movement, or an area which is not flat or hairy, creates conditions unsuitable for cupping.
2. Cups of different sizes are used according to the requirements of the area. Manipulation must be quick enough to make the cup suck tightly.
3. Take care not to burn the skin—small blisters may be dressed with sterilized gauze to avoid them being broken. Large blisters should be punctured by a sterilized needle to let the fluid out, then apply gentian violet or dress them with sterilized gauze to keep them clean.
4. It is not advisable to apply cupping to a patient with skin ulcers, oedema, or on an area overlying large blood vessels. It is unsuitable for patients with high fever and convulsions, or on abdominal or sacral regions in pregnant women.

NOTES

1. *Miraculous Pivot*, Ch. 51, "Back-Shu Points".

Other needling methods 6

THE THREE-EDGED NEEDLE METHOD

The three-edged needle was known as the *feng zhen* (锋针), or "sharp-edged needle" in ancient times.

In the *Miraculous Pivot* it states that, "for stubborn stagnation, or blockage of the meridians, or for diseases of the five zang organs with long-term stagnancy, the sharp-edged needle is selected . . . it is made in the form of a needle with a round handle, triangular head and sharp tip, and causes bleeding by pricking so as to eliminate heat and treat stubborn diseases which occur through stasis; and is also indicated for carbuncles and fever".[1]

These were the earliest records of treating diseases with three-edged needles.

MANIPULATION

Hold the handle with the thumb and index finger of one hand. Support the triangular head with the middle finger, with 0.1–0.2 inch exposed to control the depth of pricking. Hold and squeeze tightly the end of the patient's finger or toe with the other hand (by pinching up or stretching the skin), and then perform the needling.

The following manipulations are commonly used:

— spot pricking,
— collateral pricking,
— clumpy pricking,
— pinching and pricking.

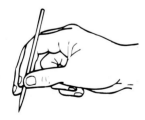

Fig. 164   Holding the three-edged needle.

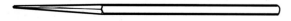

Fig. 165   The three-edged needle.

Spot pricking

Heavy massage is given to the area around the point to encourage the bloodletting through local congestion. Routine disinfection is given, then hold the handle of the needle with the right hand, prick swiftly about 0.3 cm deep, accurately at the point, and withdraw the needle immediately. Then squeeze out a few drops of blood and press the puncture hole with a sterilized dry cotton ball to stop the bleeding.

Collateral pricking

Puncture slowly with the three-edged needle into the superficial veins at the sterilized area to obtain a little blood, and then press the puncture hole with a sterilized dry cotton ball to stop bleeding.

Clinically this method is often used, for example, in pricking collaterals or superficial veins at the cubital and popliteal fossa to treat heatstroke, or else for multiple pricking at the red lines which appear in acute lymphangitis, to let out a small amount of blood.

Clumpy pricking

The *Miraculous Pivot* states that "Clumpy pricking means giving multiple punctures around the affected site to obtain blood from the jingluo".[2]

There are two methods of application according to differing conditions of the disease: either puncture around the sterilized lesion in order to cause bleeding for treating stubborn ringworm, carbuncles or swellings in an early stage (not yet purulent), or else clumpy pricking given onto the sterilized areas of a haematoma in order to let blood in the treatment of sprains and contusions.

Pinching and pricking

Pinch up the skin, or press both sides of the site with the left hand, and then prick superficially the sterilized point or reactive areas with the needle in the right hand. Use the left hand to let out a small amount of blood. Alternatively, puncture further about 0.5 cm deep and tip the three-edged needle obliquely and very slightly upward to break apart some of the fibrous tissues underneath the skin. Then again give local sterilization and apply dressings.

Reactive areas look like skin eruptions, usually brown, pink, grey or dark brown in colour, and should be differentiated from folliculitis and pigmental maculae. If the reactive areas are not distinctive, massage or rubbing can be applied to make them stand out. For example, in haemorrhoids, a reactive area often appears at the lumbar-sacral region or at the Baliao points (UB 31–34, Shangliao, Ciliao, Zhongliao and Xialiao).

In styes, reactive areas may appear at the apex of the ear, Dazhui (Du 14) or the shoulder. In scrofula there may be reactive areas at the neck, and on the vertebral sides of the scapula.

Such pinching up and pricking can be done once every 3–7 days, and 3–5 treatments comprise one course of treatment. After 10–14 days start the second course.

INDICATIONS

The three-edged needle restores consciousness, purges heat, activates blood circulation and removes obstruction from the jingluo. It is indicated for excess syndromes, heat syndromes or cold excess syndromes.

At the present time, it is frequently applied in the treatment of both acute and chronic conditions, such as unconsciousness (coma), hyperpyrexia, heatstroke, the tense syndromes of *feng* stroke, acute congested or sore throat, congested and swollen eyes, stubborn ringworms, carbuncles in their initial stage, sprains, contusions, malnutrition, indigestion, haemorrhoids, long-term Bi syndromes, headaches, erysipelas, or numbness of the fingers or toes.

PRECAUTIONS

1. The three-edged needle produces a strong intensity of stimulation, and should be applied only when the patient is in a comfortable position and cooperating with the operator. Attention should be paid to avoid the patient fainting during treatment.

2. The three-edged needle leaves open a large puncture hole after needling, therefore strict aseptic technique should be applied prior to needling in order to prevent infection.
3. For spot-pricking and clumpy pricking, the operation should be applied superficially and rapidly, to avoid injuring the large arteries, and the bleeding should not be excessive (a few drops will do).
4. Pricking must in no case be applied to those with a weak constitution, deficiency of both qi and blood, or those susceptible to bleeding.
5. Pricking can be applied once every day or every other day, 3–5 treatments constituting one course; in acute cases it can be given twice a day; if more bleeding is required, it is advisable to apply pricking 1–2 times a week.

THE CUTANEOUS NEEDLE METHOD

The cutaneous needle is also known as the plum-blossom needle or seven-star needle, as it is made of five to seven stainless steel needles in the shape of the seedpod of a lotus inlaid into one end of a handle.

The *Plain Questions* states that "The collaterals and vessels of the 12 meridians supply the cutaneous regions superficially, so the occurrence of various diseases always starts in the skin and pores".[3] The twelve cutaneous regions are closely related to the jingluo and zangfu organs, and the cutaneous needle is applied to prick these regions superficially by tapping, which activates and regulates the functions of the zangfu organs and jingluo in order to treat the disease.

MANIPULATION

Hold the posterior part of the handle with the index finger pressing on the handle (see Fig. 166).

After routine sterilization of the local area, tap vertically on the prescribed area of the skin with a light, flexible movement of the wrist.

Mild, moderate or strong stimulation is applied according to differing constitutions, ages,

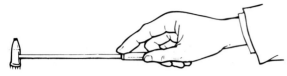

Fig. 166 Holding the cutaneous needle.

the conditions of the disease and the area to be tapped.

Mild stimulation is applied by light tapping until the local skin becomes slightly congested but without pain; it is indicated for the aged or senile, women and children, deficiency cases, disorders on the head, face, eye, ear, mouth, and nose, or on places where the muscles are thin.

Strong stimulation is applied by heavy tapping until slight bleeding and pain appears; it is indicated for patients with strong constitutions and in excess cases, and for disorders on the shoulders, back, lower back, and buttocks, and on places where there are thick muscles.

Moderate stimulation is applied by moderate tapping, until there is local congestion and slight pain but no bleeding. It is indicated for most patients and diseases, except those located on the head and face and on places with thin muscle.

AREAS TO BE TAPPED

The area to be tapped may be along the course of the meridian, or over the points prescribed, or over an affected local area.

Tapping along the course of the meridian

This is a method of tapping which is most often applied on the nape, back and lumbosacral regions along the Du and bladder meridians, as the Du meridian has the function of regulating the yang qi of the whole body and the Back-Shu points of the zangfu organs, which have a wide scope of indications, are distributed along the bladder meridian.

It is also applied along the jingluo on the lower limbs below the elbow and knee joints, where the *yuan*, *luo*, Xi-Cleft and 5 Shu points are located. Thus it is indicated for diseases of their corresponding zangfu organs and jingluo.

Tapping the prescribed points

Tapping the prescribed points is a method based on the main therapeutic properties of the points. The points frequently used in the clinic are specific points, the Huatuojiaji (Extra 19) and Ashi points.

Local tapping

Local tapping means tapping over an affected area or just over the lesion. For instance in treating local congestion, swelling or pain after sprain, or in treating stubborn ringworm, clumpy or surrounding tappings can be applied locally.

INDICATIONS

Cutaneous needling tapping is often used for treatment of headache, flank pain, back pain along the spinal column, lumbar pain, skin numbness, nervous dermatitis, hypertension, insomnia, chronic gastrointestinal diseases, indigestion, dysmenorrhoea, alopecia areata, stubborn ringworm-type diseases and myopia.

PRECAUTIONS

The tips of the needles should be level with each other and not hooked, and the head and handle of the needle should be firmly jointed to avoid possible movement of the head during tapping.

When tapping, the tips of the needles should strike the skin at right angles to the surface to avoid causing any pain.

When giving treatment along the meridian, a single tapping is given at about each centimetre, and generally 8–16 tappings given along the meridian constitute one treatment.

Sterilize the needles and the local area to be tapped; after heavy tapping, the blood should be cleared and the skin surface cleaned and sterilized again to prevent infection. Tapping is contraindicated for places where there are ulcers or wounds.

THE INTRADERMAL NEEDLE METHOD

The intradermal needle is also known as the

"embedded needle" (埋针). It has developed from the ancient method of retaining needles which is recorded in the *Plain Questions*, where it says "the needle is retained there statically for a long time".[4]

A needle shaped like a thumbtack, or piece of grain, is inserted into the skin and fixed or retained there for a certain period of time in order to give the cutaneous regions a weak, but long-term, stimulation. This regulates the functions of the jingluo and zangfu organs with the purpose of preventing and treating disease (see Fig. 167).

MANIPULATION

Firstly, make sure that the intradermal needles, forceps and areas where the needles are to be embedded are strictly sterilized. Hold the body of the grain-like needle with forceps and insert it horizontally into the point for about 0.5–1 cm, then embed the needle there by placing the handle so that it lies flat against the skin surface, fixing it there with a piece of adhesive tape.

Alternatively, hold the ring of the thumbtack needle with forceps and insert the needle accurately into the prescribed point, with the ring-shaped handle lying flat on the skin. Then fix it with a piece of adhesive tape. This particular type of embedded needle is often used in auricular points.

The duration of implant varies with different seasons—in summer the needles are embedded and retained generally for 1–2 days, and on cold days for 3–7 days, during which time manipulation by pressing the needle for 1–2 minutes is given every 4 hours. This increases the stimulation and potentiates the therapeutic effect.

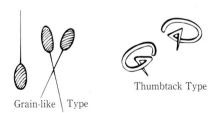

Grain-like Type

Thumbtack Type

Fig. 167 Intradermal needles.

INDICATIONS

The embedded needling method is often used in the treatment of protracted disease, or painful diseases with repeated attacks in which long-term retention of the needle is required. For example, headache, Bi syndromes of the shoulder, trigeminal neuralgia, toothache, gastric pain, irregular menstruation, dysmenorrhoea, nocturnal enuresis, insomnia, hypertension, asthma and coughing.

PRECAUTIONS

1. Needles are not embedded at the joints, or on regions of the chest or abdomen in order to prevent pain on motion or during respiration.
2. After embedding, if pain or difficulty in movement is felt, the needles should be taken out and embedded again at other selected points.
3. During the embedding period, keep the area around the needle free from contact with water, and avoid long periods of implantation during hot weather in order to prevent infection due to the patient sweating.

THE ELECTRONEEDLING METHOD

Electroneedling is a particular kind of therapeutic method in which a small electrical charge, similar to the biological electricity of the human body, is applied to needles already in points where the *de qi* has already been found. This has the advantage of combining the stimulation of both needling and electricity, and thus can potentiate the effect of the treatment.

Furthermore, with electroneedling the intensity of the stimulation can be properly controlled and a tiring manipulation by hand avoided.

THE SELECTION OF ELECTROSTIMULATORS

There are different sorts of electrostimulators. At present those most commonly used include those which incorporate buzzers, valves and semiconductors. These use an oscillator which sends out a pulsating current, of low frequency, which is similar to that of the bioelectricity charge produced within the human body.

The electrostimulator can be used for electroneedling by setting the spot or plate electrodes directly onto the selected points on the skin, or onto the area of the disease. Those machines which have a variable power control, are well-insulated and safe in use, have a choice of power source (such as dry batteries), low power consumption, and a small size (which makes them portable), and also are silent, are the best ones to use.

MANIPULATION

Point-prescriptions

Generally the points used are similar to those used in filiform needling. However the points selected should be in pairs and generally 1–3 pairs of points (with 1–3 pairs of wires), unilaterally on the same side, are selected.

Selecting too many points would produce too strong a stimulation which may become intolerable to the patient.

Method of application

Electroneedling is applied after the needling sensation is obtained (except in patients with mental disorders or numbness, or in children). Then turn the output to zero, apply the negative electrode onto the main point and the positive electrode onto the secondary point (or any random point). Turn the power on, select a desired wave-form and slowly increase the output until it reaches the desired level. Apply electricity generally for 5–20 minutes, although this can be extended during acupuncture anaesthesia.

To prevent the needling sensation gradually reducing, a certain increase in the output can be made. Otherwise the electricity can be cut off for 1–2 minutes and then applied again to ensure an adequate intensity of stimulation.

If only one point is needed for the treatment, apply one of the paired wires onto the handle of the needle which is in the point, and the other wire onto a thin aluminium plate about 25 cm² in size, which is then wrapped around with several layers of gauze and placed flat, fixed to the skin some distance from the needle. In this way a marked stimulation at the point and a weak stimulation at the plate is obtained.

Intensity of the electricity

The numb and pricking sensation caused by the electricity is known as the "sensory threshold". The painful sensation caused by increasing the intensity of the electrical charge is known as the "pain threshold". Both will vary with the individual and the condition of the disease.

Generally speaking, those charges which cause a sensation between the sense threshold and the pain threshold are the intensities most suitable to treatment. But this is a narrow range and it needs careful regulation. An intensity greater than the pain threshold is difficult for the patient to bear, and an intensity which the patient can tolerate is the best choice.

THE FUNCTION OF THE PULSATING CURRENT

The body's tissues consist of water, inorganic salts and charged bio-colloids, forming together a complex electrolytic conductor. When the human body is acted on by a pulsating current, in which wave-form and frequency are constantly changing, the ions in the tissues will acquire directional motion, eliminating the polarized state of the cell membrane, which further affects the functions of the body's tissue.

Changes in ion concentration and distribution are the most basic electrophysiological changes in the treatment with an electric current. Low frequency electricity is applied through the needle, stimulating the point to obtain an effect which regulates the general functioning of the human body, potentiates analgesic and tranquillizing effects, promotes the circulation of qi and blood and regulates muscle tone.

The effect of a low-frequency pulsating electric charge varies with different wave-forms and frequencies. Those waves with a high frequency (50–100 times per second) are called dense waves, those with low frequency (2–5 times per second) are called sparse waves. Some stimulators have a means of varying a continuous wave so that sparse and dense waves can be selected at will. Some stimulators have separate means of producing dense waves, sparse waves, dense-sparse waves, intermittent waves, etc., all in order to provide a clinical selection best suited to the conditions of the disease, and in order to potentiate the therapeutic effect.

The dense wave

This can reduce the stressed functioning of the nervous system via, firstly, its inhibitive action on sensory nerves and, secondly, its inhibitive action on motor nerves. It is often applied for relieving pain, encouraging tranquillity, relieving muscular and vascular spasms, and acupuncture anaesthesia.

The sparse wave

Along with a strong stimulation, this can cause contraction of the muscles, and increase muscle tone and the strength of the ligaments. Its inhibitive action on sensory and motor nerves is rather slow. It is often used in treating Wei syndromes, injuries of the joints, ligaments and tendons, and muscles.

The dense-sparse wave

This is a wave-form with the alternate appearance of dense waves and sparse waves, each of which lasts for about 1.5 seconds, thus avoiding the disadvantages of a single wave which can easily be adapted to by the patient. It has a strong dynamic action and its excitative effect is best during treatment, when it promotes the body's metabolism and the circulation of qi and blood, improves the nourishment of the tissues and eliminates inflammatory oedema.

It is often used to relieve pain, for sprains, bruising, peripheral shoulder arthritis, disturbance of qi and blood circulation, sciatica, facial paralysis, myasthenia and local cold injuries.

The intermittent wave

This occurs at regular intervals—the interval lasting for 1.5 seconds—and then the dense wave starting to work for 1.5 seconds. It is difficult for the organism to adapt to this effect, and its dynamic action is great. It can enhance the excitation of muscular tissue and produce a good contraction of striated muscle.

It is often used in treating Wei syndrome, paralysis and in electromuscular gymnastic training.

The serrated wave

This has an undulating wave-form with a serrated change in amplitude. Its frequency is 16–20 or 20–25 times per minute which is similar to the respiratory rhythm in humans, and so can be used to stimulate the phrenic nerve (corresponding to point Tianding, LI 17) for artificial electrorespiration in emergency treatment of respiratory failure (where there is still a weak heartbeat).

It can enhance the excitation of the nerves and muscles, regulate the functions of the jingluo and improve the circulation of qi and blood.

INDICATIONS

Electroneedling has the same range of indications as filiform needling and thus a wide scope. Clinically it is often used in treating all kinds of pain, Bi syndromes, Wei syndromes, dysfunctions of the heart, stomach, intestines, gallbladder, urinary bladder and uterus, depressive-manic psychosis, injuries to the muscles, ligaments and joints, and in acupuncture anaesthesia.

PRECAUTIONS

1. Check the electrostimulator before use. Attention should be paid to the contact made by the wires, and batteries should be renewed when necessary.
2. If the output electric potential is over 40 volts, the maximum output current should be controlled within one milliampere to avoid accidental electrical shocks. A direct or pulsating direct current may easily cause broken needles or burn

the tissues, so it cannot be used as the output current for electrostimulators.

3. When regulating the intensity of the electrical charge, it is necessary to increase it slowly and gradually; a sudden rapid increase would cause a sudden muscular contraction which the patient could not tolerate, and which may cause bent or broken needles or fainting.

4. When electroneedling is applied for heart diseases, avoid the current loop passing the heart. When applying electroneedling near the medulla and spinal cord, the output should be small to avoid accidents. It can be used in pregnant women only with great caution.

5. When applying electricity to needles in which the conductivity of the handle of the needle has been impaired by its use as a warming needle (owing to the oxidation of the surface), or onto needles where the handles have been gilded a golden yellow colour by oxidization (for various reasons), the wires can be connected directly to the body of the needle.

POINT-INJECTION THERAPY (HYDRO-ACUPUNCTURE THERAPY)

This is a method of injecting liquid medicine into acupoints in order to prevent and treat disease. It combines the permeating and stimulating functions of needles and medicine, and can enhance both their therapeutic effects in treating disease.

COMMONLY USED MEDICINES

All the drugs that can be used for muscular injection can be used in (point-injection therapy). The most frequently used herbal medicines are: Danggui (Chinese angelica root), Honghua (Carthamus), Chinese angelica in compound prescription, Banlangen (Isatis root), Xuchangqing (Cynanchi Paniculati), Dengzhanhua (Erigerontis herb), Buguzhi (Psoralea), Zhongjiefeng (Sarcandra), Chaihu (Bupleurum root), Yuxingcao (Houttuynia), Salvia in compound prescription, and Chuanxiong (Cnidium).

Western medicines which can be used are: 25% magnesium sulphate, Vitamin B1, B12, Vitamin C and K3, 0.25–2% Novocain, atropine, reserpine, ephedrine, antibiotics, fluid from placental tissue, normal saline, etc.

THERAPEUTIC METHODS

Instruments

Syringes of 1, 2, 5, 10 and 20 ml capacity, with No. 5 needles for dental use, No. 7 for general medical use, or No. 5–6° for use when injecting generally. Use No. 9 long needles for deep injections.

Selection of points

The fewer points the better, generally 2–4, are selected as the main points for treatment according to the conditions of the disease. Points at places where there is thick muscle are often selected. "Ashi points" (tender spots), where there is a positive reactive area, with nodules or cord-like nodules, can also be selected.

Dosage of injection

The injection should be applied according to the dose stipulated in the medicine instructions; overdosage should be avoided. If the amount is small, then $\frac{1}{5} - \frac{1}{2}$ of the original dosage can be applied; generally, on the head and face 0.3–0.5 ml can be used, 0.1 ml in auricular points, 1–2 ml in points on the limbs, 0.5–1 ml in points on the chest and back, 2–5 ml in points on the lumbar and gluteal regions. If 5–10% glucose solution is also injected, the dosage can be as much as 10–20 ml.

Manipulation

Ask the patient to take a comfortable position, get the strictly sterilized syringe with needle ready, and suck up the medicinal fluid. Sterilize the local area of the points selected. Puncture rapidly into the points (or positive reactive areas) and insert the needles slowly.

After the *de qi*, suck back a little and, if no blood is seen, inject the medicine into the point.

The speed of injection varies with the demands of the treatment: rapid injection in excess heat syndromes, slow injection in deficiency cold syndromes.

Duration of treatment

For acute cases, treatment is given once or twice a day; for chronic cases, once a day or every other day. Six to ten treatments constitute one course.

PRECAUTIONS

1. Attention should be paid to the properties, pharmaceutical action, dosage, expiry date, contraindications and incompatibility, side-effects and hypersensitive reactions of the medicines. Patients with hypersensitive reactions to such medicines as penicillin, streptomycin and procaine should undergo a skin test before point injection. Avoid using medicines with severe side-effects and be careful when using those with strong stimulating actions.

2. Over-deep puncture should be avoided in points on the neck and nape, chest and back, and the dosage should be controlled and the speed of injection slow in these places.

When injecting near nerve trunks, be careful to avoid them or puncture only superficially (not too deep), or else manoeuvre the needle in deeper than the location of the nerve trunks if they are superficial.

If the tip of the needle touches a nerve (manifest by an electric shock in the patient), draw the needle back and change direction to avoid the nerve, and then apply the injection. Thus you may manage to avoid causing injuries or unfavourable side-effects.

3. Avoid an injection of medicinal fluid into the blood vessels (suck back and if there is blood, withdraw the needle and try in another direction so as to avoid the vessels).

Avoid injection into a joint cavity or spinal cavity, otherwise a reaction of redness, swelling or pain in the joint, or injury to the spinal cord would result. Great attention should be paid to this.

4. Point-injection therapy is contraindicated for points on the lower abdomen, lumbosacral regions, Sanyinjiao (Sp 6) and Hegu (LI 4) in pregnant women. When using point-injection therapy with aged and senile patients the points selected should be fewer and the dosage of the medicine reduced somewhat.

5. The syringe, needle and the sites for injection should be strictly sterilized. Avoid using syringes which leak air or needles which are hooked.

6. Pay attention to the prevention of fainting, and avoid bent needles and broken needles during injection. If such accidents do occur, their management is the same as that for filiform needles.

NOTES

1. *Miraculous Pivot*, Ch. 78, "Discussion on the 9 Needles".
2. *Miraculous Pivot*, Ch. 7, "The Just Choice of Needle".
3. *Plain Questions*, Ch. 56, "Discussion on the Cutaneous Regions".
4. *Plain Questions*, Ch. 27, "The Interrelationship of the Pathogenic and Antipathogenic Qi".

Scalp acupuncture and ear acupuncture

Scalp acupuncture

Scalp acupuncture is a therapeutic method which uses acupuncture on specific stimulating areas of the scalp. Clinically it is often applied in the treatment of disease with a cerebral or encephalic origin.

LOCATIONS AND ACTIONS OF THE AREAS

In order to determine the stimulating areas, two standard lines should be fixed beforehand as guidelines.

These are the anterior–posterior midline of the head, which is a line linking the glabella (the anterior end of the midline) and the lower border of the external occipital protuberance (the posterior end of the midline), via the vertex of the head; and the eyebrow–occiput line, which links the upper border of the midpoint of the eyebrow and the tip of the external occipital protuberance (see Fig. 168).

MOTOR AREA

Location

Draw a line starting from the "upper point", which is a point 0.5 cm posterior to the midpoint of the anterior–posterior midline of the head, and stretching diagonally across to the juncture of the eyebrow–occiput line and the anterior border of the corner of the temporal hairline.

If the temporal hairline is indistinct, draw upwardly a vertical line from the midpoint of the zygomatic arch to cross the eyebrow–occiput line—the point 0.5 cm anterior to the crossing point of this line from the zygomatic arch and the eyebrow–occiput line is the "lower point" of the Motor Area; the line joining the "upper point" and the "lower point" delineates the Motor Area.

The Motor Area is divided into three regions, upper, middle and lower:

a) Upper region—upper one-fifth, for disorders of the lower limbs and trunk.
b) Middle region—middle two-fifths, for disorders of the upper limbs.
c) Lower region—lower two-fifths, for facial disorders; it is also the Speech Area I.

Indications

a) Upper region—paralysis of the lower limb of the opposite side and the trunk.
b) Middle region—paralysis of the upper limb on the opposite side.
c) Lower region—central nerve facial paralysis on the opposite side, motor aphasia, dribbling saliva and aphonia.

SENSORY AREA

Location

A line parallel with and 1.5 cm posterior to the

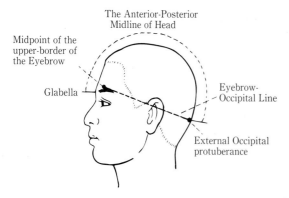

Fig. 168 Standard lines of measurement.

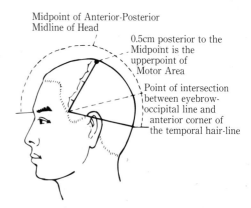

Fig. 169 Location of motor area.

Motor Area. It is divided into three regions, upper, middle and lower:

a) Upper region—upper one-fifth, the area of the lower limbs, head and trunk.
b) Middle region—middle two-fifths, the area of the upper limbs.
c) Lower region—lower two-fifths, the area of the face.

Indications

a) Upper region—low back and leg pain of the opposite side, numbness and paraesthesia, occipital headache, pain in the nape, vertigo and tinnitus.
b) Middle region—pain, numbness and paraesthesia of the upper limb of the opposite side.
c) Lower region—facial numbness, migraine and temporomandibular arthritis on the opposite side.

CHOREA/TREMOR CONTROL AREA

Location

A line parallel with and 1.5 cm anterior to the Motor Area line (see Fig. 170).

Indications

Chorea, Parkinson's disease (shaking palsy) and parkinsonian syndromes.

VERTIGO/AUDITORY AREA

Location

With a point 1.5 cm directly above the apex of the ear as the midpoint, draw a horizontal line 4 cm in length (see Fig. 170).

Indications

Vertigo, tinnitus and impaired hearing.

SPEECH AREA II

Location

A vertical line 3 cm in length, which is 2 cm posterior and inferior to the parietal tubercle and parallel with the anterior–posterior midline (see Fig. 170).

Indications

Nominal aphasia (disturbance in naming).

SPEECH AREA III

Location

A line parallel to, and overlapping the Vertigo/Auditory Area. It is 4 cm in length and extends posterior to the midpoint of the Vertigo/Auditory Area line (see Fig. 170).

Indications

Sensory aphasia (disturbance in understanding speech).

PRAXIS AREA

Location

Three lines each 3 cm in length; one is drawn vertically from the parietal tubercle, the other two are drawn also from the parietal tubercle but anteriorly and posteriorly to the former vertical line, forming a 40 degree angle respectively to the vertical line (see Fig. 170).

Indications

Apraxia (in which there is normal muscular tone

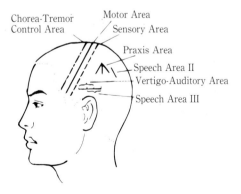

Fig. 170 Stimulating areas (side view).

and performance of basic muscular movements, but disturbance in complex activities such as unbuttoning clothes or picking up a coin).

FOOT MOTOR-SENSORY AREA

Location

From a point 1 cm lateral to the midpoint of the anterior–posterior line of the head, draw a line posteriorly 3 cm in length and parallel with the midline; the line is bilateral (see Fig. 171).

Indications

Paralysis, pain or numbness of the lower limb of the opposite side, acute lumbar sprain, nocturnal enuresis, cortical polyuria and prolapse of the uterus.

VISUAL AREA

Location

A bilateral line, which is parallel with, and 1 cm lateral to the anterior–posterior midline of the head, 4 cm in length and extending upwards from the horizontal line of the external occipital protuberance (see Fig. 172).

Indications

Cortical vision problems.

BALANCE AREA

Location

A bilateral line, which is parallel with, and 3.5 cm lateral to the anterior–posterior midline of the head, 4 cm in length and extending downwards from the horizontal line of the external occipital protuberance (see Fig. 172).

Indications

Disturbance in balance, ataxia and vertigo due to disorders of the cerebellum; numbness or paralysis of the limbs due to functional disturbance of the brain stem.

GASTRIC AREA

Location

A line 2 cm in length, parallel with the anterior–posterior midline of the head, running posteriorly from the hairline directly above the pupil of the eye (see Fig. 173).

Indications

Gastric pain and epigastric distress caused by gastroenteritis and gastric ulcers.

THORACIC CAVITY AREA

Location

A bilateral line, drawn midway between, and parallel to the Gastric Area line and the anterior–posterior midline of head, 4 cm in length (2 cm superior and 2 cm inferior to the anterior hairline respectively) (see Fig. 173).

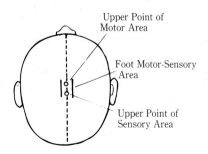

Fig. 171   Stimulating areas (top view).

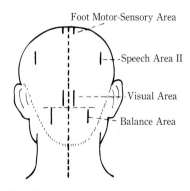

Fig. 172   Stimulating areas (back view).

Indications

Bronchial asthma, discomfort or disorders in the chest, etc.

GENITAL AREA

Location

A line 2 cm in length, parallel with the anterior–posterior midline of the head, running upwards from the corner of the head (see Fig. 173).

Indications

Functional uterine bleeding, pelvic inflammation, prolapse of the uterus, etc.

METHODS OF SELECTING AREAS

For diseases of only one side, select areas on the opposite side. For diseases located on both sides, bilateral areas are selected. For diseases of the internal organs and constitutional diseases, bilateral corresponding areas are selected with the related areas selected in combination; for example, in paralysis of the lower limbs, the Motor Area of the lower limb in combination with the Foot Motor Area can be selected.

MANIPULATION

After a correct diagnosis has been made and the

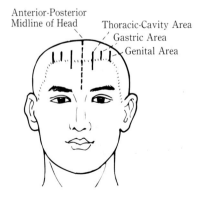

Fig. 173 Stimulating areas (front view).

Anterior-Posterior Midline of Head
Thoracic-Cavity Area
Gastric Area
Genital Area

stimulating areas selected, ask the patient to co-operate with the treatment and apply routine sterilization onto the local scalp. Then select stainless steel filiform needles No. 26–30 in gauge and 1.5–2.5 cun in length. Needling must accord with the following:

Rapid insertion

Insert the needle rapidly into the subcutaneous or muscle layer at an angle of 30 degrees (formed between the needle tip and the scalp), then push rapidly (without rotation) along the stimulating area selected to the required distance and depth (and then perhaps rotate the needle).

High frequency of needle rotation

The swift rotation method proceeds as follows. First, have a settled position for the shoulder, elbow, wrist joint and thumb in order to stabilize the needle shaft. Then hold the handle of the needle with the radial aspect of the distal phalanx of the index finger and the distal phalanx of the thumb. The metacarpal-phalangeal joint of the index finger is constantly flexed and extended making the needle rotate rapidly at a frequency of 200 times per minute (moving back and forth during each movement). Keep rotating the needle for 30–60 seconds, and then after an interval of 5–10 minutes, repeat the same manipulation again twice. Finally withdraw the needle.

A swift rotation can produce a strong needling sensation and thus enhance the therapeutic effect in treating certain diseases.

During manipulation, movement of the affected sites or limbs helps to enhance the effect. In general, after 3–5 minutes, sensations of heat, numbness, distension, coolness or twitching may appear at the affected sites (limbs or internal organs) in patients where good therapeutic effects may result. Electroneedling can be applied instead of manual manipulation (see Fig. 174 and Fig. 175).

Withdrawal of the needle

Withdraw the needle rapidly if there is no tight

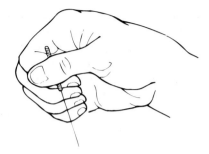

Fig. 174   Holding the needle for scalp acupuncture.

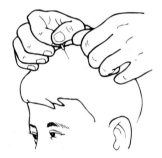

Fig. 175   Rotating the needle in scalp acupuncture.

sensation underneath, otherwise bring back the needle slowly. Press the puncture hole with a sterilized dry cotton ball for a while after withdrawing the needle to avoid bleeding.

Duration of treatment

Treatment is given once a day or every other day; 10–15 treatments constitute one course. A second course can be started after 5–7 days interval.

INDICATIONS

Scalp needling is indicated mainly in cerebral or encephalic diseases, such as paralysis, numbness, aphasia, vertigo, tinnitus, chorea, etc.

In addition, it is also indicated in commonly seen and frequently encountered diseases such as low back and leg pain, nocturnal enuresis, trigeminal neuralgia, peripheral shoulder arthritis and various kinds of neuralgia. Scalp needling can also be applied during surgical operations under acupuncture anaesthesia.

Scalp acupuncture has only a short history of application and there is progress to be made in developing its scope of indications in clinic practice.

PRECAUTIONS

1. Strict sterilization should be applied over the hair of the scalp to prevent infection.
2. If the needle is obstructed or pain is felt by the patient whilst pushing in the needle, bring back the needle to the superficial region, change the angle of needling and push it forward again.
3. Scalp needling gives a strong needling sensation and requires a long period of stimulation. Attention should be paid to the expression and feelings of the patient during treatment in order to prevent fainting.
4. In cases of cerebral haemorrhage scalp acupuncture can be applied only when the disease has stabilized and the blood pressure become stable. Scalp acupuncture is contraindicated in acute cases complicated by high fever or heart failure.

Ear acupuncture

The therapy of ear acupuncture treats and helps prevent disease by stimulating certain points on the auricle with needles. It has the advantage of a wide scope of indications, and is convenient to apply. Furthermore it can also be employed during surgical operations under acupuncture anaesthesia. The observation and examination of the ear also has a definite significance in the diagnosis of disease.

Ear acupuncture has long been used in China, and it is recorded in the *Miraculous Pivot* that "a *jue* headache with symptoms of acute pain in the head, and a hot sensation in the preauricular and retroauricular vessels, should be treated by blood-letting in order to reduce the heat, and then be followed by needling points of the meridian of foot Shaoyang".[1]

In a later chapter it states that "When pathogenic factors attack the liver, it causes pain in the flanks... the blue veins in the ear can be selected and needled to relieve the dragging pain".[2] In the *Prescriptions Worth A Thousand Gold Coin* there are records of selecting auricular points in treating jaundice, and in conditions where cold or hot toxins have caused disease. It also speaks of selecting the point "at the hairline above the ear" when treating goitre.

In other classical medical literature of the past there are descriptions of stimulating certain auricular areas with needles, moxibustion, massage, herbal suppositories or blowing on the ear, to treat and help prevent disease; and also information on inspection and palpation of the ear in diagnosing disease. These methods are still used as folk remedies, and all suggest a long history of auricular therapy in China.

THE RELATIONSHIP BETWEEN THE EAR, THE JINGLUO AND THE ZANGFU

The ear has a very close relationship with the jingluo. In the *Miraculous Pivot*[3] it is recorded that a branch luo of the hand Yangming meridian enters into the ear, the foot Yangming meridian ascends to the preauricular region, the hand Taiyang meridian enters into the ear, a branch of the foot Taiyang meridian reaches the upper corner of the ear, the hand Shaoyang meridian winds around the back of the ear and emerges from the upper corner while a branch enters into the ear, the foot Shaoyang meridian descends via the retroauricular region while a branch reaches the inside of the ear and emerges in front.

These few examples indicate that every one of the three yang meridians of the hands and feet relates to the ear. The yin meridians communicate with the ear via their divergent meridians which connect with the yang meridians.

Among the extra meridians, the Yinqiao and Yangqiao run to the retroauricular region, and the Yangwei runs along the head and enters into the ear. This is why it is recorded in the *Miraculous Pivot* that "the ear is the place where all the various major meridians converge".[4] Besides this, the muscle regions of the hand Taiyang meridian also enter into the ear.

Therefore it can be seen that the relationship between the ear and the jingluo throughout the body is very close.

The ear also has a close relationship with the zangfu because all the jingluo which enter into the ear have a relationship with the zangfu. In the *Miraculous Pivot* it is stated that "the kidney qi communicates with the ear and a harmonized kidney ensures sound hearing".[5] It also states in the *Plain Questions* that "in liver disease,... deficiency leads to impaired hearing,... and rebellion of the qi leads to headaches and deafness".[6] And in *A Plumbline for Treatment* it states that "lung qi deficiency leads to qi deficiency in the body... resulting in deafness".

All these indicate that the ear and the zangfu organs are very closely related to each other, both in physiology and pathology.

The close relationship between the ear and the zangfu shows that the ear is not only an organ of hearing, but also an integral part of the whole body. Ear-points may be used as acupoints for acupuncture and moxibustion in treating disease at various other sites in the body, and examination and inspection of positive reactive areas on the auricular surface may also be used as reference in the diagnosis of disease.

ANATOMICAL TERMINOLOGY OF THE AURICULAR SURFACE

To facilitate the location of ear-points, it is necessary to become familiar with the anatomical terminology of the auricular surface (see Fig. 176)

Helix. The prominent rim of the ear. The transverse ridge of the helix continuing backward into the ear cavity is the "helix crus"; the small tubercle at the posterior-inferior aspect of the helix is the "helix tubercle"; the inferior part of the helix, at the junction of the helix and the ear-lobe is the "helix cauda".

Antihelix. The elevated ridge anterior and opposite to the helix is the principal part of antihelix; its upper part branches out into the superior and inferior antihelix crura.

Triangular fossa. The triangular depression between the superior antihelix crus and the inferior antihelix crus.

Scapha. The narrow curved depression between

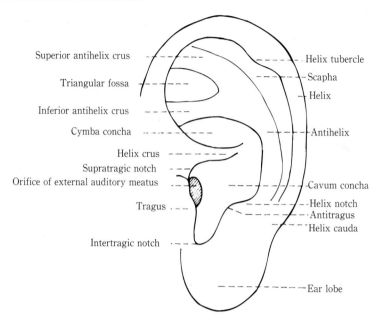

Fig. 176   Anatomical structure of the auricular surface.

the helix and the antihelix; it is also known as the scaphoid fossa.

Tragus.   The small, curved flap or prominence in front of the ear.

Supratragic notch.   The depression between the upper border of the tragus and the helix crus.

Antitragus.   The small tubercle inferior to the antihelix and opposite to the tragus.

Intertragic notch.   The depression between the tragus and the antitragus.

Antitragus helix notch.   The slightly depressed part between the antitragus and antihelix.

Ear lobe.   The lowest part of the ear without cartilage.

Cymba concha.   The concha superior to the helix crus.

Cavum concha.   The concha inferior to the helix crus.

Orifice of the external auditory meatus.   The opening in the cavum concha.

THE DISTRIBUTION OF EAR-POINTS

When disease occurs in different parts of the human body, various positive reactions may appear in corresponding areas on the ear. These reactions may be a sensation of tenderness, morphological change, discoloration, blisters, nodules, papules, depressions, exfoliations or decreased cutaneous electric resistance.

These sites are the stimulating spots for auricular acupuncture, which are used in the treatment and prevention of disease, and thus are known as "ear-points".

Ear-points are distributed on the ear in a certain pattern, like the points on the picture of an upside-down fetus. Points located on the lobe are related to the head and facial region, those on the scapha are related to the upper limbs, those on the antihelix and its two crura to the trunk and lower limbs, those in the cymba and cavum conchae to the internal organs, while those around the helix crus are related to the digestive tract (see Fig. 177).

THE LOCATIONS OF COMMONLY USED EAR-POINTS AND THEIR INDICATIONS

Ear-points have been discovered gradually during clinical practice, and at present a total of 180 ear-points has been reached. The locations and main indications of the 81 most commonly used points are as follows:

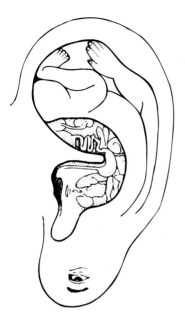

Fig. 177 The fetal image schematic distribution of auricular points.

1. AT THE SCAPHA

"Finger"

Location. Superior to the helix tubercle, at the top of the scapha.

Indications. Numbness and pain in the fingers.

"Wrist"

Location. At the scapha, level with the helix tubercle.

Indications. Sprain, swelling and pain in the wrist.

"Elbow"

Location. Between the points of "Wrist" and "Shoulder".

Indications. Bi syndromes of the elbow.

"Shoulder"

Location. At the scapha, level with the supratragic notch.

Indications. Bi syndromes of the shoulder.

"Shoulder joint"

Location. Between "Shoulder" and the antitragus helix notch.

Indications. Shoulder arthritis.

"Clavicle"

Location. On the scapha, level with the antitragus helix notch.

Indications. Pain at the corresponding area and peripheral shoulder arthritis.

2. SUPERIOR ANTIHELIX CRUS

"Toe"

Location. At the superior and lateral angle of the superior antihelix crus.

Indications. Numbness and pain in the toes.

"Ankle"

Location. At the superior and medial angle of the superior antihelix crus.

Indications. Arthritis of ankle, sprain and contusion of the ankle.

"Knee"

Location. Initial part of the superior antihelix crus, at the level with the upper border of the inferior antihelix crus.

Indications. Arthritis of the knee joint.

3. INFERIOR ANTIHELIX CRUS

"Buttocks"

Location. At the lateral half of the inferior antihelix crus.

Indications. Sciatica.

"Ischium"

Location. At the medial half of the inferior antihelix crus.

Indications. Sciatica.

"Tip of the inferior antihelix crus" (sympathetic nerve)

Location. At the junction of the terminal of

the inferior antihelix crus and the medial aspect of the helix.

Indications. Dysfunction of the digestive or circulatory system, acute infantile convulsions, asthma, dysmenorrhoea, etc.

4. ANTIHELIX

"Abdomen"

Location. On the antihelix, level with the lower border of the inferior antihelix crus.

Indications. Diseases of the abdominal cavity, the digestive system and gynaecological diseases.

"Chest"

Location. On the antihelix, level with the supratragic notch.

Indications. Pain in the chest and flanks, and mastitis.

"Neck"

Location. At the antitragus helix notch, near the scapha.

Indications. Neck sprain or stiffness, and simple goitre.

"Spinal vertebrae"

Location. On the concha aspect of the antihelix, a line between the point level with "Lower region of Rectum" and a point level with "Shoulder joint" is divided, as are the vertebrae of the spine, into 3 sections. The upper third represents the lumbosacral vertebrae, the middle third the thoracic vertebrae, and the lower third the cervical vertebrae.

Indications. Disorders of the corresponding areas.

5. TRIANGULAR FOSSA

"Uterus" (*seminal palace*)

Location. In the triangular fossa and the depression close to the midpoint of the helix.

Indications. Irregular menstruation, morbid leucorrhoea, dysmenorrhoea, pelvic inflammation, impotence and seminal emission.

"Ear-shenmen"

Location. At the lateral third of the triangular fossa, anterior to the bifurcating point between the superior and inferior antihelix crura.

Indications. Insomnia, dream-disturbed sleep, irritability, inflammation, asthma, cough, vertigo and urticaria; sedative and analgesic.

6. TRAGUS

"External nose"

Location. In the centre of the lateral aspect of the tragus.

Indications. Nose furuncles and rhinitis.

"Throat"

Location. Upper half of the medial aspect of the tragus.

Indications. Congested and sore throat, and tonsillitis.

"Internal nose"

Location. Lower half of the medial aspect of the tragus, inferior to "Throat".

Indications. Rhinitis, maxillary sinusitis and common cold.

"Supratragic apex"

Location. At the tip of the upper protuberance on the border of the tragus.

Indications. Inflammatory and painful diseases.

"Infratragic apex" (*adrenal gland*)

Location. At the tip of the lower tubercle on the border of the tragus.

Indications. Hypotension, syncope, pulseless disease, cough, asthma, common cold, heatstroke, malaria, and mastitis.

"Auricle"

Location. In the depression slightly anterior to the supratragic notch.
Indications. Tinnitus, deafness and vertigo.

7. ANTITRAGUS

"Mid-border" (brain point)

Location. Midway between the antitragic apex and the antihelix tragic notch.
Indications. Nocturnal enuresis, massive uterine bleeding and acute infantile convulsions.

"Soothing asthma" (parotid gland)

Location. At the tip of the tragus.
Indications. Asthma, cough, mumps, nocturnal enuresis and acute infantile convulsions.

"Brain" (subcortex)

Location. At the medial aspect of the antitragus.
Indications. Insomnia, dream-disturbed sleep, painful diseases; mental retardation, asthma, vertigo and tinnitus.

"Testes" (ovary)

Location. Anterior and inferior to the medial aspect of the antitragus; it comprises part of the "Brain" (subcortex) point.
Indications. Diseases of the genital system and headache.

"Occiput"

Location. Posterior and superior to the lateral aspect of the antitragus.
Indications. Diseases of the nervous system, skin diseases, syncope, occipital headache and insomnia.

"Forehead"

Location. Anterior and inferior to the lateral aspect of the antitragus.
Indications. Frontal headache, dizziness, insomnia and vertigo.

"Temple"

Location. On the lateral aspect of the antitragus, between "Forehead" and "Occiput".
Indications. Migraine.

8. INTERTRAGIC NOTCH

"Eye 1"

Location. Anterior and inferior to the intertragic notch.
Indications. Glaucoma and myopia.

"Eye 2"

Location. Posterior and inferior to the intertragic notch.
Indications. Ametropia and inflammatory external eye diseases.

"Intertragus" (endocrine)

Location. At the base of the cavum concha and in the intertragic notch.
Indications. Dysfunctions of the genital system, menopause or climacteric syndromes and skin disease.

9. PERIPHERY OF THE HELIX CRUS

"Mouth"

Location. Close to the posterior and superior border of the orifice of the external auditory meatus.
Indications. Facial paralysis and stomatitis.

"Oesophagus"

Location. At the medial two-thirds of the inferior aspect of the helix crus.
Indications. Nausea, vomiting and dysphagia.

"Cardia"

Location. Lateral third of the inferior aspect of the helix crus.
Indications. Nausea, vomiting and cardiac spasm.

"Stomach"

Location. Where the helix crus disappears.
Indications. Gastric pain, hiccup, vomiting, indigestion, gastric ulcer and insomnia.

"Duodenum"

Location. At the lateral third of the superior aspect of the helix crus.
Indications. Diseases of the biliary tract, duodenal ulcer and pylorospasm.

"Small intestine"

Location. At the middle third of the superior aspect of the helix crus.
Indications. Indigestion and palpitations.

"Large intestine"

Location. At the medial third of the superior aspect of the helix crus.
Indications. Dysentery, diarrhoea and constipation.

"Appendix"

Location. Between "Small intestine" and "Large intestine".
Indications. Appendicitis and diarrhoea.

10. CYMBA CONCHA

"Bladder"

Location. At the lower border of the antihelix crus, directly above "Large intestine".
Indications. Cystitis, retention of urine and nocturnal enuresis.

"Ureter"

Location. Between "Bladder" and "Kidney".
Indications. Calculi and colic of the ureter.

"Kidney"

Location. At the lower border of the antihelix crus, directly above "Small intestine".

Indications. Diseases of the urinary-genital system, gynaecological diseases, lumbar pain, tinnitus, insomnia, vertigo, hypertrophy of cervical and lumbar vertebrae.

"Pancreas" (Gallbladder)

Location. Between "Liver" and "Kidney"; the point is "Pancreas" on the left ear and "Gallbladder" on the right ear.
Indications. Pancreatitis, diabetes, diseases of the biliary tract, migraine and malaria.

"Liver"

Location. Posterior to "Stomach" and "Duodenum".
Indications. Stagnant liver qi, eye diseases, malaria, flank pain, irregular menstruation and dysmenorrhoea.

11. CAVUM CONCHA

"Spleen"

Location. Inferior to "Liver", lateral and superior to the cavum concha.
Indications. Indigestion, abdominal distension, chronic diarrhoea, gastric pain, stomatitis, massive uterine bleeding and blood diseases.

"Heart"

Location. In the central depression of the cavum concha.
Indications. Cardiovascular diseases, heatstroke and acute infantile convulsions.

"Lung"

Location. Superior, inferior and lateral to "Heart".
Indications. Diseases of the respiratory system, skin diseases and the common cold.

"Trachea"

Location. Between "Mouth" and "Heart".
Indications. Cough and asthma.

"Sanjiao"

Location. Superior to "Intertragus".
Indications. Constipation and oedema.

12. HELIX

"Lower region of rectum"

Location. At the helix, level with "Large intestine".
Indications. Constipation, dysentery, prolapse of the anus and haemorrhoids.

"Urethra"

Location. At the helix, level with the lower border of the inferior antihelix crus.
Indications. Frequent and urgent urination.

"External genitalia"

Location. At the helix, level with the upper border of the inferior antihelix crus.
Indications. Impotence, inflammation of the external genitalia and skin diseases of the perineum.

"Ear apex"

Location. At the superior apex of the ear when the helix is folded towards the tragus.
Indications. Fever, hypertension, congested eye with swelling and pain, or stye.

"Liver yang"

Location. At the helix tubercle.
Indications. Stagnant liver qi or hyperactivity of liver yang.

"Helix 1–6"

Location. The region from the lower border of the auricular tubercle to the midpoint of the lower border of the lobe is divided into five equal parts. The points marking the divisions are respectively (top to bottom) Helix 1, Helix 2,... to Helix 6.
Indications. Fever, tonsillitis and hypertension.

13. HELIX CRUS

"Middle ear" (diaphragm)

Location. On the helix crus.
Indications. Hiccup, jaundice, indigestion, and skin pruritus.

14. EAR LOBE

"Antihypotensive point"

Location. Inferior to the intertragic notch.
Indications. Hypotension and prostration (shock).

"Tooth 1"

Location. The lateral inferior corner of Section 1 of the ear lobe.
Indications. Tooth extraction and toothache.

"Tongue"

Location. In the centre of Section 2 of the ear lobe.
Indications. Swelling and pain in the tongue, aphasia due to stiffness of the tongue.

"Tooth 2"

Location. In the centre of Section 4 of the ear lobe.
Indications. Tooth extraction and toothache.

"Maxilla"

Location. In the middle of Section 3 of the ear lobe.
Indications. Upper toothache and pain in the mandibular joint.

"Mandible"

Location. Midpoint of the transverse line at the superior part of Section 3 of the ear lobe.
Indications. Lower toothache and pain in the mandibular joint.

"Eye"

Location.   In the centre of Section 5 of the ear lobe.

Indications.   Acute conjunctivitis, electric ophthalmia and myopia.

"Cheek"

Location.   Around the junction of Sections 5 and 6 of the ear lobe.

Indications.   Trigeminal neuralgia, deviation of the mouth and eye, and facial diseases such as acne.

"Internal ear"

Location.   Slightly superior to the middle of Section 6 of the ear lobe.

Indications.   Tinnitus, impaired hearing, otitis media, insomnia and auditory vertigo.

"Tonsil"

Location.   In the middle of Section 8 of the ear lobe.

Indications.   Throat disorders and acute tonsillitis.

15. BACK OF THE EAR

"Upper auricular root"

Location.   At the upper border of the auricular root.

Indications.   Headache, abdominal pain and asthma.

"Antihypertensive groove"

Location.   On the back of the ear, in the groove running from the medial superior region to the lateral inferior region.

Indications.   Hypertension.

"Upper auricular back"

Location.   At the cartilage protuberance at the superior back of the ear.

Indications.   Skin diseases, headache, sciatica and lumbar pain.

"Middle auricular back"

Location.   At the highest point between the upper back of the ear and the lower back of the ear.

Indications.   Skin diseases, backache, abdominal distension diarrhoea and indigestion.

"Lower auricular back"

Location.   At the cartilage protuberance in the inferior part of the back of the ear.

Indications.   Skin diseases, backache, cough and asthmatic breathing.

"Root of the auricular vagus nerve"

Location.   At the junction of the back of the ear and the mastoid, level with the helix crus.

Indications.   Gastric pain, biliary ascariasis, diarrhoea, asthmatic breathing and nasal obstruction.

"Lower auricular root"

Location.   On the lower border of the juncture between the ear-lobe and the cheek.

Indications.   Headache, toothache, sore throat and asthma.

Refer to Figure 178 for the location of the ear-points.

THE CLINICAL APPLICATION OF EAR ACUPUNCTURE

Ear acupuncture can be applied either in the prevention or treatment of disease, and furthermore is in common use during acupuncture anaesthesia. It is also significant in diagnosis.

Its main use in the prevention and treatment of disease may be introduced as follows.

SELECTION OF POINTS

Points may be selected in four main ways:

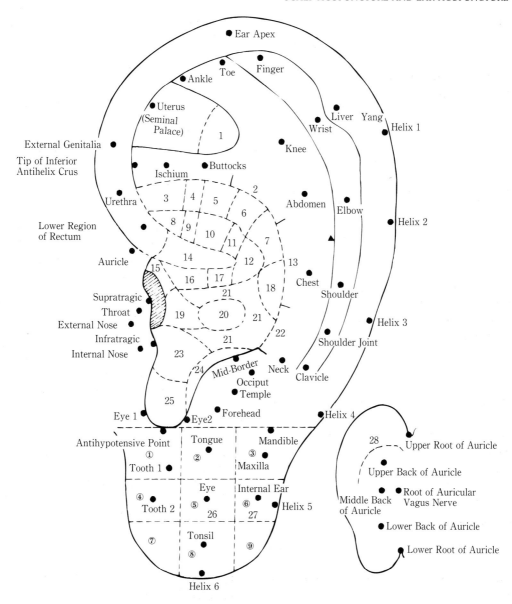

Fig. 178 Distribution of the auricular points. According to the Standard Nomenclature of Auricular Points stipulated by the China Acupuncture and Moxibustion Association, the nomenclature of the following auricular points has been changed from: "Diaphragm" to "Middle Ear", "Tragic apex" to "Upper Apex of Tragus", "Adrenal" to "Lower Apex of Tragus", "Brain Point" to "Mid-Border", "Subcortex" to "Brain", "Taiyang" to "Temple", "Endocrine" to "Intertragus", and "Sympathetic (nerve)" to "End of Inferior Antihelix Crus". 1 Ear-Shenmen, 2 Sacrolumbar Vertebrae, 3 Bladder, 4 Ureter, 5 Kidney, 6 Pancreas (Gallbladder), 7 Liver, 8 Large intestine, 9 Appendix, 10 Small Intestine, 11 Duodenum, 12 Stomach, 13 Thoracic Vertebrae, 14 Middle Ear, 15 Mouth, 16 Oesophagus, 17 Cardiac Orifice, 18 Spleen, 19 Trachea, 20 Heart, 21 Lung, 22 Cervical Vertebrae, 23 Sanjiao, 24 Brain, 25 Intertragus, 26 Cheek, 27 Face, 28 Antihypertensive Groove.

— according to disease location,
— according to TCM theory,
— according to a knowledge of modern medicine,
— according to clinical experience.

The selection of points according to disease location

For example, "Stomach" is selected for stomach disease, "Lung" for lung disease, "Appendix" for appendicitis, "Shoulder" for shoulder pain, and "Throat" for sore throat.

The selection of points according to TCM theory

For example, "Kidney" is selected for tinnitus as the kidney opens into the ear, "Liver" for eye disease as the liver opens into the eye, "Heart" for insomnia as the heart houses the mind and insomnia is usually related to restlessness of mind, and "Lung" for skin disease as the lung dominates the skin.

The selection of points according to a knowledge of modern medicine

For example, "Antihypertensive groove" is selected for hypertension, "Duodenum" or "Tip of inferior antihelix crus" for duodenal ulcer, "Heart" for cardiac arrhythmia, "Uterus" for irregular menstruation, and "Infratragic apex" for reactions to transfusion.

The selection of points according to clinical experience

For example, "Ear apex" for a congested eye with swelling and pain, "Ear-Shenmen" for depressive-manic psychosis, "Tooth" for toothache, etc.

The fewer points selected the better, about 2–3 in general.

For disease on one side of the body, points on the same side are selected. For disease on both sides, or of the internal organs, points are selected bilaterally. Alternatively, if the left side is sick select the right, if the right side is sick select the left.

Table 7.1 Examples of prescriptions for common diseases:

Common cold	"Lung", "Internal nose" and "Infratragic apex"
Heatstroke	"Heart", "Occiput" and "Brain"
Cough	"Trachea", "Lung" and "Ear-Shenmen"
Asthma	"Soothing asthma", "Lung", "Tip of inferior helix crus" and "Infratragic apex"
Vertigo	"Kidney", "Ear-Shenmen" and "Internal ear"
Gastric pain	"Stomach", "Ear-Shenmen", "Brain" and "Tip of inferior antihelix crus"
Irregular menstruation	"Uterus", "Ovary" and "Tragic apex"
Dysmenorrhoea	"Uterus", "Kidney", "Intertragus" and "Tip of inferior antihelix crus"
Acute infantile convulsions	"Heart", "Ear-Shenmen", "Mid-border" and "Tip of inferior antihelix crus"
Nocturnal enuresis	"Kidney", "Bladder", "Mid-border" and "Brain"
Sprain	Corresponding affected areas, "Ear-Shenmen" and "Brain"
Transfusion reactions	"Soothing asthma" and "Infratragic apex"

METHODS OF MANIPULATION

(i) Detection and observation of ear-points

There are three methods:

— observation by the naked eye,
— detection of the tender spot,
— detection by electrical resistance.

Observation by the naked eye

Pull the ear by holding the posterior and superior portion of the helix with the thumb and index finger. Observe with the naked eye, from top to bottom, any morphological changes, discoloration, papules, scaling, nodules, congestion, depressions or blisters. Such positive reactive areas are where obvious tenderness and lowered electrical resistance often appear.

Detection of the tender spot

After diagnosis of the disease is made, probe with a probing needle, or a matchstick, or the handle of a filiform needle in the corresponding affected areas on the ear. Use gentle and even pressure to find the tender or sensitive spot—the spot with most obvious tenderness can be selected for treatment. If a tender spot cannot be detected, just give treatment exactly on the ear-points as prescribed.

Detection by electrical resistance

In most cases, where there is disease, lowered electrical resistance may be observed in the corresponding affected areas on the ear. The cutaneous conductivity of these points with lowered electrical resistance will inevitably increase, so they are known as "conductive" points. They can be used as stimulating points for ear acupuncture.

In order to detect these points, the earphone of an electrodetector is applied to the operator's ear, one electrode is placed in the patient's hand, or on the patient's Neiguan (P 6), and the operator moves over the corresponding affected areas on the patient's ear with a probing electrode in a gentle even manner. When an increased sound is heard in the operator's earphone (and a burning pain will also be felt by the patient in the ear), the conductive spot, or ear-point, has been found.

(ii) Sterilization

With 75% alcohol, or with 2% iodine (to mark the point as well) and then 75% alcohol.

(iii) Methods of needling

A short filiform needle, thumbtack needle, electroneedling or point injection may be applied, according to the demands of the treatment for different kinds of diseases.

Stabilize the ear with the left hand and insert the needle into the cartilage with the right hand, avoiding penetrating the ear. In point injection, 0.1–0.3 ml of medicinal fluid is injected into the site, between the skin and cartilage at each point. A small cutaneous prominence usually results afterwards. When using thumbtack needles, electroneedling or point injection, refer to their corresponding sections respectively.

As well as the above, small magnets, mung beans, rape or mustard seeds may also be used, by affixing them with adhesive tape and pressing them from time to time.

During the stimulation of the ear-points, there may appear local pain or a distending pain, or a burning sensation, soreness and numbness, or a propagated needling sensation along the course of the meridians in the patient.

(iv) Retention of the needle

Filiform needles are often retained for 10–30 minutes, or 1–2 hours or even longer in cases of pain, during which manipulation of needles is often required.

Embedded needles may be retained for 2–3 days in spring and autumn, 7–10 days in winter, but avoid embedding needles for a long time in the summer to prevent possible infection caused by sweating. Press the embedded needles with fingers 2–3 times a day, 1–3 minutes each time, to increase the stimulation and potentiate the therapeutic result.

(v) Withdrawal of the needle

After withdrawing the needle, press the hole with a sterilized dry cotton ball for a while to prevent bleeding, or sterilize the punctured site again with iodine or alcohol to prevent infection.

(vi) Duration of treatment

One or two treatments a day for acute diseases. Once a day or every other day for chronic diseases. Eight to twelve successive treatments are considered one course, and five to seven days should be the interval between courses.

PRECAUTIONS

1. Strict sterilization of the stimulating areas is especially required to prevent infection. Inflamed or frostbitten regions are contraindicated for needling. If redness of the puncture hole, distending pain in the ear and a slight infection of the ear are observed after needling, 2.5% iodine or anti-inflammatory drugs should be prescribed immediately.

Serious attention must be paid to preventing possible infections as they may lead to purulent perichondritis of the ear.

2. The electrical resistance of different ear-points varies, even in normal subjects, so these findings should be analysed in combination with a clinical examination and other clinical manifestations.

3. Usually pain is expected during needling the ear. Attention should be paid to the possibility of the patient fainting during needling, and if it does occur due management is required.

4. Ear acupuncture is contraindicated for pregnant women where there is a history of spontaneous abortion. It can be used in the aged, senile, severely anaemic or those who are tired, only with the greatest caution.

5. For cases of sprain and motor impairment, after the burning sensation is felt during needling, the patient is asked to move the affected site, and massage and moxibustion (with a moxa stick) are given to the affected site to enhance the therapeutic effect.

6. Ear acupuncture has its limitations although it is widely indicated, so it is necessary sometimes to combine it with other therapies.

NOTES

1. *Miraculous Pivot*, Ch. 24, "On Jue Disease".
2. *Miraculous Pivot*, Ch. 20, "The 5 Evil Pathogens".
3. *Miraculous Pivot*, Ch. 10 "Meridians".
4. *Miraculous Pivot*, Ch. 28, "On Questioning the Patient".
5. *Miraculous Pivot*, Ch. 17, "Dimensions of the Meridians".
6. *Plain Questions*, Ch. 22, "Seasonal Rules of the Zang Qi".

Acupuncture anaesthesia 8

Acupuncture anaesthesia (abbreviated to AA) is a method of anaesthesia which works through stimulating certain acupoints with needles, while the patient undergoes an operation in full consciousness.

It is an invention based on the effectiveness of acupuncture in relieving pain and regulating the physiological functions of the human body. It is considered a significant achievement, as it is a new development of the science of acupuncture and moxibustion, made through inheriting and developing TCM by means of modern medicine, through the joint efforts of medical workers of both TCM and Western medicine.

The integration of acupuncture and surgery has resulted in enhanced manipulative techniques and better results from surgical operations. Furthermore AA has set new targets for theoretical research and promoted research into the correlation between the jingluo, the acupoints and the zangfu organs, the physiology of pain and the basic mechanism of analgesia.

THE CHARACTERISTICS OF ACUPUNCTURE ANAESTHESIA

1. The patient under acupuncture anaesthesia is mentally alert, with various sensory and motor functions normal (except for the sense of pain which becomes dulled), and he is able to cooperate with the surgeons, which greatly facilitates the operation.

For instance, in cutting the sensory branches of the trigeminal nerve, the degree and areas of absence of feeling can be found through communication with the patient, thus avoiding overcutting or inadequate cutting of the nerve root. In a goitre operation, through communication with the patient, his phonation can be examined, thus avoiding unnecessary injury to the recurrent laryngeal nerve.

Furthermore, as there is no temporary paralysis as is normally seen in drug anaesthesia, AA is especially useful during postoperative care and transportation.

2. AA is safe in application; it does not produce any side-effects, and avoids the occurrence of accidents which might happen in drug anaesthesia owing to overdosage or allergic reactions of patients.

AA is safe for patients with a functional insufficiency of the heart, lungs or kidney, or a weakened constitution (as in the aged) or shock, and for those for whom drug anaesthesia is unsuitable.

3. Owing to the effect of acupuncture in regulating various functions of the body, the patient's blood pressure, pulse and respiration are kept relatively stable during the operation. And furthermore, no postoperative sequelae result, the pain of the incision is mild, and all these are conducive to an early recovery being made by the patient.

4. AA does not require any sophisticated medical equipment, nor is it constrained by a preferential environment, so it is easily mastered and can be applied at any time, even in battle conditions, or in isolated or rural communities.

Although AA has the advantages of safety in use, efficacy, reduced physiological disturbance, quick recovery, and convenience in application, it still has some drawbacks. In some instances and during certain stages of some operations, it does not produce complete analgesia, and fails to give complete or satisfactory relaxation of the abdominal muscles, resulting in unpleasant sensations due to retraction of the internal organs.

Small amounts of adjuvants, sedative or anaesthetic drugs can be prescribed or applied at the sites of the incision to potentiate the anaesthetic effect.

METHODS OF ACUPUNCTURE ANAESTHESIA

PREOPERATIVE PREPARATIONS

A thorough investigation of the condition of the patient's disease, history and psychological state should be made. The plan for the operation under AA and any measures to be taken in case of possible unfavourable results should be fully discussed beforehand.

As the patient under AA is mentally alert during any surgical procedures, it is essential to let him know in detail the characteristic methods, process and effects of AA, and any possible uncomfortable feelings or reactions he might experience during the operation. Again, he can be instructed on how to cooperate with the surgeons (e.g. by practising deep breathing in thoracotomy) to ensure the successful result of the operation.

Needling can be applied to some selected points on the patient 1–3 times before the operation to test his condition of *de qi* and endurance of pain during needling, so that the proper methods of AA can be applied and the proper intensity of stimulation reached.

PRINCIPLES FOR THE SELECTION OF POINTS

For AA the points selected should be those where a needling sensation is found easily, (especially the sense of soreness, distension and heaviness), but they should also be not painful, not bleed easily, be comfortable for the patient and convenient for the operator.

The selection of points for body needling and ear needling may be either points on the body or ear-points.

Points (mainly from 14 meridians) for body needling

Selecting points according to the theory of the jingluo

According to jingluo theory, "where a meridian traverses, there is a place amenable to treatment". Meridional points that have a close relationship with the operative incision sites and zangfu organs being operated on, are selected.

For example, in tooth extraction, Hegu (LI 4) and Sanjian (LI 3) from the hand Yangming are selected; in gastrotubal ligation, Sanyinjiao (Sp 6) and Taichong (Liv 3).

Selecting local points

Points are selected from areas adjacent to the operative sites, e.g. Jiache (St 6) and Daying (St 5) for extracting lower teeth; Daimai (GB 26) for caesarean section.

Selecting points according to nerve theory

One way is to select the same or adjacent segmental points, e.g. Neck-Futu (LI 18), Hegu (LI 4) and Neiguan (P 6) are selected for thyroidectomy. Another way is to select points according to nerve-trunks or directly stimulate the nerve-trunks; this method is often used in orthopaedic operations. For example, Jiquan (H 1) or various points on the arm (puncture from both sides where the axillary artery throbs) for some operations on the upper limbs; stimulating the 3rd and 4th lumbar nerves, femoral and sciatic nerves for some operations on the lower limbs, and stimulating the 2nd branch of the trigeminal nerve from the point Quanliao (SI 18) for some operations on the head or cranium.

The above three methods can be applied singly or in combination.

The three methods of selecting ear-points

There are three methods of selecting ear-points, namely:

— according to theories of the zangfu,
— according to the operative sites,
— according to nerve innervation and the physiology of the points.

Selecting points according to theories of the zangfu organs

For example, "the lung dominates the skin and hair", so "Lung" is often used when the skin is incised or a wound is sutured. "The kidney dominates the bones" so "Kidney" is used in orthopaedic operations, and thoracic surgery when cutting the ribs. "The liver opens into the eyes", so "Liver" is selected in ophthalmic operations.

Selecting points according to the operative sites

"Appendix" for appendectomy, "Lung" for lung operations, and "Gallbladder" for operations on the gallbladder.

Selecting points according to nerve innervation and the anatomical physiology of the ear-points

"Mouth" and "Root of auricular vagus nerve" are selected for operations on viscera in the abdominal cavity with innervation of the vagus nerve. "Brain" and "Tip of inferior antihelix crus" are commonly used, as they can potentiate the analgesic effect and reduce the reflex movement of the viscera, according to the usual physiological theory.

The above three methods can be applied singly or in combination.

The points used for body or ear acupuncture anaesthesia are often selected from the affected side, but they may also be selected bilaterally.

TECHNIQUES OF MANIPULATION

Hand manipulation

In body needling, rotation or rotation in combination with lifting-thrusting of the needles is often adopted. In ear needling, rotation alone (no lifting-thrusting) is employed. The frequency of manipulation is about 120–200 times per minute and the amplitude of rotation about 90–360 degrees. The amplitude for lifting-thrusting needles is about 5–10 mm. It is necessary to have a "needling sensation" all the time during the operation. Manual manipulation should be done evenly and stably.

This basic technique of AA is very important as it is by this that the intensity of stimulation can be adjusted, according to the sensation under the fingers of the operator. It is in such a manner that AA can be applied in remote rural areas with only simple equipment, even in battle conditions.

Electrical stimulation

The manipulation is the same as that in electroneedling. In AA dense wave stimulation is often used and the intensity of stimulation should be moderate—one which the patient can tolerate.

Point-injection therapy

The same points are selected as those used when body needling. Drugs often used are Vitamin B1, 10% glucose injection, pethidin, Chinese angelica injection, and Corydalis injection. This method is often applied in combination with manipulation by hand, or electroneedling.

Besides the above, there are also the methods of finger-pressure anaesthesia, mechanical blockage anaesthesia and anaesthesia through the use of electrode-plates. All these can be used in place of acupuncture.

Induction and retention of the needle

Needling or electroneedling performed on selected points for a desirable length of time prior to the operation is known as induction, and it generally lasts 20–30 minutes. It can be a general induction on all prescribed points—which needs a longer length of time—or a concentrated induction on the main points, which is applied 5 minutes before the operation.

During the operation the stimulation is generally mild, but for an operation on a sensitive area the intensity of stimulation should be increased during the operation. During some operations which need only gentle stimulations, the manipulation of the needles or electroneedling can be ceased temporarily with only the retention of the needles.

For instance, in cerebral operations, after the incision has been made on the meninges, the needles are retained for a period of time without manipulation.

ADJUVANTS

In order to enhance the anaesthetic effect and to guarantee that the operation goes smoothly, some adjuvants (most often small doses of sedatives, analgesics and anticholinergics) should be given in almost every case of AA.

Usual preoperative adjuvants

0.1 g phenobarbital sodium given muscularly one hour before the operation, or else 50 mg pethidin given muscularly or intravenously 15–30 minutes before the operation (may not be used in some patients). In order to reduce the secretions from the respiratory and digestive tracts, 0.5 mg atropine or 0.3 mg scopolamine can be given subcutaneously or muscularly 30–60 minutes before the operation.

Adjuvants during operations

Some adjuvants are given according to different stages of the operation and according to the different reactions of the patient; adjuvants for sedation, analgesia, or local anaesthesia, or muscle relaxants are given or added respectively. For instance, before incising the peritoneum, ligating the big blood vessels or severely lifting or pulling the viscera, 1% procaine as a local infiltration anaesthetic is given to prevent possible severe reactions in the patient.

Adjuvants should be applied at the proper time, according to the stage of the operation, i.e. just before a severe reaction may possibly occur; and the dosage should be regulated. Overdosage may cause a hypnopompic state in patients during operations, and they may lose the ability to cooperate with the surgeon.

Muscle relaxants should be used with great care and under strict observation, with provision for emergency action if an accident should occur.

INDICATIONS

Acupuncture anaesthesia has a comparatively wide scope of indications, for example in general surgery, neurosurgery, ophthalmology, ENT surgery, stomatology, thoracic surgery, orthopaedics, gynaecology, urological surgery and paediatrics.

Generally speaking, AA has a better effect in operations of the head and facial regions, neck and chest, where it may be widely used. Owing to muscular tension and reactions during visceral lifting and pulling in operations on the abdomen, cases indicated for AA in this field are comparatively few, and require further study.

SOME EXAMPLES OF POINT PRESCRIPTIONS

a) Operations for trichiasis or entropion

Points. Jingming (UB 1) and Hegu (LI 4).

Manipulation. Concentrated induction on Jingming (UB 1) before the operation, without retention of needle. Apply a dense wave at Hegu (LI 4).

b) Tooth extraction

Points. Hegu (LI 4) towards Laogong (P 8), or use the ear-point "Toothache".

Manipulation. 20 minutes needling induction which can be slightly increased just before the extraction of the tooth.

c) Tonsillectomy

Points. Hegu (LI 4).

Manipulation. 20 minutes of needling induction, continue the hand manipulation or electroneedling during the operation.

d) Thyroidectomy

Points. Neck-Futu (LI 18) bilaterally, or Hegu (LI 4) and Neiguan (p 6), or ear-points "Lung", "Ear-Shenmen", "Intertragus" and "Neck".

Manipulation. 20 minutes induction, continue hand manipulation or electroneedling during the operation.

e) Operations on the cranium (cerebral hemisphere, sellae, forehead and parietal craniotomy)

Points. Quanliao (SI 18) on the affected side, and add Jinmen (UB 63) or Taichong (Liv 3); or ear-points "Lung", "Ear-Shenmen" towards "Kidney", and "Tip of inferior antihelix crus" or "Brain".

Manipulation. 20–30 minutes needling induction; continue the hand manipulation or electroneedling during the operation; after incising the meninges retain the needle for a period of time; manipulate the needles by hand or apply electric stimulation again before the suture of the incised meninges.

f) Pneumonectomy

Points. Either Hegu (LI 4) and Neiguan (P 6); or Sanyangluo (SJ 8) towards Ximen (P 4); or Binao (LI 14) towards Jianyu (LI 15); or Waiguan (SJ 5) towards Neiguan (P 6). One or two groups of points are employed at a time. Ear-points "Lung", "Ear-Shenmen", "Tip of inferior antihelix crus" and "Soothing asthma".

Manipulation. 20–30 minutes induction, continue the hand manipulation or electroneedling during the operation; the patients are asked to cooperate by practising slow, deep abdominal breathing.

g) Mitral commissurotomy

Points. Hegu (LI 4), Neiguan (P 6), Zhigou (SJ 6), or ear points "Lung", "Ear-Shenmen", "Chest", "Heart" and "Tip of inferior antihelix crus".

Manipulation. 20–30 minutes induction, continue hand manipulation or electroneedling during operation; the patients are asked to practise slow, deep abdominal breathing.

h) Subtotal gastrectomy

Points. Either Zusanli (St 36), Shangjuxu

(St 37) and Sanyinjiao (Sp 6) all bilaterally; or Zusanli, Yifeng (SJ 17) and Shousanli (LI 10) all bilaterally; and points on both sides of the incision. One group of points is selected, then used in combination with the ear-points "Lung", "Ear-Shenmen", "Stomach" and "Tip of inferior antihelix crus".

Manipulation. 20–30 minutes induction. A needle 5 cun long is applied subcutaneously and parallel with the incision on each side of the incision, a 6 cm distance being kept between the two needles. A pulsating electric dense wave is applied on to the two needles.

i) Tubal ligation (gastro-type)

Points. Sanyinjiao (Sp 6), Ciliao (UB 32), Gongsun (Sp 4) and Taichong (Liv 3), or ear-points "Lung", "Ear-Shenmen", "Intertragus" and "Genitalia".

Manipulation. 15 minutes "general induction", and 10 minutes "concentrated induction". Keep up the hand manipulation or electroneedling during the operation.

j) Caesarean section

Points.   Daimai (GB 26), Zusanli (St 36) and Sanyinjiao (Sp 6), or ear-points "Lung", "Ear-Shenmen", "Abdomen", "Uterus", or body and ear-points used in combination.

Manipulation.   20–30 minutes induction; continue hand manipulation or electroneedling during the operation.

PRECAUTIONS

1. The manual or electric manipulation should be of a moderate intensity, one which the patient can tolerate. Too strong a manipulation causes the patient distress and affects the AA effect.
2. The patient under AA remains mentally alert, so it is necessary to perform the operation with a precise, light and deft technique, and maintain a quiet environment to avoid causing unnecessary disturbance to the patient which may affect the results of the operation.
3. Adjuvants during operations should be applied at the proper stage and their dosage strictly controlled to avoid side-effects of these drugs.
4. AA can only be applied with great care in cases with complicated foci and extensive adhesions, or needing extensive exploration, especially in some difficult operations of the abdominal cavity where the effect of AA is still unstable.

ACUPUNCTURE AND MOXIBUSTION TREATMENT

This part deals in detail with the treatment of disease with acupuncture and moxibustion, founded on the basis of a study of the jingluo, the acupoints and the various acupuncture and moxibustion techniques.

It consists of two parts, of which the first, the *General Introduction to Treatment*, deals primarily with the main symptoms of the zangfu organs and jingluo, the general principles of treatment, the principles for prescribing points and the application of specific points; while the second, the *Treatment of Common Diseases*, deals with the treatment of commonly seen diseases.

General introduction 9
to treatment

The whole capacity for life within the human body cannot be separated from the zangfu organs and the jingluo. The development of disease, although it displays complex clinical manifestations, is basically due to a dysfunction in the zangfu and the jingluo.

Treatment with acupuncture and moxibustion should proceed by adopting the *si zhen* (四诊) or "4 diagnostic methods", and through the *bian zheng* (辨证) or "differentiation of syndromes" according to the *ba gang* (八纲) or "8 principles", all in accordance with the theories of the zangfu and jingluo. Thus you can analyse and generalize various clinical manifestations, so as to ascertain the aetiology and pathogenesis of the disease, the location of the disease (at a zang organ, at a fu organ, exterior or interior), the nature of the disease (cold or hot, deficiency or in excess) and the condition of the disease (primary or secondary, acute or chronic).

Then, according to the differentiation of syndromes, you select acupoints, form prescriptions and give treatment with either acupuncture or moxibustion, or both in combination, employing either a reinforcing or reducing method of manipulation, or else using both in combination. Thus you remove the obstruction from the jingluo, regulate the circulation of qi and blood, and restore a relative balance between yin and yang.

This is just as is stated in the *Miraculous Pivot*, when it says, "the essentials of acupuncture lie in the regulation of yin and yang. If yin and yang are balanced, essence and qi are brilliantly harmonized".[1] In this way, the functions of the zangfu are regulated and harmonized, and the goal of preventing and treating disease is achieved.

Clinical manifestations of the zangfu and jingluo, and their treatment

All functional activities in the human body are based on those of the zangfu and the jingluo, and thus all clinical manifestations are the manifestations of pathological changes within the zangfu and jingluo. Furthermore, owing to their different physiological functions, these pathological changes and manifestations within the individual zang and fu organs, and the jingluo, will vary.

Thus, if general and specific manifestations of the zangfu and jingluo are analysed, the aetiology, pathogenesis and location of disease can be ascertained, which facilitates making a correct diagnosis and treatment.

In the *Plain Questions*, it states that "the activity of the 5 zang organs appears in the passage of the meridians, circulating the qi and blood; and a disharmony in the qi and blood leads to various diseases. Therefore treatment is always concentrated on the passage of the meridians."[2] Yu Jiayan,[3] a famous physician from the end of the Ming, held that "if you treat disease without understanding clearly the zangfu and jingluo, whenever you open your mouth or touch the patient, you go wrong".

The differentiation of syndromes should always be guided by the theories of the zangfu organs and jingluo, and this is especially significant in treatment with acupuncture and moxibustion.

The chief pathogeneses of the zangfu organs and the jingluo, the general principles of treatment, and the selection of acupoints from the different meridians are now briefly introduced in what follows.

THE LUNGS AND LARGE INTESTINE

THE LUNGS

The lungs are situated in the chest, open into the nose, take charge of the respiration and dominate the qi throughout the whole body, externally joining with the skin and body-hair. They communicate with the throat and nose and their meridian is externally-internally related to the large intestine meridian. The lungs are known as the "delicate" organs, as an invasion of the body by exogenous pathogens often first attacks the lungs via the mouth, nose or skin-pores, leading to an impairment in the dispersing function of the lungs, resulting in disease.

Exogenous affection by *feng* cold, leading to an impairment in the dispersion of the *wei* qi by the lungs, is marked by chilliness and fever, headache, general aching, anhidrosis, nasal obstruction and discharge, coughing with dilute sputum or saliva, a thin and white tongue coating, and a superficial, tight pulse. It should be treated by selecting points mainly from meridians of the hand Taiyin and hand Yangming with a reducing method of needling, as well as moxibustion.

Accumulation of pathogenic heat in the lungs, or *feng* cold, turning into heat, is marked by symptoms of coughing, shortness of breath, profuse yellow and sticky sputum, stuffiness in the chest, chest pain, general feverishness and thirst. It may lead to rhinorrhoea, epistaxis and Bi syndrome of the throat, a dry red tongue with a yellowy coating, and a rapid pulse, and should be treated by selecting points mainly from the meridians of the hand Taiyin and hand Yangming with a reducing method of needling, or bloodletting with the three-edged needle.

Retention of damp *tan*, or *tan* turbidity accumulated in the lungs, is marked by coughing, asthmatic breathing, gurgling of sputum in the throat, profuse thick sputum, fullness and pain in the chest and costal region, with difficulty in lying flat, a white, greasy or yellowy thick tongue coating, and a slippery, or slippery-rapid pulse. It should be treated by selecting points mainly from the meridians of the foot Taiyin and foot Yangming with a reducing method of needling.

Pathogenic heat affecting and consuming the lung yin is marked by coughing, dry throat, blood-tinged sputum, a hectic tidal fever and night sweating, a red tongue with little coating, and a thready and rapid pulse. It should be treated by selecting points mainly from the meridians of the hand Taiyin and foot Shaoyin, and the

Back-Shu points, with a reinforcing method of needling. Moxibustion is contraindicated.

A deficiency of lung qi is marked by coughing and shortness of breath, dilute sputum, aversion to cold and spontaneous sweating, general lassitude and a disinclination to speak, pallor, a pale tongue with a white coating and a pulse of a deficient type. It should be treated by selecting points mainly from meridians of the hand and foot Taiyin, and the Back-Shu points, with a reinforcing method of needling, or needling combined with moxibustion.

If pathogenic *feng*, cold or damp invade the lung meridian, soreness and pain, or spasm, weakness and numbness, and pain of the shoulder and arm will appear along the course of the meridian. They should be treated by selecting points from the meridian of the hand Taiyin and its *luo* point, with both needling and moxibustion.

An upward attack of pathogenic heat in the lungs gives rise to epistaxis, Bi syndrome of the throat, and pain in the supraclavicular fossa, which should be treated by selecting points mainly from meridians of the hand Taiyin and Yangming, with a reducing method of needling, as well as bloodletting by pricking.

THE LARGE INTESTINE

The large intestine is situated in the abdomen and its meridian is externally-internally related to that of the lungs. It is the organ in charge of the transportation of food wastes which turn into stools, to be discharged out of the body via the large intestine. Therefore its dysfunction will result in disease.

Affection of the large intestine by exogenous pathogenic cold, or cold and raw food, is marked by abdominal pain, borborygmus, diarrhoea, a white and slippery tongue coating, and a deep and slow pulse. It should be treated by selecting mainly the Front-Mu and lower He-Sea point of the hand Yangming meridian, using both acupuncture and moxibustion.

The large intestine affected by pathogenic heat is marked by foul-smelling stools, a burning pain of the anus, stools with fresh blood, or dys-

entery with red and white mucus. If the pathogenic heat accumulated in the large intestine leads to carbuncles, it is marked by abdominal pain which is aggravated by pressure, a flexed right leg, a yellowy dry tongue coating, and a slippery and rapid pulse. Both of these should be treated by selecting points from meridians of the hand and foot Yangming, and the Front-Mu and lower He-Sea points of the large intestine, with a reducing method of needling.

If the diarrhoea or dysentery becomes protracted and lingers, leading to incontinence of the stools and prolapse of the anus, a pale tongue with a thin coating, and a thready and weak pulse, it should be treated by selecting points mainly from the meridians of the foot Taiyin and Yangming, and the Ren and Du, with both needling and moxibustion.

For stagnancy or accumulation of pathogens in the large intestine, marked by constipation, abdominal pain aggravated by pressure, or diarrhoea with tenesmus, a yellowy thick tongue coating, and a deep excess-type pulse or a wiry rapid pulse, points mainly from the meridians of the hand and foot Yangming are used, along with a reducing method of needling only (without moxibustion).

For *feng* cold obstructing the jingluo of the large intestine, marked by aching and soreness, motor impairment, numbness, and pain of the arm along the course of the meridian, points from the involved meridian are used along with a reducing method of needling, or else both needling and moxibustion.

For upward rebellion of pathogenic heat along the course of the meridian, marked by headache, yellow sclera, toothache and swelling of the cheek, twitching of the lips, deviation of the mouth, epistaxis, sore throat, foul breath, a yellowy tongue coating, and a wiry and rapid pulse, points mainly from the meridians of the hand and foot Yangming are selected, with a reducing method of needling, or else pricking to cause bleeding.

SPLEEN AND STOMACH

THE SPLEEN

The spleen and stomach are situated in the

abdomen and their meridians are externally-internally related; within the body they take charge of the muscles and open into the mouth. The spleen and stomach have the function of receiving, decomposing and digesting food, and absorbing and distributing the essentials of nutrition. They are the source of manufacture of the qi and blood, which nourishes the 5 zang and 6 fu, and all parts of the body. Hence they are considered the source of acquired health.

The spleen dominates transportation and transformation, and functions mainly in ascending; while the stomach dominates the reception of foodstuffs and functions mainly in descending. Together they function by sending upwards what is lucid and clear within the body, and sending downwards what is turbid and unclear.

An impairment in the spleen qi leads to impaired transportation and transformation, marked by vomiting, abdominal distension, loose stools, pallor, lassitude, a weak voice or disinclination to speak. If severe it may lead to cool limbs, oedema in the feet, diarrhoea with undigested food, a pale tongue with a white coating, and a soft and weak pulse. It should be treated by selecting points mainly from the meridians of the foot Taiyin and Yangming, and their Front-Mu and Back-Shu points, using a reinforcing method of needling, or both needling and moxibustion.

For retention of damp-heat obstructing the middle-jiao, marked by epigastric and abdominal fullness or pain, heaviness and weakness of the limbs, a yellowish complexion and dark yellow urine, a white greasy tongue coating and a slippery-rapid or soft-rapid pulse, select points mainly from the meridians of the foot Taiyin and Yangming, and the Front-Mu point of the small intestine, with a reducing method of needling.

For deficiency of spleen yang and retention of fluid and damp, marked by undigested food in the stools, dilute urination increased in volume, cold limbs, or haematochezia, or uterine bleeding or leucorrhoea, a pale tongue with a white coating and a deep-slow pulse, select mainly the Back-Shu and Front-Mu points of the involved zang organs, and points from the foot Taiyin and Yangming, and Ren meridians, with a reinforcing method of needling, or both needling and moxibustion.

For feng, cold or damp affecting the jingluo, marked by swelling and pain, difficulty in flexion and extension of the limbs, motor impairment or numbness, aphasia due to tongue stiffness, and hemiplegia along the course of the meridian, select points from this meridian, using a reducing method of needling, or both needling and moxibustion.

THE STOMACH

The stomach and spleen communicate with each other via certain membranes and are situated in the middle-jiao. The meridian of the stomach Yangming connects with that of the spleen Taiyin.

In cases of an impairment in the receiving function of the stomach, marked by anorexia, epigastric fullness, hiccup, vomiting, lassitude, a slightly red tongue and lips, and a weak pulse, select points from meridian of the foot Yangming, and its Front-Mu and Back-Shu points, using a reinforcing method of needling, or both needling and moxibustion.

For insufficiency of stomach yang and excessive pathogenic cold, marked by a distending pain in the epigastrium, watery regurgitation, a preference for hot food, a white and slippery tongue coating, and a deep slow pulse, select points from the meridians of the foot Yangming, foot Taiyin, hand Jueyin and the Front-Mu and Back-Shu points. Apply a reinforcing method of needling, or both needling and moxibustion.

For pathogens affecting the Yangming meridian, with heat accumulated in the stomach, marked by general feverishness, a strong thirst, preference for cold but aversion to heat, getting easily frightened on seeing people, delirium, mania, eruptions on the lips, vomiting on eating, or constipated stools, a yellowy dry tongue coating, and an overflowing and forceful pulse, select points mainly from the meridians of the hand and foot Yangming, with a reducing method of needling, but no moxibustion.

When the meridian is affected by feng, cold or damp, or accumulated heat in the spleen and stomach attacking upwards along the course of the meridian, it is marked by ulcers of the mouth and lips, foul breath, a swollen neck, sore throat, toothache and swelling of gums, rhinorrhoea, epistaxis, pain in the supraclavicular fossa, a breast swelling and pain, hemiplegia, and numbness or motor impairment of the lower limbs which the meridian supplies. Then points should be selected mainly from the involved meridian, using a reducing method of needling, or both needling and moxibustion.

HEART AND SMALL INTESTINE

THE HEART

The heart is situated in the chest and surrounded by the pericardium. The heart and small intestine meridians are externally-internally related; within the body they take charge of the blood vessels and open into the tongue. The heart dominates the whole body and mind, and is the centre maintaining its vital activity, including mental activity. Therefore affection of the heart by exogenous or endogenous pathogenic factors may lead to disease.

In cases of too many ideas and thoughts impairing the heart and mind, leading to an insufficiency of heart yang, marked by palpitations, stuffiness in the chest, shortness of breath, cardiac pain, pallor, a pale tongue with a white coating, and a thready and weak, or empty-big and forceless pulse, points should be selected mainly from the Front-Mu and Back-Shu points of the involved zang organ, and the meridian of the hand Jueyin, treated with a reinforcing method of needling, or both needling and moxibustion.

In cases of deficiency of heart yin due to consumption of the nourishing blood and yin essence, marked by palpitations, irritability, insomnia or somnolence, and in severe cases amnesia, nocturnal emission, a dry red tongue with little coating and a thready rapid pulse, points mainly from the meridians of the hand Jueyin and foot Shaoyin are selected with a reinforcing method of needling, or both reinforcing and reducing.

Mental depression or emotional disturbance turning into fire and *tan* heat which disturb the heart, marked by palpitations, insomnia, irritability and heat in the chest, or depressive-manic psychosis or dementia, or a flushed face, thirst, or haematemesis, epistaxis, red and hot urination, stranguria with blood and pain, a red tongue with a yellowy coating, and a slippery and rapid pulse, can be treated by selecting points mainly from the meridians of the hand Shaoyin and Jueyin, and foot Yangming, and their Back-Shu points, with a reducing method of needling. Moxibustion is contraindicated.

If heart fire flares up along the course of its meridian, marked by erosions of the mouth cavity, irritability, sore throat, congested and painful eyes, headache, or epistaxis, a red tongue with a yellowy coating, and a wiry and rapid pulse, it can be treated by selecting points mainly from the meridian of the hand Shaoyin with a reducing method of needling.

If exogenous *feng*, cold or damp affect the heart meridian leading to obstruction in its course, marked by pain and numbness in the area the meridian supplies, and cold and pain in the scapular regions, it should be treated by selecting points mainly from the meridians of the hand Shaoyin and Taiyang, with a reducing method of needling, as well as both needling and moxibustion.

THE SMALL INTESTINE

It is situated in the abdomen, connecting above with the pylorus and the stomach, and below with the large intestine. The meridians of the small intestine and heart are externally-internally related. It functions mainly in separating out the lucid and clear, and secreting the turbid within the body.

If invaded by pathogenic cold, there are symptoms such as a dull pain in the lower abdomen, borborygmus, loose stools, frequent urination, a pale tongue with a thin white coating, and a thready and slowed-down pulse, which should be treated by selecting mainly the Front-Mu, Back-Shu and lower He-Sea points of the small intestine, using a reinforcing method of needling, or else both needling and moxibustion.

If the heart transmits its heat to the small intestine, or there is accumulated heat in the small intestine, it is marked by irritability, ulcers of the tongue and mouth, scanty and dark yellow urination or bloody urination, pain in the penis, a distending pain in the lower abdomen, a red tongue with a yellowy coating, and a slippery-rapid pulse. It can be treated by using points from the meridians of the hand Shaoyin and Taiyang and the Front-Mu and lower He-Sea points of the small intestine, along with a reducing method of needling.

Affection of this meridian by pathogens may result in a congested eye, sore throat, swollen neck, deafness, tinnitus, occipital stiffness and headache, pain in the lower abdomen affecting the lower back and umbilical region, or pain, numbness or motor impairment at the area the meridian supplies. It can be treated by selecting points mainly from the meridian of the hand Taiyang, along with its lower He-Sea and Back-Shu points, using a reducing method of needling, or both acupuncture and moxibustion.

KIDNEYS AND URINARY BLADDER

THE KIDNEYS

The kidneys are situated in the lumbar region, one on the left and the other on the right. They dominate water metabolism, storing the yin essence, and take charge of the bones, producing bone marrow. The meridians of the kidneys and the bladder are externally-internally related.

The kidneys open into the ear, and take the external urethral orifice and anus as their opening; they are the congenital source of health, and the organs which bring harmony between the "water" and "fire" of the body. They are the source of growth and development of life. Therefore exogenous pathogens or over-indulgence in sexual activity may injure the kidneys, leading to disease.

Overwork, or a protracted illness in which nourishment is being withheld, may lead to a deficiency of kidney qi and impairment of its storing function. This gives rise to pallor, soreness and weakness of the lower back and knees, impotence and premature ejaculation, urination increased in volume or more frequent, dizziness, tinnitus, impaired hearing, aversion to cold and cold urination, a pale tongue with a

white coating, and a weak pulse, which can be treated by selecting points from the Front-Mu and Back-Shu points of the kidneys and the meridians of the Ren, Du and foot Shaoyin, mainly with moxibustion, as well as using a reinforcing method of needling.

If the kidney qi is injured, it fails in receiving the qi from the lungs, and this is marked by shortness of breath and asthmatic breathing aggravated by slight exertion, spontaneous sweating, vertigo, aversion to cold, cold feet, a puffy pale face, a pale tongue with a thin coating, and a thready-weak or superficial-forceless pulse. It should be treated by selecting points mainly from the Front-Mu and Back-Shu points of the kidneys, and the Ren, Du and foot Shaoyin meridians, using a reinforcing method of needling, or both acupuncture and moxibustion. Strong moxibustion is especially suitable.

The kidney yang being consumed in a protracted illness means it fails to warm and vaporize fluid, which leads to general oedema, which is worse in the lower limbs, loose stools or coughing and asthmatic breathing due to upward rebellion of the fluid and qi, profuse dilute sputum, a moist and slippery tongue with a whitish coating, and a deep and slippery pulse. It should be treated by selecting points mainly from the Ren, Du and foot Shaoyin meridians with a reinforcing method of needling, or both acupuncture and moxibustion. Moxibustion is especially suitable.

Over-indulgence in sexual activity consumes the kidney yin, which is marked by asthenia, vertigo and dizziness, tinnitus, insomnia, amnesia, dream-disturbed sleep, nocturnal seminal emissions, soreness and weakness of the lower back and knees; or a flush in the malar region and lips, a hectic tidal fever and night sweating, dry mouth and throat, seminal emission; or a dry cough, blood-tinged sputum, a red tongue with little coating, and a thready-rapid pulse. It should be treated by selecting points mainly from the foot Taiyang and foot Shaoyin meridians, or in combination with points from the meridians of the hand Taiyin and Shaoyin, with a reinforcing method of needling.

Pathogens affecting this meridian give rise to pain, soreness and heaviness, numbness and motor impairment in areas the meridian supplies. They should be treated by selecting points from the involved meridian, with needling, moxibustion or both, in combination with cutaneous needling.

THE BLADDER

Situated in the lower abdomen, the meridian of the bladder is externally-internally related to that of the kidneys. It functions in storing body fluid, activating qi circulation and transforming water within the body.

Deficiency and cold of the lower-jiao causes the bladder's function of transforming qi to fail, giving rise to frequent urination, or nocturnal enuresis, a white slippery tongue coating and a thready weak pulse. It should be treated with points mainly from the Front-Mu and Back-Shu points of the bladder and the meridians of the foot Taiyang and Shaoyin, with both needling and moxibustion.

Accumulated heat of the excess type in the bladder leads to scanty and unsmooth urination which is dark yellow and turbid, or in severe cases retention of urine, or stranguria with pus, blood and stones, burning pain in the penis, a red tongue with a yellowy coating, and a slippery and rapid pulse. It should be treated with points mainly from the three yin meridians of the foot and the meridian of the foot Taiyang and the Ren meridian, using a reducing method of needling.

The bladder meridian affected by exogenous *feng* and cold gives rise to pain, soreness, spasm or numbness and motor impairment of the nape, back and lumbosacral regions which the meridian supplies. It should be treated with points mainly from this meridian using needling or moxibustion, or both, or used in combination with other therapies such as cutaneous needling.

PERICARDIUM AND SANJIAO

THE PERICARDIUM

The pericardium is situated in the chest, surrounding the heart and protecting the heart and mind. Its meridian is externally-internally related with that of the Sanjiao. Its pathogenesis and clinical manifestations are similar to those of the heart meridian of the hand Shaoyin.

Affection of this meridian by exogenous *feng*, cold and damp gives rise to pain in the cardiac and chest regions radiating to the axilla, irritability, swelling in the axilla, pain, numbness or motor impairment in the area the meridian supplies, and a feverish feeling in the palms. It should be treated with points mainly from the involved meridian, with a reducing method of needling, or with both acupuncture and moxibustion.

THE SANJIAO

This is a collective term for the three *jiao*, the upper, middle and lower heating-spaces within the body. Its meridian is externally-internally related with that of the pericardium, and it has a close relationship with the lungs, spleen, kidneys and bladder.

The normal distribution and metabolism of fluid in the human body depends on the qi-transforming function of the Sanjiao. Impaired qi transformation gives rise to retention of fluid and damp in the interior, marked by a swelling of the muscles and skin, distension and fullness in the abdomen, qi rebellion and abdominal coldness, or nocturnal enuresis, incontinence of urine, a white slippery tongue coating, and a deep-thready or slippery pulse. It should be treated with mainly the Front-Mu, Back-Shu and lower He-Sea points of the Sanjiao and points from the Ren meridian, using both acupuncture and moxibustion.

Retention of damp-heat in the bladder leading to retention of fluid gives rise to general feverishness, qi rebellion, swelling or distension of the muscles and skin, dysuria, a red tongue with a yellowy greasy coating, and a slippery-rapid pulse. It should be treated with the Front-Mu, Back-Shu and lower He-Sea points of the Sanjiao and points from the 3 yin meridians of the foot, with a reducing method of needling.

Retention of pathogenic *feng*, cold and damp obstructs the course of the Sanjiao meridian and gives rise to soreness, distension, pain, numbness and motor impairment in the area which the meridian supplies. Being affected by exogenous *feng* and heat, or an upward attack of interior heat may lead to obstruction of the meridian and give rise to dizziness and vertigo, tinnitus, sudden deafness, a congested eye and canthus, swelling of the cheek, Bi syndromes of the throat, scrofula, flank pain, or in severe cases constipation, dark yellow urine, a red tongue with a yellowy coating and a wiry and rapid pulse. This should be treated with points mainly from the meridians of the hand and foot Shaoyang, with a reinforcing or reducing method, using needling or moxibustion, or by bleeding with a three-edged needle.

LIVER AND GALLBLADDER

THE LIVER

The liver is situated within the hypochondrium; it takes charge of the tendons, stores the blood, and opens into the eyes. Its meridian is externally-internally related to that of the gallbladder; it connects with the eyes and the vertex. It is an organ whose nature is said to be forceful, which tends to promote the free passage of the qi and be disinclined to stagnation. The regulation of the emotions is closely related with the liver.

Emotional disturbance leading to stagnant liver qi is marked by costal or hypochondriacal pain, stuffiness in the chest, a quick temper, poor appetite, dry vomiting, rebellion of the qi with the sensation of a foreign body obstructing the throat, or sour regurgitation, yellow watery vomiting, abdominal pain and diarrhoea, a slightly yellow tongue coating, and a wiry long pulse. It can be treated with points mainly from the foot Jueyin, Shaoyang, Yangming and Taiyin meridians, using a reducing method of needling.

Stagnated liver qi turning into fire, and flaring upward of the liver fire, leads to a distending pain of head and eye, vertigo and blurred vision, congested and swollen eyes, irritability and insomnia, a quick temper, tinnitus, deafness, haematemesis or epistaxis, a red tongue with a yellowy coating, and a wiry-rapid or wiry-forceful pulse. It should be treated mainly with points from the meridians of the foot Jueyin and Shaoyang, using a reducing method of needling, or bloodletting with a three-edged needle.

A sudden attack of liver yang, or liver *feng* being stirred up within, often leads to a sudden loss of consciousness, high fever, coma, delirium, convulsions of limbs, opisthotonos, or deviation of the mouth, hemiplegia, slurred speech or deviation and tremor of tongue, a white thick or yellow-greasy tongue coating, a wiry-slippery or superficial pulse. It should be treated with points from the meridians of the foot Jueyin and Du, and the 12 Jing-well points, with a reducing method of needling, or bloodletting with a three-edged needle.

Kidney yin insufficiency or liver fire consuming yin (fluids) often leads to vertigo, headache, tinnitus, deafness, blurred vision, night-blindness, a tendency to be easily frightened, twitching of muscles in the limbs, a dry mouth and throat, afternoon tidal fever, a red tongue with little moisture, and little coating, and a thready-wiry or wiry-rapid pulse. It should be treated mainly with points from the meridians of the foot Jueyin Shaoyang and Shaoyin, with both reinforcing and reducing methods of needling, or a method of even movement.

Affection of this meridian by pathogenic cold is marked by cold and pain in lower abdomen, hernia, a pulling down sensation and pain of the testes which is worsened by cold and alleviated by warmth, or pain, numbness, cramps and contracting pain of the area which this meridian supplies. It should be treated with points of the involved meridian, with both acupuncture and moxibustion.

THE GALLBLADDER

The gallbladder is attached to the liver, and their meridians are externally-internally related. It is an organ said to have the character of "hardness" and "boldness", and it stores the refined product of bile within.

Impaired function of the gallbladder in the distribution of bile, due to it being affected by damp-heat, is marked by headache, bitter taste in the mouth and dry throat, tinnitus, deafness, flank distension, fullness and pain, alternate chilliness and fever, jaundice, vomiting of bitter tasting fluid, a red tongue with a yellowy greasy coating, and a wiry-rapid or wiry-slippery pulse. It should be treated with the Front-Mu and Back-Shu points of the gallbladder and those from the meridian of the foot Shaoyang, with a reducing method of needling.

Weakness of gallbladder qi often leads to a tendency to be easily frightened, fear and timidity, a preference for sighing, or restless sleep, blurred vision, vertigo and nausea, a thin and slippery tongue coating and a thready-wiry pulse. It should be treated with points mainly from the Back-Shu point of the gallbladder and those points from the meridians of the foot Shaoyang and both the hand and foot Jueyin, using a reinforcing method of needling, or both needling and moxibustion.

Exogenous *feng* cold affecting the meridian, or the retention of damp in the course of the meridian, often gives rise to pain and numbness of the area which the meridian supplies. It should be treated with points from the involved meridian, using needling or moxibustion.

General principles of treatment

The general principles of acupuncture and moxibustion treatment are determined according to the nature of the development and change of the disease, which, although complex and variable, can be classified within the "8 principles". These consist of *yin/yang* (阴/阳), *biao/li* (表/里) or exterior/interior, *xu/shi* (虚/实) or deficiency/ excess, and *han/re* (寒/热) or cold/heat .

In the *Miraculous Pivot* it states that "in treatment with acupuncture, deficiency should be reinforced, fullness should be reduced, stasis should be removed and excess of pathogens should be eliminated".[4]

Also in the *Miraculous Pivot*, it says "excess should be reduced, deficiency should be reinforced, heat should be cleared by swift needling, cold should be treated by retaining the needles, prolapse should be corrected by moxibustion, while those syndromes neither excess nor

deficient in nature should be treated on the basis of the meridians".[5]

These both show that, in the case of excess or fullness of the pathogen, a reducing method is used to eliminate the excess; in the case of a deficiency, a reinforcing method is used to reinforce and strengthen the antipathogenic qi. In the case of pathogenic heat, swift needling or pricking to cause bleeding is applied to clear the heat, while in the case of excessive cold and stagnation of the qi in the zangfu organs and jingluo, retaining the needle is used to await the recovery of the yang qi and dispel the cold pathogens, or moxibustion is applied to promote yang and dispel the cold. If a stasis of qi and blood is obstructing the jingluo, it should be eliminated by bloodletting. In the case of a yang qi deficiency, leading to a prolapse of the meridional qi, moxibustion is applied to uplift the yang and raise up the prolapse. Finally, if other meridians are not affected by the disorder, then only points of the involved meridian are selected in order to regulate its qi and blood.

Therefore, acupuncture and moxibustion treatment should be applied in the clinic according to the basic theories of TCM, through adopting the 4 classical diagnostic methods of inspection, auscultation and olfaction, inquiring, and palpation (in combination with other methods) and the 8 principles of the differentiation of syndromes, in order to determine the general principles of treatment.

1. YIN/YANG

Yin and yang are the basic theoretical core of TCM and the most pervasive of the 8 principles.

In the *Plain Questions* it states that "one who is good at diagnosing disease, in the first case, often observes the complexion, palpates the pulse, and differentiates yin and yang".[6] Generally speaking, those disorders of the exterior, at the fu organs, or of an excess or heat type are yang disorders; while those on the interior, at the zang organs, or of a deficient or cold type, pertain to yin.

As it states in the *Miraculous Pivot*, "with yin and yang differentiated, the method of needling may be selected; and with the origin of the disease ascertained, the principle behind the needling can be understood".[7] Clinically speaking, yang syndromes are usually excess or hot syndromes, in which case the reducing or swift method of needling, or pricking to cause bleeding can be applied. Yin syndromes are usually deficiency or cold syndromes, in which case the reinforcing method of needling, or moxibustion, or retention of the needle is applied.

These are the basic principles of the acupuncture and moxibustion treatment of disease.

2. EXTERIOR/INTERIOR

Exterior and interior refer to the depth of the location of the disease, which is closely related to the depth of needling. In the *Plain Questions* it states that "there are the superficial and deep diseases, there are the various depths in needling".[8]

Disease in the jingluo, the skin or muscles, pertains to the exterior, and superficial needling with swift withdrawal of the needle is applied; disease in the zang and fu organs, tendons and bones, is interior, and deep needling and long-term retention of the needle is required.

Exterior syndromes caused by exogenous pathogens should be treated with a reducing method, with needling or moxibustion. Those syndromes transmitting into the interior and the zangfu organs should be treated according to their differing conditions with needling or moxibustion, or both in combination, along with the methods of reinforcing or reducing.

3. COLD/HEAT

These terms refer to the nature of the disease. Generally cold syndromes are due to an excess of yin qi, or deficiency of yang qi which fails to resist the cold pathogen. Treatment should be applied according to the differing conditions. Cold pathogens may be either exterior or interior, of a deficiency or excess type, in which case the methods of retaining the needle, or reinforcing, or moxibustion, or both needling and moxibustion are applied.

Heat syndromes are due to an excess of yang qi, or deficiency of yin which fails to resist the heat pathogen. They can be seen in syndromes of the zang and fu organs, or throughout the whole course, or part of the course, of a certain meridian. Furthermore they can be exterior syndromes or interior syndromes. In treatment, generally the swift method of needling for reducing is used, or pricking to cause bleeding. Moxibustion is not used.

Complicated cold and heat syndromes involving genuine cold or pseudo-heat, and genuine heat or pseudo-cold should each be differentiated carefully. Genuine cold and pseudo-heat syndromes should be treated as cold, while genuine heat and pseudo-cold should be seen as hot. These complicated cold and heat syndromes are both treated by warming or clearing methods in their individual ways.

4. DEFICIENCY/EXCESS

These terms refer to the condition of the antipathogenic qi in the human body and to the growth and decline in the disease.

Deficiency is due to insufficiency of antipathogenic qi, as it states in the *Plain Questions*— "when essence and qi are consumed, it leads to deficiency".[9] This refers, in general, to diseases caused by insufficiency of yin or yang in the zangfu organs, the jingluo, or the qi and blood within the body. The method of reinforcing in needling, or both acupuncture and moxibustion, is applied in treating deficiency syndromes. It also states in the *Plain Questions* that "reinforcing is applied in any case of deficiency, until the deficiency is corrected and regulated".[10]

Excess refers to an excess of pathogens or hyperactivity of functioning within the body. In the same chapter of the *Plain Questions* it is recorded that "a preponderance of pathogenic qi leads to excess". In the *Miraculous Pivot* it is recorded that, "an excess in the body qi and the pathogenic qi, should be reduced at once, this is the meaning of 'reducing the excess'".[11] Usually, in excess syndromes, needling with a reducing method or bleeding is applied to eliminate the excess pathogens.

For deficiency complicated with excess or excess complicated with deficiency, reinforcing first and reducing second, or reducing first and reinforcing second, or both reinforcing and reducing are applied, according to the severity of the deficiency and excess.

The composition of acupoint prescriptions

Acupuncture and moxibustion treatment is applied through needling or applying moxibustion to certain acupoints. Therefore the selection of points and the composition of their prescriptions is closely related to the therapeutic results.

Clinically, forming point-prescriptions should be done in accordance with the basic theories of TCM, under the guidance of the principles of differentiating syndromes. By combining the actions and properties of the points, point-prescriptions can be made through a careful matching and selection, by considering the principles and methods of treatment and through being flexible about their application.

The composition of a prescription also consists of *jun* (君) "monarch", *chen* (臣) "minister", *zui* (佐) "assistant" and *shi* (使) "guide" points, with a difference being made between main and secondary points, as is done in the formation of herbal formulae. At the same time, attention should be paid to the possible selection of other therapies, or to the application of acupuncture and moxibustion along with other therapies.

BASIC PRINCIPLES FOR PRESCRIBING POINTS

The basic principle for prescribing and combining points is to select points according to the course of the meridian. Within this, there may be differentiated three ways in which points may be selected:

— local points,
— distant points,
— symptomatic points.

Selecting local points

This is based on the universal law that each acupoint is indicated for diseases of the local area, or adjacent area to which it is located. This method is applied for the treatment of disease within a superficial region of body and is limited to a local effect—for example, selecting Yingxiang (LI 20) for nose disorders, Jiache (St 6) and Dicang (St 4) for deviation of the mouth, and Zhongwan (Ren 12) and Liangmen (St 21) for gastric pain.

This method is widely used in the clinic and rich experience has been accumulated in this field. There are many examples in classical medical literature, for example "a headache with stagnated blood, or wounds with severe pain should be treated by puncturing the site beside them, but not remote points".[12] And, "in tinnitus, the preauricular artery is selected",[13] or "Xuanlu (GB 5) and Hanyan (GB 4), are good for relieving migraine".[14]

Selecting distant points

This method of selection is based on the basic theories of yin and yang, the zangfu and jingluo, and the therapeutic properties of the acupoints. It entails the selection of points far from the diseased area, e.g. Chize (Lu 5) and Yuji (Lu 10) for coughing and haemoptysis, Weizhong (UB 40) and Kunlun (UB 60) for lumbar pain, Hegu (LI 4) for oral and tooth pain. In practice, those points of the involved meridian, or of the externally-internally related meridian, or any other related meridian, can be selected, e.g. Zusanli (St 36) from the involved meridian, Gongsun (Sp 4) from the externally-internally related meridian, or Taichong (Liv 3) and Neiguan (P 6), both from related meridians, can be selected for gastric pain.

Examples of this method are recorded in the *Miraculous Pivot*, where it says "select points below for a disease above and vice versa, select points in the feet for a disease in the head, and points in the popliteal fossa for a disease in the lower back".[15]

Selecting symptomatic points

This can also be considered as selecting points

according to the differentiation of syndromes. It is based on the theories of TCM and the therapeutic properties of acupoints. It is different from the selection of local or distant points as these are based on the location of disease, which excludes diseases such as fever, spontaneous sweating, night sweating, prostration (shock), insomnia and dream-disturbed sleep.

The *Classic on Medical Problems* states that "the Influential point of the fu organs is Taicang (another name for Zhongwan, Ren 12), the Influential point of the zang organs is Jile (another name for Zhangmen, Liv 13), that of the tendons is Yanglingquan (GB 34), that of the marrow is Juegu (another name for Xuanzhong, GB 39), that of the blood is Geshu (UB 17), that of bone is Dashu (UB 11), that of the vessels is Taiyuan (Lu 9) and that of the qi is Shanzhong (Ren 17)".[16] These points are closely related to diseases with certain aspects and can be conveniently selected in the clinic. For instance, in stuffiness of the chest due to qi problems, Shanzhong is selected, for blood deficiency or chronic bleeding Geshu is used, and for disorders in the tendons or muscles Yanglingquan is often selected. Or again, in exogenous diseases accompanied by fever, Dazhui (Du 14), Hegu (LI 4) and Quchi (LI 11) are selected to clear heat and relieve exterior symptoms. In cases of coma, Renzhong (Du 26), Suliao (Du 25) and Neiguan (P 6) restore consciousness and promote resuscitation. Also, for yin deficiency leading to fever and night sweating, Yinxi (H 6) and Fuliu (K 7) are selected to nourish yin, clear heat and check sweating.

The above three methods can be applied singly or in combination in the clinic. For example, in the *Miraculous Pivot* it is recorded that "for borborygmus and severe asthmatic breathing, due to upward rebellion of the qi and pathogens in the large intestine, give needling to Qihai (Ren 6), Shangjuxu (St 37) and Zusanli (St 36)".[17] In this case, these are the local point Qihai, along with the distant and symptomatic points Shangjuxu and Zusanli. This is a typical example of a point-prescription which combines local, distant and symptomatic points together.

VARIATION IN PRESCRIBING POINTS

A single point-prescription may result in a variety of effects, owing to a different reinforcing or reducing method, the order or timing of the treatment, whether points are added to, or omitted from the prescription, the depth of the needling and the period of needle retention.

Differing effects of reinforcing and reducing

Reinforcing and reducing are two basic techniques, used in clinical treatment, with opposing effects. It is recorded in the *Miraculous Pivot* that "needling aims at regulating the qi; by tonifying yin or reducing yang, hoarseness is relieved and ear and eye diseases cured, otherwise the blood and qi would stagnate".[18] In other words, with differing manipulations, prescriptions with the same points may have exactly opposite effects. For example, clinically reinforcing Hegu (LI 4) and reducing Sanyinjiao (Sp 6) has the effect of activating the circulation of qi and blood, and removing blood stasis, and it is used for amenorrhoea due to stagnant blood, although these points are contraindicated in pregnancy. Contrariwise, reducing Hegu and tonifying Sanyinjiao has the effect of regulating the qi, nourishing blood and consolidating the normal menses, and they are used in menorrhagia or massive uterine bleeding. To give another example, Hegu and Fuliu (K 7) can be used for inducing or checking sweating, depending on the manipulative method applied.

Therefore, in the *Miraculous Pivot* it says, "the disease will be aggravated by treatment with the wrong reinforcing or reducing method of manipulation, that is, reinforcing in excess syndromes and reducing in deficiency syndromes".[19]

Effects varying with the depth of needling

Clinically, the same point-prescription varies in its effects with different depths of needling.

The effects of prescriptions are very closely related to the depth of needling, as it states in the *Miraculous Pivot* "deep needling applied for superficial diseases would only injure the healthy muscles, while superficial needling for deeply

situated diseases would have no effect in eliminating the pathogen."[20] When treating disease
according to prescriptions, not only the depth of
needling but also the condition of the disease,
the climate and the individual should be considered. It states in the *Miraculous Pivot* that,
"the spring qi is at the hair and pores, the summer qi at the skin and flesh, the autumn qi at
the muscles and the winter qi at the tendons
and bone. In treating these diseases, the depth
of needling should be varied accordingly. Furthermore, when needling fat patients the depth
should be that of autumn and winter, when
needling thin patients the depth should be that
of the spring and summer".[21]

These factors are very important in clinical
practice.

The selection of main and secondary points, and the proper order of needling or manipulation

In the *Miraculous Pivot* it is recorded that, "for
interior diseases, treat yin first and yang second,
otherwise the disease will be aggravated; for
disease located at the yang, treat the exterior first
and the interior second, otherwise the disease
will be aggravated".[22] Also in the *Miraculous
Pivot* it states that, "for pain running from above
to below, puncture below first to stop it and
above second to eliminate it; for pain running
from below to above, puncture above first to
stop it and below second to eliminate it".[23]

Generally, the order of needling in the clinic
is from above to below, and from yang to yin
regions of the body. But under any special conditions, the specific order of the needling and
manipulation should be further considered so as
to facilitate the treatment.

Moxibustion is applicable when needling will not do

For excess heat syndromes, generally, needling
only is applied without moxibustion. And, generally, in cold and deficiency syndromes, moxibustion is applied often and needling less often.
Clinically the decision of whether to use needling or moxibustion, or both, and whether there
should be more needling and less moxibustion,
or more moxibustion and less needling, should
be made according to the concrete condition of
the disease so that a satisfactory and desirable
therapeutic effect can be achieved.

Variation of the point-prescription can greatly affect the therapeutic effect

Generally, the main point(s) are kept unchanged,
while other points are varied along with changes
in the condition of the disease.

For example, the prescription of Hegu (LI 4) as
main point and Quchi (LI 11) as secondary point
is used for regulating the upper-jiao. If it is combined with Sanyinjiao (Sp 6) then the prescription has the function of activating the circulation
of qi and blood, and regulating menstruation; if
combined with Fuliu (K 7) it can induce sweating or alternatively check sweating; if combined
with Taichong (Liv 3) it functions in treating
Bi syndromes and promoting resuscitation, pacifying the liver and subduing *feng*, and can be
used as an important formula in *feng* stroke
(apoplexy) or deviation of the mouth.

BASIC PRINCIPLES FOR COMBINING POINTS

Combining points means matching together
points with the same or similar therapeutic properties, so that they can cooperate with each
other, in order to potentiate their therapeutic
effect. There are various ways of combining
points:

— combining points of the involved meridian,
— combining points of externally-internally
   related meridians,
— combining points in front and behind,
— combining points above and below,
— combining contralateral points.

Combining points of the involved meridian (of the diseased zangfu organ or meridian)

For instance, for coughing, Zhongfu (Lu 1) as the
local point and Front-Mu point of the lungs,
Chize (Lu 5) and Taiyuan (Lu 9) as the distant

points of the involved meridian, are used. In the *Miraculous Pivot* it states, "for firstly a *Jue* headache with aching in vertex, and next a pain in the lower back, select first Tianzhu (UB 10) and then points on the urinary bladder foot Taiyang".[24]

Combining points of externally-internally related meridians

This is based on the yin and yang, and exterior-interior relationships between the zangfu and the jingluo.

When a certain zangfu organ or meridian is diseased, points from its externally or internally related meridian are selected (possibly from one or both of them). For instance, again in the *Miraculous Pivot*, it says "for *Jue* cardiac pain with an ache radiating into the back, with cramps and severe pain in the back as in renal cardiac pain, select first Jinggu (Lu 8) and Kunlun (UB 60)".[25] The urinary bladder foot Taiyang is externally-internally related to the kidney meridian. This gives an example of selecting points from the externally related meridian for an interior disorder.

The *Miraculous Pivot* again says, "for pathogens affecting the kidneys, the bones aching and *Bi* syndromes of yin type, select Yongquan (K 1) and Kunlun (UB 60)",[26] which shows the combination of points from externally-internally related meridians.

The *Miraculous Pivot* again says, "for *Jue* cardiac pain (cardiac pain coming from the gastric region) with abdominal distension, fullness in the chest and severe cardiac pain, select Dadu (Sp 2) and Taibai (Sp 3)".[27] This shows the selection of points from an internally related meridian for the treatment of an exterior disease. The combination of *yuan* and *luo* points is also an application of this method.

Combining points in front and behind

This is also known as the "Method of Combining Back and Belly, Yin and Yang points". The "Even-number Method of Needling" and the "Method of Combining Front-Mu and Back-Shu points", both mentioned in the *Miraculous Pivot*, are included. This method is applied in treating disorders of zangfu organs, e.g. Zhongwan (Ren 12) and Jianli (Ren 11) for epigastric pain, with Pishu (UB 20) and Jizhong (Du 6) on the back used in combination; or just select its Front-Mu point Zhongwan and its Back-Shu point Weishu (UB 21) for epigastric pain.

Combining points above and below

In the *Lyric of the Hundred Diseases* (see Appendix 2), it states that "Qiangjian (Du 18) which is located above, and Fenglong (St 40) located below are selected for severe headaches; for night blindness due to problems of the liver qi, select Jingming (UB 1) above and Xingjian (Liv 2) below". Both the prescription in *The Rhymes of Grand Number One*[28] where it says, "for cardiac pain with tremor in the hands use Shaohai (H 3), and if you wish to dispel it select Yinshi (St 33)", and combining points according to the "Confluent Points of the 8 Extra meridians" (see Ch. 2, and below) are applications of this method.

Combining contralateral points

In this method, points can be selected either bilaterally, or else points on the left can be selected for disorders on the right, and vice versa; or again, when selecting points along the meridian (on the jing) you also select the *luo* point (on the luo) according to the condition of the diseases. Alternatively, bilateral points are used in treating diseases of the zangfu and jingluo, when both sides are involved. For example, in a case of pathogenic *feng* affecting the jingluo, marked by hemiplegia, contralateral points can be used (for a disorder on the opposite side) or else points bilaterally selected.

THE APPLICATION OF SPECIFIC POINTS

These specific points are groups of points, on the 14 meridians, which have a specific therapeutic function, but which, owing to their dissimilar distribution and use, are grouped under separate classifications. This has been previously mentioned in Part I, the *General Introduction to Jingluo and Acupoints*.

These points may be differentiated into:

(i)   5 Shu points,
(ii) Front-Shu and Back-Mu points,
(iii) *Yuan* and *luo* points,
(iv) 8 Extra Meridians' Confluent points,
(v)   8 Influential points,
(vi) Xi-cleft points,
(vii) Lower He-Sea points,
(viii) Crossing points.

What follows is a further exploration into their particular characteristics.

(I) THE 5 SHU POINTS

The 5 Shu (输) points are the 5 points of each of the 12 regular meridians (totalling 60 in all) below the elbow and knee: namely, the Jing-well (井), Ying-spring (荥), Shu-stream (输), Jing-river (经) and He-sea (合). They were imagined by the ancients to function as if controlling a stream of flowing water, representing the volume of the qi in the meridians and the depth of the qi flowing within the body, exerting its different functions.

They are described in the *Miraculous Pivot* where it says that, "the points from which qi wells up are called Jing-well points, the points where the qi flows on copiously are called Ying-spring points, the points where the qi pours in like a stream are called Shu-stream points, the points where the qi passes on through are called Jing-river points, and the points where the qi converges are called He-sea points".[29]

The 5 Shu points of the 12 regular meridians can be referred to in Tables 9.1 and 9.2.

The 5 Shu points have a function in treating pathological changes of the 5 zang and 6 fu organs and the meridians and collaterals.

In the *Miraculous Pivot* it is recorded that "for disorders in the 5 zang organs Jing-well points are used, for pathological changes manifesting in the face and complexion, Ying-spring points are used, diseases varying in severity, from time to time, can be treated by using Shu-stream points, in cases when the voice is affected by disease, Jing-river points are selected, for excess and fullness of the meridional qi, stomach disorders and injury through eating, He-sea points can be selected".[30]

The chapter in the *Classic on Medical Problems* states that "Jing-well points are indicated for fullness in the chest, Ying- spring points for febrile diseases, Shu-stream points for a heavy sensation in the body and painful joints, Jing-river points for coughs and asthma due to pathogenic cold and heat, and He-sea points for diarrhoea due to rebellion of the qi".[31] This is also one method of using the 5 Shu points in clinical practice.

Besides this, the *Classic on Medical Problems* also puts forward the method of "reinforcing the mother in deficiency and reducing the son in excess", according to combining the therapeutic properties of the 5 Shu points with the 5 Elements and the classification of zangfu organs

Table 9.1 Yin meridians' 5 Shu points

| | Five Shu points | | | | |
	Well (wood)	Spring (fire)	Stream (earth)	River (metal)	Sea (water)
Yin meridians					
Lung hand Taiyin	Shaoshang (Lu 11)	Yuji (Lu 10)	Taiyuan (Lu 9)	Jingqu (Lu 8)	Chize (Lu 5)
Pericardium hand Jueyin	Zhongchong (P 9)	Laogong (P 8)	Daling (P 7)	Jianshi (P 5)	Quze (P 3)
Heart hand Shaoyin	Shaochong (H 9)	Shaofu (H 8)	Shenmen (H 7)	Lingdao (H 4)	Shaohai (H 3)
Spleen foot Taiyin	Yinbai (Sp 1)	Dadu (Sp 2)	Taibai (Sp 3)	Shangqiu (Sp 5)	Yinlingquan (Sp 9)
Liver foot Jueyin	Dadun (Liv 1)	Xingjian (Liv 2)	Taichong (Liv 3)	Zhongfeng (Liv 4)	Ququan (Liv 8)
Kidney foot Shaoyin	Yongquan (K 1)	Rangu (K 2)	Taixi (K 3)	Fuliu (K 7)	Yingu (K 10)

Table 9.2 Yang meridians' 5 Shu points

| | Five Shu Points | | | | |
	Well (metal)	Spring (water)	Stream (wood)	River (fire)	Sea (earth)
Yang meridians					
Large intestine hand Yangming	Shangyang (LI 1)	Erjian (LI 2)	Sanjian (LI 3)	Yangxi (LI 5)	Quchi (LI 11)
Sanjiao hand Shaoyang	Guanchong (SJ 1)	Yemen (SJ 2)	Zhongzhu (SJ 3)	Zhigou (SJ 6)	Tianjing (SJ 10)
Small intestine hand Taiyang	Shaoze (SI 1)	Qiangu (SI 2)	Houxi (SI 3)	Yanggu (SI 5)	Xiaohai (SI 8)
Stomach foot Yangming	Lidui (St 45)	Neiting (St 44)	Xiangu (St 43)	Jiexi (St 41)	Zusanli (St 36)
Gallbladder foot Shaoyang	Foot-Qiaoyin (GB 44)	Xiaxi (GB 43)	Foot-Linqi (GB 41)	Yangfu (GB 38)	Yanglingquan (GB 34)
Bladder foot Taiyang	Zhiyin (UB 67)	Tonggu (UB 66)	Shugu (UB 65)	Kunlun (UB 60)	Weizhong (UB 40)

into the 5 Elements. For example, the lungs pertain to the metal element, and so for an excess syndrome of the lung meridian, the point from among the 5 Shu points which pertains to the water element, Chize (Lu 5), can be selected, as "metal" promotes "water" and "water" is the son of "metal". Therefore Chize is selected according to the idea of "reducing the son in excess". In a deficiency syndrome of the lung meridian, Taiyuan (Lu 9), which is the point which pertains to "earth" and is the mother of "metal", can be selected, according to the idea of "reinforcing the mother in deficiency" (cf. the method of "Ziwu Liuzhu Acupuncture Therapy", in Appendix 3).

The application of "mother" and "son" points for reinforcing and reducing can be referred to in Table 9.3.

(II) THE FRONT-MU AND BACK-SHU POINTS

The Front-Mu (募) points are places on the chest and abdomen where the qi of the zangfu organs converges, while the Back-Shu (俞) points are places on the back where the qi of the zangfu organs is infused. Front-Mu points are on the yin aspect of the body (chest and abdomen), which is an important place for yang diseases running into the yin, while Back-Shu points are located on the yang aspect of the body (on the Bladder meridian), which is an important place where yin diseases run into the yang. Each zang and each fu organ has its own Front-Mu and Back-Shu points (see Table 9.4).

These points are closely related to the zangfu

Table 9.3 Mother and Son points for reinforcing and reducing

Five elements	Zangfu	Mother point	Son point
Metal	Lung	Taiyuan (Lu 9)	Chize (Lu 5)
	Large intestine	Quchi (LI 11)	Erjian (LI 2)
Water	Kidney	Fuliu (K 7)	Yongquan (K 1)
	Bladder	Zhiyin (UB 67)	Shugu (UB 65)
Wood	Liver	Ququan (Liv 8)	Xingjian (Liv 2)
	Gallbladder	Xiaxi (GB 43)	Yangfu (GB 38)
Fire (ruler)	Heart	Shaochong (H 9)	Shenmen (H 7)
	Small intestine	Houxi (SI 3)	Xiaohai (SI 8)
Fire (minister)	Pericardium	Zhongchong (P 9)	Daling (P 7)
	Sanjiao	Zhongzhu (SJ 3)	Tianjing (SJ 10)
Earth	Spleen	Dadu (SP 2)	Shangqiu (Sp 5)
	Stomach	Jiexi (St 41)	Lidui (St 45)

Table 9.4 The Back-Shu points and Front-Mu points

	Back-Shu point	Front-Mu point
Zang organs		
Lung	Feishu (UB 13)	Zhongfu (Lu 1)
Pericardium	Jueyinshu (UB 14)	Shanzhong (Ren 17)
Heart	Xinshu (UB 15)	Juque (Ren 14)
Liver	Ganshu (UB 18)	Qimen (Liv 14)
Spleen	Pishu (UB 20)	Zhangmen (Liv 13)
Kidney	Shenshu (UB 23)	Jingmen (GB 25)
Fu organs		
Stomach	Weishu (UB 21)	Zhongwan (Ren 12)
Gallbladder	Danshu (UB 19)	Riyue (GB 24)
Bladder	Pangguangshu (UB 28)	Zhongji (Ren 3)
Large intestine	Dachangshu (UB 25)	Tianshu (St 25)
Sanjiao	Sanjiaoshu (UB 22)	Shimen (Ren 5)
Small intestine	Xiaochangshu (UB 27)	Guanyuan (Ren 4)

Table 9.5 The 12 meridians' yuan and luo points

Meridian	Yuan-source	Luo-connecting
Lung hand Taiyin	Taiyuan (Lu 9)	Lieque (Lu 7)
Large intestine hand Yangming	Hegu (LI 4)	Pianli (LI 6)
Stomach foot Yangming	Chongyang (St 42)	Fenglong (St 40)
Spleen foot Taiyin	Taibai (Sp 3)	Gongsun (Sp 4)
Heart hand Shaoyin	Shenmen (H 7)	Tongli (H 5)
Small intestine hand Taiyang	Wangu (SI 4)	Zhizheng (SI 7)
Bladder foot Taiyang	Jinggu (UB 64)	Feiyang (UB 58)
Kidney foot Shaoyin	Taixi (K 3)	Dazhong (K 4)
Pericardium hand Jueyin	Daling (P 7)	Neiguan (P 6)
Sanjiao hand Shaoyang	Yangchi (SJ 4)	Waiguan (SJ 5)
Gallbladder foot Shaoyang	Qiuxu (GB 40)	Guangming (GB 37)
Liver foot Jueyin	Taichong (Liv 3)	Ligou (Liv 5)

organs to which they respectively pertain. Furthermore, when pathological change occurs in a certain zang or fu organ, tenderness or sensitivity may appear at its own Front-Mu or Back-Shu point. So then the Front-Mu or Back-Shu points of that zangfu organ are often selected for treatment.

In the *Plain Questions* it states that "deficiency of the gallbladder with a bitter taste in the mouth is treated with the Front-Mu and Back-Shu points of the gallbladder",[32] showing the way to apply the Front-Mu and Back-Shu points. Clinically, they are not only used in combination for disorders of the zang or fu organs, but also singly for disorders of the tissues and organs related to their respective zangfu and jingluo. For example, the liver opens into the eye, and eye disease can be treated with Ganshu (UB 18) the Back-Shu point of the liver; the kidneys open into the ear and deafness can be treated with Shenshu (UB 23), the Back-Shu point of the kidneys.

(III) THE YUAN AND LUO POINTS

The *yuan* (原) points are sites where the *yuan* (source or original) qi pours into the body and returns. The *yuan* points are closely related to the Sanjiao (or three heating areas of the body) through which the *yuan* qi travels. The *yuan* qi, originating below the umbilicus and between the kidneys, is dispersed to the zangfu organs

and further on to the whole body via the Sanjiao; thereby it regulates exterior and interior, above and below, affecting the qi-transforming function of the zangfu organs. Hence the popular saying, "for diseases of the zangfu organs, the *yuan* points are selected". Each of the 12 regular meridians has a *yuan* point which is located on the limbs around the wrist and ankle joints.

Clinically, the *yuan* points can be used to treat diseases of the zangfu organs to which they pertain, and in deducing the conditions of their respective zangfu via the observation of changes at these points. As it states in the *Miraculous Pivot*, "Disorders of the 5 zang should manifest at the 12 *yuan* points, observing changes at these points helps in deducing the particular sickness of the 5 zang".[33]

The *luo* (络) points are sites where a divergent meridian branches off and where the meridian connects with its externally-internally related meridian. The *luo* points are indicated for diseases related to the externally-internally related meridians (see Table 9.5).

Yuan points and *luo* points can be used independently or in combination. Their combination is termed "host and guest combination" and is applied according to the occurring order of the disorders in the externally-internally related meridians. When a first meridian is diseased, its *yuan* point is used, with the *luo* point of the secondly diseased meridian.

For example, when both the lung and large intestine meridians are diseased, with the former (lung) being affected first, its *yuan* point Taiyuan (Lu 9) is selected as host point, with the *luo* point of the large intestine meridian Pianli (LI 6) as guest. Alternatively, if the large intestine meridian is diseased first and the lung meridian second, the *yuan* point Hegu (LI 4), should be used as host point, while the *luo* point Lieque (Lu 7) is used as guest. This is what is known as "combining exterior-interior points".

(IV) THE 8 EXTRA MERIDIANS' CONFLUENT POINTS

The 8 extra meridians' Confluent (交会) points are the 8 points on the limbs where the regular meridians communicate with the 8 extra meridians (which were found by the ancients according to the therapeutic properties of these 8 points). These 8 points are indicated in the treatment of disease of the corresponding 8 extra meridians. Each point can be used either singly in treating diseases of the particular extra meridian it communicates with, or in combination with the point from its related meridian. For example, Houxi (SI 3), which communicates with the Du meridian, can be used alone for stiffness and pain along the Du meridian and spinal column, or opisthotonos; or again, rebellious qi and problems of the chest and abdomen along the Chong meridian can be relieved by using Gongsun (Sp 4), which communicates with the Chong meridian.

Alternatively, these points can be used in combination with the point from their related meridian according to their connections. Gongsun communicates with the Chong meridian and Neiguan (P 6) communicates with the Yinwei meridian, and these two can be used in combination for treating diseases in the stomach, heart

and chest. Houxi (SI 3) communicates with the Du meridian and Shenmai (UB 62) with the Yangqiao meridian, so these two can be used in combination to treat diseases of the inner canthus, neck (nape), ear and shoulder. This latter use of combined points is also included in the category of the so-called "matching of upper and lower points".

The ways of combining the Confluent points and their therapeutic applications can be referred to in Table 9.6.

Appendix: Classical Poem

Song of the 8 Extra Meridians and 8 Confluent Points

Gongsun (Sp 4), the Chong meridian, stomach, heart and chest,

Neiguan (P 6), the Yinwei below, collectively they are all together.

Linqi (GB 41), the Gall meridian links to the Dai,

The Yangwei, and outer canthus of the eye, along Waiguan's (SJ 5) seam.

Houxi (SI 3), the Du meridian—the inner canthus and neck,

Shenmai (UB 62), the Yangqiao, they all join and communicate.

Lieque (Lu 7), by the Ren meridian, travels to the lungs,

The Yinqiao, and Shaohai (K 6) for diaphragm and throat.

(V) THE 8 INFLUENTIAL POINTS

The 8 Influential (会) points are the sites where the essential qi of the qi, blood, tendons, bone,

Table 9.6 The eight Confluent points of the eight Extra meridians

Confluent point	Extra meridian	Indications
Gongsun (Sp 4) Neiguan (P 6)	Chong Yinwei	{ Heart, chest, stomach.
Houxi (SI 3) Shenmai (UB 62)	Du Yangqiao	{ Inner canthus, neck (nape), ear, shoulder.
Waiguan (SJ 5) Zulinqi (GB 41)	Yangwei Dai	{ Outer canthus, retroauricle, cheek, neck, shoulder.
Lieque (Lu 7) Zhaohai (K 6)	Ren Yinqiao	{ Lung system, throat, chest, and diaphragm.

Table 9.7 The 8 Influential points

Tissue	Influential point
Zang organs	Zhangmen (Liv 13)
Fu organs	Zhongwan (Ren 12)
Qi	Shanzhong (Ren 17)
Blood	Geshu (GB 17)
Tendons	Yanglingquan (GB 34)
Pulse, vessels	Taiyuan (Lu 9)
Bone	Dashu (UB 11)
Marrow	Xuanzhong (GB 39)

marrow, vessels, zang and fu organs converges. The *Classic on Medical Problems* states that, "for interior febrile diseases, the Influential points are selected".[34]

While clinically the indications of the Influential points cover a broader area than just febrile diseases, as mentioned in the *Classic on Medical Problems*, what is more important is that these points are indicated for diseases of their corresponding tissues and zangfu organs.

So, for example, in diseases of the tendons the Influential point of the tendons, Yanglingquan (GB 34), is used; for vessel disorders, the Influential point of the vessels, Taiyuan (Lu 9), is used; for diseases of the fu organs, the Influential point of the fu organs Zhongwan (Ren 12) is selected, and so on (see Table 9.7).

(VI) THE XI-CLEFT POINTS

Xi-Cleft (郄) points are the sites where the qi and blood of the meridians is deeply converged. Each of the 12 regular meridians and the 4 extra meridians (Yinwei, Yangwei, Yinqiao and Yangqiao) has a Xi-Cleft point on the limbs, amounting to 16 in all.

Clinically, the Xi-Cleft points are used in treating acute diseases of their corresponding meridians. For example, haemoptysis is a disorder of the lungs, and the Xi-Cleft point of the Lung meridian Kongzui (Lu 6) can be selected. In acute gastric diseases, the Xi-Cleft point of the stomach meridian Liangqiu (St 34) is selected (see Table 9.8).

(VII) THE LOWER HE-SEA POINTS

The lower He-Sea (下合) points are the six He-Sea

Table 9.8 The Xi-Cleft points

Meridian	Xi-Cleft point
Lung hand Taiyin	Kongzui (Lu 6)
Pericardium hand Jueyin	Ximen (P 4)
Heart hand Shaoyin	Yinxi (H 6)
Large intestine hand Yangming	Wenliu (LI 7)
Sanjiao hand Shaoyang	Huizong (SJ 7)
Small intestine hand Taiyang	Yanglao (SI 6)
Spleen foot Taiyin	Diji (Sp 8)
Liver foot Jueyin	Zhongdu (Liv 6)
Kidney foot Shaoyin	Shuiquan (K 5)
Stomach foot Yangming	Liangqiu (St 34)
Gallbladder foot Shaoyang	Waiqiu (GB 36)
Bladder foot Taiyang	Jinmen (UB 63)
Yinwei meridian	Zhubin (K 9)
Yangwei meridian	Yangjiao (GB 35)
Yinqiao meridian	Jiaoxin (K 8)
Yangqiao meridian	Fuyang (UB 59)

points pertaining to the six fu organs, along the three yang foot meridians which travel along the lower limbs.

In the *Miraculous Pivot* it states that "disorders of the six fu organs can be treated by selecting their lower He-Sea points."[35] For instance, the large intestine communicates with Shangjuxu (St 37), so when the large intestine is diseased point Shangjuxu is used; the gallbladder communicates with Yanglingquan (GB 34), and Yanglingquan is selected when the gallbladder is diseased (see Table 9.9).

(VIII) THE CROSSING POINTS

Crossing (交会) points refer to those points located at the intersection of two or more meridians.

Clinically these points are indicated in diseases of intersecting meridians. For example, Sanyinjiao (Sp 6) pertains to the spleen meridian and is also the crossing point of the three yin meridians, so it can be used not only in treating

Table 9.9 The Lower He-Sea Points

Lower He-Sea points	Three yang meridians of hand	Taiyang—Xiajuxu (St 39)
		Shaoyang—Weiyang (UB 39)
		Yangming—Shangjuxu (St 37)
	Three yang meridians of foot	Taiyang—Weizhong (UB 40)
		Shaoyang—Yanglingquan (GB 34)
		Yangming—Zusanli (St 36)

diseases of the spleen meridian, but also in diseases of the liver and kidney meridians. Guanyuan (Ren 4) is a point on the abdomen and the crossing point of the Ren meridian and the three yin meridians of foot, so it can be used not only in treating diseases of the Ren meridian, but also in those of the three yin meridians of foot.

Crossing points are given in Table 9.10 according to how they are recorded in *A Classic of Systematic Acupuncture and Moxibustion*.

Table 9.10   The crossing points of meridians

Point	Foot Taiyin (SP)	Hand Taiyin (LU)	Foot Jueyin (LV)	Hand Jueyin (PC)	Foot Shaoyin (K)	Hand Shaoyin (HT)	Foot Taiyang (UB)	Hand Taiyang (SI)	Foot Shaoyang (GB)	Hand Shaoyang (SJ)	Foot Yangming (ST)	Hand Yangming (LI)	Ren meridian	Chong meridian	Du meridian	Dai meridian	Yinwei meridian	Yangwei meridian	Yinqiao meridian	Yangqiao meridian	Remarks
Chengjiang (Ren 24)											√	√	○		√						from *Compendium of Acupuncture & Moxibustion*
Lianquan (Ren 23)													○				√				
Tiantu (Ren 22)													○				√				
Shangwan (Ren 13)								√			√		○								
Zhongwan (Ren 12)								√		√	√		○								promoted by hand Taiyang, hand Shaoyang and foot Yangming
Xiawan (Ren 10)	√												○								
Yinjiao (Ren 7)													○	√							
Guanyuan (Ren 4)	√		√		√								○								
Zhongji (Ren 3)	√		√		√								○								
Qugu (Ren 2)			√										○								
Huiyin (Ren 1)													○	√	√						
Sanyinjiao (Sp 6)	○		√		√																
Chongmen (Sp 12)	○		√																		
Fushe (Sp 13)	○		√														√				
Duheng (Sp 15)	○																√				
Fuai (Sp 16)	○																√				
Zhongfu (Lu 1)	√	○																			
Zhangmen (Liv 13)			○						√												
Qimen (Liv 14)	√		○														√				
Tianchi (P 1)				○					√												
Henggu (K 11)					○									√							
Dahe (K 12)					○									√							
Qixue (K 13)					○									√							
Siman (K 14)					○									√							
Zhongzhu (K 15)					○									√							
Huangshu (K 16)					○									√							
Shangqu (K 17)					○									√							

Table 9.10 The crossing points of meridians (*contd*)

Point	Foot Taiyin	Hand Taiyin	Foot Jueyin	Hand Jueyin	Foot Shaoyin	Hand Shaoyin	Foot Taiyang	Hand Taiyang	Foot Shaoyang	Hand Shaoyang	Foot Yangming	Hand Yangming	Ren meridian	Chong meridian	Du meridian	Dai meridian	Yinwei meridian	Yangwei meridian	Yinqiao meridian	Yangqiao meridian	Remarks
Shiguan (K 18)					○									√							
Yindu (K 19)					○									√							
Tonggu (K 20)					○									√							
Youmen (K 21)					○									√							
Zhaohai (K 6)					○														√		
Jiaoxin (K 8)					○														√		
Zhubin (K 9)					○												√				
Shenting (Du 24)							√				√				○						
Shuigou (Du 26)											√	√			○						
Baihui (Du 20)							√								○						
Naohu (Du 17)							√								○						
Fengfu (Du 16)															○			√			
Yamen (Du 15)															○			√			
Dazhui (Du 14)							√		√		√				○						
Taodao (Du 13)							√								○						from *Illustrated Manual on Points for Acu. & Moxi. on A Bronze Figure*
Changqiang (Du 1)					√		√								○						*– ditto –*
Changqiang (Du 1)					√										○						
Jingming (UB 1)							○	√			√								√	√	from *Plain Questions*
Dashu (UB 11)							○	√													
Fengmen (UB 12)							○								√						
Fufen (UB 41)							○	√													
Fuyang (UB 59)							○													√	
Shenmai (UB 62)							○													√	
Naoshu (SJ 10)								○										√		√	
Bingfeng (LI 12)								○	√	√		√									
Pucan (UB 61)							○													√	
Jinmen (UB 63)							○											√			
Quanliao (SI 18)								○	√												
Tinggong (SI 19)								○	√	√											
Tongziliao (GB 1)								√	○	√											
Shangguan (UB 6)									○	√	√										
Hanyan (GB 4)									○	√	√										
Xuanli (GB 6)									○	√	√										

Table 9.10   The crossing points of meridians (*contd*)

Point \ Meridian	Foot Taiyin	Hand Taiyin	Foot Jueyin	Hand Jueyin	Foot Shaoyin	Hand Shaoyin	Foot Taiyang	Hand Taiyang	Foot Shaoyang	Hand Shaoyang	Foot Yangming	Hand Yangming	Ren meridian	Chong meridian	Du meridian	Dai meridian	Yinwei meridian	Yangwei meridian	Yinqiao meridian	Yangqiao meridian	Remarks
Qubin (GB 7)							√		○												
Shuaigu (UB 8)							√		○												
Fubai (GB 10)							√		○												
Touqiaoyin (GB 11)							√		○												
Wangu (GB 12)							√		○												
Benshen (GB 13)									○									√			
Yangbai (GB 14)									○									√			
Toulinqi (GB 15)							√		○									√			
Muchuang (GB 16)									○									√			
Zhengying (GB 17)									○									√			
Chengling (GB 18)									○									√			
Naokong (GB 19)									○									√			
Fengchi (GB 20)									○									√			
Jianjing (GB 21)									○	√								√			
Riyue (GB 24)	√								○									√			
Huantiao (GB 30)							√		○												
Daimai (GB 26)									○							√					
Wushu (GB 27)									○							√					
Weidao (GB 28)									○							√					
Juliao (GB 29)									○											√	
Yangjiao (GB 35)									○									√			
Tianliao (SJ 15)										○								√			
Yifeng (SJ 17)									√	○											
Jiaosun (SJ 20)									√	○	√										
Heliao (SJ 22)								√	√	○											
Chengqi (St 1)											○		√							√	
Juliao (St 3)											○									√	
Dicang (St 4)											○	√								√	
Xiaguan (St 7)									√		○										
Touwei (St 8)									√		○							√			
Qichong (St 30)											○			√							where the Chong Meridian originates
Binao (LI 14)												○									meeting with collateral of hand-Yangming
Jianyu (LI 15)												○								√	
Jugu (LI 16)												○								√	
Yingxiang (LI 20)											√	○									

NOTES

1. *Miraculous Pivot*, Ch. 5, "Origins and Terminations".
2. *Plain Questions*, Ch. 62, "Discussion on Regulating the Meridians".
3. Yu Jiayan lived from 1585-1664. He was a famous physician from the end of the Ming and beginning of the Qing dynasties.
4. *Miraculous Pivot*, Ch. 1, "On the 9 Needles and 12 Yuan-sources".
5. *Miraculous Pivot*, Ch. 10, "Meridians".
6. *Plain Questions*, Ch. 5, "Great Discourse on the Responding Imagery of Yin and Yang".
7. *Miraculous Pivot*, Ch. 6, "Longevity or Early Death, the Firm and the Yielding".
8. *Plain Questions*, Ch. 53, "Discourse on Needling Essentials".
9. *Plain Questions*, Ch. 28, "A Penetrating Discussion on Deficiency and Excess".
10. Ibid.
11. *Miraculous Pivot*, Ch. 5, "Origins and Terminations".
12. *Miraculous Pivot*, Ch. 24, "On Jue Diseases".
13. Ibid.
14. From the *Lyric of the Hundred Diseases*, see Appendix 2.
15. *Miraculous Pivot*, Ch. 9, "Looking to Endings and Beginnings".
16. *The Classic on Medical Problems*, 45th problem.
17. *Miraculous Pivot*, Ch. 19, "Variation in Seasonal Qi".
18. *Miraculous Pivot*, Ch. 9, "Looking to Endings and Beginnings".
19. *Miraculous Pivot*, Ch. 4, "The Shape of Disease in the Zangfu according to the Evil Qi".
20. *Miraculous Pivot*, Ch. 7, "The Just Choice of Needle".
21. *Miraculous Pivot*, Ch. 9, "Looking to Endings and Beginnings".
22. *Miraculous Pivot*, Ch. 49, "The Five Facial Colours".
23. *Miraculous Pivot*, Ch. 27, "Total Bi Syndrome Disease".
24. *Miraculous Pivot*, Ch. 24, "On Jue Diseases".
25. Ibid.
26. *Miraculous Pivot*, Ch. 20 "The Five Evil Pathogens".
27. *Miraculous Pivot*, Ch. 24, "On Jue Diseases".
28. The *Heavenly Rhymes of Grand Number One* is contained within the Ming *Classic on Spiritual Resonance* (see Bibliography).
29. *Miraculous Pivot*, Ch. 1, "On the 9 Needles and 12 Yuan-sources".
30. *Miraculous Pivot*, Ch. 44, "Following the Daily Qi divided as if Seasonally".
31. *The Classic on Medical Problems*, 68th problem.
32. *Miraculous Pivot*, Ch. 47 "Various Other Diseases".
33. *Miraculous Pivot*, Ch. 1, "On the 9 Needles and 12 Yuan-sources".
34. *The Classic on Medical Problems*, 68th problem.
35. *Miraculous Pivot*, Ch. 4, "The Shape of Disease in the Zangfu according to the Evil Qi".

Treatment of common diseases

10

A. Internal diseases

1. FENG STROKE

Feng stroke (中风) is a commonly seen acute disease occurring often in both elderly and middle-aged people. The disease is manifested by falling down in a fit with loss of consciousness, hemiplegia or slurred speech and a deviated mouth. In classical Chinese medical literature it was named *zu-zhong* (卒中), "sudden inner attack", *jue* syndrome (厥), or *pian-ku* (偏枯), meaning hemiplegia, and noted because of the severity of its attack and symptomology.

Clinically, there are two types of *feng* stroke according to the severity and depth of the location of the disease. The severe type, or what is known as "the zangfu being attacked", shows signs and symptoms in the jingluo and viscera. The mild type, or "the jingluo being attacked" shows signs and symptoms pertaining to the jingluo. Treatment is based on this classification.

Feng stroke refers to cerebral vascular accidents (CVAs), including cerebral haemorrhage, thrombosis, or embolism, etc.

AETIOLOGY AND PATHOGENESIS

As for the causative factors of this disease, since ancient times different schools have presented different arguments. They can be summed up as follows: the main causative factors in *feng* stroke are related to *feng*, fire and *tan*, and pathological changes which may be observed in the heart, liver, spleen and kidney.

The occurrence of this disease may be due to accidental exasperation, agitation, overstrain or stress, or sexual indulgence which uncoordinates yin and yang. Any of these may cause the stirring of *feng* arising from hyperactivity of the liver yang and hyperactivity of heart-fire, consequently the confrontation of *feng* and fire leading to an upward rebellion of qi and blood.

Alternatively, it may be due to alcoholic indulgence, or a fatty diet, which results in asthenia of the spleen complicated by *tan* heat leading to fire which stirs up the *feng*, and the *feng* and yang go upwards accompanied by turbid *tan*, to disturb the mind and cause an abrupt dysfunction of the zangfu organs.

Uncoordination and derangement of yin and yang will result in *feng* stroke of the tense type; deficiency of antipathogenic qi and separation of yin and yang will result in *feng* stroke of the flaccid type.

If the *feng* and *tan* attack the jingluo, the normal activity of vital energy and blood will be impeded. In this case dysfunctions of the jingluo may occur.

DIFFERENTIATION

Feng stroke is caused by the upward flowing of qi and blood, therefore there may appear such prodromal signs as dizziness, palpitations, numb extremities, weak limbs and stiff tongue.

When the jingluo are being attacked, symptoms and signs show the dysfunction of the jingluo. This often happens without afflicting the zangfu organs, or during a slow restoration of the function of zangfu organs, and can be seen while the vital energy and blood of the jingluo are still impeded. Manifestations are hemiplegia, numbness, slurred speech due to stiff tongue and deviation of the mouth, wiry and slippery pulse, etc.

When the zangfu are being attacked this is the severe type of *feng* stroke. It is marked by falling down, fits with loss of consciousness, hemiplegia, aphasia due to a stiff tongue and deviation of the mouth. It must be classified into either a tense or flaccid syndrome according to its causative factors.

Tense. A tense syndrome is due to upward rushing of qi and fire leading to stagnation of blood in the upper part of the body, liver *feng* being stirred up and *tan* turbidity in excess. Manifestations are loss of consciousness, clenched fists and jaw, a flushed face and coarse breathing, rattling in the throat, retention of urine and stool, and a wiry, rolling and forceful pulse.

Flaccid. A flaccid syndrome is caused by prostration of the vital yang and true kidney qi. Manifestations are loss of consciousness with mouth agape and eyes closed, flaccid paralysis of limbs, incontinence of urine, snoring but feeble breathing, cold limbs, and thready and weak pulse. In critical cases, there may be oily sweating and malar flush, and a fading and floating big pulse indicating the outward floating of the kidney-yang.

TREATMENT

Needling and moxibustion

1. The jingluo being attacked

a) *Hemiplegia*

Method. Points of the hand and foot Yangming meridians are selected as the main points, and points of the Taiyang and Shaoyang meridians as supplementary ones. For prolonged cases the affected side is punctured. It is also a common practice to puncture the true side first and then the affected side.

Prescription.
— Upper limbs: Jianyu (LI 15), Quchi (LI 11), Shousanli (LI 10), Waiguan (SJ 5), Hegu (LI 4).
— Lower limbs: Huantiao (GB 30), Yanglingquan (GB 34), Zusanli (St 36), Jiexi (St 41), Kunlun (UB 60).

Explanation. A *feng* disease usually attacks the yang meridians and so points from the yang meridians are selected as the main ones.

The Yangming meridians are full of qi and blood, with which a smooth circulation of qi and blood, sufficient antipathogenic qi and the restoration of vital function are maintained.

Points of the Yangming meridians are selected separately, according to the different routes of the meridians in the upper and lower limbs. This promotes a free circulation of qi and blood throughout the body to regulate the jingluo.

Modification. Besides the above prescription, pricking to cause bleeding in the Jing-well points of the affected side can be used for hemiplegia.

Jianyu (LI 14), Yangchi (SJ 4), and Houxi (SI 3) can be employed alternately on the upper limbs and Fengshi (GB 31), Yinshi (St 34), and Xuanzhong (GB 39) on the lower limbs.

In chronic cases, supplementary points Dazhui (Du 14), and Jianwaishu (SJ 14) for the upper limbs, and Yaoyangguan (Du 3) and Baihuanshu (UB 30) for the lower limbs can be used.

For stiffness on the affected side, Quze (P 3) at the elbow, Daling (P 7) at the wrist, Ququan (Liv 8) at the knee, and Taixi (K 3) at the ankle can be used. This is the therapy of "treating yang from yin".

In addition, Yamen (Du 15), Lianquan (Ren 23) and Tongli (H 5) may be added for slurred speech. For numbness, cutaneous needling can be applied by tapping the affected side.

b) *Deviated mouth*

Method. Choose points mainly from the hand and foot Yangming meridians. Puncture the affected side in acute cases and both sides in chronic cases.

Prescription. Dicang (St 4), Jiache (St 6), Hegu (LI 4), Neiting (St 44), Taichong (Liv 3).

Explanation. The hand and foot Yangming meridians traverse the head. Dicang and Jiache are used to regulate qi in the local area, while Hegu, Neiting and Taichong, being distal points, are used to regulate the qi of the involved meridians.

Modification. Shuigou (Du 26), Qianzheng (Extra 10), Sibai (St 2) and Xiaguan (St 7) are used according to the affected part.

2. The zangfu being attacked

a) *Tense syndrome*

Method. Points of the Du meridian and the 12 Jing-well points are selected as the main points. The reducing method of needling or pricking is applicable.

Prescription. Shuigou (Du 26), the 12 Jing-well points, Taichong (Liv 3), Fenglong (St 40), Laogong (P 8).

Explanation. This prescription is formulated to pacify the liver and subdue *feng*, purge fire and resolve *tan*, and restore consciousness.

The tense syndrome is caused by an upsurge of liver yang and upward flowing of qi and blood, so pricking the twelve Jing-well points and puncturing Shuigou can dispel heat and restore consciousness. Taichong is reduced to subdue the upsurging of qi in the Liver meridian and pacify the liver yang.

The spleen and stomach are the source of *tan* production. A stagnation of turbid *tan* impairs the qi passage, so Fenglong of the foot Yangming is used to invigorate the functions of the spleen and stomach and to help resolve the turbid *tan*.

Ying-spring points are often indicated for fever, so Laogong, being a Ying-spring point in the pericardium meridian of the hand Jueyin, is used to clear away heat from the heart.

Points according to symptoms and signs. Clenched teeth: Jiache (St 6) and Hegu (LI 4). Slurred speech: Yamen (Du 15), Lianquan (Ren 23) and Guanchong (SJ 1).

b) Flaccid syndrome

Method. Points of the Ren meridian are selected. Moxibustion with large moxa-cones is applied to Shenque (Ren 8).

Prescription. Shenque (Ren 8) (indirect moxibustion with salt), Guanyuan (Ren 4).

Explanation. The Ren meridian is the sea of the Yin meridians. Guanyuan is the meeting point of the Ren meridian and the three yin meridians, and a point where the vital qi of Sanjiao originates. It connects with the "gate of life", close to the Mingmen (Du 4), and the true kidney yang, where the "yang is shadowed within the yin". Guanyuan is used to aid the true yang and restore it, preventing it from floating outwards.

Shenque is located at the umbilicus where the *zhen* qi dwells. So, by applying moxibustion with large moxa-cones to these two points, the waning yang can be restored.

Scalp needling

Select mainly the Motor Area on the true side, and the Foot Motor-Sensory Area as well. The Speech Area is used for slurred speech.

Good results can be obtained in treating cerebral thrombosis.

Electroneedling

Select 2–3 pairs of the above points on the limbs. After insertion, the needles are manipulated by lifting and thrusting to make the needle sensation extend to distal areas. The electricity is applied with a machine which emits sparse or intermittent waves for half a minute, during which the intensity of stimulation is increased gradually.

This can be repeated 3–4 times, with intervals in between, till the patient has a numb sensation and regular contraction of the muscles. The method is indicated for hemiplegia.

Point-injection therapy

Inject 2–4 ml Dengzhanhua (*Herba Erigerontis* solution) or Danggui (*Radix Angelicae sinensis* solution) into 2–4 of the above points, 1 ml for each point. The treatment is given once every other day. Ten treatments make a course. When the course has finished, wait 7–10 days, then continue a second time. This therapy is indicated in hemiplegia.

Cupping

Cupping with small cups is applied onto Jianyu (LI 15), Quchi (LI 11), Yangchi (SJ 4), Huantiao (GB 30), Binao (LI 14), Fengshi (GB 31), Zhibian (UB 54), Futu (St 32), Yanglingquan (GB 34), and Qiuxu (GB 40), etc., which are divided into groups and used alternately. This treatment is indicated for hemiplegia.

REMARKS

1. Elderly people who have a deficiency of qi and manifestations of the upsurge of liver yang may present with dizziness and numbness of the fingers, which may be prodromes of *feng* stroke. Attention should be paid to a regular life style and diet. Moxibustion and needling applied to Zusanli (St 36) and Fengshi (GB 31) may prevent an attack of *feng* stroke.
2. The patient should be instructed to practise functional exercises of his paralytic limbs in combination with massage and physiotherapy.
3. Comprehensive treatment should be given if the patient is at the acute stage.

2. DIZZINESS AND VERTIGO (INCLUDING HYPERTENSION)

Dizziness or vertigo is a common disease in the

clinic. A mild bout lasts only a short time and can be relieved by closing one's eyes, while a serious case causes the illusion of bodily movement with a rotary sensation like sitting in a sailing boat or a moving car, and a tendency to fall.

The case can sometimes be mild and sometimes severe, accompanied by other symptoms, which makes it lingering. The symptom can manifest as high blood pressure.

AETIOLOGY AND PATHOGENESIS

The disease is related to a weak constitution, poor health after disease, exasperation, or indulgence in a fatty or spicy diet.

The disease may be due to deficiency of the heart and spleen and deficiency of qi and blood, which fails to fill up "the sea of marrow" in the head.

It may be induced by the kidney water, as a yin deficiency fails to nourish the liver which leads to an upward attack of the liver yang, affecting the head.

Alternatively, it is due to a constitutional excess of damp, or indulgence in greasy or spicy food which gives rise to *tan*, which mists the head and mind.

DIFFERENTIATION

The main symptoms are dizziness and blurring of vision, in which the patient feels that his surroundings are whirling around, accompanied by nausea and a tendency to fall.

If the dizziness is accompanied by pallor and general weakness, palpitations, insomnia, pale tongue proper, and a thready and weak pulse, it results from deficiency of qi and blood.

An upward attack of hyperactivity of the liver yang, due to exasperation, may result in lumbar soreness and weakness of the legs, a red tongue proper, a wiry and rapid pulse, headache and feeble legs, and dizziness accompanied by nausea and vomiting.

A suffocating sensation in the chest, thick fur over the tongue proper, anorexia, irritability, a thick greasy tongue coating and slippery pulse result from the interior retention of *tan* damp.

TREATMENT

Needling and moxibustion

a) Deficiency of qi and blood

Method. Mainly to invigorate the function of the spleen and stomach. Apply the reinforcing method of needling. Moxibustion is applicable.

Prescription. Pishu (UB 20), Zusanli (St 36), Qihai (Ren 6) and Baihui (Du 20).

Explanation. The disease is caused by a deficiency of qi and blood. Treatment should begin with invigorating the spleen and stomach.

Pishu and Zusanli are used to invigorate the spleen and stomach, the sources of qi and blood, so as to promote qi and blood production.

Baihui and Qihai belong to the Ren and Du meridians. They are used to make the qi and blood supply the head, and to nourish "the sea of marrow" in the head. Thus the dizziness or vertigo can be relieved automatically.

b) Hyperactivity of the liver yang

Method. Mainly to pacify the liver yang. Apply the reducing method of needling.

Prescription. Fengchi (GB 20), Ganshu (UB 18), Shenshu (UB 23), Xingjian (Liv 2) and Xiaxi (GB 43).

Explanation. This syndrome is caused by deficiency of kidney yin and hyperactivity of liver yang.

The reducing method is applied to Fengchi and Xiaxi from the gall-bladder meridian, and Xingjian from the liver meridian. This pacifies the yang of the liver and gallbladder, and relieves the acute symptom.

The reinforcing method is applied to Ganshu and Shenshu to nourish the kidney water (yin) in order to treat the primary cause.

c) Interior retention of tan *damp*

Method. Mainly to resolve *tan* and invigorate the spleen. Apply the even method of needling and also moxibustion.

Prescription. Fenglong (St 40), Zhongwan (Ren 12), Neiguan (P 6), Touwei (St 8), and Jiexi (St 41).

Explanation. Zhongwan and Fenglong are needled for resolving damp and *tan*. Neiguan is for harmonizing the stomach and checking vomiting.

Touwei is for blurred vision. Jiexi is to make stomach qi descend and resolve the damp and *tan*, so as to relieve vertigo.

Point-injection therapy

Prescription. Hegu (LI 4), Taichong (Liv 3), Yiming (Extra 11), Neiguan (P 6), Fengchi (GB 20) and Sidu (SJ 9).

Method. Select 2–3 points in each treatment. Apply 1–2 ml of 5–10% glucose solution, or 0.5 ml of Vitamin B12 (100 micrograms) into each point once every other day.

Ear needling

Points. Kidney, Ear-Shenmen, Occiput, Inner-ear, Brain.

Method. Select 2–3 points in each treatment. Manipulate the needles intermittently with a strong and moderate stimulation. Retain the needles for 20–30 minutes.

Scalp needling

Areas to be selected. Vertigo-Auditory Area on both sides.

Method. Treatment is given once a day. Ten treatments make a course.

REMARKS

1. During the attack of Ménière's disease, a simple diet and less water intake are recommended. For vertigo the primary cause of disease should be treated.
2. Patients should keep quiet and avoid noise. For those with excess *tan* damp, fatty or phlegm-producing food should be avoided.

APPENDIX: HYPERTENSION

Hypertension refers to conditions where there is

a systolic pressure above 140 mm of mercury and a diastolic pressure above 90 mm of mercury at a state of rest.

Clinically it is divided into primary (essential) hypertension and secondary hypertension. At an early stage, the disease may not present any symptoms or it may present with headache, dizziness or vertigo, a sense of distension in the head, tinnitus, palpitations, and insomnia. At the later stage, apart from the above manifestations, it may affect the heart, brain and kidney, leading to symptoms in these affected organs.

TREATMENT

Prescription. A: Quchi (LI 11), Zusanli (St 36). B: Fengchi (GB 20), Taichong (Liv 3).

Modification.
— Headache: Yintang (Extra 2), Taiyang (Extra 5).
— Insomnia: Shenmen (H 7).
— Palpitations: Ximen (P 4), Neiguan (P 6).

Method. The above two prescriptions are used alternately in combination with the supplementary points. One treatment is given daily or every other day. Ten treatments make a course.

3. HEADACHE (INCLUDING TRIGEMINAL NEURALGIA)

A headache, or pain in the upper half of the head, is a subjective symptom often seen in various acute and chronic diseases. As it covers a wide sphere, this section only deals with headaches caused by an attack of the jingluo due to pathogenic *feng* affection, hyperactivity of the liver yang, deficiency of both qi and blood and retarded circulation of blood in the meridians that traverse the head. Headache as an accompanying symptom in the development of other diseases will not be discussed.

The occurrence of a headache is often seen in various diseases such as hypertension, migraine and functional headaches, infective fever, and ear, nose and throat diseases.

AETIOLOGY AND PATHOGENESIS

A headache may be due to pathogenic *feng*

affecting the jingluo which causes derangement of qi and blood and obstruction of the meridians in the upper part of the body. This leads to stagnation of blood in the collaterals, and a headache is evoked by a sudden change in the weather, or exposure to pathogenic *feng*.

It may also be due to hyperactivity of liver yang caused by long-term depression of the liver qi, owing to an emotional disturbance, which results in an upward attack by the liver and gallbladder, as the liver "wood" strives to "grow freely"—the liver regulates the activities of the vital energy and this function should be carried out smoothly.

Alternatively it is due to a congenital deficiency, or long-term deficiency of the "sea of marrow" caused by overstrain or mental stress.

It may also be due to stagnation of blood and obstruction of the luo, derived from damage to the "sea of marrow" caused by trauma, leading to a lingering and repeated headache.

DIFFERENTIATION

A headache due to invasion of pathogenic *feng* into the jingluo is marked by an unfixed, boring headache accompanied by a sensation of distension or tightening. The pain is either at the vertex or over the whole head. Such symptoms are also called "head *feng*".

A headache due to upsurge of liver yang is manifest by a headache with blurred vision, severe pain on both sides of the head, irritability, hot temper, flushed face, bitter taste in the mouth, a wiry and rapid pulse and a reddened tongue with a yellow coating.

A headache due to deficiency of both qi and blood is manifest by it being lingering, by dizziness, blurred vision, lassitude and pallor, which are all aggravated by overstrain or mental stress, a weak and thready pulse, and a pale tongue with a thin and white coating.

A headache due to obstruction of the jingluo derived from stagnation of blood is manifest as a lingering headache, dizziness, fixed boring pain accompanied by mental retardation, amnesia, palpitations, and a dark purple tongue proper or one with purplish spots and a wiry pulse. There may be a past history of trauma.

TREATMENT

Needling and moxibustion

a) Invasion of pathogenic feng *into the jingluo*

Method. Select points according to the painful areas. Apply the reducing method of needling with retention of the needles.

Prescription.
— Parietal headache: Baihui (Du 20), Tongtian (UB 7), Xingjian (Liv 2), Ashi points.
— Frontal headache: Shangxing (Du 23), Touwei (St 8), Hegu (LI 4), Ashi points.
— Temporal headache: Shuaigu (GB 8), Taiyang (Extra 5), Xiaxi (GB 43), Ashi points.
— Occipital headache: Houding (Du 19), Tianzhu (UB 10), Kunlun (UB 60), Ashi points.

Explanation. The above prescriptions are set by combining local points with distal points, according to the location of the headache and the affected meridians. The aim is to remove obstruction of the qi in the jingluo on the head. When the obstruction is removed the pain is relieved.

b) Upsurge of the liver yang

Method. Select points mainly from the Jueyin and Shaoyang meridians of the hands and feet. Puncture the points with a reducing method.
Prescription. Fengchi (GB 20), Baihui (Du 20), Xuanlu (GB 5), Xiaxi (GB 43) and Xingjian (Liv 2).
Explanation. The Jueyin meridians of the feet and hands supply the vertex. The Shaoyang meridian runs up both sides of the head. Selecting points in the affected area, in combination with local and distal points, can pacify the liver yang.

c) Deficiency of both qi and blood

Method. Select mainly from the Du and Ren meridians and corresponding Back-Shu points. Puncture the points with a reinforcing method. Moxibustion is applicable.
Prescription. Baihui (Du 20), Qihai (Ren 6), Ganshu (UB 18), Pishu (UB 20), Shenshu (UB 23), Hegu (LI 4) and Zusanli (St 36).

Explanation. Qihai is chosen to tonify the *yuan* qi. Baihui is for lifting up the clear yang.

Hegu and Zusanli are used in combination to regulate the qi of the Yangming meridians.

Ganshu, Pishu and Shenshu are Back-Shu points of the liver, spleen and kidney. Since the liver stores blood, the spleen controls blood, the kidney stores and produces marrow, and the head is the "sea of marrow", these three points can be used to strengthen the kidney essence and tonify qi and blood.

This treatment concentrates mainly on relieving the primary symptoms and neglecting the secondary ones.

d) Headache due to stagnation of blood in the meridians of the head

Method. Refer to the treatment of headache due to invasion of pathogenic *feng* into the jingluo. Select points according to the course of the meridians and affected area. Puncture with the reducing method. The needles are retained. Tapping with needles is applicable.

Explanation. For blood stasis in the collaterals caused by trauma, Shangxing (Du 23), Touwei (St 8), Shuaigu (GB 8), Taiyang (Extra 5) and Houding (Du 19) are to be tapped. This causes bleeding which can remove the blood stagnation in the meridians and dredge the meridional passage.

Warming needling

Puncture Fengfu (Du 16), Yamen (Du 15) and Fengchi (GB 20) with thick silver needles. Select 1–2 points in each treatment, with moxa burnt and replaced 3–5 times on each needle. 2–3 points may be selected in each treatment, which is given once daily or every other day. This therapy is applied to headache due to pathogenic *feng* and cold.

Cutaneous needling

Apply heavy tapping to Taiyang (Extra 5), Yintang (Extra 2) and the area of the headache to cause bleeding and then apply cupping. This treatment is applied for headache due to invasion of pathogenic *feng* into the meridians and an upsurge of the liver yang.

Point-injection therapy

Inject a mixed solution of procaine and caffeine (3.5 ml of 0.25% procaine and 0.5 ml of caffeine) into Fengchi (GB 20), 0.5–1 ml into each point. Or else inject 0.1 ml into any tender points. This therapy is applicable to obstinate headaches.

Ear needling

Points. Occipital, Forehead, Brain, Ear-Shenmen.

Method. Select 2–3 of the above points in each treatment. The needles can be retained for 20–30 minutes and manipulated every 5 minutes, or embedded for 3–7 days. For obstinate headaches blood-letting should be applied to the veins at the back of the ear.

REMARKS

Needling and moxibustion give gratifying results in treatment of headache either short-term or long-term. If the headache fails to respond to treatment or is continuous and aggravating, the causes should be found out and the primary disease treated.

APPENDIX: TRIGEMINAL NEURALGIA

This is a transient paroxysmal severe pain on the facial region where it is traversed by the trigeminal nerve. Clinically the 2nd and 3rd branches of the trigeminal nerve are often involved. The disease can be divided into two types: primary and secondary. It often occurs in people after middle age and most frequently in females.

The disease is marked by sudden onset, evoked by a touch on the face, which makes the patient dare not wash the face, brush the teeth or take food. This presents as a paroxysmal electric shock, a burning, boring or cutting pain accompanied by a contracture of the facial muscles on the affected side, lacrimation, nasal discharge and salivation. The attack lasts for only a few seconds or minutes and then will subside. No symptom will present between attacks.

TREATMENT

Needling and moxibustion

Method. Local points and distal points along the meridians are selected together. The reducing method of needling is applied with continuous manipulation and retention.

Prescription. The prescription is divided into adjacent points and distal points. Adjacent points are:

1st branch: Zanzhu (UB 2), Yangbai (GB 14), Yuyao (Extra 3).
2nd branch: Sibai (St 2), Juliao (St 3), Quanliao (SI 18).
3rd branch: Jiachengjiang (Extra 9), Jiache (St 6), Xiaguan (St 7).

The distal points, Hegu (LI 4), Sanjian (LI 3) and Neiting (St 44) are the same for all three branches.

Point-injection therapy

Method. Use 0.5–1 ml of Vitamin B12 (100 micrograms) or Vitamin B1 (100 mg) or 1% procaine solution, injected into the painful points. The injection is given every 2–3 days.

REMARKS

Needling is effective in checking the pain. For secondary trigeminal neuralgia, treatment should be aimed at the primary cause.

4. FACIAL PARALYSIS

Facial paralysis can occur in patients of any age, but mostly at the age of 20–40, and more frequently in males and in spring and autumn.

Clinically it is divided into two patterns: peripheral facial paralysis and central paralysis. Their causative factors and symptoms are quite different. This section only deals with peripheral facial paralysis.

AETIOLOGY AND PATHOGENESIS

The disease is due to flaccidity of facial muscles caused by an attack of pathogenic *feng* and cold on the Yangming and Shaoyang meridians. This leads to stagnation of the qi in the meridians and malnutrition of the muscle regions of the meridians.

MANIFESTATION

Sudden onset, usually upon waking up, one-sided flaccidity and numbness of the facial muscles, inability to frown, raise the eyebrow, close the eye, blow out the cheek, show the teeth etc., and drooping of the angle of the mouth to the true side, lacrimation, incomplete closure of the eye on the affected side, disappearance of wrinkles, flattened philtrum.

In some cases, pain in the mastoid and facial regions may be accompanied by an impaired sense of taste of two-thirds of the tongue on the affected side and hypersensitivity of hearing. In longstanding cases, drooping of the angle of the mouth to the affected side may appear due to contraction of the muscles.

TREATMENT

Needling and moxibustion

Method. Select those points from the Yangming meridians of the hands and feet as principal points, supplemented by those from the Shaoyang meridians. Also combine local points and distal points.

At the beginning use shallow puncture. A week later horizontal penetration of two points with oblique insertion may be applied.

Prescription. Fengchi (GB 20), Yifeng (SJ 17), Jiache (St 6), Dicang (St 4), Hegu (LI 4) and Taichong (Liv 3).

Explanation. The disease is caused by an attack of pathogenic *feng* on the Shaoyang and Yangming meridians. Thus Fengchi and Yifeng are selected to eliminate *feng*. Yifeng is for eliminating *feng* and relieving pain, and is suitable for retroauricular pain at the onset of the disease.

Jiache and Dicang belong to the Yangming, and penetration of Jiache horizontally towards Dicang has the effect of invigorating the qi in the meridians.

Hegu and Taichong are distal points. Hegu is good at treating diseases on the facial and head regions, whilst the reducing method applied to Taichong is effective in treating deviation of the mouth.

Modification.
— Flattened philtrum: Yingxiang (LI 20), Heliao (SJ 22).
— Deviation of the philtrum: Shuigou (Du 26).
— Deviation of mental-labial groove: Chengjiang (Ren 24).
— Difficulty in closing eyes: Zanzhu (UB 2),
— Yangbai (GB 16) or Shenmai (UB 62), Zhaohai (K 6).
— Flaccidity of the face: Sibai (St 2), Juliao (St 3).

Points are selected in groups and are used alternately according to the location of the affected area.

Point-injection therapy

Inject Vitamin B1 (100 mg) or B12 (100 micrograms) into Yifeng (SJ 17), Qianzheng (Extra 10) etc., 0.5–1 ml into each point once a day or every other day. The above points are to be used alternately.

Electroneedling

Select points on the affected side. Electricity is applied for 10–15 minutes with an intermittent or dense-sparse wave until contraction of the muscles appears.

Cutaneous needling

Tap Yangbai (GB 14), Taibai (Sp 3), Sibai (St 2) and Taiyang (Extra 5) to cause slight bleeding and then apply cupping for 5–10 minutes, once every other day. The therapy is indicated in the early stage of the disease for numb sensations of the facial region and sequelae of facial paralysis.

External herbal applications

Scatter 1–2 mg of ground Maqianzi (*Semen* *Strychni*, nuxvomica) on a medicated plaster or adhesive tape and then apply to Xiaguan (St 7). The plaster is to be changed 4–5 times, every 2–3 days.

REMARKS

1. Facial paralysis occurs in two forms: peripheral facial paralysis and central paralysis. Careful differentiation should be made between them.
2. Strong stimulation should be avoided at the onset.
3. During the treatment the patient should avoid cold and wind. Massage and a hot compress can be applied.
4. To prevent inflammation of the eyes, eye covers and eye drops are to be used.

5. BI SYNDROMES (INCLUDING PERIPHERAL SHOULDER ARTHRITIS, SCIATICA)

Bi syndromes (痹) are characterized by obstruction of the qi and blood in the jingluo due to invasion of pathogenic *feng*. They are manifested by soreness, pain, numbness and a heavy sensation in the limbs and joints, and limitation of movement. Bi syndromes can be classified into wandering Bi, painful Bi, fixed Bi and heat Bi according to their aetiology and manifestations.

The disease includes rheumatoid arthritis, rheumatic fever, fibrositis, osteoarthritis and neuralgia.

The causative factors are weakened *wei* qi, poor function of skin pores or invasion of *feng*, cold and damp when one is wet through with perspiration, exposed to the wind, dwelling in damp places or wading in water. These result in Bi syndromes due to *feng*, cold or damp.

In the *Plain Questions* chapter on "Bi Syndromes"[1] it says that when *feng*, damp and cold come together to attack the body, they agglomerate together to Bi syndromes. Besides this, constitutionally an exuberant Yang qi and accumulated heat, invasion of pathogenic *feng*, cold and damp can also give rise to heat Bi.

DIFFERENTIATION

A Bi syndrome due to *feng*, cold or damp manifests as arthralgia, muscular soreness or numbness. In prolonged cases, contracture of the extremities and swelling of the joints as the main symptoms may present. Since different body constitutions vary in response to the attack, the symptoms differ: there is wandering Bi (in which *feng* dominates), fixed Bi (in which damp dominates) and painful Bi (in which cold dominates). The three symptoms are differentiated as follows.

1. Wandering Bi is caused by pathogenic *feng* which is characterized by constant movement. Manifestations are wandering pain in the joints or general pain, with perhaps chills, fever, a yellow greasy tongue, and superficial and slippery pulse.
2. Painful Bi is marked by general or local aching which is alleviated by warmth and aggravated by the cold, a white tongue coating, and wiry and tight pulse.
3. Fixed Bi is caused by the damp which is characterized by symptoms of agglomeration. Manifestations are numbness of the muscles, fixed pain, heaviness and soreness in the joints which is liable to occur on cold, rainy or windy days, a white and greasy tongue coating and soft pulse.
4. Heat Bi manifests as soreness in one or several joints, local redness, swelling, hotness or excruciating pain with limitation of movement, accompanied by fever and thirst, a yellow dry tongue coating, and a slippery and rapid pulse.

TREATMENT

Needling and moxibustion

Method. Select points along the meridians supplying the diseased areas, according to the nature and location of the disease.

Wandering Bi and heat Bi are treated by the reducing method of superficial needling. Tapping with the cutaneous needle may also be applied.

For painful Bi it is better to use moxibustion and deep insertion, with prolonged retention of the needles. For severe pain, intradermal needles or indirect moxibustion with ginger may be used.

Fixed Bi may be also treated by both needling and moxibustion, or together with the warming needle, tapping and cupping.

Prescription.
— Wandering Bi: Geshu (UB 17), Xuehai (Sp 10).
— Painful Bi: Shenshu (UB 23), Guanyuan (Ren 4).
— Fixed Bi: Zusanli (St 36), Shangqiu (Sp 5).
— Heat Bi: Dazhui (Du 14), Quchi (LI 4).
— Pain in the shoulder: Jianyu (LI 15), Jianliao (SJ 14) and Naoshu (SI 10).
— Pain in the elbow: Quchi (LI 11), Hegu (LI 4), Tianjing (SJ 10), Waiguan (SJ 5), Chize (Lu 5).
— Pain in the wrist: Yangchi (SJ 4), Waiguan (SJ 5), Yangxi (LI 5), Wangu (SI 4).
— Pain in the back: Shuigou (Du 26), Shenzhu (Du 12), Yaoyangguan (Du 3).
— Pain in the hip joints: Huantiao (GB 30), Juliao (GB 29), Xuanzhong (GB 39).
— Pain in the thigh region: Zhibian (UB 54), Chengfu (UB 36), Fengshi (GB 31), Yanglingquan (GB 32).
— Pain in the knee joints: Dubi (St 35), Liangqiu (St 34), Yanglingquan (GB 34), Medial Xiyan (Extra 39).
— Pain in the ankle: Shenmai (UB 62), Zhaohai (K 6), Kunlun (UB 60), Qiuxu (GB 40).

Explanation. The above prescriptions are set according to the nature of the syndromes.

For example, wandering Bi is due to domination by pathogenic *feng* so Geshu and Xuehai are selected to regulate and nourish the blood. This selection is based on the principle that *feng* will be naturally eliminated if blood circulates smoothly.

Fixed Bi is due to stagnation of damp derived from dysfunction of the spleen. Zusanli and Shangqiu are taken to strengthen the function of the spleen and stomach since regulating the spleen is a prerequisite in treating diseases caused by the damp.

Prolonged painful Bi will result in deficiency of the Yang qi, so Guanyuan and Shenshu are employed to strengthen the source of fire, invigorate Yang qi and dispel cold.

Dazhui and Quchi, which can clear away heat and expel exterior symptoms, are used to treat heat Bi.

Prescriptions according to location, based upon the meridional routes, aim at removing the obstruction of qi and blood in the jingluo and regulating the *ying* qi and *wei* qi. Thus the *feng*, damp and cold will have no place to attach to and the Bi syndromes can be relieved.

Differing treatments and manipulations should be applied according to the differing locations and severity of the disease.

Pricking and cupping

Heavy tapping to induce slight bleeding along the sides of the spine or the local area of the affected joints, followed by cupping, is often used for the treatment of painful swollen joints caused by heat Bi.

Point-injection therapy

Use Danggui (Chinese angelica solution), Weilingxian (*Radix Clematidis* solution) and paenol (tree peony bark in solution).

Inject into the points in the shoulder, elbow, hip joints and knees, 0.5–1 ml for each point. Avoid injecting into the joint cavity. Injection is given once every 1–3 days. Ten treatments make a course. Do not select too many points at one time. For frequently occurring joint diseases, key lesions can be selected for injection and used alternately.

Electroneedling

Select 4–6 points from the above prescription. When the qi arrives after insertion, electricity is applied for 10–20 minutes, during which a dense-sparse wave is applied after stimulation with the dense wave for 5 minutes. Treatment is given once every other day, 10 treatments make a course. A one-week interval follows and then the electroneedling may be continued or another therapy applied, according to the condition of the disease.

REMARKS

1. Needling is effective in treating Bi syndrome.

For lingering rheumatoid arthritis, the result is usually slow.

2. Differentiation should be made between Bi syndromes and bone tumours or bone TB, to prevent delay in the treatment of the latter two.

3. Attention should be paid to keeping warm.

PERIPHERAL SHOULDER ARTHRITIS

Peripheral shoulder arthritis refers to degenerative and inflammatory pathological changes of the peripheral soft tissues of the shoulder joint. It is held that this disease is related to exposure of the shoulder to cold, overstrain or chronic overloading. The disease occurs in people after middle age, a little more frequently in females. It may be termed "frozen shoulder", or "50-year-old shoulder", etc., according to the particular circumstances.

At an early stage, the disease is manifest mainly as soreness and aching in one shoulder, occasionally both, which radiates to the neck and back, presenting a diffuse pain. The disease is characterized by pain which is static, alleviated during the daytime and aggravated at night. The patient may be woken at night by the pain, which may be alleviated in the morning after slight exercise of the joint. Because of the pain, an obvious limitation in the movement of outwardly stretching and inwardly rotating the shoulder may be present. Local pressure gives rise to wide-ranging pain.

At a later stage, adhesion of the diseased tissues ensues, with functional disturbance being aggravated and pain alleviated. In short, the disease is manifest mainly as pain in the early stages and functional disturbance later.

Peripheral shoulder arthritis is subject to the following clinical differentiation in terms of anatomy and aetiology:

DIFFERENTIATION

(i) Tendinitis of the supraspinatus muscle

With tenderness around the mid-brachial joint, the disease is marked by pain which occurs when stretching and raising the arm at an angle of 60–120 degrees. In any movement less than 60 degrees or beyond 120 degrees, no pain will present in the shoulder joint.

(ii) Subacromial bursitis

Pain in the lateral aspect of the shoulder. Outward stretching and rotating of the arm gives rise to pain and limitation of use. In acute cases a spheroidal bulge of the anterior border of the deltoid muscle may be present and the affected shoulder may appear enlarged.

(iii) Tenosynovitis of the longer head of the biceps brachii

Swelling and tenderness in the area of the longer head of the biceps brachii. The pain is aggravated when flexing the elbow. A slight local sensation of warmth and aching may be felt when palpating the painful area.

TREATMENT

Needling and moxibustion

Method. Select both local and distal points according to the location of the disease. The reduction method of needling is applied with retention of the needles.

Prescription. Jianyu (LI 15), Jianliao (SJ 14), Jianqian (Extra 34), Ashi points, Tiaokou (St 38) and Yanglingquan (GB 34).

Modification.
— Pain in the upper limb: Binao (LI 14), Quchi (LI 11).
— Pain in the scapular region: Quyuan (SI 13), Tianzong (SI 11).

Point-injection therapy

Method. Inject 5 ml of 10% glucose solution into the tender points. The injection is given once every other day. Ten treatments make a course. If the tender points are extensive, 2–3 of the most painful tender points may be chosen for the injection.

Pricking and cupping

Tapping is applied to the tender points and diseased areas to cause bleeding; then apply cupping.

REMARKS

1. In the treatment, diseases such as shoulder joint tuberculosis and tumours should be excluded.
2. After alleviation of the pain in the shoulder-joint and disappearance of the swelling, functional exercises should be taken under the guidance of the doctor.

SCIATICA

Sciatica refers to pain along the route of the sciatic nerve. It is symptomatic of a common peripheral neuritis often seen in adults, and most frequently in males. It is clinically divided into two patterns: primary and secondary.

Primary sciatica is related to exposure to cold, damp, trauma or infection.

Secondary sciatica is caused by mechanical pressure or adhesions produced by pathological changes of the tissues around or near the route of the nerve, for example, prolapse of the lumbar intervertebral disc, spinal tumour, pathological changes in the intervertebral or sacro-iliac joints or pelvis, and strain of the lumbosacral soft tissue. According to the affected part, the disease can be classified as either radical sciatica or trunk sciatica.

The disease is mainly manifest as paroxysmal or continuous pain on one side of the waist and thigh. The main symptom is a radiating and burning or stabbing pain in the hips, the back of the thigh, or posterior and lateral side of the foot and calf, which is aggravated when walking. A straight-leg raising test is positive and the knee-jerk reflex weakened.

Primary sciatica presents with an acute or subacute onset, along with radiating pain and remarkably tender points along the sciatic nerve. The most violent pain appears within a few days after onset, the disease is gradually alleviated within weeks and months. Exposure to cold and damp may induce attacks.

In secondary sciatica, the primary disease may be traced. Coughing, sneezing and exertion during defaecation may aggravate the pain. There is tenderness and pain on percussion beside the lumbar vertebrae and motor impairment. Radiating pain in the lower limbs may present during movement.

TREATMENT

Needling and moxibustion

Select from the foot Shaoyang and Taiyang meridians for the main points. The reducing method of needling is applied in combination with moxibustion or cupping.

Prescription. Shenshu (UB 23), Qihaishu (UB 24), Huatuojiaji (Extra 19, L3–5), Ciliao (UB 32), Zhibian (UB 54), Huantiao (GB 30), Ashi points.

Points on the meridians.
— Taiyang meridian: Yinmen (UB 37),
   Weizhong (UB 40), Chengshan (UB 57).
— Shaoyang meridian: Yanglingquan (GB 34),
   Yangjiao (GB 35), Juegu (GB 39).

4–5 of the above points are selected according to the sites where the pain appears to radiate from. After inserting the needle into points in the lumbar and hip areas, it is necessary to let the needling sensation extend downwards. But this should not be done repeatedly in case the nerve is damaged.

A few days after contracting the disease, Houxi (SI 3), Wangu (SI 4), Yemen (SJ 2) and Zhongzhu (SJ 3) on the upper limbs, which are from meridians with the same names (Taiyang and Shaoyang), should be selected for those with severe pain caused by obstruction of the qi in the meridians.

Point-injection therapy

Method. Use a mixed solution of 10–20 ml 10% glucose and Vitamin B1 (100 mg), or else Vitamin B12 (100 micrograms). The solution is to be injected into Zhibian (UB 54) and the Jiaji (Extra 19, L2–4), 5–10 ml into each point and 2–3 points selected in each treatment.

After a strong needling sensation radiating downwards appears, lift the syringe a little and inject the solution quickly into the point. The treatment is given once every other day.

You may also inject 5–10 ml of 1% procaine solution into any Ashi point or Huantiao (GB 30), when there is severe pain.

Electroneedling

Points.
— Radical sciatica: Jiaji (Extra 19, L4–5),
   Yanglingquan (GB 34) or Weizhong (UB 40).
— Trunk sciatica: Zhibian (UB 54) or Huantiao
   (GB 30), Yanglingquan (GB 34) or Weizhong
   (UB 40).

After the needles are inserted, electricity is applied with a dense, or dense and sparse wave. The stimulation is increased gradually from moderate to strong. Treatment is given for 10–15 minutes, once every day. Ten days make up a course of treatment.

Pricking collaterals and cupping

Tap the lumbo-sacral region and tender points, to cause bleeding, and then apply cupping.

REMARKS

1. For sciatica caused by tumour, tuberculosis, etc., the primary disease should be treated. For that caused by prolapse of an intervertebral disc, the treatment should be combined with traction or massage and manipulation.
2. During the acute stage, the patient should be confined to bed.
3. Keep warm and adopt a correct posture when working. A broad belt should be used for fastening the waist.

6. LUMBAR PAIN

The lumbar region is where the kidneys are located and the area the kidney meridian supplies, therefore lumbar pain is closely related to the kidneys. Lumbar pain is a commonly seen disease in the clinic. Disorders and injuries of the meridians, muscle regions and collaterals supplying the lumbar region may also lead to lumbar pain.

This disease is often seen in injuries of the soft tissue of the lumbar region, muscular rheumatism and pathological changes of the spine and internal organs. This section deals only with lumbar pain due to cold-damp, lumbar strain and kidney deficiency.

AETIOLOGY AND PATHOGENESIS

Lumbar pain due to cold-damp is often caused by being affected by *feng* and cold, or dwelling in wet places. The jingluo are affected by the *feng*, cold, wet and damp, which leads to obstruction of the qi in the meridians.

Lumbar strain caused by unhealed or old injuries, trauma or contusions, leads to injuries of the muscle regions of the jingluo and vessels, and consequently stagnation of blood.

Lumbar pain due to kidney deficiency is caused by long-term fatigue or impairment, standing or sitting for too long, or over indulgence in sexual activities in which the kidney essence and kidney qi are consumed and become deficient.

DIFFERENTIATION

Lumbar pain due to cold-damp (*feng*, cold and damp) is marked by heaviness, pain, soreness, numbness, or stiffness and motor impairment of the lumbar region, or pain radiating to the buttock and leg, or a cold sensation at the affected sites, all of which are aggravated by cloudy, rainy, windy or cold weather, and are protracted and lingering.

Lumbar strain due to old injuries is often evoked by impairment or fatigue. It is marked by a stiff or contracting sensation in the lumbus and fixed pain which is aggravated by movement.

Lumbar pain due to kidney deficiency is marked by chronic onset, dull pain, or a soreness which is more obvious than a lingering pain,

and soreness and weakness of the lower back and the leg. If it is accompanied by listlessness, lumbar coldness, spermatorrhoea and a thready pulse, it is due to kidney yang deficiency; if accompanied by restlessness of the deficiency type, yellow urine, a thready and rapid pulse, and a red tongue, it is due to kidney yin deficiency.

TREATMENT

Needling and moxibustion

Method. Points are selected mainly from the foot Taiyang and Du meridians. Reinforcing, reducing or even methods of needling, or both acupuncture and moxibustion, can be applied according to the condition of deficiency or excess in the disease.

Prescription. Shenshu (UB 23), Weizhong (UB 40), Huatuojiaji (Extra 19) and Ashi points.

Modification.
— Cold-damp: add Fengfu (Du 16) Yaoyangguan (Du 3).
— Lumbar strain: add Geshu (UB 17) and Ciliao (UB 32).
— Kidney deficiency: add Mingmen (Du 4), Zhishi (UB 52) and Taixi (K 3).

Explanation. The kidney meridian supplies the lumbar region which is the "dwelling house of the kidney". Shenshu is used to regulate and replenish kidney qi and, with moxibustion, it eliminates cold and damp.

The bladder meridian runs alongside the spine, reaches the lumbus and connects with the kidney; the distal point along this meridian, Weizhong, is used to remove obstruction and regulate qi in the foot Taiyang meridian.

The Huatuojiaji points and Ashi points are adjacent points for activating the circulation of qi and blood in the local muscle regions of the jingluo and vessels.

Fengfu is for dispelling *feng* and cold, and, together with Yaoyangguan, for promoting the circulation of yang qi as both are from the Du meridian.

Geshu is the Influential point of blood. Together with Weizhong and Ciliao, these points act to remove obstruction from the Bladder meridian and stagnant blood from the collaterals, facilitating the treatment of lumbar strain.

Applying moxibustion to Mingmen and reinforcing Zhishi tonifies the genuine yang of the kidney.

Taixi is selected according to the principle of *yuan* points being selected for diseases of the zang organs.

Bloodletting with a three-edged needle at Weizhong can be applied in cases of acute and severe lumbar pain.

Cutaneous needling and cupping

Apply heavy tapping with cutaneous needles and then cupping on the local tenderness over the point Weizhong (UB 40). This method is indicated for lumbar pain due to cold and damp, and chronic lumbar strain.

Point-injection therapy

5–10 ml of 10% glucose injection plus Vitamin B1 (100 ml), or a compound prescription of Danggui (Chinese Angelica), injected into the muscular layer of the tender area. One treatment every other day, 10 treatments as one course. This is indicated for chronic lumbar strain.

REMARKS

1. Needling and moxibustion have a good therapeutic effect in lumbar pain except in those cases due to vertebral tuberculosis and tumour.
2. Frequent massage applied twice a day (morning and evening) onto the low back, helps alleviate and prevent lumbar pain.

7. FLANK PAIN

Flank pain refers to pain in the hypochondriacal or costal regions on one or both sides. The *Miraculous Pivot* states that "pathogens in the liver give rise to pain in the flanks",[2] showing that the flank pain is closely related to the liver (as its meridian supplies the flank), and the gallbladder (as its meridian is externally-internally related to that of the liver).

This disease is often seen in acute and chronic diseases of the liver, gallbladder or pleurae, trauma of the chest or flank, or intercostal neuralgia.

AETIOLOGY AND PATHOGENESIS

The liver is situated at the flank and its meridian supplies the flank on both sides. Emotional disturbances impairing the free-going of qi of the liver, or damp-heat accumulated in the liver and gallbladder, leading to retarded circulation or obstruction of qi in jingluo, may cause flank pain.

Alternatively, retention of exogenous pathogens in the chest and flank consuming blood and yin, which fail to nourish the liver meridian, may cause flank pain.

Also sprain or contusion of the hypochondriacal and costal regions, injuring the jingluo and giving rise to stagnant qi and blood, may cause flank pain.

DIFFERENTIATION

Flank pain is often one-sided. Hypochondriacal distension and pain, stuffiness in the chest, poor appetite, a wiry pulse or emotional disturbance may be due to stagnant liver qi.

Flank pain due to damp-heat accumulated in the liver and gallbladder is marked by flank distension and pain, nausea and vomiting, a bitter taste in the mouth, and a red tongue with a yellow greasy coating.

If due to trauma or sprain, it is marked by a fixed stabbing pain owing to stagnant qi and blood in the jingluo. The above three conditions are all of the excess type.

If there is a deficiency of essence and blood which fails to nourish the liver, leading to a lingering dull pain, a red tongue with little coating and a thready and rapid pulse, the flank pain is of the deficiency type.

TREATMENT

Needling and moxibustion

a) Excess type

Method. Points are mainly selected from the

foot Jueyin and Shaoyang meridians. Use a reducing method of needling.

Prescription. Qimen (Liv 14), Zhigou (SJ 6), Yanglingquan (GB 34), Zusanli (St 36) and Taichong (Liv 3).

Explanation. The liver and gallbladder are externally-internally related to each other and their meridians supply the flank region.

Therefore Qimen and Taichong are used, with Zhigou and Yanglingquan as distal points, selecting along the meridians to promote the free flowing of the liver and gallbladder qi, and activate and regulate the circulation of qi and blood so as to relieve the pain.

Zusanli is added to pacify the stomach qi and relieve fullness and distension.

b) Deficiency type

Method. Select mainly Back-Shu points and points from the foot Jueyin meridian. Use a reinforcing or even method of needling.

Prescription. Ganshu (UB 18), Shenshu (UB 23), Qimen (Liv 14), Xingjian (Liv 2), Zusanli (St 36) and Sanyinjiao (Sp 6).

Explanation. Ganshu and Shenshu with a reinforcing method can nourish the qi and blood of the liver and kidney.

The Front-Mu point of the liver, Qimen, is used to regulate liver qi.

The Ying-spring point, Xingjian, is used with an even reducing method to clear heat of the deficiency type from the collaterals.

Zusanli and Sanyinjiao are used in combination to strengthen the spleen and stomach as they are the source of the manufacture of qi and blood.

Cutaneous needling

Apply tapping with cutaneous needles onto the painful sites on the chest and hypochondrium and then apply cupping. This method is indicated in flank pain due to impairment or fatigue, and has the effect of relieving pain and removing stagnant blood.

Point-injection therapy

Inject with 10 ml of 10% glucose, or with 100 micrograms of Vitamin B12 (1 ml injected), into the Huatuojiaji (Extra 19) point of the corresponding segment. The needle is inserted perpendicularly into the area of the root of the intercostal nerve, withdrawn a little when an obvious needling sensation is obtained, and then the medicine is injected. The injection can be made into several points. This method is indicated for intercostal neuralgia.

Ear needling

Points. Chest, Occiput, Ear-Shenmen and Liver.

Method. 2–3 points on the affected side are stimulated with moderate or strong stimulation along with rotation of needles, and 20–30 minutes retention of the needles. The needling is given during attacks of the flank pain.

REMARKS

Acupuncture has a good effect in treating flank pain. During the treatment corresponding examinations are required and, if necessary, aetiological treatment can be applied.

8. WEI SYNDROME

Wei syndrome (痿) is marked by flaccidity, atrophy or numbness of the limbs with motor impairment, and since the leg is usually involved it is also called "flaccid lameness". These kind of syndromes are often seen in multiple neuritis, the early stages of acute myelitis, the sequelae of poliomyelitis, myodystrophy, periodic paralysis and hysterical paralysis.

AETIOLOGY AND PATHOGENESIS

Wei syndrome may be caused by burning heat in the lung consuming body fluid, owing to the lung being affected by exogenous pathogenic heat or mild heat which consumes body fluids so the tendons and muscles are deprived of nourishment, and this leads to muscular flaccidity or atrophy.

Alternatively it may be caused by accumulation of damp-heat in the Yangming meridian which fails to moisten and nourish the tendons and muscles or control and facilitate the movement of the tendons and joints.

It may also be caused by deficiency resulting from long-term illness, or deficiency of kidney essence and blood due to over-indulgence in sexual activity, by which the tendons and muscles and meridians are deprived of nourishment, which leads to Wei syndrome.

DIFFERENTIATION

Wei syndromes are marked mainly by flaccidity or muscular atrophy of the limbs, along with motor impairment. They should be differentiated from Bi syndromes which are marked by soreness, distension, and pain along with motor impairment. Initially there may be fever or no fever, then weakness or flaccidity of the upper limb(s) or lower limb(s), and finally complete motor impairment. This is gradually accompanied by emaciation, with a numb or cool sensation in the affected areas.

Wei syndromes due to lung heat are accompanied by fever, coughing, irritability, thirst, scanty dark yellow urination, constipation, a red tongue with yellow coating, and a thready and rapid pulse.

Those due to damp-heat are accompanied by general heaviness, stuffiness in the chest, turbid urine, or hot feet which are relieved by the cold, a yellow and greasy tongue coating and a soft and rapid pulse.

Wei syndromes due to yin deficiency of the liver and kidney are accompanied by lumbar soreness or weakness, seminal emission or premature ejaculation, dizziness, vertigo, blurred vision, a red tongue with little coating, and a thready and rapid pulse.

TREATMENT

Needling and moxibustion

Method. Points are selected mainly from the Yangming meridians: those from hand Yangming for the upper limbs and those from the foot Yangming for the lower limbs (refer to the treatment of *feng* stroke and hemiplegia).

For conditions due to lung heat or damp-heat, only needling without moxibustion is given, with a reducing method, or in combination with tapping by cutaneous needles. For those conditions due to yin deficiency of liver and kidney, a reinforcing needling method is employed.

Prescription.
— Upper limb: Jianyu (LI 15), Quchi (LI 11), Hegu (LI 4) and Yangxi (LI 5).
— Lower limbs: Biguan (St 31), Liangqiu (St 34), Zusanli (St 36) and Jiexi (St 41).

Modification.
— Lung heat: Chize (Lu 5), Feishu (UB 13) and Dazhui (Du 14).
— Damp-heat: Yinlingquan (Sp 9), Pishu (UB 20).
— Yin deficiency of liver and kidney: Ganshu (UB 18), Shenshu (UB 23), Xuanzhong (GB 39) and Yanglingquan (GB 34).

Explanation. The prescription is formed according to the principle laid down in the chapter "On Wei Syndromes" in the *Plain Questions*: "In treating Wei syndromes, points are mainly selected from the Yangming".[3] Those from the hand and foot Yangming meridians are used alternately.

The Yangming meridians are full of qi and blood, and function by "nourishing the tendons" so a reducing method is applied to clear the heat. Only when the heat is cleared can moxibustion or needling in combination with moxibustion be applied.

Chize, Feishu and Dazhui are used to clear the lung heat, with Yinlingquan and Pishu used in combination to eliminate damp-heat, to clear the "upper source of the water" (lung), and strengthen the middle-jiao to clear heat and damp.

Ganshu and Shenshu are used to replenish the essence and qi of the liver and kidney. The liver dominates the tendons and the kidney dominates marrow, so Yanglingquan and Xuanzhong are selected, as they are Influential points of tendon and bone. These four points used together have the effect of strengthening the tendons and bones.

Cutaneous needling

Tap the above-mentioned points from the Yangming meridians. Add the Huatuojiaji (Extra 19), along the vertebrae T3–5 for upper limbs and vertebrae L1–S4 for the lower limbs. Tap the points on the affected areas repeatedly.

Point-injection therapy

Points. Jianyu (LI 15), Quchi (LI 11), Shousanli (LI 10), Waiguan SJ 5), Biguan (St 31), Zusanli (St 36), Yanglingquan (GB 34) and Juegu (GB 39).

Method. Vitamin B1 (100 mg), Vitamin B6 (50 mg), and Vitamin B12 (100 micrograms) are injected into the above points, 2–4 points each time, with 0.5–1 ml into each point; treatment is given once every other day, 10 treatments as one course.

REMARKS

1. The duration of treatment for Wei syndrome is usually long and patience is required. Needling and moxibustion have effects of differing degrees in treating certain aspects of Wei syndrome.
2. Examinations are required to ascertain the focal location and the aetiology.
3. Herbal treatment, massage and physiotherapy may also be considered to help potentiate the therapeutic effect.
4. Functional exercises under the guidance of a doctor are also important.

9. EPILEPSY

Epilepsy is a kind of paroxysmal mental disorder marked by sudden, short and repeated attacks, manifested by falling down in a fit, loss of consciousness, foam on the lips, and screaming and convulsions of the limbs. After some time, consciousness returns and the patient's condition becomes normal.

There are various types which may be classified in primary or secondary categories. In this section only grand mal epilepsy is discussed.

AETIOLOGY AND PATHOGENESIS

It usually congenital and often attacks occur during childhood. It may be due to *tan* caused by accumulation of damp, due to dysfunction of the spleen and stomach.

Alternatively it is due to dysfunction of the qi of the liver, spleen and kidney owing to emotional disturbance and stagnant liver qi, so that the yang ascends suddenly stirring up *feng*, which, associated with the stagnant *tan* and qi, obstructs the jingluo leading to sudden seizures.

DIFFERENTIATION

It is of excess type generally, but long-term repeated attacks may result in deficiency of antipathogenic qi. There could be precursors such as vertigo, stuffiness in the chest and lack of spirit before the attack. It manifests as sudden falling down and unconsciousness, pallor, clenched teeth with eyes staring upward, convulsions of the limbs, foam from the mouth, perhaps incontinence of urine and stool, a thin greasy tongue coating and a wiry-slippery pulse. After the seizures, there may be dizziness, lassitude, a sleepy sensation and a thready pulse.

TREATMENT

Needling and moxibustion

Method. To promote resuscitation by subduing the *feng* and dispelling the *tan*.

Prescription.
— During seizures: Baihui (Du 20), Renzhong (Du 26), Houxi (SI 3) and Yongquan (K 1).
— Between seizures: Jiuwei (Ren 15), Dazhui Du 14), Yaoqi (Extra, see below), Jianshi (P 5) and Fenglong (St 40).

Explanation. Baihui and Renzhong both pertain to the Du meridian, and are used to subdue *feng* and restore consciousness. Houxi communicates with the Du meridian and is an important point for epilepsy.

Yongquan is the Jing-well point of the kidney meridian and is punctured to "pacify yang by nourishing yin" (滋水潜阳).

During intervals between seizures, Jiuwei from the Ren meridian and Dazhui where the yang meridians meet are used to regulate yin and yang. Fenglong is used to regulate the spleen and stomach and promote their transportation and transformation functions, so as to resolve *tan* and prevent its production.

Jianshi is used to regulate qi of the pericardium meridian, together with Yaoqi (below the spinous process of the 2nd sacral vertebra, 2–2.5 cun). They are both the empirical points for treating epilepsy and are often used in combination with Jiuwei. A good therapeutic effect can be expected.

Point-injection therapy

Points.   Zusanli (St 36), Neiguan (P 6), Dazhui (Du 14) and Fengchi (GB 20).

Method.   Inject 0.5–1 ml Vitamin B1 (100 mg) or 0.5–1 ml Vitamin B12 (100 micrograms); each day use 2–3 points.

Electroneedling

Points.   A: Shenting (Du 24) and Neiguan (P 6). B: Taiyang (Extra 5) and Zusanli (St 36). C: Fengchi (GB 20) and Pucan (UB 61).

Method.   The above three groups of points are used alternately, with a pulsating dense wave for 10–20 minutes. This method is indicated for epilepsy during intervals between attacks.

REMARKS

1. Needling and moxibustion can improve the symptoms of epilepsy and can be used as supplementary treatment.
2. As for epilepsy in the secondary category, a detailed past history and examination by a specialist is required so as to give treatment to the primary disease.

10. MANIC-DEPRESSIVE SYNDROMES

Manic-depressive syndromes are mental disorders seen mainly in young and middle-aged people. Depressive disorders are marked by mental dejection and reticence, and pertain to the yin type; manic disorders are marked by restless and violent behaviour, and pertain to the yang type. These have been summarized in classical medical literature as "extreme yin leading to depression, extreme yang leading to mania".

AETIOLOGY AND PATHOGENESIS

Depressive syndromes are often due to overthinking or failure to succeed in some matter which one most anxiously attempts to carry out, which causes impaired free-flowing of liver qi and failure in the normal transporting and transforming function of the spleen and stomach, giving rise to stagnant fluid which is condensed into *tan*. Then there is *tan* misting the heart and mind, leading to depressive syndromes.

Manic syndromes are, in most cases, caused by anger, mental depression, and excessive fire of the liver and stomach which are associated with *tan* attacking upwardly leading to mental disorders and mania.

DIFFERENTIATION

Depressive syndromes are marked by reticence and dullness, mental depression and apathy, or murmuring to oneself or incoherent speech, grief and crying or laughing without any reason, loss of the sense of shame or tidiness, loss of appetite, a thin and greasy tongue coating and a wiry-thready or wiry-slippery pulse.

Manic syndromes are marked by irritability, headache, insomnia, a flushed face and eyes and an angry look in the eyes at the beginning, then by shouting and cursing others, not recognizing one's relatives and friends, beating others and damaging objects, abnormally energetic or forceful behaviour, going without food for a few days, a deep red tongue with a yellow coating, and a wiry and slippery pulse.

TREATMENT

Needling and moxibustion

a) Depressive syndrome

Method.   Mainly to remove depression, resolve

tan and calm the mind. Use an even method of needling.

Prescription. Xinshu (UB 15), Ganshu (UB 18), Pishu (UB 20), Shenmen (H 7) and Fenglong (St 40).

Explanation. This disease is caused by stagnant liver qi with failure of the spleen qi to ascend. Thus the body fluid turns into *tan* with its turbidity misting the mind.

Ganshu, Pishu and Fenglong are used to treat the primary cause of the disease by soothing the liver qi depression, invigorating the transporting function of the spleen qi and resolving *tan*. At the same time, Shenmen and Xinshu promote resuscitation and clear the mind.

b) Manic syndrome

Method. Mainly to clear the heart, reduce heat and promote resuscitation. Use a reducing method of needling.

Prescription. Shuigou (Du 26), Shaoshang (Lu 11), Yinbai (Sp 1), Fengfu (Du 16), Daling (P 7), Quchi (LI 11) and Fenglong (St 40).

Explanation. Manic syndromes are caused by an upward disturbance of the associated qi, fire, *tan* and turbidity, so Daling and Quchi are used to clear pathogenic heat from the pericardium and the Yangming meridians.

Shuigou, Shaoshang, Yinbai and Fengfu are used to promote resuscitation. Fenglong pacifies the stomach, resolves *tan* and eases the mind.

Electroneedling

Points. A: Shuigou (Du 26), Baihui (Du 20). B: Dazhui (Du 14), Fengfu (Du 16).

Method. One group of points is used each time. The electricity is applied onto the needles for 5–20 minutes, with a continuous wave and long-term stimulation for manic disorders, or an intermittent wave and short-term strong stimulation. One treatment is given per day, and after the symptoms are relieved, treatment is given once every other day.

Point-injection therapy

Points. Xinshu (UB 15), Juque (Ren 14), Jianshi (P 5), Zusanli (St 36) and Sanyinjiao (Sp 6).

Method. 25–50 mg of Lubingqin (Wintermine) injected into 1–2 points each time. The treatment is given once a day and the points are used alternately. This method is indicated for manic syndromes.

REMARKS

1. Special nursing care of the patient and cooperation from the patient's relatives is required during treatment.
2. Needling and moxibustion have a definite effect in treating these kinds of syndromes and if ideological or psychological therapy can be applied alongside, the effect will be even better.

11. INSOMNIA

Difficulty in falling asleep, short-term sleep (with early awakening), or difficulty in falling asleep again after awakening, intermittent waking through the period of attempted sleep, dream-disturbed sleep and even inability to sleep all night are the commonly seen patterns of insomnia. This syndrome is seen often in neurasthenia.

AETIOLOGY AND PATHOGENESIS

It may be due to over-thinking, anxiety and overwork damaging the heart and spleen, in which the manufacture of qi and blood is impaired and the heart and mind are deprived of nourishment.

It may be due to emotional fright or fear, or over-indulgence in sexual activities damaging the kidney and giving rise to hyperactivity of the heart fire, disharmony between the heart and kidney and restlessness of the mind.

It may also be due to a congenital deficiency in the constitution, the heart and gallbladder.

Otherwise, it is due to mental depression and disturbance of the hyperactive liver yang.

Alternatively, it is due to irregular food intake which leads to disharmony between the spleen and stomach, giving rise to insomnia.

DIFFERENTIATION

Different patterns of insomnia have different accompanying symptoms.

Damage of the heart and spleen is accompanied by palpitations, amnesia, vertigo, blurred vision, easy sweating and a thready-weak pulse.

In kidney deficiency, it is accompanied by vertigo, tinnitus, seminal emission, lumbar soreness, a red tongue and a thready-rapid pulse.

In deficiency of the heart and gallbladder, it is accompanied by palpitations, dream-disturbed sleep, being easily frightened and afraid, a pale tongue and a wiry-thready pulse.

In cases of mental depression and upward disturbance of liver yang, it is accompanied by irritability and a quick temper, vertigo, headache, and distending flank pain.

In disharmony of the spleen and stomach, it is accompanied by stuffiness in the epigastrium, belching, foul and sour regurgitation, a thick greasy tongue coating and a slippery pulse.

TREATMENT

Needling and moxibustion

Method. Mainly to nourish the heart and calm the mind. Select the *yuan* or Back-Shu points of the involved meridians, on the basis of differentiation of syndromes. Use a reinforcing or even method of needling, or both needling and moxibustion.

Prescription. Shenmen (H 7) and Sanyinjiao (Sp 6).

Modification.
— Deficiency of heart and spleen: Xinshu (UB 15), Jueyinshu (UB 14), Pishu (UB 20).
— Disharmony between the heart and kidney: Xinshu (UB 15), Shenshu (UB 23), Taixi (K 3), Daling (P 7), Qiuxu (GB 40).
— Upward disturbance of liver yang: Ganshu (UB 18), Jianshi (P 5), Taichong (Liv 3).
— Disharmony of spleen and stomach: Weishu (UB 21), Zusanli (St 36).

Explanation. This syndrome is mainly caused by deficiency of the heart, spleen and kidney, and the prescription is mainly to nourish the

heart and calm the mind. Therefore the *yuan* point of the heart meridian, Shenmen, is selected to nourish and regulate the qi of the heart meridian so as to calm the heart and mind.

Sanyinjiao is used to regulate the qi passage of the spleen and kidney.

According to different aetiological factors, the *yuan* or Back-Shu points of the involved meridians are selected, e.g. Xinshu and Pishu with a reinforcing or moxibustion method to nourish the heart and kidney and restore the harmony between the fire (heart) and water (kidney), or else Ganshu and Taichong to purge the liver in cases of a restless mind due to upward disturbance of liver yang. Weishu and Zusanli harmonize the stomach and the middle-jiao in cases of insomnia due to disharmony of the spleen and stomach.

Cutaneous needling

Method. Tap the sites 0.5–3 cun lateral to the spinal column on both sides of the sacral and temporal regions, with cutaneous needles until the local skin gets congested. Treatment is given once a day or every other day.

Ear needling

Points. Ear-Shenmen, Heart, Spleen, Kidney, Brain and tip of inferior antihelix crus.

Method. 2–3 points are used each time. Use moderate or strong stimulation by rotating the needles, with 20 minutes retention of the needles.

REMARKS

1. Needling and moxibustion have a good therapeutic effect in treating insomnia. It is better to give the treatment in the afternoons.
2. If insomnia is caused by other diseases, the primary cause should be treated at the same time.
3. Give advice to the patients about getting rid of worries, and having a reasonable life-style, proper physical exercise and entertainment.

12. ZANGZAO

Zangzao (脏躁) is an hysterical disorder due to

the zang organs. It corresponds to hysteria in modern medicine and is a kind of neurosis, seen often in adults and young people and in females. It has various clinical manifestations, and those patterns mentioned in classical medical literature such as "piglet running qi", "globus hystericus", *jue* syndrome (厥) or syncope, and other related depressive syndromes, are included in this syndrome.

AETIOLOGY AND PATHOGENESIS

This disease is often caused by emotional disturbance. Emotional injuries such as grief, worry, repressed anger or mental depression may affect the heart and the *ying* qi, so then insufficient *ying* qi and blood leads to excessive heart qi and fire, giving restlessness of the heart and mind.

Otherwise, it is caused by heat and fire consuming and condensing the body fluid into *tan*, and the *tan* fire upwardly disturbing the mind, resulting in restlessness.

DIFFERENTIATION

It is marked mainly by emotional disorders such as capricious joy or anger, grief, singing; moaning, or dullness and reticence; or sudden aphasia, blindness, sudden distress in the chest, hiccup, dysphagia or even syncope in severe cases; or else numbness, pain, paralysis and tremor in the limbs.

TREATMENT

Needling and moxibustion

Method. Mainly to calm the heart and mind and promote resuscitation, and treat the accompanying symptoms with modified points. Use an even or reducing method of needling.

Prescription. Renzhong (Du 26), Neiguan (P 6), Shenmen (H 7), Fenglong (St 40) and Yongquan (K 1).

Modification.
— Aphasia: Yamen (Du 15), Tongli (H 5).

— Dysphagia: Tiantu (Ren 22), Lianquan (Ren 23).
— Blindness: Jingming (UB 1), Guangming (GB 37), (refer to prescriptions for *feng* stroke).

Explanation. Renzhong from the Du meridian is used to promote resuscitation.

The heart houses the mind and the pericardium surrounds the heart, so Neiguan and Shenmen are used to clear heart fire so as to calm the mind. In cases of fire and heat giving rise to *tan*, the *luo* point of the Stomach meridian is used to subdue fire and resolve *tan*. The Jing-well point of the kidney meridian Yongquan is also used to nourish the kidney water so as to check heart fire.

The above five points can be applied during the attacks of hysteria. The modified points are selected according to the combination of local points and points along the meridians; they have the action of promoting resuscitation, easing the throat and restoring eyesight respectively.

Ear needling

Points. Ear-Shenmen, Occiput, Heart, Stomach and Brain.

Method. 2–3 points are selected each time. Use a moderate or strong stimulation with rotation of needles and 15 minutes needle retention. The "Throat" and "Oesophagus" points are added for globus hystericus, and "Kidney" and "Brain" for aphasia.

Electroneedling

Method. Points on the limbs are selected according to symptoms. A dense wave is applied, with electrical stimulation for 10–20 minutes which can generally be used in treatment over 3–7 successive days. It is indicated for hysteria manifesting with mental, sensory and motor inhibition.

REMARKS

1. This disease is complex and changeable in its clinical manifestations. Attention should be paid

to the possibility of confusing it with other organic pathological changes.

2. Explanatory ideological work with the patient and the patient's confidence in the treatment are required.

13. PALPITATIONS

Palpitations refers to an unduly rapid action of the heart which is felt by the patient and accompanied by nervousness and restlessness. In the classical Chinese medical literature palpitations are divided into *jingji* (惊悸) or mild palpitations, and *zhengzhong* (怔忡) or serious palpitations.

Mild palpitations are mostly due to sudden fright and overstrain, the general condition is comparatively good and the symptoms are of short duration; serious palpitations are not related to fright or fear, but are often due to prolonged internal injury, the general condition is comparatively poor and the symptoms severe. As these two kinds of palpitations are quite similar in aetiology and treatment with acupuncture and moxibustion, they are discussed together.

This disease is often seen in cardiac arrhythmia, cardiac neurosis, coronary heart disease, hyperthyroidism and anaemia.

AETIOLOGY AND PATHOGENESIS

This disease is often due to constitutional deficiency, deficiency of heart and gallbladder, repressed anger, or being frightened by surprising objects or dangerous environments.

It may be due to insufficiency of heart blood in which the heart is deprived of nourishment.

It may also be due to retention of harmful fluid and deficiency of heart yang.

Otherwise it is due to upward disturbance of *tan* heat leading to restlessness of heart qi.

DIFFERENTIATION

This condition is often marked by intermittent palpitations, nervousness, being easily fright-

ened, restlessness, dream-disturbed sleep, and sleeping but being easily woken.

If due to insufficiency of heart blood, there may also be pallor, vertigo, blurred vision, a slightly red tongue, a thready-weak or knotted and intermittent pulse.

If due to *tan* fire being stirred up in the interior, there may also be restlessness, trance or dream-disturbed sleep, a yellow tongue coating and a rapid pulse.

If due to retention of fluid in the interior, there may also be stuffiness and fullness in the chest and epigastrium, vertigo and excessive salivation, spiritlessness, cold limbs, a white tongue coating and a thready and slippery pulse.

TREATMENT

Needling and moxibustion

Method. Select points mainly from the hand Shaoyin and Jueyin meridians; also use the Back-Shu points. Use an even method of needling. In case of yang deficiency, moxibustion can be applied.

Prescription. Ximen (P 4), Shenmen (H 7), Xinshu (UB 15) and Juque (Ren 14).

Modification.
— Insufficiency of heart blood: Geshu (UB 17), Pishu UB 20), Zusanli (St 36).
— *Tan* fire stirred up in the interior: Chize (Lu 5), Neiguan (P 6), Fenglong (St 40).
— Fluid retention in the interior: Pishu (UB 20), Weishu (UB 21), Sanjiaoshu (UB 22).

Explanation. The principle of treatment in this disease is mainly to calm the mind and tranquillize the palpitations.

Ximen is the Xi-Cleft point of the pericardium meridian and Shenmen the *yuan* point of the heart meridian. Both are used to calm the mind and ease the palpitations, and are especially indicated for sudden attacks of cardiac pain with palpitations.

Xinshu and Juque are respectively the Back-Shu and Front-Mu points of the heart meridian. They are used in combination to regulate the qi passage along the heart meridian, and tranquillize the mind or any fear due to the palpitations.

In case of insufficiency of heart blood, the Influential point of blood, Geshu, and Pishu and Zusanli are used with a reinforcing method to replenish the heart blood.

In cases of *tan* fire in the interior, Chize and Fenglong with a reducing method are used to clear heat, resolve *tan* and clear the lung.

Neiguan, communicating with the Yinwei meridian, is used to treat restlessness and palpitations.

In cases of interior retention of fluid, Pishu, Weishu and Sanjiaoshu are used to facilitate the qi passage and the downward excretion of water and fluid, so as to check the palpitations.

Point-injection therapy

Points. Neiguan (P 6), Ximen (P 4), Xinshu (UB 15) and Jueyinshu (UB 14).

Method. An injection of Danshen (Salvia) is applied into the above points, 1–2 points a time, 0.5–1 ml into each point. Treatment is given once a day or every other day, 10 treatments as one course. This method is indicated for palpitations, stuffiness in the chest and angina pectoris.

Ear needling

Points. Heart, Brain, tip of inferior antihelix crus, Ear-Shenmen and Small intestine.

Method. 2–3 points are used each time, with a mild rotation of the needles, and 20–30 minutes retention.

REMARKS

1. Needling and moxibustion have a good effect in treating palpitations. A definite diagnosis is required before treatment as the syndrome can occur in various diseases.
2. Give advice about quitting smoking or alcohol if the patients have such habits.

14. MALARIA

Malaria is an infectious disease caused by malarial parasites; it is mostly seen in summer and autumn. It is stated in the *Elementary Medical Studies* that "when malarial pestilent factors prevail in an area, they give similar manifestations both in adults and children", indicating that the disease can be endemic.

Clinically it is marked by paroxysms of shivering chills and high fever, sweating and regular attacks.

AETIOLOGY AND PATHOGENESIS

Malaria is caused by malarial pestilential factors together with an invasion of pathogenic *feng*, cold, summer-heat or damp which affect the half-exterior and half-interior region of the body (the Shaoyang), where the *ying* and *wei* qi and pathogenic and antipathogenic qi are engaged in a severe struggle leading to the symptoms of malarial attacks.

The Shaoyang meridian lies halfway between the exterior and interior, and when pathogenic factors move inward to struggle with the yin there appear chills, and when they move outward to fight with the yang there appears fever. This is the reason for the presence of alternate chills and fever, and the regularity of the attacks.

Protracted malaria consumes qi and blood, and damp blocks the passage of the qi, giving rise to stagnant *tan* in the Shaoyang meridian which manifests as a mass in the hypochondrical region, which is known as "malaria with splenomegaly".

DIFFERENTIATION

This disease is marked by alternate chills and fever and regular attacks, preceded by a reaction at the skin pores, yawning and lassitude. Then there appear chills, soreness of the limbs, general hotness, intolerable headache, flushed face and lips, polydipsia; after sweating a reduction in the fever; a white greasy tongue coating, a wiry-tight pulse during chills and a slippery-rapid pulse during fever.

The recurrence of chills and fever varies—it may be once a day, every second or every third day. Those cases with attacks gradually appearing earlier than expected indicate that the pathogenic factors are moving outward to the yang region and the case is improving; while those cases with attacks gradually appearing later than expected indicate that the pathogenic factors are moving into the yin, and the case will be aggravated.

If, in a case of protracted malaria, there is a mass appearing in the left hypochondriacal region, either painful or not to pressure, it is called "malaria with splenomegaly".

TREATMENT

Needling and moxibustion

Method. Mainly to promote and regulate the yang qi and relieve the exterior symptoms. Use a reducing needling method, given about 2 hours before the attacks.
Prescription. Dazhui (Du 14), Houxi (SI 3), Jianshi (P 5).

Modification.
— Excessive heat: Shangyang (LI 1), Guanchong (SJ 1).
— Malaria with splenomegaly: Zhangmen (Liv 13), Pishu (UB 20).

Explanation. Dazhui is the meeting point of the hand and foot yang meridians of the Du meridian, and is used to activate the yang qi and eliminate pathogenic factors. It is an important point for the treatment of malaria. Houxi is from the Taiyang meridian and communicates with the Du meridian; it is used to eliminate pathogens from these meridians. Jianshi, from the hand Jueyin, is an empirical point for the treatment of malaria.

These three points used together can regulate yang and eliminate the pathogenic factors.

Shangyang and Guanchong respectively are the Jing-well points of the hand Yangming and Shaoyang meridians. In excessive heat cases the three-edged needle is applied at these points to cause bleeding, in order to clear the pathogenic heat.

Moxibustion is applied to Zhangmen and Pishu to warm and resolve *tan* and damp, and relieve the mass in the area around the flank.

Blister-inducing method

Method. Pound fresh buttercup, wild mint or large cloves of garlic into pieces. Apply them externally 1–2 hours before the attacks onto the points Neiguan (P 6) or Jianshi (P 5) for 3–4 hours, fixing them with adhesive tape.

Ear needling

Points. Brain, Intertragus, Infratragic apex, Liver and Spleen.
Method. Needling is given 1–2 hours before the attacks; retain the needles for 20–30 minutes, during which manipulation is applied from time to time. Treatment is given over three successive days.

REMARKS

1. Needling and moxibustion have a good effect in treating tertian malaria. Herbal therapy should be applied in combination with acupuncture and moxibustion when treating malignant malaria.
2. It is generally held that treatment given 2–3 hours before the attacks exerts better results. According to clinical observations, needling given during the attacks may be as effective as that given before.

15. COMMON COLD

A common cold is a frequently seen exogenous disease occurring all the year round, but especially in spring and autumn with sudden changes in the weather. According to differences in severity, mild attacks are called *shangfeng* (伤风), meaning *feng* injury, while severe attacks are put down to epidemic causes.

AETIOLOGY AND PATHOGENESIS

The disease is often due to a weakened resistance and enfeebled *wei* qi which makes the body unable to adapt to the sudden change in the weather, when there is abnormal cold or heat.

Then the exogenous pathogenic *feng* invades the body through the pores, the skin, mouth and nose, leading to manifestations relating to the lung meridian.

Very often pathogenic *feng* combined with other pathogenic factors, like pathogenic cold, causes a *feng* cold syndrome, or combining with pathogenic heat causes a *feng* heat syndrome.

Pathogenic *feng* cold may impair the dispersing function of the lung and block the yang qi and skin pores; while pathogenic *feng* heat may impair the lung's dispersing and descending function by the evaporating heat leading to an abnormal function of the skin pores.

DIFFERENTIATION

Feng cold is marked by headache, soreness and aching of the limbs, nasal obstruction and watery discharge, itching in the throat and cough with dilute sputum, chills and fever (or absence of fever), anhidrosis, a superficial-tight pulse and a thin-white tongue coating.

Feng heat manifests as fever, sweating, a slight aversion to the cold, distending headache, cough with thick sputum, sore throat, thirst, dryness in the nose, a superficial-rapid pulse and a thin and slightly yellow tongue coating.

TREATMENT

Needling and moxibustion

a) Feng *cold*

Method. Points are selected mainly from the hand Taiyin and Yangming, and foot Taiyang meridians. Use a reducing method of superficial needling. Use an even movement in patients with a weak constitution, where moxibustion is applicable.

Prescription. Lieque (Lu 7), Fengmen (UB 12), Fengchi (GB 20), Hegu (LI 4).

Explanation. The prescription is mainly to disperse pathogenic *feng* cold from the exterior.

The *luo* point of the lung meridian is punctured superficially to promote the dispersing function of the lung qi and to check coughing.

Fengmen is used to regulate the qi of the Taiyang meridians which dominate the yang qi of the whole body, to disperse *feng* cold and relieve the chills and fever, headache and aching limbs.

The Yangwei meridian dominates the yang and exterior, so Fengchi, the crossing point of the foot Shaoyang and Yangwei meridians, is selected to relieve exterior symptoms.

The Taiyin and Yangming meridians are externally-internally related, so the *yuan* point of the Yangming meridian, Hegu, is used to dispel pathogens and relieve the exterior.

All these four points used together can dispel *feng* cold and promote the dispersion of lung qi.

b) Feng *heat*

Method. Points are selected mainly from the hand Taiyin, Yangming and Shaoyang meridians. Use a reducing method of superficial needling.

Prescription. Dazhui (Du 14), Quchi (LI 11), Hegu (LI 4), Yuji (Lu 10), Waiguan (SJ 5).

Explanation. The prescription aims at dispelling *feng* heat and restoring the normal dispersing and descending of lung qi.

The Du meridian is the sea of the yang meridians. Dazhui, from the Du meridian, is a converging point of the various yang meridians. It is used to dispel yang pathogens and relieve heat.

Hegu and Quchi respectively are the *yuan* and He-sea points of the hand Yangming meridian, which is externally-internally related to the hand Taiyin. They are used to clear the lung and subdue fever (heat).

Yuji is the Ying-spring point of the lung meridian and it is used to purge the lung fire, ease the throat and relieve pain.

Waiguan, the *luo* point of the hand Shaoyang meridian communicates with the Yangwei. It is used to relieve fever by dispelling yang pathogens from the exterior.

Together these five points disperse *feng* heat and restore the normal function of dispersing and descending of the lung qi.

Cupping

Apply cupping onto Dazhui (Du 14), Shenzhu

(Du 12), Dashu (UB 11), Fengmen (UB 12) and Feishu (UB 13). This method is indicated for a common cold due to invasion of *feng* and cold.

Ear needling

Points. Lung, Internal nose, Infratragic apex, Forehead.

Method. Moderate or strong stimulation is applied by rotating the needles for 2–3 minutes and retaining them for 20–30 minutes. Add "Throat" and "Tonsils" if there is a sore throat.

REMARKS

1. A common cold is similar to early symptoms of some infectious diseases, and they should be differentiated from each other.
2. During an epidemic period of common cold, needling Zusanli (St 36) bilaterally once a day, for three successive days, has the effect of preventing an attack.

16. COUGHING

Coughing is the chief symptom of disorders of the respiratory system. According to its causative factor it can be classified into two categories—due either to exogenous affection or else due to internal injuries, all caused through a dysfunction of the zangfu organs.

Coughing is often seen in an infection of the upper respiratory tract, acute and chronic bronchitis, bronchiectasis and pulmonary tuberculosis.

AETIOLOGY AND PATHOGENESIS

Coughing may be caused by exogenous pathogenic *feng* cold or *feng* heat invading the lung and the *wei* qi system via the mouth, nose, or skin pores, impairing the normal function of the lung qi in dispersing and descending.

Otherwise it is due to the lung being affected by disorders of other internal organs, leading to coughing, e.g. spleen deficiency gives rise to *tan*

damp which affects upwardly the lung, impairing the normal descending of the lung qi.

Alternatively, stagnant liver qi turning into fire burns the lung, impairing the normal dispersing and descending function of the lung and resulting in coughing.

DIFFERENTIATION

a) Exogenous pathogenic factors

Feng heat manifests as coughing with yellow sputum, general feverishness, headache, a superficial and rapid pulse, and a thin yellow tongue coating.

Feng cold manifests as coughing, itching of the throat, thin and white sputum, headache, fever, aversion to cold, anhidrosis, a superficial and tight pulse, and a thin and white tongue coating.

b) Endogenous pathogenic factors

Tan damp invading the lung manifests as coughing with sticky sputum, stuffiness in chest and epigastrium, impaired appetite, a white and greasy tongue coating and a soft and slippery pulse.

Liver fire burning the lung manifests as coughing with pain affecting the chest and hypochondrium, rebellion of qi leading to coughing with a small amounts of sticky sputum, a flushing of the face, dryness in the throat, a yellow tongue coating with little moisture, and a wiry and rapid pulse.

TREATMENT

Needling and moxibustion

a) Exogenous affection

Method. Points are selected mainly from hand Taiyin and hand Yangming meridians. Use a reducing method of superficial needling, with swift needling in the case of *feng* heat, and retaining the needle or cupping on the back (such as on Feishu) in *feng* cold.

Prescription. Feishu (UB 13), Lieque (Lu 7), Hegu (LI 4).

Modification.
— Sore throat: Shaoshang (Lu 11), Chize (Lu 5).
— Fever: Dazhui (Du 14), Waiguan (SJ 5).

Explanation. The lung dominates the skin pores and the exterior of the body, so superficial needling is given.

The hand Taiyin and Yangming meridians are externally-internally related. The *luo* and *yuan* points Lieque and Hegu are used, in combination with Feishu, to strengthen the dispersion of lung qi and relieve the exterior symptoms, and to restore the normal functions of the lung.

In cases of a sore throat due to *feng* heat, bleeding Shaoshang and reducing Chize can clear the lung heat and relieve the sore swollen throat.

In cases of fever, Dazhui and Waiguan are used with a reducing needling method to eliminate pathogenic heat from the exterior.

b) Endogenous affection

In the case of *tan* damp invading the lung, points are selected mainly from the foot Taiyin meridian. Use an even method of needling or add moxibustion.

Prescription. Feishu (UB 13), Taiyuan (Lu 9), Zhangmen (Liv 13), Taibai (Sp 3), Fenglong (St 40).

Explanation. Taiyuan (*yuan* point of the lung) and Taibai (*yuan* point of the spleen) are used. In combination with Feishu and Zhangmen, they strengthen the transporting function of the spleen and facilitate the lung qi.

As the spleen is the source of *tan* production, treating the spleen and lung is treating both the symptoms and the cause.

Fenglong, the *luo* point of the foot Yangming, is used to promote the qi of the middle-jiao so that fluid is dispersed along with the circulation of the qi, and thus *tan* and damp resolved.

In the case of liver fire burning the lung, points are selected mainly from the hand Taiyin and foot Jueyin meridians. Use a reducing needling method in points from the foot Jueyin and an even method in points from the hand Taiyin. No moxibustion is applied.

Prescription. Feishu (UB 13), Chize (Lu 5), Yanglingquan (GB 34) and Taichong (Liv 3).

Explanation. Feishu is used to regulate lung qi, and Chize (He-sea point of the lung) to clear lung heat.

Yanglingquan and Taichong clear pathogenic heat from the liver and gallbladder meridians and prevent the lung yin from being burnt and injured.

Point-injection therapy

Points. Dingchuan (Extra 17), Dashu (UB 11), Fengmen (UB 12), Feishu (UB 13).
Method. Vitamin B1 (100 mg), or placental tissue fluid, is injected into points on the back (such as Feishu); each time bilateral points are used and 0.5 ml is injected into each point. Points are used alternately in order from above to below. Treatment is given once every other day, 20 treatments as one course. This method is indicated for chronic bronchitis.

Moxibustion

Points. Dazhui (Du 14), Feishu (UB 13) or Fengmen (UB 12), Gaohuang (UB 43).
Method. Small-sized moxa cones are applied; treatment is given every 3–5 days, 5 treatments as one course. Or use moxa sticks, once a day, each time for 5–10 minutes, until the skin gets locally red. This can be used in combination with needling. This method is indicated in chronic bronchitis.

REMARKS

1. Coughing can be seen in various diseases of the respiratory system; a definite diagnosis is required so that herbal therapy can also be applied in certain cases.
2. Ask the patient to keep warm, to avoid the cold and wind, and to quit smoking and alcohol.

17. ASTHMA

Asthma is a common illness marked by repeated attacks of paroxysmal dyspnoea, or *chuan* (哮), and wheezing, *xiao* (喘). The classic,

Orthodox Medical Problems, states that *xiao* depicts the sound of the wheezing, while *chuan* describes a problem with the breathing. They may attack together and have a similar aetiology, thus they are discussed together.

Asthma, as described here, can be seen in bronchial asthma, asthmatic bronchitis and obstructive pulmonary emphysema.

AETIOLOGY AND PATHOGENESIS

Asthma is basically due to retention of *tan* fluid in the interior. It results in children repeatedly being affected by exogenous pathogens at differing seasons, while in adults it is often due to a long-term illness which involves coughing.

Otherwise it is due to impaired transportation by the spleen which leads to retention of damp and *tan*.

It may also be due to a preference for salty or greasy food, or seafood like shrimps, crabs or fish, or food with a strange smell.

It may be due to emotional disturbance, overstrain or stress.

Alternatively, the dormant *tan* fluid in the lung meridian is stirred up, which blocks the passage of the qi and impairs the dispersing and descending function of the lung qi, leading to a gurgling in the throat, asthma and coughing.

During attacks, there may be depressed qi and an accumulation of *tan*, blocking the qi passage, which manifests as an excess syndrome. If there are repeated attacks, lung qi will be consumed and the spleen and kidney also affected, so during the remission period a deficiency syndrome is also often seen.

DIFFERENTIATION

The main symptoms are shortness of breath, a gurgling in the throat, perhaps dyspnoea with an open mouth, raised shoulders and an inability to lie flat. It is divided into excess and deficiency syndromes, according to either an excess in the form of the pathogen or a deficiency in the antipathogenic qi.

Excess syndromes arise from being affected by exogenous *feng* and cold, and are marked by coughing, dilute sputum, aversion to cold, anhidrosis, headache, absence of thirst, a superficial and tight pulse, and a thin and white tongue coating.

If due to *tan* and heat, there is coughing with sticky yellow sputum which it is difficult to spit out, distress and stuffiness in the chest, coughing affecting the chest and flank, or general feverishness, thirst, constipation, a slippery and rapid pulse, and a yellow greasy tongue coating.

A deficiency syndrome is due to insufficiency of lung qi owing to long-term illness. It is marked by shortness of breath, a weak speaking voice, sweating upon slight exertion, a pale or slightly red tongue, and a thready-rapid or forceless pulse.

Protracted asthmatic breathing leads to failure in the kidney receiving the qi, and there will be listlessness, shortness of breath, asthmatic breathing aggravated upon any slight exertion, sweating, cold limbs, and a deep and thready pulse.

TREATMENT

Needling and moxibustion

a) Excess syndrome

Method. Points are selected mainly from the hand Taiyin meridian, with a reducing method of needling. In *feng* cold cases moxibustion is applicable. In cases of *tan* heat, points from the foot Yangming are used in combination, and moxibustion is unsuitable.

Prescription. Shanzhong (Ren 17), Lieque (Lu 7), Feishu (UB 13), Chize (Lu 5).

Modification.
— *Feng* cold: Fengmen (UB 12).
— *Tan* heat: Fenglong.
— Severe asthmatic breathing: Tiantu (Ren 22), Dingchuan (Extra 17).

Explanation. Lieque and Chize are used to promote the dispersion of the lung qi.

Fengmen and Feishu from the bladder meridian are near the lung, and are used to promote the dispersion of lung qi and dispel *feng*.

Shanzhong is the Influential point of qi, and

Fenglong is where the branch of the stomach meridian joins on, so reducing the two points can regulate qi and resolve *tan*, and they are indicated for *tan* heat.

Tiantu and Dingchuan are effective points for checking the abnormal ascent of the lung qi and for soothing asthma. They are local points.

b) Deficiency syndrome

Method. Mainly to regulate and nourish the spleen and kidney qi. Use a reinforcing method of needling; moxibustion is applicable.

Prescription. Feishu (UB 13), Gaohuang (UB 43), Qihai (Ren 6), Shenshu (UB 23), Zusanli (St 36), Taiyuan (Lu 9), Taixi (K 3).

Explanation. Reinforcing the *yuan* points of the lung and kidney, Taiyuan and Taixi, replenishes the *zhen* qi. Moxibustion on Feishu and Gaohuang strengthens the lung qi.

Shenshu and Qihai are used with a reinforcing method to receive the kidney qi, so that the normal function of the lung and kidney qi, and ascent and descent of the passage of the qi, can be restored.

Zusanli is used to regulate the stomach qi and promote the manufacture of qi and blood, so that the nourishment from food can be distributed to the lung. This enables there to be sufficient lung qi supporting the *wei* qi.

Cutaneous needling

Method. During the asthma attack, tapping the point Yuji (Lu 10) and the course of the hand Taiyin meridian on the forearm for 15 minutes, or tapping the sternocleidomastoid muscles, both sides for 15 minutes, may relieve the symptoms.

Point-injection therapy

Method. Select Huatuojiaji (Extra 19, T1–6). Inject placental tissue fluid into a pair of points (on both sides), 0.5–1 ml into each point at a time. Use these points alternately, in order, from above to below, once a day. This method is indicated during the remission period of bronchial asthma.

Moxibustion

Points. Dazhui (Du 14), Fengmen (UB 12), Feishu (UB 13), Shanzhong (Ren 17).

Method. Small-sized moxa-cones are applied, 3–5 cones on each point, and moxibustion is given once every 10 days; 3 times constitute one course. This method is indicated for the remission period of bronchial asthma, and treatment is often given in the summer.

External herbal applications

Method. Grind white mustard seed, Gansui (*Euphorbiae Kansui* root), Xixin (Asarum, wild ginger) and Yanhusuo (Corydalis tuber), 15 g of each, into a fine powder, and mix it with fresh ginger juice. Form it into six small flat pieces, to which is then added some *Ding Gui San* powder (Powder of Cloves and Cinnamon).

Apply this externally onto Bailao (Extra), Feishu (UB 13) and Gaohuang (UB 43) and keep it there for 2 hours and then remove. There may be a hot, numb and painful sensation during the herbal application on these points, or redness of the local skin, sometimes even blistering.

This method is applied during the "three months of summer" (one treatment at each month) and treatments can be given over three successive years. The method is indicated for children.

Ear needling

Points. Soothing asthma, Infratragic apex, Lung, Ear-Shenmen, Brain, tip of inferior antihelix crus.

Method. 2–3 points are used each time, a moderate or strong stimulation with needle rotation, and retention of the needles for 20–30 minutes. This method is indicated during asthma attacks; it has a soothing effect.

Scalp needling

The Thoracic Cavity Area is selected, with intermittent manipulation of the needle, and 15 minutes retention of the needle. This method is indicated for bronchial asthma.

REMARKS

1. Asthma can be seen in various diseases. After the attack is relieved, treatment of the cause should be given.
2. When there are severe attacks or persistent states of asthma, the treatment should be combined with herbal treatment.
3. Ask patients to keep warm, to avoid contact with objects to which they are sensitive, and to avoid eating things to which they have an allergic reaction.

18. PULMONARY TUBERCULOSIS

Pulmonary tuberculosis is a chronic consumptive disease. It was known in medical classics as *guzhen* (骨蒸)—the "bone-steaming disease", or *chuanshi* (传尸)—"the passing-from-door-to-door disease". In the *Prescriptions for Relieving the Sick* it states that "this disease is infectious and protracted, and even the members of a whole family may die of it", showing that it is both chronic and infectious.

AETIOLOGY AND PATHOGENESIS

This disease is often due to a weak inherited constitution and weakened body resistance, which occurs in patients who are susceptible to invasion by, or who come into contact with someone suffering from, this disease. The location of the disease is the lung. The lung yin is consumed first and the lung is deprived of nourishment and moistening, which leads to dryness of the throat and a dry cough.

After a long time the kidney is affected and both the lung and kidney are sick, giving rise to yin deficiency, hyperactivity of fire and manifestation of a hectic fever and flushed face.

If there is empty fire (fire due to yin deficiency) it consumes the body fluid and causes haemoptysis. A lung disorder may also affect the spleen, leading to spiritlessness, lassitude, poor appetite, and loose stools, which are manifestations of a deficiency of both qi and yin.

DIFFERENTIATION

This disease is marked mainly by coughing, haemoptysis, hectic fever and night sweating; generally syndromes of yin deficiency are often seen. Initially there may be a persistent cough, spiritlessness, impaired appetite, progressive emaciation, dull pain in the chest, and blood-tinged sputum.

Then the cough becomes aggravated into a dry cough with little sputum, afternoon fever, malar flush, night sweating, even haemoptysis to a large extent, irritability, insomnia, seminal emission in men and amenorrhoea in women, a red tongue, and a thready and rapid pulse.

In severe cases there may be severe emaciation, hoarseness of the voice, loose stools, oedema of the face and limbs, a glossy and deep red tongue, and a feeble and thready pulse.

TREATMENT

Needling and moxibustion

Method. Points are selected mainly from the Back-Shu points. Needling is used mainly in yin deficiency cases; moxibustion is used mainly in yang deficiency cases.

Prescription. Chize (Lu 5), Feishu (UB 13), Gaohuang (UB 43), Zusanli (St 36).

Modification.
— Poor appetite: Pishu (UB 20), Zhongwan (Ren 12).
— Hectic fever: Dazhui (Du 14), Taixi (K 3).
— Night sweating: Yinxi (H 6), Fuliu (K 7).
— Haemoptysis: Yuji (Lu 10), Geshu (UB 17).
— Seminal emission: Zhishi (UB 52), Guanyuan (Ren 4), Sanyinjiao (Sp 6).
— Amenorrhoea: Xuehai (Sp 10), Pishu (UB 20).

Explanation. Pulmonary tuberculosis is due to empty fire (fire due to yin deficiency) consuming body fluid, which leads to yin deficiency and lung dryness. Therefore the treatment is mainly to clear the empty heat, nourish fluids and moisten the dryness of the lung, and at the same time strengthen the middle-jiao and consolidate the source of health.

The He-sea point of the lung meridian, Chize,

is used in combination with Feishu to clear heat from the lung meridian and treat yin deficiency and lung dryness.

Gaohuang is an important point for tuberculosis—it is used to regulate and nourish the lung qi.

Tonifying the He-sea point of the stomach meridian, Zusanli, strengthens the acquired source of health.

For impaired appetite in tuberculosis, Pishu and Zhongwan are used to promote the transportation by the middle-jiao and invigorate the spleen.

In a hectic fever, Dazhui and Taixi are added to nourish yin and clear heat.

Yinxi and Fuliu are effective points for treating night sweating.

Yuji is the Ying-spring point of the hand Taiyin, Geshu is the Influential point of blood, and they are both used to clear heat from the lung and treat haemoptysis.

In the case of seminal emission and amenorrhoea, points are selected according to their therapeutic properties.

Point-injection therapy

Points. Jiehexue (Extra 18), Zhongfu (Lu 1), Feishu (UB 13), Dazhui (Du 14); also Gaohuang (UB 43), Quchi (LI 11) and Zusanli (St 36) can be used in combination.

Method. 100 mg of Vitamin B1, or 0.2 g streptomycin are injected into 2–3 points each time. The points are used alternately.

REMARKS

1. The patient should pay attention to having sufficient and reasonable nutrition, and avoid irritative and pungent foods, alcohol and smoking.
2. Vessels or objects used by the patient should be sterilized to avoid cross-infection.
3. Herbal and antitubercular drugs should be used in combination with acupuncture and moxibustion to potentiate the therapeutic effect.

19. VOMITING

Vomiting is a common clinical symptom and an accompanying symptom in various diseases. It can be caused by pathogens like *feng*, cold, warmth (mild heat) and heat, or by *tan* fluid, food stagnancy or stagnant liver qi.

Vomiting can be seen in acute gastritis, hepatitis, cardiospasm, pyloric spasm or obstruction, pancreatitis and cholecystitis.

AETIOLOGY AND PATHOGENESIS

Exogenous pathogens affecting the stomach impair the normal harmony and descending function of the stomach (together with the spleen, they function in sending the clear above and the turbid below) and induce the upward rebellion of stomach qi, which gives rise to vomiting.

Retention of *tan* and damp in the spleen and stomach, or an over-intake of raw and cold or greasy food, gives rise to impaired movement within the middle-jiao and obstruction of food, which leads to vomiting.

It may also be due to deficiency of the middle-jiao with impaired transformation and transportation, and impaired digestion.

Alternatively it is due to emotional depression, in which the stomach is affected by the depressed liver qi and the stomach qi fails to descend.

DIFFERENTIATION

Cold affecting the stomach and epigastrium manifests as dilute or watery vomiting, vomiting attacking only long after the food intake, a white tongue coating, a slow pulse, a preference for warmth but aversion to cold, or loose stools.

Retention of pathogenic heat in the interior manifests as vomiting attacking shortly after the food intake, sour, bitter, or hot and foul vomiting, thirst, a preference for cold but aversion to heat, constipation, a rapid pulse and a yellow tongue coating.

Retention of *tan* fluid manifests as stuffiness in the chest, vertigo, vomiting of salivary substances, or palpitations, a white tongue coating and a slippery pulse.

In the case of retention of food, there is epigastric and abdominal distension and fullness or pain, which are aggravated by food intake, belching, anorexia, constipation, breaking of wind, a thick and greasy tongue coating, and a slippery pulse of the excess type.

In the case of liver qi affecting the stomach, there is flank pain, sour regurgitation, and a wiry pulse.

Deficiency of stomach qi manifests as vomiting from time to time, no sense of taste and a poor appetite, slightly loose stools, listlessness, weakness of the limbs, a forceless pulse and a thin and greasy tongue coating.

TREATMENT

Needling and moxibustion

Method. Points are selected mainly from the foot Yangming meridian. Use retention of needles and moxibustion in cold syndromes, and swift needling without retention of needles and without moxibustion in hot syndromes.

In cases of liver qi affecting the stomach, points from the foot Jueyin meridian are reduced and points from the foot Yangming meridian are reinforced. In cases of deficiency of the middle-jiao, the principle of treatment is to tonify the spleen qi.

Prescription. Zhongwan (Ren 12), Weishu (UB 21), Zusanli (St 36) and Neiguan (P 6).

Modification.
— Vomiting due to heat: Hegu (LI 4), Jinjin and Yuye (Extra 8).
— Vomiting due to cold: Shangwan (Ren 13), Weishu (UB 21).
— Vomiting due to *tan* fluid: Shanzhong (Ren 17), Fenglong (St 40).
— Vomiting due to food stagnancy: Xiawan (Ren 10), Xuanji (Ren 21).
— Vomiting due to liver qi affecting the stomach: Yanglingquan (GB 34), Taichong (Liv 3).
— Vomiting due to deficiency of middle-jiao: Pishu (UB 20), Zhangmen (Liv 13).

Explanation. Zhongwan and Weishu are a combination of Back-Shu and Front-Mu points. Together with Zusanli, the He-sea point of the foot Yangming meridian, they regulate and restore the normal descent of the stomach qi.

Neiguan, the *luo* point of the hand Jueyin meridian and also crossing point of the Yinwei meridian, promotes the qi passage in the upper and middle-jiao.

Gongsun, from the Spleen meridian which is externally-internally related to the stomach meridian and also the crossing point of the Chong meridian, is used to regulate the middle-jiao and check qi rebellion in the Chong meridian.

Moxibustion applied to Shangwan on the superior epigastrium can warm the stomach and dispel cold.

Hegu is used to reduce the qi of the hand Yangming meridian so as to clear heat. Jinjin and Yuye are used to produce fluid and check vomiting and are indicated for vomiting due to heat.

Fenglong promotes the transporting function of the spleen and stomach, and Shanzhong regulates qi circulation so as to resolve *tan*.

Xiawan and Xuanji disperse the qi passage and resolve food stagnancy.

Yanglingquan and Taichong reduce the qi of the liver and gallbladder meridians and check the liver qi in afflicting the stomach.

Pishu and Zhangmen are Back-Shu and Front-Mu points used to regulate and nourish the spleen qi, in its transporting function through the middle-jiao, to restore its normal ascent and descent.

Point-injection therapy

Points. Zusanli (St 36), Zhiyang (Du 9), Lingtai (Du 10).

Method. Two points are used each time; the points are used alternately. 2 ml normal saline is injected into each point, once a day.

Ear needling

Points. Stomach, Liver, tip of inferior antihelix crus, Brain, Ear-Shenmen.

Method. 2–3 points are selected each time, with a strong stimulation by rotating the needle; retain the needles for 20–30 minutes. Treatment is given once every day or every other day.

REMARKS

1. Needling and moxibustion have a good effect

in treating vomiting. As for the treatment of morning sickness or vomiting due to drug reaction, refer to the therapies mentioned above.

2. The patient should pay attention to a regular and proper food intake and avoiding over-eating or drinking, or raw and cold, or sour or pungent foods.

20. EPIGASTRIC PAIN

Epigastric pain, or gastric pain, is a common symptom characterized by its repeated recurrence. Since the pain is close to the heart, it was sometimes referred to as "cardio-abdominal pain" or "cardiac pain" in ancient times, but it is different from the true cardiac pain recorded in the "Discussion on Jue Diseases" in the *Miraculous Pivot*.[4]

This disease is often seen in gastritis, gastric ulcers and gastroneurosis.

AETIOLOGY AND PATHOGENESIS

The spleen and stomach are externally-internally related, and the liver affects the spleen and stomach with regard to the free-flowing of its qi; therefore epigastric pain is closely related to the liver and spleen.

For instance, liver qi affecting the stomach is often due to an emotional upset, which gives rise to stagnant liver qi and impaired free-flowing of the qi. This affects the stomach, leading to obstruction of passage of the qi.

Alternatively, deficiency and coldness of the spleen and stomach is due to a congenital deficiency and yang deficiency, which gives rise to internal cold and is evoked by irregular food intake, over-strain and stress, or by cold pathogenic factors.

DIFFERENTIATION

Liver qi affecting the stomach is marked by a distending pain in the epigastrium radiating to the hypochondrium, belching, or sour or bitter regurgitation, a thin and white tongue coating, a deep and wiry pulse.

Deficiency and coldness of the spleen and stomach is marked by a dull pain in the epigastrium, watery regurgitation, a preference for warmth and aversion to cold, pain which is aggravated by pressure, listlessness, lassitude, a white tongue coating, and a soft pulse of the deficiency type.

TREATMENT

Needling and moxibustion

a) Liver qi affecting the stomach

Method. Points are selected mainly from the foot Jueyin and Yangming meridians. Use a reducing method of needling.

Prescription. Zhongwan (Ren 12), Qimen (Liv 14), Neiguan (P 6), Zusanli (St 36), Yanglingquan (GB 34).

Explanation. Zhongwan and Zusanli are used to regulate the stomach qi and restore the normal function of ascent and descent.

Neiguan relieves symptoms of distress in the chest.

Qimen is the Front-Mu point of the liver and is used in combination with Yanglingquan to pacify the rebellious qi of the liver and gallbladder so that the liver and stomach qi are harmonized and the stomach qi descends as normal.

b) Deficiency and coldness of spleen and stomach

Method. Points are selected mainly from Back-Shu points and the Ren meridian. Use a reinforcing method of needling in combination with moxibustion.

Prescription. Pishu (UB 20), Weishu (UB 21), Zhongwan (Ren 12), Zhangmen (Liv 13), Neiguan (P 6), Zusanli (St 36).

Explanation. Since the pain is due to deficiency of yang in the middle-jiao, Back-Shu and Front-Mu points are selected as the main ones, with those below the elbow and knee as secondary ones.

For example, Weishu and Zhongwan, Pishu and Zhangmen, are a combination of Back-Shu and Front-Mu points. Neiguan and Zusanli are secondary points, used to harmonize the stomach qi and relieve pain.

Cupping

Apply cupping onto the selected points on the abdomen and back after the acupuncture and moxibustion treatment. This method is indicated for epigastric pain due to deficiency and cold of the stomach.

Point-injection therapy

Points.   Weishu (UB 21), Pishu (UB 20), the corresponding Jiaji (Extra 19), Zhongwan (Ren 12), Neiguan (L 6), Zusanli (St 36).

Method.   An injection of Honghua (Carthamus), Danggui (Chinese Angelica), atropine (0.5 mg) or 1% procaine is applied into the above points. 1–3 points each time, 1–2 ml into each point.

Ear needling

Points.   Stomach, Liver, tip of inferior anti-helix crus, Ear-Shenmen, Brain.

Method.   2–3 points are selected each time. Use strong stimulation by rotating the needles and 20–30 minutes retention of the needles. This method is indicated for gastroneurosis.

REMARKS

1. Epigastric pain is sometimes similar to symptoms of liver and gallbladder diseases and pancreatitis. Differentiation should be made to avoid confusion.
2. If there is a haemorrhage or perforation, as in the case of an ulcer, surgical management is needed.
3. Ask the patient to eat regularly and to avoid irritating foods.

21. ABDOMINAL PAIN

Abdominal pain is a frequently encountered symptom in the clinic, often accompanying many disorders of the zangfu organs, of which dysentery, epigastric pain, hernia, appendicitis and gynaecological diseases will be discussed separately. In this section only accumulation of cold in the interior, deficiency of spleen yang and retention of food are discussed.

AETIOLOGY AND PATHOGENESIS

Accumulation of cold in the interior is often due to over-eating of raw and cold food which injures the yang of the spleen and stomach.

It may be due to invasion of the body (the abdomen via the umbilicus) by pathogenic cold.

It may also be due to constitutional yang deficiency and spleen yang deficiency impairing the transportation by the spleen and stomach.

Alternatively it may be due to irregular food intake or over-indulgence in greasy and spicy food which gives rise to impaired decomposition and transportation, and failure to divide the clear and turbid, which leads to blockage of the passage of the qi.

All the above can result in abdominal pain, either acute or chronic.

DIFFERENTIATION

Accumulation of cold in the interior leads to a sudden onset of violent abdominal pain which responds to warmth and gets worse through cold, loose stools, cold limbs, a pale tongue with a white and moist coating, and a deep and tight pulse.

Deficiency of spleen yang may give rise to an intermittent dull pain which can be alleviated by pressure, loose stools, listlessness and aversion to cold, a thin and white tongue coating, and a deep and thready pulse.

Retention of food is marked by epigastric and abdominal distension and fullness and pain which is aggravated by pressure, anorexia, foul or sour regurgitation, or abdominal pain which is alleviated by passing loose stools, a greasy tongue coating, and a slippery pulse.

TREATMENT

Needling and moxibustion

a) Accumulation of cold

Method.   Points are selected mainly from the

foot Taiyin and Yangming meridians. Use a reducing method of needling, in combination with moxibustion over a layer of salt on point Shenque (Ren 8).

Prescription. Zhongwan (Ren 12), Shenque (Ren 8), Guanyuan (Ren 4), Zusanli (St 36), Gongsun (Sp 4).

Explanation. Zhongwan is used to bring the clear above and send the turbid below. It warms and regulates the stomach qi, and in combination with Zusanli and Gongsun strengthens the transportation function of the spleen and stomach.

Moxibustion applied onto Shenque and Guanyuan warms the lower-jiao and dispels stagnant cold.

b) Deficiency of spleen yang

Method. Mainly the Back-Shu point and points from the Ren meridian are selected. Use a reinforcing method of needling with moxibustion.

Prescription. Pishu (UB 20), Weishu (UB 21), Zhongwan (Ren 12), Qihai (Ren 6), Zhangmen (Liv 13), Zusanli (St 36).

Explanation. Pishu, Weishu and the Influential point of the fu organs, Zhongwan, are used together to invigorate the yang of the spleen and stomach. In combination with Qihai and Zusanli, they promote digestion and transportation.

c) Retention of food

Method. Points are selected mainly from the Ren and foot Yangming meridians. Use a reducing method of needling with moxibustion.

Prescription. Zhongwan (Ren 12), Tianshu (UB 25), Qihai (Ren 6), Zusanli (St 36) and Lineiting (Extra 44).

Explanation. Zhongwan, Zusanli, Tianshu and Qihai are used to regulate the function of the stomach and intestines. Lineiting is an empirical point for the treatment of food stagnancy.

If these points are used together, the normal function of digestion and transportation is restored.

Cupping

Method. Large cups are applied onto points on the abdomen and back as selected in the above prescription, 3–4 points each time. 1–2 treatments are given every day. This method is indicated for abdominal pain due to accumulated cold in the abdomen and retention of food.

Ear needling

Points. Large intestine, tip of inferior antihelix crus, Small intestine, Liver, Brain, Spleen.

Method. 2–3 points are used each time, with a strong stimulation by rotating the needles; needles are retained for 20–30 minutes. This method is indicated for abdominal pain due to acute or chronic enteritis.

REMARK

Needling and moxibustion have a good therapeutic effect in treating abdominal pain. During the treatment of acute abdominal pain with acupuncture and moxibustion, strict observation of condition of the disease is required, or else it can be transferred for surgery.

22. JAUNDICE

Jaundice is mainly manifested by a yellow discoloration of the sclera, skin and urine. Its aetiology varies in exogenous and endogenous affections but the pathological changes of the zangfu generally occur in the liver, gallbladder, spleen and stomach. It may be classified as either yin jaundice or yang jaundice.

This disease includes hepatogenic jaundice, obstructive jaundice and haemolytic jaundice.

AETIOLOGY AND PATHOGENESIS

Jaundice is mainly caused by pathogenic damp, such as exogenous pathogenic damp, heat and pestilential factors which invade and accumulate in the spleen and stomach. The liver and gallbladder are heated from the heat in the spleen and stomach, leading to an overflow of bile into the skin surface, thus resulting in "yang jaundice".

Alternatively, an irregular diet and over-strain give rise to deficiency of the spleen and stomach, and impaired functioning of the yang of the middle-jiao, which further leads to internal formation of dampness obstructing the normal passage of bile. Therefore the bile overflows to the surface of skin, and "yin jaundice" appears.

DIFFERENTIATION

Yang jaundice. A lustrous yellow skin and sclera, fever, thirst, scanty and yellow urine, abdominal distension, constipation, stuffiness in the chest, nausea, a yellow and greasy tongue coating, a slippery and rapid pulse.

Yin jaundice. A dim yellow skin and sclera, spiritlessness, lassitude, poor appetite, loose stools, aversion to cold, epigastric fullness and abdominal distension, a pale tongue with greasy coating, a deep and slow pulse.

TREATMENT

Needling and moxibustion

a) Yang jaundice

Method. To promote the free-flowing of the liver and gallbladder qi, to clear heat and resolve damp. Use a reducing method of needling.

Prescription. Danshu (UB 19), Yanglingquan (GB 34), Yinlingquan (Sp 9), Neiting (St 44), Taichong (Liv 3).

Modification.
— Stuffiness in the chest and nausea: Neiguan (P 6), Gongsun (Sp 4).
— Abdominal distension and constipation: Dachangshu (UB 25), Tianshu (St 25).

Explanation. Danshu and Yanglingquan are used to clear heat from the gallbladder. Taichong is used in combination to regulate qi of the liver meridian.

Yinlingquan is the He-sea point of the foot Taiyin meridian, and Neiting is the Ying-spring point of the foot Yangming. They are used together to promote diuresis, and clear the damp-heat from the spleen and stomach.

Neiguan and Gongsun are Confluent points used to harmonize the stomach and check the abnormal upward rebellion of qi. Dachangshu and Tianshu are used as a combination of Back-Shu and Front-Mu points; they are reduced with needling to bring down the qi and remove obstruction from the fu organs so as to relieve abdominal distension and constipation.

b) Yin jaundice

Method. To strengthen the spleen, ease the gallbladder, warm the cold and resolve damp. Use an even movement method of needling in combination with moxibustion.

Prescription. Zhiyang (Du 9), Pishu (UB 20), Danshu (UB 19), Zhongwan (Ren 12), Zusanli (St 36), Sanyinjiao (Sp 6).

Modification.
— Listlessness and aversion to cold: Mingmen (Du 4), Qihai (Ren 6).
— Loose stools: Tianshu (St 25), Guanyuan (Ren 4).

Explanation. Yin jaundice is due mainly to cold-damp, so the principle of treatment is to strengthen the spleen in its transporting function and give warmth.

Zhiyang is a site where the qi of the Du meridian is infused; needling and moxibustion at this point can warm and promote the yang qi. It is an important point for jaundice.

Zhongwan is the Influential point of the fu organs, and is used in combination with Zusanli and Pishu, with reinforcing needling, to strengthen the spleen and stomach and resolve damp.

Danshu is used to ease the gallbladder, and Sanyinjiao to induce the damp downward. They are used together to treat jaundice. Mingmen and Qihai are tonic points—with moxibustion they warm and strengthen the kidney yang.

Tianshu and Guanyuan are the Front-Mu points of the large and small intestines respectively, and with moxibustion they are used to treat diarrhoea due to deficiency and cold.

Point-injection therapy

Points. Ganshu (UB 18), Pishu (UB 20), Zhongdu (GB 32).

Method. Injection of Banlangen (Isatis root), Tianjihuang (*Hypericum japonicum*), Danshen (Salvia) or Vitamin B1, B12 solution is applied into 2–4 points at a time, 0.5–1 ml into each point. Apply once every other day; 10 treatments constitute one course.

REMARKS

1. Needling and moxibustion have a good therapeutic effect in treating acute icteric hepatitis, and strict sterilization and isolation should be performed during the acute stage.
2. As for jaundice due to other causes, synthesized treatment combining Chinese herbal and Western medical therapies should be given, while acupuncture and moxibustion can be applied in cooperation.

23. DIARRHOEA

Diarrhoea refers to abnormally frequent and liquid or watery faecal discharge. It can be seen in various diseases, but the internal organs involved are mainly the spleen, stomach, large and small intestine. It is clinically classified into the acute and chronic types since in ancient times it had many names and classifications.

This syndrome refers to acute and chronic enteritis, indigestion, allergic colitis and intestinal tuberculosis.

AETIOLOGY AND PATHOGENESIS

Acute diarrhoea. Due to raw and cold, or unclean food intake, or also being affected by pathogenic cold, damp or summer-heat, which accumulate in the intestines and stomach blocking the passage of the qi and impairing the transporting function of the spleen and stomach and intestines, which further gives rise to failure in dividing the clear and turbid, thus resulting in diarrhoea.

Chronic diarrhoea. Due to constitutional deficiency of the spleen and stomach. It may be due to qi deficiency after a long-term illness which impairs the transporting function of the middle-jiao, the digestive functions. Alternatively, it is due to deficiency of kidney yang, known as the fire of "the gate of life", and failure in the decomposition of food, which leads to diarrhoea.

DIFFERENTIATION

Acute diarrhoea. Acute onset, increased frequency and volume of faecal discharges.

If due mainly to cold-damp, there may be dilute diarrhoea with undigested food in it, borborygmus, abdominal pain, absence of thirst, aversion to cold and a preference for warmth, a slow pulse, and a pale tongue with a white and slippery coating.

If mainly due to damp-heat, there may be hot, yellow and foul diarrhoea, abdominal pain, burning sensation at the anus, scanty and dark yellow urine, a soft and rapid pulse, and a yellow and greasy tongue coating, and it may be accompanied by general feverishness and thirst.

Chronic diarrhoea. Chronic onset, or turning from acute to chronic, with less frequent diarrhoea.

If due to spleen deficiency, there may be sallowish complexion, listlessness and weak limbs, poor appetite, and a thin and white tongue coating.

If due to kidney deficiency, there will be slight abdominal pain at dawn with diarrhoea ensuing, or borborygmus without abdominal pain, diarrhoea once or several times every morning, aversion to cold at the abdomen and lower limbs, a deep thready pulse, and a pale tongue with white coating.

TREATMENT

Needling and moxibustion

a) Acute diarrhoea

Method. Mainly to regulate the qi passage of the intestine and stomach. If due to cold, retention of needles and moxa sticks or moxibustion over a layer of ginger can be applied. If due to heat, needling with a reducing method is applied.

Prescription. Zhongwan (Ren 12), Tianshu (St 25), Shangjuxu (St 37), Yinlingquan (Sp 9).

Explanation. Zhongwan is the Front-Mu point of the stomach and Tianshu that of the large intestine, where the qi of zangfu organs is infused, so these two points are used to regulate the transporting function of the stomach and intestines.

The lower He-Sea point of the hand Yangming meridian, Shangjuxu, is used to regulate the qi passage of the stomach and intestines.

The spleen and stomach are externally-internally related, so Yinlingquan is used to regulate the qi of the spleen meridian. This restores the transporting function of the spleen qi: water and essence are distributed, diuresis promoted, stagnant damp resolved and solid stools again formed.

b) Chronic diarrhoea

Method. Mainly to strengthen the spleen and stomach and warm the kidney yang. Use also a reinforcing method of needling and moxibustion.

Prescription. Pishu (UB 20), Zhangmen (Liv 13), Zhongwan (Ren 12), Tianshu (St 25), Zusanli (St 36).

Modification. Diarrhoea due to kidney deficiency: Mingmen (Du 4), Guanyuan (Ren 4).

Explanation. Pishu and Zhangmen are a combination of the Back-Shu and Front-Mu points of the spleen meridian which are used to strengthen the spleen and replenish qi.

The reinforcing method of needling and moxibustion is applied to the Front-Mu point of the large intestine, Tianshu. The Front-Mu of the stomach, Zhongwan, and He-sea point of the stomach meridian, Zusanli, are used with a reinforcing method of needling and moxibustion to invigorate the spleen yang and promote transportation and transformation.

Moxibustion applied to Mingmen and Guanyuan tonifies the fire of the "gate of life" and strengthens the kidney yang, so as to warm and nourish the spleen and kidney and promote their decomposing function. This is to treat the root cause.

Cupping

Points. Tianshu (St 25), Guanyuan (Ren 4), Zusanli (St 36), Shangjuxu (St 37), Xiajuxu (St 39), Dachangshu (UB 25), Xiaochangshu (UB 27).

Method. Cupping is applied onto the selected points with cups of differing sizes according to the location of points. This method is indicated for chronic diarrhoea due to deficiency and cold.

Ear needling

Points. Large intestine, Small intestine, tip of inferior antihelix crus, Lung, Spleen.

Method. 2–3 points are used each time, with a moderate or strong stimulation by needle rotation, with 20–30 minutes needle retention. This method is indicated for diarrhoea seen in enteritis.

REMARKS

1. During the treatment of acute diarrhoea, control of the diet is required.
2. If dehydration due to frequent diarrhoea occurs, fluid transfusion is needed.
3. Avoid an improper or unclean diet.

24. DYSENTERY

Dysentery is a commonly seen infectious disease of the intestinal tract; it often occurs in summer and autumn and is marked by its main symptoms of abdominal pain, tenesmus, and frequent stools containing blood and mucus. In ancient medical literature, the strongly infectious and severe type of dysentery was known as "seasonal pestilential dysentery".

In the clinic, common patterns are damp-heat dysentery, cold-damp dysentery, food-retained dysentery and intermittent dysentery.

AETIOLOGY AND PATHOGENESIS

Dysentery is due to exogenous affection either by summer-heat and damp, or pestilential factors, or unclean food intake, or over-eating of raw and cold food. The exogenous pathogens or food stagnate and block the intestines, impairing the transportation by the large intestine.

Damp and heat cause the qi and blood to stagnate and the zangfu and collaterals are injured, thus giving rise to dysentery with pus and blood. If heat is more predominant than damp, there will be more red mucus than white; if damp is more predominant than heat, there will be more white mucus than red.

Dysentery may also be due to a constitutional deficiency of the spleen and stomach, and weakness of the qi of the zangfu organs, and then being affected by exogenous cold, *feng* or summer damp, in which the stagnant cold and damp leads to dysentery.

Otherwise it is due to accumulation of damp-heat in the middle-jiao and turbid obstruction within the intestines in which the ascending and descending function of the spleen and stomach is impaired, leading to food-retained dysentery.

Alternatively it is due to protracted dysentery with a deficiency of qi within the middle-jiao, and lingering pathogens, recurrence often being evoked by the cold or an improper diet, leading to intermittent dysentery.

DIFFERENTIATION

In damp-heat dysentery there may be abdominal pain, with red and white mucus in stools and tenesmus, accompanied by a burning sensation in the anus, scanty dark yellow urine, a slippery and rapid pulse, a yellow and greasy tongue coating, or chilliness and fever, irritability and thirst.

In cold-damp dysentery there may be white mucus in the stools, a preference for warmth and aversion to cold, stuffiness in the chest, absence of thirst, a white and greasy tongue coating, a soft and retarded or slow pulse.

In the case of food-retained dysentery, it is marked by red or white mucus in the stools, total loss of appetite, nausea and vomiting.

In the case of intermittent dysentery, there are protracted and repeated attacks with intervals between, spiritlessness, with abdominal pain and tenesmus before passing stools, a pale tongue with a greasy coating, and a soft and thready, or empty (deficiency) and large pulse.

TREATMENT

Needling and moxibustion

Method. Points are selected mainly from the foot Yangming meridian. Use a reducing method of needling; moxibustion can be added in cold cases. In cases of protracted dysentery, the spleen and stomach should also be treated.

Prescription. Hegu (LI 4), Tianshu (St 25), Shangjuxu (St 37).

Modification.
— Damp-heat dysentery: Quchi (LI 11), Neiting (St 44).
— Cold-damp dysentery: Zhongwan (Ren 12), Qihai (Ren 6).
— Food-retained dysentery: Zhongwan (Ren 12), Neiguan (P 6), Neiting (St 44).
— Intermittent dysentery: Pishu (UB 20), Weishu (UB 21), Guanyuan (Ren 4), Shenshu (UB 23).

Explanation. The *yuan* point of the Yangming meridian, Hegu, the Front-Mu point of the large intestine, Tianshu, and the lower He-Sea point, Shangjuxu, are used to regulate the qi of the Large Intestine meridian and resolve damp.

Quchi and Neiting are the He-sea point of Large Intestine meridian and Ying-spring point of the stomach meridian respectively, and they are used to clear damp-heat from the intestines and stomach.

Zhongwan harmonizes the stomach qi so as to resolve damp and bring down turbidity.

Qihai activates and regulates qi circulation, and it is used with moxibustion to give warmth and dispel cold.

Neiguan connects with the hand Jueyin meridian and it is used to check the qi rebellion in the Sanjiao. Pishu and Weishu regulate and nourish the qi of the middle-jiao, and promote the manufacture of qi and blood.

Guanyuan and Shenshu, with a reinforcing method of needling or moxibustion, are used to tonify the vital yang of the kidney so as to remove the stagnation.

In cases of anal prolapse due to chronic dysentery, moxibustion can be applied to Baihui (Du 20). With tenesmus and frequent loose stools, needling at Zhonglushu (UB 29) can be added.

Point-injection therapy

Method. A 50 mg injection of 25% glucose solution or Vitamin B1 is applied bilaterally into Tianshu (St 25), 1 ml into each point, once a day.

REMARKS

1. Needling and moxibustion have a good effect in treating dysentery. But for toxic bacillary dysentery, which is a critical condition, emergency treatment in a synthesized way should be given.
2. Dietary control and environmental isolation are necessary; avoid unclean food.

25. BERIBERI

Beriberi is marked by numbness, soreness, aching and weakness of the foot and calf. According to its clinical manifestations, it is divided into dry beriberi, wet beriberi and beriberi affecting the heart. Detailed descriptions concerning this disease were found in the ancient medical classic *General Treatise on the Causes and Symptoms of Diseases*.

This disease refers mainly to beriberi caused by the lack of vitamin B1 in the diet, and also to diseases such as malnutrition and multiple neuritis with similar symptoms.

AETIOLOGY AND PATHOGENESIS

This disease is due to affection of the lower limbs by water (fluid), cold and damp-heat which overflow into the skin, muscles and tendons.

It may also be due to irregular diet injuring the spleen and stomach in which damp-heat flows to the foot and calf.

Otherwise it is due to constitutional weakness after disease, giving rise to deficiency of qi and blood and undernourishment of the jingluo, the muscles and tendons.

Alternatively it is due to upward affection by damp-toxins which disturb the heart and mind leading to palpitations and irritability; or else they invade the lung and stomach along the course of the meridians leading to asthmatic breathing, fullness in the chest and nausea.

DIFFERENTIATION

Initially only forcelessness in the feet is felt, then soreness, heaviness, numbness and flaccidity are gradually observed, and later weakness and muscular atrophy or oedema of the lower limbs ensues.

Wet beriberi manifests as an excess type, with symptoms such as swelling of the foot and calf, a soft and retarded pulse, and a white and greasy tongue coating.

Dry beriberi is mainly a deficiency syndrome marked by muscular atrophy of the foot and calf worsening gradually, worsening sensations of cold, numbness, soreness and heaviness in the lower limbs, listlessness, accompanied by constipation, yellow urine, a slightly red tongue with yellow coating, and a wiry or wiry-rapid pulse.

If there is asthmatic breathing, fullness in the chest, palpitations and irritability, cloudiness of mind or unconsciousness, it is "beriberi affecting the heart" which is a critical case.

TREATMENT

Needling and moxibustion

Method. Points are selected mainly from the foot Shaoyang, Yangming and Taiyin meridians A reducing method of needling is used for excess cases while reinforcing is used for deficiency cases.

Prescription. Yanglingquan (GB 34), Zusanli (St 36), Xuanzhong (GB 39).

Modification.
— Beriberi affecting the heart: Juque (Ren 14), Neiguan (P 6), Ximen (P 4).
— Deficiency of spleen and stomach: Pishu (UB 20), Weishu (UB 21).
— Swelling and numbness of foot: Bafeng (Extra 42), Taibai (Sp 3).

Explanation. In case of damp, the lower part of the body is first affected, so Zusanli and Sanyinjiao are used to eliminate damp from Yangming and Taiyin meridians.

The Influential point of marrow, Xuanzhong, and of the tendons, Yanglingquan, are used to nourish the bones and tendons to facilitate walking.

In cases of beriberi affecting the heart, the Front-Mu point of the heart, Juque, and Neiguan and Ximen from the pericardium meridian are used to relieve palpitations, irritability and fullness in the chest.

The reinforcing method of needling applied to Pishu and Weishu strengthens the transporting of the spleen and stomach, and resolves damp.

Bafeng and Taibai are effective points for the treatment of beriberi. Used with a reducing method they can clear the damp-heat and relieve oedema in the feet.

Electroneedling

Points. Fengshi (GB 31), Zusanli (St 36), Femur-Futu (St 32), Xuanzhong (GB 39).

Method. Electricity is applied for 10–15 minutes, with the sparse wave or dense-sparse wave and an intensity of stimulation and frequency within the tolerance of the patient. Two pairs of points are used each time, and treatment is given once a day or every other day.

Point-injection therapy

Points. Quchi (LI 11), Waiguan (SJ 5), Yinlingquan (Sp 9), Zusanli (St 36), Xuanzhong (GB 39).

Method. Vitamin B1 (100 mg) or Vitamin B12 (100 micrograms) are used, 2–4 points each time, 0.5–1 ml being injected into each point. Treatment is given once every other day; 10 treatments constitute one course.

REMARKS

1. In treating this disease, acupuncture and moxibustion can be used in combination with herbal and massage therapies, to potentiate the therapeutic effect.
2. Beriberi "affecting the heart" has an acute onset and rapid development, and treatment by both TCM and Western medicine combined should be applied.

3. It is advisable to eat more red beans, Coix seeds, peanuts and red dates (jujube) to regulate the spleen and stomach.

26. CONSTIPATION

Constipation refers to the condition in which the faeces are hard and elimination from the bowels is difficult and infrequent (every two days or more). This disease can be divided into two types: constipation due to deficiency and that due to excess.

AETIOLOGY AND PATHOGENESIS

Excess syndrome. Mainly due to constitutional yang hyperactivity, or else indulgence in alcohol and spicy greasy food which leads to accumulation of heat in the stomach and intestines.

Or it is due to excessive endogenous pathogenic heat consuming the body fluid, giving rise to dryness of the intestines and obstruction of qi in the fu organs.

Alternatively it is due to emotional disturbance which leads to stagnation in the passage of the qi, and failure of the body fluid to distribute, and impaired transportation by the intestines resulting in constipation.

Deficiency syndrome. Mostly due to deficiency of qi and blood after disease or childbirth.

Or it is due to deficiency of qi and blood in aged or asthenic patients in whom transporting is impaired by qi deficiency and the intestines are deprived of moisture owing to a deficiency of blood.

Alternatively it is due to insufficient yang qi in the lower-jiao which causes the yin and cold to stagnate and obstruct the qi in the intestines and fu organs, giving rise to constipation.

DIFFERENTIATION

Due to excess. The main manifestations are infrequent and difficult defaecation, perhaps every three to five days or even longer.

If due to accumulation of heat, there is general

feverishness, excessive thirst, foul breath, a preference for a cold diet, a slippery pulse of the excess type, and a yellow and dry tongue coating.

If due to stagnation of qi, it is marked by fullness and a distending pain in the flank and abdomen, frequent belching, loss of appetite, a wiry pulse and a thin greasy tongue coating.

Due to deficiency. If due to deficiency of qi and blood, it is marked by a pale and lustreless complexion, lips and nails, dizziness, palpitations, listlessness and lassitude, a pale tongue with thin coating, and a thready pulse of the deficiency type.

If due to stagnation of yin cold, it is marked by abdominal cold pain, a preference for warmth and aversion to cold, a deep and slow pulse, and a pale tongue with a white and moist coating.

TREATMENT

Needling and moxibustion

Method. Points are selected mainly from the Back-Shu, Front-Mu and lower He-Sea points of the large intestine meridian. Use a reducing method of needling for excess conditions, or a reinforcing method for deficiency conditions. Moxibustion is added for constipation due to cold.

Prescription. Dachangshu (UB 25), Tianshu (St 25), Zhigou (SJ 6), Shangjuxu (St 37).

Modification.
— Accumulation of heat: Hegu (LI 4), Quchi (LI 11).
— Stagnation of qi: Zhongwan (Ren 12), Xingjian (Liv 2).
— Deficiency of qi and blood: Pishu (UB 20), Weishu (UB 21).
— Constipation due to cold: moxibustion is applied to Shenque (Ren 8) and Qihai (Ren 6).

Explanation. Impaired transportation by the large intestine is the common cause of constipation of different types, so its Front-Mu point Tianshu, and Back-Shu point Dachangshu, and its lower He-Sea point Shangjuxu are used to regulate the qi of the fu organs and restore the transportation function of the large intestine.

Zhigou is used to regulate the qi in the Sanjiao and the qi of the fu organs.

Quchi and Hegu are used to reduce and clear the qi and heat in the fu organs. The Influential point of the fu, Zhongwan, is used to regulate and bring down their qi.

Xingjian is used to regulate liver qi and relieve its depression.

Tonifying Pishu and Weishu strengthens the qi of the middle-jiao so as to promote the manufacture of qi and blood. This is the basic treatment for constipation due to deficiency.

Moxibustion applied to Shenque and Qihai warms and regulates the yang qi of the lower-jiao so as to eliminate the stagnation of yin cold.

Electroneedling

Points. A: Daheng (Sp 15), Xiajuxu (St 39). B: Shimen (Ren 5), Zhigou (SJ 6).

Method. Electricity is applied for 10–20 minutes with a dense-sparse wave. Treatment is given every other day, and the two groups of points can be used alternately.

Ear needling

Points. Lower region of rectum, Large intestine, Brain.

Method. Apply stimulation of moderate or strong intensity, with 20–30 minutes retention of needle.

REMARKS

1. Needling and moxibustion have a good effect in treating this disease. If many treatments have been given but without effect, it is necessary to find out the real causative factor.
2. Give the patients advice to encourage regular physical exercise and more vegetables in the diet, and cultivate the habit of regular defaecation.

27. PROLAPSE OF THE RECTUM

A prolapse of the rectum or anus is likely to happen to the elderly, infants or women who have had many children.

AETIOLOGY AND PATHOGENESIS

This disease is often due to prolonged diarrhoea or dysentery, or else it occurs in women after having many children; alternatively it occurs after protracted coughing or constipation which gives rise to a deficiency of the lower-jiao and prolapse of the qi of the middle-jiao. This leads to failure in the qi to uplift and contract the rectum.

DIFFERENTIATION

It has a slow onset, with initially only a pulling down and distending sensation at the anus, and occasional prolapses of the anus which can be restored spontaneously.

If treatment is delayed it becomes chronic and usually is evoked by slight fatigue, when the prolapse can be corrected only with the help of the hand. It may be accompanied by spiritlessness and lassitude, sallowish complexion, vertigo and palpitations, a soft and thready pulse, and a pale tongue with a white coating.

TREATMENT

Needling and moxibustion

Method. Points are selected mainly from the Du meridian. Use a reinforcing method of needling. Moxibustion is applicable.

Prescription. Baihui (Du 20), Changqiang (Du 1), Dachangshu (UB 25).

Explanation. Reinforcing Dachangshu strengthens the qi of the large intestine and the fu organs.

Baihui is the crossing point of the Du meridian and the three yang meridians. Moxibustion on Baihui can promote yang qi and its action of uplifting and contracting the prolapsed organ.

Changqiang, from the Du meridian and near the anus, is punctured to strengthen the controlling function of the anus.

These three points used together uplift the prolapsed organ; Qihai (Ren 6), Zusanli (St 36) and Pishu (UB 20) are selected according to the differentiation of syndromes.

Needle pricking and picking

Method. Apply the "needle pricking and picking" method, using a three-edged needle to break some fibrous tissue on any of the points along a vertical line 1.5 cun lateral to, and parallel with the midline of the spinal column, between the 3rd lumbar and 2nd sacral vertebrae.

Cutaneous needling

Points. Dachangshu (UB 25), Tianshu (St 25), Baihui (Du 20), Kongzui (Lu 6), Zhongliao (UB 33), Changqiang (Du 1), Zhongwan (Ren 12), Liangqiu (St 34), Jizhong (Du 6), Huatuojiaji (T9–L5, Extra 19).

The following points can also be used: Guanyuan (Ren 4), Qihai (Ren 6), Chengshan (UB 57), Huiyin (Ren 1), Hegu (LI 4), and Chengfu (UB 36).

REMARK

Needling and moxibustion have a good effect in treating a prolapse of the anus. In cases with a constitutional deficiency herbal medicine taken orally should be used in combination.

28. RETENTION OF URINE

Retention of urine is a disease manifest mainly by difficult urination or even blockage of the urine. The mild case has difficulty in urination and dripping of urine, while the severe case refers to failure of urination.

It may involve organic and functional pathological changes in the bladder and urethra, and difficult urination and urinary retention can be caused by impaired renal function.

AETIOLOGY AND PATHOGENESIS

This disease is due to dysfunction of the qi transformation within the Sanjiao, while the dysfunction is located in the bladder. Accumulated heat in the lung and accumulated damp-heat in the middle-jiao shift to the bladder, impairing the transformation of qi in the bladder and blocking the passage of water.

Otherwise, damage of the kidney qi and decline of the fire of the "gate of life" result in failure of the yang qi to resolve yin fluid, impairing the transformation of qi in the bladder and leading to retention of urine.

Alternatively, following a traumatic injury or surgical operation, the passage of qi in the bladder is impaired, leading to retention of urine.

DIFFERENTIATION

Insufficiency of kidney qi is marked by dribbling urination, pallor, listlessness, lumbar and knee-joint soreness and weakness, a pale tongue, and a deep and thready pulse which is especially weak in the most proximal position.

In the case of accumulated heat pouring down to the bladder, there is scanty hot urine, dark yellow in colour, or retention of urine, distension in the lower abdomen, thirst, a red tongue with a yellow coating, and a rapid pulse.

If there is traumatic injury, there is difficult or dribbling urination and distension and fullness in the lower abdomen, with a past history of traumatic injury or surgical operation.

TREATMENT

Needling and moxibustion

a) *Insufficiency of kidney qi*

Method. Points are selected mainly from the foot Shaoyin meridian, in combination with the Back-Shu point of the bladder meridian. Use a reinforcing method of needling, or else moxibustion.

Prescription. Yingu (K 10), Shenshu (UB 23), Sanjiaoshu (UB 22), Qihai (Ren 6), Weiyang (UB 39).

Explanation. The principle of treatment for insufficiency of kidney qi and decline of the fire of "the gate of life" is mainly to replenish the kidney qi. Therefore the He-sea point of the kidney meridian, Yingu, is used in combination with the Back-Shu of the kidney, Shenshu. Use a

reinforcing method, to invigorate the qi passage along the kidney meridian.

Sanjiaoshu and the lower He-Sea point of the Sanjiao meridian, Weiyang, are used to regulate the qi passage of the Sanjiao, on the basis of replenishing the kidney qi.

Moxibustion applied to Qihai on the Ren meridian warms and tonifies the lower-jiao, so as to replenish the kidney qi, regulate the Sanjiao and relieve the retention of urine.

b) *Damp-heat pouring down to the bladder*

Method. Select points mainly from the foot Taiyin meridian. Use a reducing method of needling. Moxibustion is not applied.

Prescription. Sanyinjiao (Sp 6), Yinlingquan (Sp 9), Pangguangshu (UB 28), Zhongji (Ren 3).

Explanation. Sanyinjiao and Yinlingquan are used to clear damp-heat from the Spleen meridian. At the same time, Pangguangshu and Zhongji are used according to the combination of Back-Shu and Front-Mu points, to regulate the qi of the Sanjiao and eliminate damp-heat.

c) *Traumatic injuries*

Method. Mainly to regulate the qi passage of the bladder. Use needling, or moxibustion, applied according to the concrete condition of the disease.

Prescription. Zhongji (Ren 3), Sanyinjiao (Sp 6), Xuehai (Sp 10).

Explanation. The retention of urine is due to a traumatic injury or surgical operation impairing the qi passage of the bladder. Therefore the Front-Mu point of the bladder meridian, Zhongji, in combination with the crossing point of the three yin meridians of foot, Sanyinjiao, is used to regulate the qi passage of the Sanjiao to ease urination.

In cases of traumatic injury leading to stagnant blood blocking the collaterals, a reducing method of needling is applied to Xuehai. This resolves the stagnant blood and removes the obstruction to ease urination.

Electroneedling

Puncture point Weidao (GB 28, bilaterally) in a

direction towards Qugu (Ren 2). About 2–3 cun into the point apply an intermittent wave and increase the intensity of electric stimulation gradually. Apply electricity for 15–30 minutes.

REMARKS

1. When the bladder is full, points on the lower abdomen should be punctured superficially, or obliquely or transversely. Deep perpendicular puncture is contraindicated.
2. If the retention is due to mechanical obstruction or to nerve injury it is necessary to ascertain the cause and manage accordingly.

29. OEDEMA

Oedema refers to subcutaneous retention of fluid which leads to puffiness of the head, face, eyelids, limbs, abdomen, back or even the whole body. According to the differentiation of deficiency and excess conditions of the disease, oedema is divided into two patterns: yin oedema and yang oedema.

Oedema is often seen in acute and chronic nephritis, congestive heart failure, hepato-cirrhosis and dystrophy.

AETIOLOGY AND PATHOGENESIS

Since the circulation of fluid within the body is related to regulation by the lung, transportation by the spleen, vaporizing by the kidney, drainage by the Sanjiao and transformation by the bladder, the derangement or impairment of the normal functions of either the lung, spleen, kidney, Sanjiao or bladder may lead to accumulated fluid in the body. This then overflows into the body surface leading to oedema.

Exogenous affection by pathogenic *feng* may impair the function of the lung qi in dispersing and in regulating the passage of water leading to an overflow of water and damp, which is termed "yang oedema".

Alternatively, over-strain injures the spleen and kidney so that yang deficiency of the spleen

and kidney fails to vaporize the water and fluid, leading to "yin oedema". Protracted oedema may also lead to oedema of the yin type.

DIFFERENTIATION

Yang oedema. Acute onset with a slightly puffy face and eyelids and then anasarca, lustrous skin, extremely enlarged scrotum, stuffiness and distress in the chest, even asthmatic breathing, scanty and yellow urine, a superficial and slippery or slippery-rapid pulse, and a white and slippery or greasy tongue coating.

Yin oedema. Insidious onset with mild oedema in the feet at first, and then oedema in the calf, abdomen and face gradually, with sallowish complexion, dilute, scanty or difficult urination, loose stools, a preference for warmth and aversion to cold, a deep thready or slow pulse, and a pale tongue with white coating.

TREATMENT

Method. Mainly to regulate the passage of qi within the Sanjiao. Also to regulate the functions of the lung and bladder in yang oedema, with a reducing method of needling (moxibustion is generally not applied). Otherwise, to regulate the function of the spleen and kidney in yin oedema, with a reinforcing method of needling and, often, moxibustion.

Prescription. Shuifen (Ren 9), Qihai (Ren 6), Sanjiaoshu (UB 22), Zusanli (St 36).

Modification.
— Yang oedema: Feishu (UB 13), Hegu (LI 4), Renzhong (Du 26).
— Yin oedema: Pishu (UB 20), Shenshu (UB 23), Yinlingquan (Sp 9).

Explanation. This prescription aims mainly at regulating and strengthening the qi in its transformation or vaporization of fluid.

Sanjiaoshu is used to regulate the qi-transforming function of the Sanjiao. Qihai is used in combination to promote the qi-transforming function of the Sanjiao.

Shuifen from the Ren meridian, near the small

intestine, has the function of separating the clear and turbid, and is an effective point for disorders of water metabolism.

Zusanli is the He-sea point of the stomach meridian and is externally-internally related to the spleen meridian. It is used to invigorate the function of the spleen and stomach so as to relieve oedema.

Yang oedema is due to impaired dispersion of the lung qi and distribution of body fluid. Feishu is used to promote the dispersion of the lung qi and the qi of the foot Taiyang meridian. Hegu from the large intestine meridian, which is externally-internally related to the lung meridian, is used to regulate the water circulation and ease the water's transportation to the bladder.

Renzhong is the crossing point of the hand Yangming and the Du meridians, and is used as an empirical point for puffiness in the face.

Yin oedema is due to deficiency of kidney yang, failure of water and fluids to vaporize, deficiency of spleen qi and impaired transporting of the yang qi of the middle-jiao. Therefore moxibustion is applied to Shenshu and Pishu, with a reinforcing method of needling applied to Yinlingquan, to warm and strengthen the kidney yang and the transporting function of the spleen. This warms the yang and eases diuresis.

REMARKS

1. Needling and moxibustion have a certain effect in relieving oedema. The causative factor should be ascertained beforehand and a definite diagnosis made. If necessary, herbal drugs can be applied in combination with symptomatic treatment.
2. Ask the patient to rest in bed, keep warm and avoid being affected by the cold. A salty diet should be avoided (a low-salt diet can be taken after the oedema is relieved), and less water drunk.

30. SEMINAL EMISSION

Seminal emission can be divided into two types: nocturnal emission and spermatorrhoea. Gener-ally, in unmarried males, an occasional emission is a normal physiological phenomenon and not considered pathological.

AETIOLOGY AND PATHOGENESIS

This disease is mostly due to disorders of the heart and kidney, such as excessive thinking and wanton desire, or vain attempts at love affairs in which the heart-yin is consumed, heart-fire becomes excessive and the "palace of essence" (kidney qi) is stirred up.

Otherwise it is due to over-indulgence in sexual activity by which the kidney qi is damaged and the "palace of essence" no longer solid.

Alternatively it is due to indulgence in alcohol and spicy food, giving rise to downward pouring of damp-heat.

Sometimes it is seen in patients with phimosis.

DIFFERENTIATION

Nocturnal emission with long-term and frequent emissions may manifest as dizziness, vertigo, spiritlessness, tinnitus and lumbar soreness.

Spermatorrhoea shows as frequent involuntary emission without orgasm, emaciation, a thready and weak pulse, perhaps even palpitations and impotence.

TREATMENT

Needling and moxibustion

Method. The treatment for nocturnal emission is mainly to restore harmony between the heart and kidney with an even method of needling. The treatment for spermatorrhoea is mainly to tonify the kidney, with a reinforcing method of needling, or using both needling and moxibustion.

Prescription. Guanyuan (Ren 4), Dahe (K 12), Zhishi (UB 52).

Modification.
— Nocturnal emission: Xinshu (UB 15), Shenmen (H 7), Neiguan (P 6).

— Spermatorrhoea: Shenshu (UB 23), Taixi (K 3), Zusanli (St 36).

Explanation. Guanyuan is the crossing point of the three yin meridians of the foot and the Ren meridian. It is the root of the vital qi in the human body, and is used to invigorate kidney qi. In combination with Zhishi and Dahe it consolidates the storage of essence.

In nocturnal emission, Xinshu, Shenmen and Neiguan are used in combination to subdue heart-fire and restore harmony between the heart and kidney.

In spermatorrhoea, Shenshu and Taixi are added to tonify the kidney, in combination with Zusanli, to promote the manufacture of qi and blood.

Point-injection therapy

Points. Guanyuan (Ren 4), Zhongji (Ren 3).

Method. Vitamin B1 (50 mg) or Danggui (Chinese Angelica) is injected into Guanyuan and Zhongji, 0.5–1 ml into each point. The injection of the herbal or medicinal fluid is applied only after the needling sensation radiates to the external genitalia.

Treatment is given once every other day; 10 treatments constitute one course.

Cutaneous needling

Points. Shenshu (UB 23), Xinshu (UB 15), Zhishi (UB 52), Guanyuan (Ren 4), Sanyinjiao (Sp 6), Neiguan (P 6), Shenmen (H 7), Zhongji (Ren 3), Huiyin (Ren 1) and Huatuojiaji (T11–S5, Extra 19).

Points for alternate use. Taixi (K 3), Jingmen (GB 25), Taichong (Liv 3), Zhongfeng (Liv 4), Dahe (K 12), Qihai (Ren 6).

Method. Tap the above points with cutaneous needles, each time for about 15 minutes. The treatment is given once every day or every other day.

REMARKS

1. Most cases of seminal emission are functional disorders, so psychological explanation and advice should be given along with the treatment.

2. In cases due to organic pathological change, treatment should also be given to the primary disease.

31. IMPOTENCE

Impotence refers to an inability to engage in sexual intercourse because of an inability to have an erection, or an erection that is strong enough. It occurs among men who are not yet at the age of sexual dysfunction.

AETIOLOGY AND PATHOGENESIS

Impotence is generally due to over-indulgence in sex or excessive masturbation, which injures the kidney qi leading to a decline in the fire of the "gate of life", and exhaustion of kidney essence.

Alternatively it is due to fear, fright or worry which injures the kidney, leading to impotence.

DIFFERENTIATION

Impotence is marked by a failure of the penis to erect, or by a weak erection. Often it is accompanied by dizziness or vertigo, blurred vision, listlessness, mental depression, soreness or weakness of the lumbar region and knee joints, a thready and weak pulse, and a slightly red tongue.

TREATMENT

Needling and moxibustion

Method. To tonify and replenish the kidney qi—mainly with a reinforcing method of needling, or else both needling and moxibustion.

Prescription. Shenshu (UB 23), Mingmen (Du 4), Sanyinjiao (Sp 6), Guanyuan (Ren 4).

Explanation. This disease is mainly due to deficiency of the kidney qi. Shenshu, Mingmen and Sanyinjiao are used to nourish the kidney qi and activate the function of the Kidney meridian.

Guanyuan used with a reinforcing method replenishes the vital qi, promotes kidney qi and restores normal sexual ability.

Electroneedling

Points. A: Baliao, (UB 31–34, bilaterally), Rangu (K 2). B: Guanyuan (Ren 4), Sanyinjiao (Sp 6).

Method. The two groups of points are used alternately with a low frequency electrical pulse, which is applied for 3–5 minutes.

Point-injection therapy

Points. Guanyuan (Ren 4), Zhongji (Ren 3), Shenshu (UB 23).

Method. Vitamin B1 (50 mg) or 5 mg of testosterone propionate are injected alternately into the above points, once every 2–3 days; 4 treatments constitute one course.

REMARKS

1. Most cases of this disease are due to some functional disturbance. Psychological explanation and advice should be given to the patient whilst giving treatment.
2. Ask the patient to abstain from sexual intercourse during the treatment.

32. HERNIA

A hernia in TCM refers to the protrusion of any organ in the abdominal cavity through the abdominal muscles, and a swelling or distending pain of the testes or scrotum. Its occurrence is often related to the Ren and Liver meridians. There were different names, categories, and descriptions of this disease in ancient times. Nowadays it is divided into cold hernias, damp-heat hernias and other hernias (scrotal enlargement).

AETIOLOGY AND PATHOGENESIS

Dwelling in wet places, wading in water or exposure to rain, dampness, wind and cold, in which the qi and blood of the Ren and foot Jueyin meridians becomes stagnant, leads to cold hernias. Downward pouring of damp-heat affects the Ren and foot Jueyin meridians, leading to damp-heat hernias. Over-exertion of force, overstrain and overwork cause deficiency and prolapse of qi, leading to other hernias (an enlarged scrotum).

DIFFERENTIATION

This disease is marked by lower abdominal pain affecting the testes, or else by a swelling or distending pain in the testes or scrotum.

Cold hernias manifest as scrotal coldness and pain, a contracting sensation in the testes affecting the lower abdomen, a thin white tongue coating, and a deep and thready pulse.

In damp-heat hernias, you may find scrotal swelling and hotness, distending pain in the testes, or chilliness and fever, yellow urine, constipation, a yellow tongue coating, and a wiry and rapid pulse.

Other hernias (e.g. an enlarged scrotum) are marked by a dragging and distending pain in an area from the lower abdomen (near Qichong, St 30) to the scrotum. The protrusion goes down when the patient stands up and enters the abdominal cavity when the patient lies down.

TREATMENT

a) Cold hernias

Method. Points are selected mainly from the Ren and foot Jueyin meridians. Use a reducing method of needling, and also moxibustion.

Prescription. Guanyuan (Ren 4), Sanyinjiao (Sp 6), Dadun (Liv 1).

Explanation. In a hernia, the Ren meridian is mainly involved. The liver meridian circles the external genitalia, and the three yin meridians of the foot cross over the Ren meridian, so Guanyuan from the Ren meridian, Dadun from the liver meridian and Sanyinjiao (the crossing point of the three yin meridians), are used to remove obstruction from the jingluo. Moxibustion is added to warm the meridians and dispel cold, so as to relieve the acute pain.

b) Damp-heat hernias

Method.   Points are selected mainly from the Ren, foot Jueyin and Taiyin meridians. Use a reducing method of needling.

Prescription.   Zhongji (Ren 3), Guilai (St 29), Taichong (Liv 3), Yinlingquan (Sp 9), Sanyinjiao (Sp 6).

Explanation.   Zhongji and Taichong are used in combination to clear heat accumulated in the liver and Ren meridians.

The Yangming meridians connect with the major tendons around the private parts, so Guilai is used to assist in the treatment.

Yinlingquan and Sanyinjiao are used to eliminate damp-heat via the water passages, and to relieve gradually the swelling, distension, hotness and pain of the testes and scrotum.

c) Other hernias (e.g. an enlarged scrotum)

Method.   Points are selected mainly from the Ren meridian, with moxibustion.

Prescription.   Guanyuan (Ren 4), Sanjiaojiu (Extra 14), Dadun (Liv 1).

Explanation.   Guanyuan from the Ren meridian is used to replenish the vital qi so as to uplift the protrusion.

Sanjiaojiu is used, with moxibustion applied frequently, to help the effect of Guanyuan in uplifting the collapsed qi.

Dadun from the liver meridian, which circles the private parts, is a frequently used point for hernias.

REMARK

Needling and moxibustion can improve the symptoms of a hernia. For those with frequent attacks and difficulty in returning the prolapse to its original place, an operation may be considered.

B. *Gynaecological and paediatric diseases*

1. IRREGULAR MENSTRUATION

Irregular menstruation refers to any abnormal change in the menstrual cycle, in the quantity and colour of the menstrual flow, or any other accompanying symptoms. A temporary change in the menstrual cycle due to climatic or environmental factors, life-style, or other emotional factors, is not considered pathological.

In this section, early menstruation, delayed menstruation and irregular menstruation are discussed.

AETIOLOGY AND PATHOGENESIS

Early menstruation is often due to long-term emotional depression which gives rise to fire.

Otherwise it is due to accumulation of heat in the uterus, and the fire and heat cause extravasation of blood which leads to menstruation earlier than the due date.

Delayed menstruation may be due to retention of pathogenic cold in the uterus. Or else it is due to yang and blood deficiency, affecting the Chong and Ren meridians which leads to menstruation later than the due date.

Irregular menstruation is due to multiple deliveries of children, over-indulgence in sexual activity, or protracted loss of blood due to disease.

Alternatively it is due to a constitutional weakness of the spleen and stomach, which injures the liver and kidney, leading to damage of the Chong and Ren meridians.

DIFFERENTIATION

Early menstruation is marked by menstruation earlier than the due date or even twice a month, with fresh red or purplish menstrual flow, accompanied by irritability, feverishness, thirst, and a preference for cold drinks, a rapid pulse and a red tongue with a yellow coating.

Delayed menstruation is manifest as light red

or dimly coloured menses in a delayed cycle, an aversion to cold and preference for warmth, a slow or thready pulse, and a pale and moist tongue.

Irregular menstruation is marked by an alteration of the menstrual cycle and quantity of blood flow, light or purplish coloured menses, a weak constitution, sallowish complexion, a thready and choppy pulse, and a pale tongue.

TREATMENT

Needling and moxibustion

Method. Select points mainly from the Ren and foot Taiyin meridians. It is advisable to apply needling with an even method but not moxibustion in early menstruation. In cases of delayed or irregular menstruation, both needling and moxibustion are applied.

Prescription. Qihai (Ren 6), Sanyinjiao (Sp 6).

Modification.
— Early menstruation: Taichong (Liv 3), Taixi (K 3).
— Delayed menstruation: Xuehai (Sp 10), Guilai (St 29).
— Irregular menstruation: Shenshu (UB 23), Jiaoxin (K 8), Pishu (UB 20), Zusanli (St 36).

Explanation. The prescription is mainly to regulate the Chong and Ren meridians and harmonize the qi and blood. The Ren meridian dominates the uterus and when the qi is harmonized within the Ren meridian it makes menstruation normal.

Qihai from the Ren meridian is used to regulate the qi in the whole body. Then the blood is well dominated by sufficient qi, since "qi is the commander of blood". The spleen and stomach govern the acquired source of health, and qi and blood production and sufficient spleen qi controls the blood normally, so Sanyinjiao is selected.

Early menstruation due to heat in the blood can be treated with Taichong added to clear the liver heat, and Taixi to replenish the kidney yin (water and fluids) so as to regulate the menstruation.

For delayed menstruation due to stagnant blood, the reducing method is applied to Xuehai, Guilai and Qihai to activate the circulation of qi and blood.

In cases of blood deficiency the reinforcing method with moxibustion is applied to warm the menses and nourish the blood.

Irregular menstruation due to a congenital deficiency in the kidney qi and an acquired deficiency of qi and blood, is treated by adding Shenshu and Jiaoxin to strengthen the congenital source of health, and Pishu and Zusanli to promote the function of the middle-jiao (and acquired source of health) which manufactures and transforms the qi and blood.

Ear needling

Points. Intertragus, Ovary, Uterus, Kidney, Liver.

Method. Each time 2–4 points are used, with a moderate or strong stimulation caused through rotating the needles, along with 15–20 minutes of needle retention. Embedded needles in the ear-points can also be applied.

REMARKS

1. Pay attention to personal hygiene during the period, avoid raw, cold or spicy food, avoid psychological stimulation and physical strain.
2. Usually the treatment for this disease starts 3–5 days before the period, and 3–5 treatments are given successively. The same treatments are given at about the same time before the next period.

2. DYSMENORRHOEA

Dysmenorrhoea refers to lower abdominal pain, sometimes intolerable, occurring during, before or after the menstruation. It is often seen in young women.

AETIOLOGY AND PATHOGENESIS

Dysmenorrhoea is classified into deficiency and excess types.

The excess syndrome is often due to being affected by the cold or cold drinks, during menstruation. This gives rise to stagnation of the blood in the blood vessels and uterus, which obstruct the menstrual flow leading to pain.

Or else it is due to emotional depression leading to a stagnant circulation of the qi and a retarded menstrual flow.

The deficiency syndrome is often due to insufficiency of qi and blood, because of a weak constitution, or after a severe or protracted illness. This leads to emptiness in the "sea of blood" (the uterus) and the meridians related to the uterus are deprived of nourishment.

DIFFERENTIATION

Lower abdominal pain during, before and after the menstruation is the main symptom. Then deficiency and excess are differentiated according to their causative factors, the nature and severity of the pain, and examination of the abdomen.

Excess syndrome.   Retarded menstrual flow and severe lower abdominal pain.

If the pain is aggravated by pressure, there is a purplish-red flow with clotting and the pain is alleviated after the clots are discharged, and a deep and choppy pulse, it is due to stagnant blood.

If the distension is more predominant than the pain or there is pain affecting the chest and flank, accompanied by a stuffiness in the chest, nausea, and a wiry pulse, it is due to stagnant qi.

Deficiency syndrome.   Dull pain appearing by the end of or after the menstruation; the lower abdomen is soft and the pain can be alleviated by pressure; a decreased amount of flow, often accompanied by lumbar soreness and weak limbs, impaired appetite, dizziness or vertigo, palpitations, a wiry and thready pulse, and a pale tongue.

TREATMENT

Needling and moxibustion

a) Excess syndrome

Method.   Points are selected mainly from the Ren and foot Taiyin meridians. Use a reducing method of needling. Moxibustion can be applied according to the concrete conditions of the disease.

Prescription.   Zhongji (Ren 3), Ciliao (UB 32), Diji (Sp 8).

Explanation.   This prescription is set to regulate the Chong and Ren meridians, remove stagnant blood and relieve pain.

Zhongji from the Ren meridian is used to regulate the qi of the Chong and Ren meridians. Diji, the Xi-Cleft Point of the spleen meridian, is used to regulate the qi of the spleen meridian so as to relieve pain.

Ciliao is an empirically effective point for treating dysmenorrhoea.

These three points used in combination have the function of activating menstrual flow and relieving pain.

b) Deficiency syndrome

Method.   Points are selected mainly from Ren, Du, foot Shaoyin and foot Yangming meridians. Use a reinforcing method of needling, and moxibustion.

Prescription.   Mingmen (Du 4), Shenshu (UB 23), Guanyuan (Ren 4), Zusanli (St 36), Dahe (K 12).

Explanation.   This prescription is set to regulate and nourish the qi and blood, and warm and nourish the Chong and Ren.

Mingmen, on the Du meridian, dominates the yang of the whole body, and is used to tonify the true yang.

Shenshu, the Back-Shu point of the kidney, and Dahe from the kidney meridian, are used with moxibustion to warm and strengthen the kidney yang.

Guanyuan, from the Ren meridian, is used with moxibustion to warm the lower-jiao, and to warm and nourish the Chong and Ren meridians.

Zusanli is then used to tonify the spleen and stomach, replenish qi and blood, and to nourish the meridians related to the uterus so that the qi of the Chong and Ren can be regulated or harmonized spontaneously.

Besides these points, Guilai (St 29), Pishu (UB 20), Sanyinjiao (Sp 6) and Taichong (Liv 3) may be selected according to variation in the condition of the disease.

Point-injection therapy

Method. 1 ml of 1% procaine solution is injected subcutaneously into Shangliao (UB 3) and Ciliao (UB 32), once a day.

Ear needling

Points. Uterus, Ovary, Intertragus, Kidney.
Method. 2–4 points are used each time, with a moderate or strong stimulation applied by rotating the needles, along with 15–20 minutes of needle retention. Needles can also be embedded into the ear points.

REMARKS

1. Pay attention to personal hygiene during the menstrual period. Avoid emotional stimulation, and avoid being affected by the cold or raw and cold food.
2. Dysmenorrhoea can be due to various causes. A gynaecological examination is necessary in some cases to help make a definite diagnosis.

3. AMENORRHOEA

Menstrual flow begins at about 14 in healthy girls. If menstruation does not come until 18 or there is suppression of menstruation for longer than three months (except during the period of gestation and lactation), it is known as amenorrhoea.

AETIOLOGY AND PATHOGENESIS

This disease is classified into deficiency and excess types. It may be due to many deliveries of children, over-thinking and worry, a constitutional deficiency or else deficiency after a prolonged disease. Either may impair the manufacturing and transforming functions of the spleen and stomach, and severely consume the yin blood, leading to blood depletion and thus amenorrhoea.

Otherwise it may be due to retention of cold in the uterus owing to being affected by the cold or a cold diet or cold drinks.

Alternatively it is due to emotional depression with stagnancy in the passage of the qi, leading to stagnant blood obstructing the meridians, resulting in amenorrhoea due to stagnant blood.

DIFFERENTIATION

It is classified into the following two types according to the causes, manifestations and pulse.

Blood depletion. The menstrual flow is decreased gradually in amount until it finally ceases. Often marked by impaired appetite, loose stools, pale and lustreless lips and nails, vertigo, blurred vision, spiritlessness and lassitude, a thready and choppy pulse, and a pale tongue.

Stagnant blood. There is ceasing of the menstrual flow, lower abdominal distension or distending pain, accompanied by irritability, feverishness, and stuffiness in the chest.

In severe cases, there may be abdominal masses, dry and constipated stools, squamous and dry skin and nails, a dry mouth, a dark red tongue or purplish spots, and a deep, wiry and choppy pulse.

TREATMENT

Needling and moxibustion

a) Amenorrhoea due to blood depletion

Method. Select Ren meridian points and Back-Shu points. Apply the reinforcing method of needling with moxibustion.
Prescription. Pishu (UB 20), Shenshu (UB 23), Qihai (Ren 6), Zusanli (St 36).
Explanation. This prescription is set to regulate the spleen and stomach and replenish the kidney qi.

Pishu and Zusanli are used to strengthen the spleen and stomach, so as to fill up the source of the qi and blood and restore sufficient normal menses.

Sufficient essence and blood depends on sufficient kidney qi, so Shenshu and Qihai are used to replenish kidney qi.

b) Amenorrhoea due to stagnant blood

Method. Points are selected mainly from the

Ren and foot Taiyin meridians. Use a reducing method of needling. Moxibustion is generally not used.

Prescription. Zhongji (Ren 3), Hegu (LI 4), Xuehai (Sp 10), Sanyinjiao (Sp 6), Xingjian (Liv 2).

Explanation. This prescription is mainly to soothe the qi circulation, relieve the qi stagnation, resolve stagnant blood and promote the generation of new blood.

Zhongji is used to regulate the Chong and Ren meridians and benefit the lower-jiao.

Xuehai from the spleen meridian and Xingjian from the liver meridian are used to regulate the qi of the liver and spleen, so as to activate the qi circulation and remove blood stagnation.

Hegu and Sanyinjiao are used to enable the blood to circulate downward so as to restore normal menses.

Cutaneous needling

a) Due to blood depletion. Ganshu (UB 18), Shenshu (UB 23), Pishu (20), Taichong (Liv 3), Taibai (Sp 3), Qimen (Liv 14), Zhongwan (Ren 12), Zusanli (St 36), Qihai (Ren 6), Sanyinjiao (Sp 6), Huatuojiaji (T11–T12, Extra 19).

Other points are Guanyuan (Ren 4), Weishu (UB 21), Jingmen (GB 25), Zhaohai (K 6), Gaohuang (UB 43), Xiawan (Ren 10), Hegu (LI 4).

b) Stagnant blood. Sanyinjiao (Sp 6), Xuehai (Sp 10), Tianshu (St 25), Dachangshu (UB 25), Guanyuan (Ren 4), Zhongji (Ren 3), Baliao (UB 31–34) with clumpy puncture, Hegu (LI 4), Yaoyan (Extra 22), Jiaji (T11–S5, Extra 19).

Other points are Shenshu (UB 23), Ganshu (UB 18), Shuiquan (K 5), Yinlingquan (Sp 9), Xingjian (Liv 2), Qichi (LI 11), Jianshi (P 5).

REMARKS

1. Amenorrhoea should first of all be differentiated from the early stages of pregnancy.
2. A relative examination is required whilst giving needling and moxibustion, so as to ascertain the cause and give treatment accordingly.

4. UTERINE BLEEDING

Vaginal bleeding beyond the menstrual period is called uterine bleeding. There may be either a copious discharge with a sudden onset comprising quite massive bleeding, or else a scanty discharge with a gradual onset which is more continuous.

Although these are different in appearance, they can transform into each other. Massive uterine bleeding may turn into continuous leakage of blood after emergency haemostatic treatment, and a prolonged and continuous leakage of uterine blood may finally lead to massive uterine bleeding.

This disease is often seen in patients during puberty or the menopause.

AETIOLOGY AND PATHOGENESIS

This disease is mainly due to damage to the Chong and Ren meridians and disharmony of the liver and spleen. Over-indulgence in sexual activity injures the kidney, the Chong and Ren meridians, which fail to hold together the blood in the vessels, leading to vaginal bleeding beyond the menstrual period.

Otherwise it is due to emotional depression which impairs the free-flowing of the liver qi, and the stagnation of qi and blood gives rise to heat and an impaired liver function in storing blood, thus resulting in an extravasation of blood.

Alternatively an irregular diet, prolonged thinking or worry impairs the spleen, which fails to control blood. This leads to continuous uterine leakage of blood in mild cases and massive uterine bleeding in severe cases.

DIFFERENTIATION

This disease can be differentiated as cold or hot in nature, and of deficiency or excess type, according to the amount of menstrual flow, the quality, colour and smell of the flow, the pulse, the tongue (and coating) and general other symptoms.

When due to excessive heat, there is a sudden onset of massive uterine bleeding, in a large amount, of purplish red colour, a foul smell, a thick blood flow with clots, abdominal pain aggravated by pressure, constipation, thirst, a wiry, rapid and forceful pulse, and a red tongue with a yellow coating.

If due to yin deficiency there is a fresh red menstrual flow, accompanied by vertigo, tinnitus, palpitations, insomnia, afternoon fever, a thready, rapid and forceless pulse, and a red tongue with no coating.

When due to qi deficiency, there is prolonged continuous uterine blood leakage which is light red or dim red in colour and thin, lower abdominal coldness and pain, pallor, spiritlessness, lassitude, impaired appetite, a slow and thready pulse, and a white and slippery tongue coating.

If due to prostration (shock), there is prolonged continuous uterine blood leakage, or sudden massive uterine bleeding leading to syncope or shock, accompanied by pallor, profuse and cold sweating, shortness of breath, cold limbs, and a minute pulse as if it were fading.

TREATMENT

Needling and moxibustion

Method. Points are selected mainly from Ren and foot Taiyin meridians.

In excessive heat, the reducing method of needling without moxibustion is applied; in deficiency cold conditions, the reinforcing method of needling as well as moxibustion is applied.

Prescription. Guanyuan (Ren 4), Sanyinjiao (Sp 6), Yinbai (Sp l).

Modification.
— Excessive heat: Xuehai (Sp 10), Shuiquan (K 5).
— Yin deficiency: Neiguan (P 6), Taixi (K 3).
— Qi deficiency: Pishu (UB 20), Zusanli (St 36).
— Shock: Baihui (Du 20), Qihai (Ren 6).

Explanation. This prescription is set mainly to regulate and nourish the qi of the Chong and Ren meridians, and also to clear heat and remove stagnant blood.

Guanyuan, the crossing point of the three yin meridians of the foot, the Chong and Ren meridians, is used to regulate and nourish the qi of the Chong and Ren meridians so as to draw together and check the extravasation of blood.

Sanyinjiao, the crossing point of the three yin meridians, is used to tonify the spleen and strengthen its function in controlling blood. It is an important point for treating gynaecological diseases.

Yinbai is the Jing-well point of the spleen meridian. It is often used with moxibustion to treat uterine bleeding.

Xuehai and Shuiquan are added to clear heat from the blood so as to check the extravasation of blood.

Zusanli and Pishu are added to tonify the qi of the middle-jiao so that sufficient qi can draw together the blood as normal.

Neiguan and Taixi are added to nourish the heart and kidney so as to subdue heat due to yin deficiency.

Moxibustion applied to Baihui and Qihai promotes the vital qi so as to restore the depleted yang and check the shock reaction.

Cutaneous needling

Points. Xuehai (Sp 10), Geshu (UB 17), Sanyinjiao (Sp 6), Taibai (Sp 3), Ganshu (UB 18), Yinbai (Sp 1). Xinshu (UB 15), Baihui (Du 20), Guanyuan (Ren 4), Duyin (Extra 43), Jiaji (T11–T12, Extra 19), Baliao (UB 31–34), using clumpy puncture.

Supplementary points. Shenshu (UB 23), Chengjiang (Ren 24), Gongsun (Sp 4) Neiguan (P 6), Qihai (Ren 6), Sanjiaoshu (UB 22), Dadun (Liv 1).

Point-injection therapy

Points. Guanyuan (Ren 4), Sanyinjiao (Sp 6), Zhongji (Ren 3), Xuehai (Sp 10).

Method. 5% Danggui (Chinese angelica) solution or Vitamin B12 (100 micrograms) are used; 0.5 ml is injected into each point, once a day. 15 treatments constitute one course. This method is indicated in functional uterine bleeding.

Scalp needling

The Genital Area on both sides is used, by rotating needles at the same time for 3–5 minutes. This procedure is repeated twice.

REMARKS

1. Women who have repeated uterine bleeding during the menopause should have a gynaecological examination to make a definite diagnosis.
2. Emergency treatment is required in cases of shock due to massive uterine bleeding.

5. MORBID LEUCORRHOEA

Morbid leucorrhoea refers to a persistent excessive vaginal discharge accompanied by changes in colour and quality. Clinically morbid leucorrhoea of a white colour is often seen, and is known as white leucorrhoea.

AETIOLOGY AND PATHOGENESIS

Morbid leucorrhoea is often due to unconsolidation of the Ren meridian qi, and impaired control by the Dai meridian leading to downward pouring of water, damp and turbidity.

Otherwise it is due to dietary excess or overstrain which injures the spleen and stomach in transportation and transformation, giving rise to an accumulation of damp which pours downward to result in morbid leucorrhoea.

Yellow leucorrhoea is due to damp-heat in the spleen meridian, and white leucorrhoea due to deficiency and cold.

Alternatively it is due to emotional depression and liver qi stagnation over a long time, giving rise to heat, and leading to excessive heat in the blood and downward pouring of damp-heat. This results in red leucorrhoea or red and white leucorrhoea.

DIFFERENTIATION

This syndrome is differentiated and classified into damp-heat and cold-damp categories. Among them, white leucorrhoea is often seen, then white and yellow mixed together is the next most frequent. Red leucorrhoea is often associated with white-yellow leucorrhoea.

When due to damp-heat, it is marked by acute onset of morbid leucorrhoea, which is sticky, yellow and foul, accompanied by constipation, scanty and dark yellow urine, a soft and rapid pulse, and a yellow and greasy tongue coating. Or else the leucorrhoea is tinged with red, there is a bitter taste in the mouth and dry throat, irritability and feverishness, quick temper, a wiry rapid pulse, and a yellow tongue coating.

When due to cold-damp, there is chronic morbid leucorrhoea which is dilute, white and fishy smelling, accompanied by lumbar heaviness, soreness and pain, vertigo and dizziness, listlessness, lassitude, poor appetite, a slow-soft or deep and slow pulse, and a white and slippery tongue coating.

TREATMENT

Needling and moxibustion

Method. Points are selected mainly from the Ren, Dai and spleen meridians. Use a reducing method of needling but no moxibustion in cases of damp-heat. Use an even method of needling in cases of cold-damp, often with moxibustion.

Prescription. Daimai (GB 26), Baihuanshu (UB 30), Qihai (Ren 6), Sanyinjiao (Sp 6).

Modification.
— Damp-heat: Xingjian (Liv 2), Yinlingquan (Sp 9).
— Cold-damp: Guanyuan (Ren 4), Zusanli (St 36).

Explanation. This prescription has the effect of strengthening the spleen, eliminating damp, and regulating and tonifying the Ren and Dai meridians.

Daimai is used to strengthen the qi of the Dai meridian. Baihuanshu and Qihai are used to regulate the qi of the Ren and Bladder meridians so as to resolve pathogenic damp. Sanyinjiao strengthens the spleen, eliminates damp and regulates the liver and kidney.

In excessive damp-heat, reducing the Yingspring point of the liver meridian, Xingjian, clears accumulated heat in the liver meridian, while reducing Yinlingquan clears damp-heat from the spleen meridian.

In cold-damp cases, Guanyuan and Zusanli

are added with moxibustion to warm and consolidate the lower-jiao, to strengthen the spleen and eliminate damp. Frequent application of moxibustion onto these two points can strengthen the body resistance (the antipathogenic qi) so as to eliminate pathogenic qi.

Moxibustion with a moxa stick

Points. Mingmen (Du 4), Shenque (Ren 8), Zhongji (Ren 3), Yinbai (Sp l), Sanyinjiao (Sp 6).

Method. Apply moxibustion with a moxa-stick for 5 minutes onto each point; treatment is given once every other day, 10–15 treatments constitute one course. This method is indicated in morbid leucorrhoea due to deficiency and cold.

REMARKS

1. Needling and moxibustion have a certain therapeutic effect in treating white morbid leucorrhoea. In cases of yellow and red leucorrhoea, a gynaecological examination is required.
2. Pay attention to personal hygiene and keep the external genitalia clean.

6. MALPOSITION OF THE FETUS

Among normal fetal positions, most are occiput anterior. Malposition of the fetus refers to those which are occiput posterior, breech and transverse in presentation. This is found by a prenatal examination 30 weeks after the conception.

This condition is often seen in those pregnant women who are multipara or have a lax abdominal wall.

TREATMENT

Points. Zhiyin (UB 67).

Method. Moxibustion is applied to Zhiyin on both sides for 15–20 minutes while the pregnant woman sits in a chair or lies supine on a bed with her belt unfastened. Give the treatment once or twice every day till the malposition of the fetus is corrected.

According to reports, the success rate is over 80% and more effective in multipara pregnancies. The highest success rate was observed in those who were seven months pregnant, and next in those with an eight months pregnancy.

Application of needling or electroneedling was also reported, but moxibustion was most usually applied.

REMARK

Malposition of the fetus may be due to various causative factors such as a contracted pelvis or uterine deformity. These should not be continually treated with needling and moxibustion, but referred to the obstetric department.

7. PROLONGED LABOUR

The period from the beginning of labour till the complete opening of the orifice of uterus is known as the first stage of labour. If during this period the contraction of the uterus fails to increase gradually it makes the first stage of labour prolonged.

AETIOLOGY AND PATHOGENESIS

This is often due to the nervousness of the primipara, or premature rupture of the amniotic membrane, with massive uterine bleeding. Otherwise it is due to uterine inertia, owing to a weak constitution or insufficiency of qi and blood.

Symptoms. Amniotic fluid is lost, and labour pain reduced; there is a failure to deliver the child, the patient is listless, there is emotional depression, pallor, and a deep thready pulse or even a scattered and irregular pulse.

TREATMENT

Method. Points are selected mainly from the meridians of the hand Yangming and foot Taiyin.

Prescription. Hegu (LI 4), Sanyinjiao (Sp 6), Zhiyin (UB 67), Duyin (Extra 43).

Explanation. The *yuan* point of the hand Yangming meridian Hegu is reinforced, and the crossing point of the three yin meridians Sanyinjiao is reduced, to replenish qi, regulate blood and help the delivery of the child.

The Jing-well point of the foot Taiyang meridian, Zhiyin, and the extra point Duyin, are used with moxibustion as empirical points for hastening and inducing labour.

These four points, used together, hasten and induce labour.

REMARK

Needling and moxibustion have a definite effect in hastening and inducing labour, or when treating a prolonged labour due to uterine inertia. If the delay is due to uterine deformity or a contracted pelvis, other management is needed.

8. INSUFFICIENT LACTATION

Generally, milk secretion is observed 2–3 days after labour. Insufficient lactation applies when a nursing mother's milk is insufficient to feed the baby or even when there is no secretion of milk at all.

AETIOLOGY AND PATHOGENESIS

Milk is made out of the transformation of qi and blood. A weak constitution, impaired transportation and transformation by the spleen and stomach, or a massive loss of blood during the delivery, will all give rise to an insufficiency of qi and blood, which fails to produce milk.

Alternatively, any emotional disturbance, such as worry or undue nervousness, gives rise to a disturbance in the passage of the qi and obstructs the qi circulation in the jingluo, leading to halted secretion of milk.

DIFFERENTIATION

Insufficient lactation is divided into deficiency and excess syndromes.

Deficiency syndrome. Insufficient lactation or lack of milk, no distension in the breasts, accompanied by pallor, poor appetite, shortness of breath, loose stools, pale lips and nails, a thready pulse, and a pale tongue.

Excess syndrome. Impeded milk secretion, distending pain in the breasts, or emotional depression, stuffiness in the chest, constipation, and scanty and dark yellow urine.

TREATMENT

Needling and moxibustion

Method. Points are selected mainly from Yangming meridians. Use a reinforcing method of needling in deficiency syndromes, and moxibustion. Use an even method of needling in excess syndromes.

Prescription. Rugen (St 18), Shanzhong (Ren 17), Shaoze (SI 1).

Supplementary points.
—Qimen (Liv 14) for excess syndromes.
—Pishu (UB 20) and Zusanli (St 36) for deficiency syndromes.

Explanation. Rugen, located on the breast which the foot Yangming meridian supplies, is used to regulate the qi of the Yangming meridian to promote lactation.

Shanzhong, the Influential point of qi, is punctured to regulate qi and promote lactation.

Shaoze is an empirical point for promoting lactation.

These three points, used together, promote milk secretion. In excess syndromes, Qimen is used to soothe the liver and regulate qi. In deficiency syndromes, a reinforcing method of needling is applied to Pishu and Zusanli to strengthen the spleen and stomach and promote the manufacture and transformation of milk.

Moxibustion with a moxa stick

Points. Shanzhong (Ren 17), Rugen (St 28).
Method. Moxibustion with a moxa stick is applied each time for 10–20 minutes, twice a day.

Cutaneous needling

Points. Ganshu (UB 18), Weishu (UB 21),

Shanzhong (Ren 17), Shaoze (SI 1), Zhongwan (Ren 12), Zusanli (St 36), Tianzong (SI 11), Rugen (St 28), Jiaji (T5–T9, L1–L5, Extra 19), mild puncture applied surrounding the breasts.

Method. Treatment is given once a day, with moderate stimulation. 10 treatments constitute one course.

REMARK

The treatment should be combined with an increase in nutrition, including fluids such as soup. Ask the patient to adopt the correct methods of breast-feeding.

9. PROLAPSE OF THE UTERUS

Properly the uterus lies in the centre of the pelvic cavity, with anteversion and anteflexion; its fundus is level with the symphysis pubis and the cervix level with the ischial spine. The descent of the uterus into the vagina below the level of the ischial spine, or even out of the orifice of the vagina, is known as a prolapse of the uterus.

AETIOLOGY AND PATHOGENESIS

Its occurrence is mainly due to deficiency and weakness of the qi which fails to contract up the uterus. It either results from a weak constitution, or too early physical labour or exercise after delivery before the full recovery of qi and blood, or multiple deliveries which damage the qi.

Symptoms. There is a difference between mild, moderate and severe prolapse of the uterus.

In mild cases, there is only lumbar soreness, distension and heaviness in the lower legs and a pulling-down sensation felt in the vagina.

In moderate cases, there may be prolapse of the cervix out of the vagina, while in severe cases there may be prolapse of the total uterus out of the vagina, aggravated lumbar soreness, accompanied by listlessness, a weak pulse and a pale tongue. Its recurrence is often evoked by over-strain, severe or violent coughing or too

much exertion in passing stools. The condition may become protracted if treatment is delayed.

TREATMENT

Needling and moxibustion

Method. Points are selected mainly from the Ren and Du meridians, with a reinforcing method of needling. Retention of the needles and strong moxibustion is required.

Prescription. Baihui (Du 20), Qihai (Ren 6), Dahe (K 12), Weidao (GB 28), Taichong (Liv 3), Zhaohai (K 6).

Explanation. This prescription is set to uplift the collapsed yang qi and contract up the uterus.

Baihui is selected according to the principle of "selection of points above for diseases below".

Qihai is used to replenish the qi and help it draw together. Weidao, the crossing point of the foot Shaoyang and Dai meridians, is used to retract the uterus.

Both the liver and kidney meridians supply the lower abdomen and connect with the uterus, so Taichong, Zhaohai and Dahe from these two meridians are used to regulate and nourish the liver and kidney.

Point-injection therapy

Points. Pishu (UB 20), Ganshu (UB 18), Tituo (Extra 15), Weidao (GB 28).

Supplementary points. Shanzhong (Ren 17), Qimen (see below), Sanyinjiao (Sp 6).

Method. 5% Danggui (Chinese angelica) solution is used, 0.5–1 ml into each point, and treatment is given once every other day. Points on both sides are used alternately, with 0.8–1 cun insertion of needle and then the medicinal fluid is injected. 10 treatments constitute one course.

Scalp needling

Select bilaterally the Genital Area and Foot Motor Sensory Area. Apply rotation of the needles intermittently; the needles are retained for 15–20 minutes.

REMARKS

1. Needling and moxibustion are effective in

treating a prolapsed uterus in cases of varying severity.

2. In cases of constitutional deficiency or those accompanied by a secondary infection, herbal or medical treatment should be applied in combination.

3. Avoid heavy physical labour during the treatment. Practise exercising the levator ani muscle.

4. Point Qimen is 3 cun lateral to Guanyuan (Ren 4).

10. INFANTILE CONVULSIONS

Infantile convulsions are a commonly seen emergency in the paediatric department, manifest by impairment of consciousness, tetanic contraction, clenched jaws and opisthotonos. They are termed acute infantile convulsions because of their sudden onset and severity.

The disease is most often seen below the age of three. It is often seen in infantile hyperpyrexia, cerebral meningitis, encephalitis, hypocalcaemia, and epilepsy.

AETIOLOGY AND PATHOGENESIS

Infants are endowed with "pure yang" and their skin and muscles are frail, hence they are easily attacked by external pathogenic *feng* which results in the yang qi failing to disperse.

Accumulation of excessive heat in the interior is liable to stir up liver *feng*.

The disease may also be due to accumulation of undigested food in the stomach which damages the spleen and stomach, leading to disorder in the distribution of the body fluid, which then condenses into *tan* turbidity, leading to excessive heat which turns into *feng*.

The disease is sometimes also caused by sudden fright.

Manifestations. At the beginning, the disease is manifest as fever, a flushed face, shaking head with the teeth shown in grinning, palpitations during sleep, agitation and impaired consciousness with upward gazing of the eyes, clenched jaws and continuous paroxysmal contracture of the limbs, shortness of breath, constipation, dark yellow urine and a superficial rapid and wiry, or slippery-rapid pulse.

TREATMENT

Points of the Du and hand Yangming meridians are selected as principal points and those from the foot Jueyin meridian as supplementary ones. A reducing method with shallow needling or pricking with a three-edged needle to cause bleeding is applied.

Prescription. Shuigou (Du 26), Yintang (Extra 2), Shixuan (Extra 24), Hegu (LI 4), Taichong (Liv 3).

Modification.
— Fever: Dazhui (Du 14), Quchi (LI 11).
— Excessive *tan*: Lieque (Lu 7), Fenglong (St 40).
— Clenched jaws: Jiache (St 6), Hegu (LI 4).

Explanation. The prescription is aimed at subduing *feng* and pacifying fright.

Yintang and Shuigou, points of the Du meridian, can promote relaxation and check convulsions, and are effective in promoting resuscitation.

Pricking to cause bleeding at the Shixuan eliminates heat from various meridians.

Hegu and Taichong, the *yuan* points of the liver and large intestine meridians, when used together, are effective in stopping convulsions.

In cases with excessive heat, Dazhui and Quchi are used together to clear the pathogenic heat.

An attack of convulsions is usually accompanied by turbid *tan*. Lieque and Fenglong, *luo* points of the lung and stomach meridians, are used to regulate the lung to resolve turbid *tan*.

When there are clenched jaws, Hegu and Jiache are used together to relieve them.

REMARK

Needling is effective for relieving the symptoms of convulsions. But the causative factor should be found out and treatment should be given accordingly.

11. NOCTURNAL ENURESIS

Nocturnal enuresis refers to involuntary discharge

of urine at night, in children over the age of three who usually have a normal function in the excretion of urine. If it is caused by overdrinking of water before sleep or overtiredness, it is not considered a disease.

AETIOLOGY AND PATHOGENESIS

The normal excretion of urine is mainly concerned with the activities of the kidney qi and the restraining function of the bladder. The kidney is in charge of storing essence, and qi transformation, while the bladder stores and excretes urine. If the kidney qi is insufficient, it will be unable to maintain the bladder's action in restraining the urine, thus leading to enuresis.

Manifestations. Involuntary micturition during sleep, over several nights in mild cases or several times a night, with a sallow complexion and loss of appetite in prolonged cases.

TREATMENT

Needling and moxibustion

Method. Select mainly points from the Ren meridian, and the Back-Shu point of the bladder. The reducing method of needling and moxibustion can be applied.

Prescription. Guanyuan (Ren 4), Zhongji (Ren 3), Sanyinjiao (Sp 6), Shenshu (UB 23), Pangguangshu (UB 28).

Explanation. The causative factor is a deficiency of the kidney qi, which results in impaired qi transformation.

Guanyuan and Shenshu are selected to reinforce the kidney qi in its restraining function.

Sanyinjiao, a meeting point of the three yin meridians, is taken to regulate the spleen and kidney. Since the disease is also caused by unrestraint in the bladder, Zhongji (Ren 3) and Pangguangshu (UB 28) are employed to strengthen the bladder, according to the principle of combining Back-Shu and Front-Mu points.

Point-injection therapy

Method. Use 1% procaine solution. Inject it

into Ciliao (UB 32) or Sanyinjiao (Sp 6), 1 ml for each point. The two points are used alternately. Treatment is given once every other day.

Cutaneous needling

Points. Shenshu (UB 23), Guanyuan (Ren 4), Qihai (Ren 6), Qugu (Ren 2), Sanyinjiao (Sp 6), Jiaji (T11–S5, Extra 19).

Supplementary points. Zhongji (Ren 3), Pangguangshu (UB 28), Taixi (K 3), Baliao (UB 31–34).

Scalp needling

Select the Foot Motor-Sensory Area on both sides. The needles are manipulated intermittently and retained for 15 minutes.

REMARKS

1. Needling is effective for nocturnal enuresis. As for enuresis caused by organic changes, treatment should be given to the primary cause.
2. During the treatment the child should be asked to control his intake of fluid before sleep and be woken to discharge urine regularly, so as to make him develop the habit of getting up to urinate. Furthermore the child should be encouraged to get rid of self-contempt and shyness, and to build up his self-confidence through conquering the disease.

12. INFANTILE MALNUTRITION

Infantile malnutrition, caused by a variety of chronic diseases, often occurs in babies below the age of three. Often it is due to a deficiency of body fluid. Thus it is clinically characterized by sallow complexion, sparse hair and a distended belly.

The symptom can be seen when there is improper and irregular artificial feeding, chronic diarrhoea, TB, intestinal parasitosis, etc.

AETIOLOGY AND PATHOGENESIS

Immoderate intake of food, improper feeding,

early weaning, poor nourishment after disease, overdosage of drugs and parasitosis may cause damage of the spleen and stomach, and over-consumption of body fluids. Thus food cannot be digested.

Also long-term stagnancy of undigested food will give rise to heat and ultimately to malnutrition.

DIFFERENTIATION

A gradual onset, slight fever or tidal fever in the afternoon, over-preference for sweet and sour food, dryness of the mouth, diarrhoea with an offensive odour, urine like rice-water, crying with irritability and anorexia, followed by a distended belly with protruding umbilicus due to internal stagnation, sallow complexion, emaciation, squamous and dry skin, and sparse hair.

In prolonged cases, weakness of limbs, pallor, and lassitude may appear with a deep red tongue, a dirty and sticky tongue coating or glossy tongue, and a thready and rapid, weak pulse.

TREATMENT

Needling and moxibustion

Method. Select mainly points of the Taiyin and Yangming meridians. Apply shallow needling without needle retention and also moxibustion.

Prescription. Xiawan (Ren 10), Zusanli (St 36), Sifeng (Extra 25), Shangqiu (Sp 5).

Explanation. The pathological changes of this disease are due to a dysfunction of the spleen and stomach in transformation and transportation. If the spleen and stomach are active in functioning, food stagnation can be removed and the source of essential nutrients can be regained.

Therefore Xiawan is applied to harmonize the stomach and intestines and eliminate heat.

Zusanli, the lower He-Sea point of the stomach, is used to build up the "earth" and replenish the qi of the middle-jiao.

Shangqiu, on the spleen meridian, is employed to reinforce the spleen and remove the stagnation.

The Sifeng are extra points beneficial in treating malnutrition when tapped to cause the appearance of some yellow fluid. Pishu (UB 20), Weishu (UB 21) and Shenshu (UB 23) also can be tapped in the same fashion.

Modification.
— Parasitosis: Baichongwo (Extra 37).
— Tidal fever: Dazhui (Du 14).

Cutting therapy

The area of Yuji (Lu 10) is selected and cut vertically about 0.4 mm deep. 0.3 mg of fat is taken out. After that a surgical dressing is applied.

Cutaneous needling

Tapping with cutaneous needles is applied to the lower back and sacral region, or points on the limbs, for 10–20 minutes in each case.

REMARK

Feeding should be regular and in regular quantities. Over-eating or over-eating of sweet or fatty foods, or hunger, should be avoided.

13. INFANTILE PARALYSIS

Infantile paralysis, also called the "sequelae to poliomyelitis", is an acute epidemic disease caused by the polio virus. It happens in all the seasons of the year but mostly summer and autumn. It is more frequently seen among children, especially in those below the age of five.

During the acute stage, the disease is manifest as headache, fever, sore throat, and nausea belonging to the category of epidemic febrile disease. After paralysis, it falls into the category of *wei* syndromes (see above, under *A. Internal Diseases*). This section deals mainly with the stage of paralysis.

AETIOLOGY AND PATHOGENESIS

The disease is due to an invasion of pathogenic dampness and heat. These two pathogenic factors invade the lung and stomach, get into and obstruct the meridians, and consume the yin fluid of the lung and stomach.

A long-lasting illness will affect the liver and kidney, leading to deficiency of essence and blood; the meridians and muscles are deprived of nourishment and become withered and flaccid, thus causing *wei* syndromes. Flaccid paralysis of the limbs may be present, especially in the lower limbs, or there may appear one-sided paralysis or hemiplegia.

In severe cases, paralysis of the abdominal, diaphragmatic and intercostal muscles may appear. After the acute stage is over, the paralysed limbs begin to recover within 1–2 weeks. After 6 months, recovery is obvious and then it will decrease, leaving deformity in the joints and muscular atrophy.

TREATMENT

Needling and moxibustion

Method. Points from the hand and foot Yangming meridians are selected as the main points, accompanied by points in the affected part. Apply a reducing or reinforcing method of needling or electroneedling, according to the conditions of the disease.

Prescription. Points are modified according to the affected site and symptoms:
a) Paralysis of the lower limb: Kidney Jiaji (Extra 19, L2), Huantiao (GB 30), Yinmen (UB 33), Futu (St 32), Yanglingquan (GB 34), Zusanli (St 36).

Modification:
— Difficult raising of leg: Biguan (St 31), Jianxi (see below).
— Contracted knee: Yinshi (S 33), Jianxi (see below).
— Reverse flexion of knee: Chengfu (UB 36), Weizhong (UB 40), Chengshan (UB 57).
— Foot drop: Jingxia (see below), Jiexi (St 41).
— Inversion of foot: Fengshi (GB 31), Kunlun (UB 60), Qiuxu (GB 40), Xuanzhong (GB 39), Jiuneifan (see below).
— Eversion of foot: Jixia (see below), Yanglingquan (UB 34), Sanyinjiao (Sp 6), Taixi (K 3), Jiuwaifan (see below).
— Heel-walking: Chengshan (UB 57), Kunlun (UB 60), Taixi (K 3).

b) Paralysis of the upper limb: Cervical Jiaji (Extra 19, next to the cervical vertebrae 0.5 lateral to the posterior midline), Naoshu (SI 10), Jianyu (LI 15), Jianliao (SJ 14), Quchi (LI 11), Shousanli (LI 10), Hegu (LI 4).

Modification:
— Difficult raising of arm: Tianzong (SI 11), Jubi (see below), Binao (LI 14).
— Forceless stretching and flexing of elbow: Neiguan (P 6), Waiguan (SJ 5), Bizhong (see below), Gongzhong (see below).
— Difficult turning in and out of hand: Yangchi (SJ 4), Yangxi (LI 5), Houxi (SI 3), Sidu (SJ 9), Shaohai (H 3).
— Paralysis of abdominal muscles: Jiaji (Extra 19), Liangmen (St 21), Tianshu (St 25), Daimai (GB 26).

Point-injection therapy

Points. Refer to the supplementary points of the above prescription.

Method. Use a 10% glucose solution, Vitamin B1, Vitamin B12 solution, Yansuan Funan Liuan (furane thiamine hydrochloride), or Danggui (Chinese Angelica solution).

The 10% glucose solution should be injected into an area of thick muscle such as Yinmen (UB 37), Futu (St 32) or Zusanli (St 36), 2–5 ml applied to each point.

The dosage of the other solutions should be decided by the conditions of the disease, less for mild cases and more in severe ones. Two points are to be selected for each treatment. Injection is given once a day or once every other day. 20 treatments make up one course.

Point catgut embedding

Refer to points of the above prescription.

Cutaneous needling

Refer to points of the above prescription.

LOCATIONS OF EXTRAORDINARY POINTS

Jianxi. Located 3 cun in from the middle of the superior border of the patella.

Jingxia. Located 3 cun above Jiexi (St 41) and 1 cun lateral to the laterosuperior border of the shin bone.

Jianneifan. Located 1 cun lateral to Chengshan (UB 57).

Jixia. Located 2 cun below Jimen (Sp 11).

Jiuwaifan. Located 1 cun interior to Chengshan (UB 57).

Jubi. Located 3.5 cun below the anterior acromion.

Bizhong. Located midway on the line connecting the transverse crease of the wrist and the transverse cubital crease; between the two bones.

Gongzhong. Located 5 cun below Tianquan (P 2).

REMARK

In recent years oral intake of poliomyelitis vaccine has been used for the prevention of this disease. The occurrence of the disease has decreased remarkably. The sequelae of poliomyelitis should be treated along with practice of functional exercises. An orthopaedic operation should be performed on patients with severely deformed joints.

C. *External diseases*

1. WIND WHEAL

Wind wheal, also named "urticaria" in modern medicine, is a common allergic disease. It is apt to appear after exposure to wind, so it is termed "wind wheal". It is also called "hidden rash" in ancient medical literature because it comes and goes. Acute cases subside quickly after onset while chronic cases may repeatedly occur and linger, lasting for months or years.

AETIOLOGY AND PATHOGENESIS

It is often due to a deficiency within the skin pores of the body surface and the *wei* qi resulting in an attack of pathogenic *feng* (wind).

Otherwise it is due to stagnation of toxins within the skin, caused by biting lice or insects, which affects the jingluo.

Alternatively it is due to accumulated heat in the stomach and intestines, resulting in obstruction of the qi within the fu organs, which can neither be dispersed interiorly nor removed exteriorly. Therefore pathogenic *feng* and heat accumulate in the skin and muscles, resulting in wind wheal.

The disease may also be induced by eating fish or shrimps.

DIFFERENTIATION

This is an eruption of the skin characterized mainly by itching and flat-topped wheals appearing in groups. There is an abrupt onset with itching wheals of various sizes or pimples rising one after another, which look like those caused by biting mosquitos or other insects. The wheals are often seen on the side of the thigh. When the disease subsides, it leaves no scars.

If it occurs in the throat, difficulty in breathing may be present. Nausea, vomiting, abdominal pain and diarrhoea may appear if the reaction occurs in the stomach or intestines. Obstinate wind wheals may be protracted and reoccur, and be difficult to heal.

TREATMENT

Needling and moxibustion

Method. Points of the hand and foot Yangming meridians are selected as main points. The reducing method of needling is applied.

Prescription. Quchi (LI 11), Hegu (LI 4), Weizhong (UB 40), Xuehai (Sp 10), Geshu (UB 17), Tianjing (SJ 10).

Explanation. The disease is due to the stagnation of pathogenic *feng* (wind) in the skin and muscles.

Quchi and Hegu, belonging to the Yangming meridian, are good at dispersion, and Xuehai, a point on the foot Taiyin, is effective for syndromes of the blood system. The reducing method is applied to these three points to disperse pathogenic *feng* and eliminate heat in the blood.

Weizhong, being the blood Xi-Cleft point, and

Geshu, the Influential point of the blood, are the best points for epidemic heat toxins and hidden rashes which accumulate in the blood system.

Tianjing on the hand Shaoyang meridian is taken to regulate the meridional qi of the Sanjiao and dredge out accumulated heat.

Modification.
— Difficult breathing: Tiantu (Ren 22).
— Nausea and vomiting: Neiguan (P 6).
— Abdominal aching and diarrhoea: Tianshu (St 25).

Cutaneous needling

Points. Fengchi (LI 11), Fengmen (UB 12), Fengfu (Du 16), Weizhong (UB 40), Feishu (UB 13), Hegu (LI 4), Sanyinjiao (Sp 6).

Ear-needling

Points. Lung, Infratragic apex, Occiput, Spleen, Soothing asthma.
Method. 2–3 points are punctured in each treatment with a moderate or strong stimulation. Needles are retained for 20–30 minutes.

REMARKS

1. Needling is effective for treating wind wheal. The causative factor should be found out for chronic conditions and proper treatment given accordingly.
2. People of allergic constitution should avoid shrimps and fish. The bowels should be kept open in cases with a tendency to constipation.

2. FURUNCLE OR BOIL

This is an acute disease often seen in the surgery; frequently it occurs on the face, hand and extremities. It first appears in tiny shapes with a base as hard as a nail.

AETIOLOGY AND PATHOGENESIS

A furuncle is usually caused by contamination of the skin derived from dirt, a wound made by a metal or wooden implement, or improper pricking or pressure on other lesions on the skin, which leads to an attack of toxic heat and an accumulation of heat in the skin.

Alternatively it is due to attack by endogenous toxins due to accumulation of heat in the zangfu resulting from fatty and spicy food. It would be dangerous if these excessively toxic factors affected the jingluo or zangfu organs.

DIFFERENTIATION

A furuncle first appears like a grain of millet, yellow or purple in colour. A blister or pustule with a base as hard as a nail is formed, usually accompanied by tingling. Later there is increased redness, swelling and pain with a burning sensation, often accompanied by chills and fever.

If the furuncle toxin attacks the interior there will be high fever, restlessness, vertigo, vomiting, and impaired consciousness, which is known as furunculosis complicated by septicaemia. If it occurs in the extremities with a red line extending outward from the furuncle, the disease is called "red-threaded boil".

TREATMENT

Needling

Method. Points of the Du meridian are selected as the main points. Apply the reducing method of needling, or pricking with a three-edged needle to cause bleeding.
Prescription. Shenzhu (Du 12), Lingtai (Du 10), Hegu (LI 4), Weizhong (UB 40).
Explanation. The Du meridian commands the qi of all the yang meridians. Shenzhu and Lingtai, being empirical points for the treatment of this disease, are used for dispersing yang pathogenic fire.

Since the Yangming meridian is abundant in qi and blood, Hegu, the *yuan* point of the hand Yangming, is used to remove toxic heat from the Yangming. This point is effective for the treatment of furuncles on the face and lips.

Weizhong is effective for clearing away toxins

from the blood. Points can also be chosen along meridians related to the diseased areas, e.g. furuncle on the face: Shangyang (LI 1), Quchi (LI 11); on the tip of the fingers: Quchi (LI 11), Yingxiang (LI 20); on the temporal region: Yanglingquan (GB 34), Zuqiaoyin (GB 44); on or near the fifth toe: Yanglingquan (GB 34), Tinghui (GB 21).

For a "red-threaded boil", prick with a three-edged needle to cause bleeding along the red line from the terminating end of the line towards the focus.

3. MUMPS

Mumps or epidemic parotitis refers to an acute infectious disease characterized by painful swelling in the parotid region, caused by a virus. It usually happens in winter and spring. It is more frequently seen among preschool children or sometimes in adults when the symptoms are more severe.

AETIOLOGY AND PATHOGENESIS

Mumps is due to an exogenous attack of epidemic heat. Together with *tan* fire it obstructs the Shaoyang meridians, bringing painful swelling in the parotid region accompanied by chills and fever. The liver and gallbladder are externally-internally related to each other and the foot Jueyin meridian winds around the genital organs, so the disease is usually accompanied by painful swelling of the testis.

DIFFERENTIATION

Mild cases present only with soreness and pain in the parotid region followed by swelling, which may slowly disappear in a few days if there are no other symptoms. In less severe cases, chills, fever, headache, vomiting, a congested parotid area and difficulty in chewing may occur.

In severe cases there may be high fever, polydipsia, swelling of the testis, a yellow greasy tongue coating and a superficial-rapid, or slippery-rapid pulse.

TREATMENT

Needling and moxibustion

Method. Points of the hand Yangming meridian are selected as the main points. The reducing method of needling is applied.

Prescription. Yifeng (SJ 17), Guanchong (SJ 1), Waiguan (SJ 5), Jiache (St 6), Hegu (LI 4).

Explanation. Mumps is located in an area which the Shaoyang meridians supply. Treatment is aimed at dispelling the accumulated heat in the Shaoyang.

Yifeng, the Crossing point of the hand and foot Yangming meridians, is used to remove local stagnation of qi and blood.

Since the hand and foot Yangming meridians also travel up to the face, Jiache and Hegu are applied to eliminate pathogenic heat and remove toxic material.

Distal points Guanchong and Waiguan are employed to ease the qi passage of the Shaoyang meridians, clear away heat and dissipate the conglomeration.

Taichong (Liv 3) and Ququan (Liv 8) are used for those with swelling of the testis.

Burning rush moxibustion

Method. Cut away the hair around Jiaosun (SJ 20) on the affected side and then apply routine skin sterilization. Pieces of rush pith soaked with vegetable oil are ignited held close to the point. Remove as soon as there is a crackling sound. 1–2 treatments are given.

If the swelling will not subside, the treatment can be repeated the following day.

Cutaneous needling

Points. Hegu (LI 4), Jiache (St 6), Erjian (LI 2), Yifeng (SJ 17), Lieque (Lu 7), Waiguan (SJ 5), Jiaji (T1–4, Extra 19).

Supplementary points. Shousanli (LI 10), Neiting (St 44), Xiaxi (GB 43).

REMARKS

1. Needling is effective for treating mumps. If

there are severe complications, needling should be given in combination with other treatment.

2. The patient should be in isolation from the onset until the subsidence of the swelling.

3. During the epidemic seasons of the disease, Jiache (St 6) and Hegu (LI 4) can be punctured as prevention.

4. BREAST ABSCESS (INCLUDING NODULES OF THE BREAST)

A breast abscess, or acute mastitis, is often found during the lactation period after delivery. It is rare during pregnancy. Severe conditions are similar to acute breast cellulitis.

AETIOLOGY AND PATHOGENESIS

It is due to stagnation of the liver qi, caused by mental depression and exasperation, or too much fatty or spicy food, that brings about accumulated heat in the stomach, obstructing the Yangming meridians and bringing disharmony to the *ying* qi.

Otherwise it is due to accumulated heat in the blood after pregnancy, leading to stagnation in the *ying* qi and thus an abscess.

The disease can also be caused by invasion of exogenous toxic fire into the breast through the rupture of the nipple, which agglomerates with the accumulated milk in the breast, resulting in disease.

DIFFERENTIATION

Redness and swelling of the breast, mostly within the first month after delivery.

At an early stage when the abscess has not yet been formed there is a lump in the breast accompanied by swelling, distension, pain, difficult lactation, chills, fever, headache, nausea, irritability and dire thirst. Growth of the lump accompanied by local heat, redness and a throbbing pain indicates suppuration.

If the fever does not subside within ten days, with the centre of the lump sunken in and fluctuating, an abscess may have formed. Excretion of pus through the nipple may be seen.

TREATMENT

Needling

Method. Points of the Yangming and Jueyin meridians are selected as the main points. The reducing method is applied, and moxibustion is not applicable after needling.

Prescription. Zusanli (St 36), Liangqiu (St 34), Qimen (Liv 14), Neiguan (P 6), Jianjing (GB 21).

Explanation. The disease is caused by pathogenic heat in the stomach, stagnation of liver qi and toxic fire.

Zusanli of the Stomach meridian, and Liangqiu, a Xi-Cleft point, are taken to clear away heat from the blood and eliminate the accumulation of pathogenic factors in the Yangming meridian.

Qimen and Neiguan, both belonging to Jueyin meridians, are employed to soothe the liver and remove the symptoms at the chest.

Jianjing, the crossing point of the hand and foot meridians and the hand Yangming meridian and the Yangwei meridian, is an empirical point for the treatment of breast abscess. It is effective for reducing a swelling or lump in the breast.

Moxibustion

Method. At an early stage, ground garlic and scallion stalks are used to cover the diseased area and then moxibustion with moxa sticks is applied for 10–20 minutes. Treatment is given once or twice daily. The therapy is applicable when suppuration has not occurred.

REMARKS

1. The nipple should be washed before and after breast-feeding and kept clean.

2. Needling is effective for the treatment of swelling or a lump at an early stage of mastitis, when suppuration has not yet occurred.

3. A hot compress combined with massage is useful for effective treatment at an early stage.

When suppuration appears, an operation should be performed.

APPENDIX: NODULES OF THE BREAST

Nodules of the breast are similar to lobular hyperplasia of the mammary gland or cyto-hyperplasia. They often occur in middle-aged women. The causative factor is still unknown but it is assumed to be related to an imbalance in the proportion of progestogen and oestrogen (female sex hormones) in the body. It is induced by exasperation, upset or derangement of the Chong and Ren meridians according to TCM theory.

The patient has a sensation of distending or piercing pain in the breast, accompanied by stuffiness in the chest and belching. Nodules of various sizes may appear in the breast on one or both sides. There is no clear demarcation between the nodules or tissue around them and they are movable. The condition is aggravated before the menses and alleviated after it. The nodules grow or disappear in the wake of emotional disturbance.

TREATMENT

Method.   An even method of needling is applied to points of the foot Yangming meridian.

Prescription.   Wuyi (St 15), Shanzhong (Ren 17), Zusanli (St 36), Tianzong (SI 11), Jianjing (GB 21), Shenshu (UB 23).

Modification.
— Stagnation of liver qi: Ganshu (UB 18).
— Deficiency of blood: Xuehai (Sp 10),
   Sanyinjiao (Sp 6).

Method.   The above points are all selected bilaterally. The needles are retained for 20–30 minutes after insertion and can be manipulated 2–3 times during retention. Reducing is applied for stagnation of liver qi and reinforcing for deficiency of the blood.

Eight treatments are considered one course. A second course can be given 2–3 days after the first one. A check is given after three courses.

5. INTESTINAL ABSCESS

An intestinal abscess means acute or chronic appendicitis, or peri-appendicular abscesses. It is a commonly seen disease within the category of "acute abdomen". It is related to the anatomical characteristics of the appendix, the appendicular luminal obstruction and any bacterial infection. Clinically it is marked by fixed tenderness, muscular tension and rebounding pain in the right lower abdomen.

AETIOLOGY AND PATHOGENESIS

This disease is often due to an irregular intake of food, such as over-greasy or spicy food, raw and cold food, or voracious eating and drinking, which injure the spleen and stomach and impair the function of the stomach and intestines, and the passage of the qi.

Otherwise it is due to a running or falling accident after a large meal which injures the intestinal vessels, giving rise to stagnant blood and heat in the intestines and fu organs. Then this leads further to an intestinal abscess.

DIFFERENTIATION

At the onset there is sudden paroxysmal pain in the upper abdomen or around the umbilicus but soon the pain shifts to the right lower abdomen. The pain is fixed and aggravated by pressure, accompanied with difficulty in extension of the right leg, fever, chilliness, nausea, vomiting, constipation, yellow urine, a thin greasy and yellow tongue coating, and a rapid-forceful pulse.

In severe cases, there will be contracture of the abdominal wall which is aggravated by pressure, local masses, high fever, spontaneous sweating, and an overflowing and rapid pulse.

TREATMENT

Needling and moxibustion

Method.   Points are selected mainly from the foot Yangming meridian. Use a reducing method of needling, along with 20–40 minutes of needle retention. Treatment is usually given once or twice every day, but in severe cases once every four hours.

Prescription.   Zusanli (St 36), Lanweixue (Extra 41), Quchi (LI 11), Tianshu (St 25).

Explanation.   This prescription is set mainly to regulate the qi of the foot Yangming meridian and the qi of fu organs, so as to dispel stagnant blood, relieve swelling, clear heat and relieve pain.

According the principle, "He-sea points are indicated for disorders of the fu", the He-sea point of the stomach meridian, Zusanli, is used to regulate the qi of the fu organs and remove obstructions from the foot Yangming meridian.

Lanweixue is an effective point for the treatment of appendicitis, and it lies on the stomach meridian, so it can be used to clear accumulated heat from the intestines and fu organs.

Quchi is the He-sea point of the large intestine meridian. It is used with a reducing method to purge pathogenic heat from the intestines.

The Front-Mu point of the large intestine, Tianshu, is used to regulate the qi passage of the intestines and fu organs.

Point-injection therapy

Points.   Lanweixue (Extra 41), tenderness at the abdomen.

Method.   2–5 ml of 10% glucose injection is applied, with an injection depth of 0.5–0.8 cun. The treatment is given once a day.

Ear needling

Points.   Appendix, tip of inferior antihelix crus, Large intestine, Ear-Shenmen.

Method.   Intermittent rotation of needles, 2–3 hours of needle retention.

REMARKS

1. Needling and moxibustion have a good effect in treating simple appendicitis. In severe cases with a tendency to perforate or necrose, surgical measures should be resorted to in time.

2. In chronic appendicitis, the above points can be referred to, and treatment given once every day or every other day. Also moxibustion with a moxa stick or cones over a layer of ginger-root can be applied onto the local area.

6. HAEMORRHOIDS

Haemorrhoids are a chronic disease of the anus or rectum, often seen in the young and middle-aged. They are divided into internal, external or mixed haemorrhoids according to the location of the lesions.

AETIOLOGY AND PATHOGENESIS

Its occurrence is often related to long-term sitting or standing during work, long distance walking with heavy loads or disturbance during pregnancy.

Otherwise it is due to chronic dysentery, diarrhoea and constipation.

Alternatively it is due to indulgence in a greasy and spicy diet, in which the qi of the middle-jiao is prolapsed, muscles and tendons become flaccid, qi and blood stagnant and pathogenic dryness, heat and turbid qi accumulated in the rectum and anus, thus leading to haemorrhoids.

Symptoms.   Haemorrhoids located above the anal dentate line are known as internal haemorrhoids; those below the anal dentate line are external haemorrhoids; and those located both above and below the anal dentate line are mixed haemorrhoids.

Internal haemorrhoids are mainly manifested by bleeding during passing stools; the blood is freshly red or dark red, varying in amount. A protrusion of the haemorrhoids out of the anus which are not returned to their normal position may cause local infection and severe pain. If incarceration occurs it may lead to swelling and distension, erosions or necrosis.

External haemorrhoids are marked by a feeling of a foreign body in the anus, with severe pain, or no pain, or with swelling and pain during inflammation.

Mixed haemorrhoids have symptoms of both internal and external types.

TREATMENT

Needling and moxibustion

Method. Points are selected mainly from the foot Taiyang meridian. Use a reducing method of needling and puncture the needles to a certain depth.

Prescription. Ciliao (UB 32), Changqiang (Du 1), Huiyang (UB 35), Chengshan (UB 57), Erbai (Extra 31).

Explanation. Ciliao, Huiyang and Chengshan, from the foot Taiyang meridian which has branches connecting with the anus, are used, puncturing in deep with a reducing method to regulate the qi of this meridian and remove the obstruction and stagnant blood.

Changqiang is used locally to potentiate the above effect.

Erbai is an empirical point for haemorrhoids, as described in the *Ode to the Jade Dragon* (see Appendix 2), when it says that "haemorrhoids with pain, itching or bleeding can be treated by using the point Erbai, which lies proximal to the palm". This point is effective in treating internal haemorrhoids which occur without bleeding.

Pricking and picking therapy

Method. Find the "haemorrhoids spots" on the back on both sides of vertebra T7, and in the lumbar-sacral region. One haemorrhoids spot is used each time by the method of pricking and picking the tissue fibres in the point. Treatment is given once every 7 days.

Ear needling

Points. Lower region of rectum, Large intestine, Ear-Shenmen, Brain, Spleen.

Method. 2–3 points are used each time, and the needles retained for 20–30 minutes. Treatment is given once every day.

REMARK

Needling and moxibustion can improve the symptoms of this disease. Radical or curative treatment is given especially in the haemorrhoids department of a hospital. Ask the patient to avoid a pungent or spicy diet and to keep passing stools regularly.

7. SPRAIN (INCLUDING NECK SPRAIN)

A sprain means an injury of the soft tissue, such as the skin, muscles or tendons, ligaments, blood vessels, etc., near the joints in the body, without fracture, dislocation or wound. The main clinical manifestations are swelling, distension and pain of the injured areas, and motor impairment of the joints.

AETIOLOGY AND PATHOGENESIS

Obstruction of the meridional qi and stagnation of qi and blood in the local area affected, due to an awkward posture in carrying a heavy load, violent movement, careless falling, traction or overtwisting injuring the tendons and muscles, jingluo or joints.

DIFFERENTIATION

Swelling, distension and pain appear in the affected areas, together with a red, bluish or purplish discoloration of the local skin, in which red is due to an injury of the skin, blue to an injury to the tendons and muscles, and purple due to stagnant blood.

In recently affected areas where there is slight swelling and muscular tenderness the case is mild. If the affected area is red with severe swelling and impaired joint movement the case is severe. Sprains often occur at the shoulder, elbow, wrist, lumbar region, hip, knee and ankle.

TREATMENT

Needling and moxibustion

Method. Mainly local points of the affected areas are selected, using the reducing method of

344 CHINESE ACUPUNCTURE AND MOXIBUSTION

needling. Retain the needles and add moxibustion in cases of old injuries, or apply warming needles.

Choice of points.
— Shoulder: Jianyu (LI 15), Jianliao (SJ 14), Jianzhen (SJ 9).
— Elbow: Quchi (LI 11), Xiaohai (SI 8), Tianjing (SJ 10).
— Wrist: Yangchi (SJ 4), Yangxi (LI 5), Yanggu (SJ 5).
— Waist: Shenshu (UB 23), Yaoyangguan (Du 3), Weizhong (UB 40).
— Hip: Huantiao (GB 30), Zhibian (UB 54), Chengfu (UB 36).
— Knee: Liangqiu (St 34), Xiyan (Extra 39), Yaoyangguan (Du 3).
— Ankle: Jiexi (St 41), Kunlun (UB 60), Qiuxu (GB 40).

Explanation. In a sprain, generally the local points are selected to activate the circulation of qi and blood, and remove the obstruction from the jingluo so as to restore the function of the injured tissues. In severe cases, adjacent and distal points along the course of the affected meridians can be selected in combination.

Tapping with cutaneous needles and cupping

Method. Tap heavily with the cutaneous needles on the affected areas which are tender, until they bleed slightly and then apply cupping. This method is indicated for newly affected areas when there is an obvious haematoma, old injuries with retention of stagnant blood, or when the collaterals are affected by pathogenic cold.

Point-injection therapy

Method. 10 ml of 10% glucose injection, or else the same with Vitamin B1 (100 mg), is injected into the muscles where there is tenderness. It is required that the needling sensation radiates in the same direction as the original pain. Treatment is given once every day or every other day. This method is indicated in acute lumbar sprain.

Ear needling

Points. Corresponding sensitive spots, Brain, Ear-Shenmen.

Method. Moderate or strong stimulation with rotation of needles and needle retention for 10–30 minutes are applied. Treatment is given once every day. This method is indicated for acute sprains, in which a remarkable analgesic effect is observed.

REMARKS

1. Needling and moxibustion can improve the symptoms when treating sprains in various parts. But fracture, dislocation, rupture of the ligament or bone disease should be excluded.
2. If necessary, massage therapy and herbal treatment can be applied in combination.

NECK SPRAIN

A sprain of the neck is caused by an awkward position of the neck during sleep, or twisting the neck whilst carrying heavy things, or else due to the nape and back being affected by *feng* and cold, which injure the local jingluo and lead to disharmony of meridional qi in the local area.

It is often manifested by twisting of the head towards the affected side, and a contracting or dragging pain on one side leading to the nape and back, which even radiates to the shoulder and upper arm on the same side. There is limited movement of the neck and obvious tenderness.

Method. Points are selected mainly from the Du and foot Taiyang meridians, such as Dazhui (Du 14), Tianzhu (UB 10), Jianwaishu (SI 14), Xuanzhong (GB 39), Houxi (SI 3). Use a reducing method of needling, and after needling add moxibustion in order to dispel *feng* and cold, soothe the tendons and muscles and activate the circulation of qi and blood in the collaterals.

For impaired forward bending and backward extension, Kunlun (UB 60) and Lieque (Lu 7) are added.

For impaired turning of the head to left or right, Zhizheng (SI 7) is added to remove obstruction of qi in the Taiyang meridians.

At the same time cupping can be applied onto the points around the affected areas. Besides this, Luozhenxue (Extra 28) can be used in combination.

REMARKS

1. Needling and moxibustion have a good effect in treating neck sprain. After needling, massage and a hot compress can be applied to help the treatment.
2. The thickness of the pillow should be correct during sleep, and attention should be paid to avoiding the cold.
3. In middle or old age when there are repeated attacks of neck strain, cervical vertebral disorders should also be considered.

8. TENNIS ELBOW

Tennis elbow corresponds to external humeral epicondylitis, and is categorized as an "injury to the tendons". This disease is often seen in labourers engaged in work which needs rotation of the forearm, or flexion and extension of the elbow joint, such as in carpenters, fitters, electricians, and tennis players.

AETIOLOGY AND PATHOGENESIS

This disease is mainly due to chronic strain and impairment, by over-use of the elbow and wrist joints during long-term work which injures the qi and blood.

Alternatively it is due to accumulated *feng* and cold in the elbow joint giving rise to contraction of the blood vessels, leading to disorders and disharmony in the tendons and muscles and the jingluo.

Symptoms. Chronic onset and repeated attacks, without an obvious past history of trauma. Soreness, pain and forcelessness on the lateral aspect of the elbow joint, possibly with the pain radiating to the forearm, shoulder or back. The pain and soreness can be aggravated by making a fist and twisting the forearm. There is no obvious local swelling, with tenderness around the external humeral epicondyle, and normal motor activity of the joint; testing by twisting the flexed wrist is positive.

TREATMENT

Needling and moxibustion

Method. To ease the tendons and muscles, and remove obstruction from the jingluo. Mainly local points are used, with a reducing method of needling and also moxibustion.

Prescription. Tender spots, Quchi (LI 11), Zhouliao (LI 12), Shousanli (LI 10), Hegu (LI 4).

Puncture the tender spot in different directions or with multiple needles, to remove the obstruction from the jingluo. Retain the needles for 20 minutes. Treatment is given once every day or every other day. 10–15 treatments constitute one course.

Point-injection therapy

Method. 0.5 ml of hydrocortisone acetate is injected into the tender spot, once a week, at the early state of this disease. Or 2 ml of Danggui (Chinese Angelica) is injected into a tender spot, twice a week. During a later stage of this disease, 1 ml of Weilingxian (Clematis solution) is injected into the tender spot, once every other day.

Cutaneous needling and cupping

Method. Tap the local areas with cutaneous needles until there is bleeding, then apply cupping. Treatment is given once every 2–3 days. This method is indicated for cases with local swelling.

REMARKS

1. Avoid exertion and movement of the elbow joint as much as possible during treatment.
2. External application of herbal drugs onto the local area is given to help treatment and potentiate the therapeutic effect.

9. THECAL CYST

A thecal cyst often occurs around the joints and tendon sheaths. It is often seen on the dorsum of the wrist or foot of young people (especially females). The cause of this disease is still not clear and it is generally held that it is related to traumatic injury, mechanical stimulation or chronic strain and impairment.

This disease is marked by slow progression, with a round and prominent appearance but no obvious subjective feeling or symptoms, only slight soreness, pain and lassitude. The lesion is round in shape, with a smooth surface and clear margin; it is soft and gives an undulating feeling upon palpation. When the cyst is full of fluid its wall becomes hard and locally tender.

TREATMENT

Method. Local needling is given. Firstly fix the location of the cyst, and apply routine sterilization. Then puncture from the top of the cyst into the lesion, in different directions, with a thick needle or three-edged needle, to penetrate the cyst wall. Squeeze and press the cyst heavily and allow the fluid out of the cyst via the puncture hole. Tight bandaging is applied afterwards for 3–5 days.

If the cyst is large in size, suck out fluid with a syringe, then puncture several holes in the cyst and do the same bandaging as mentioned above. If the cyst recurs, the same needling method is applied again one week later.

10. ERYSIPELAS

Erysipelas is an acute contagious and infectious disease marked by sudden onset, with a red discoloration of the skin which often takes place on the face and lower leg. It is often seen in spring and autumn, and often occurs in infants and the elderly. Acupuncture is mainly indicated for erysipelas on the lower limbs.

AETIOLOGY AND PATHOGENESIS

This disease is often due to invasion of the body by toxins via wounds in the skin, and deficiency of the *wei* qi which gives rise to heat in the blood and accumulation of heat in the superficial region of the body.

If associated with *feng*, the head and face will be affected, while if associated with damp, the lower limbs are often affected. Therefore erysipelas on the head and face is often due to *feng* heat, while that in the lower limbs is often due to damp-heat.

DIFFERENTIATION

Manifest mainly by the rapid onset of a well-demarcated patch of redness, hotness and burning pain. Initially there are chills and fever which are followed by the presence of a bright red skin area which is burning hot. Its border is prominent and higher than the normal skin and rapidly extending in size; in areas with a change in colour from bright red to dull red there may be a small patch of desquamation.

Alternatively there may be yellow blisters oozing liquid, pain and itching, and irritability, thirst, general feverishness, constipation, and dark yellow urine.

If there is high fever, vomiting, coma, delirium, or convulsions, it is due to invasion of the interior by toxins.

TREATMENT

Needling and moxibustion

Method. Points are selected mainly from the hand Yangming and foot Taiyin meridians. Use a reducing method of needling, and also clumpy needling to cause bleeding in the local area.

Explanation. This prescription is set to dispel *feng* heat and clear damp-heat so as to clear the toxins.

Hegu (LI 4) and Quchi (LI 11) are used to dispel *feng* heat from the Yangming meridians. Yinlingquan (Sp 9), the He-sea point of the foot Taiyin meridian, is used with a reducing method to clear damp-heat from the lower leg. Reducing Xuehai (Sp 10) and Weizhong (UB 40), and local clumpy needling to cause bleeding, can clear the accumulated heat in the blood.

Pricking collaterals and cupping

Method. Apply clumpy needling at the local lesions which are red or swollen with the three-edged needle, or tap with cutaneous needles to cause bleeding, then apply cupping. Treatment is given 1–2 times a day.

REMARKS

1. Needles should be strictly sterilized to prevent cross-infection. In cases where there are mixed infections leading to ulcers or septicaemia, a unified approach combining TCM and western medicine should be resorted to.
2. Prevent the skin from being unduly wounded.

11. HERPES ZOSTER

Herpes zoster refers to a kind of acute inflammatory skin disease which occurs mainly on the chest, back, face and lumbar region with small skin eruptions in the shape of a girdle around the waist. It is often seen in the spring and autumn.

AETIOLOGY AND PATHOGENESIS

It is mostly caused by accumulated damp-heat in the spleen meridian, accumulated hyperactive fire of the liver meridian in the interior and affection by exogenous toxins which affect the muscles and skin, and jingluo.

Symptoms. At the onset, there is a stabbing pain of the skin like a girdle around the waist, which soon becomes erythematous. It is accompanied by mild fever, lassitude, and poor appetite. There are patches of blisters the size of mung-beans or soybeans, in a girdle-like distribution with bloody or purulent lesions mixed in between the blisters. Most skin lesions occur unilaterally and are often seen in the intercostal spaces or the head and facial region as well.

The blisters and lesions gradually turn dry, and scab over; finally the scabs are lost after 2–3 weeks. Generally it is healed without scar formation but, in some cases, the pain may last afterwards for quite a long period.

TREATMENT

Needling and moxibustion

Method. Mainly distal points along the course of the involved meridians are selected. Local points are used as well. Use a reducing method of needling.

Prescription. A: Quchi (LI 11), Hegu (LI 4), Zhigou (SJ 6). B: Xuehai (Sp 10), Sanyinjiao (Sp 6), Taichong (Liv 3).

Method. The above two groups of points are used alternately. Use a reducing method by lifting and thrusting the needles, and retaining them for 20–30 minutes after the arrival of the qi.

The treatment is given once a day. Multiple needles are punctured obliquely along the distribution of the skin lesions and blisters locally. Adjacent points are selected for lesions on the face, with rotation of the needles used as a reducing method.

Ear needling

Points. Corresponding sensitive spots, Lung, Liver, Inferior antitragic apex, Intertragus.

Method. 2–3 points are used each time, with a strong stimulation by rotating the needles. Retain the needles for 20–30 minutes.

REMARK

Acupuncture is effective in treating herpes zoster, especially in relieving the pain. Surgical management is necessary in cases which are complicated by purulent infection.

D. Diseases of the sensory organs

1. CONGESTION, SWELLING AND EYE PAIN

Congestion, swelling and pain of the eye is an acute condition in various external eye diseases.

This disease is often seen in acute conjunctivitis, pseudomembranous conjunctivitis and epidemic conjunctivitis.

AETIOLOGY AND PATHOGENESIS

It is mostly due to exogenous pathogenic *feng* heat affecting the eye, leading to stagnation of qi in the meridians.

Otherwise it is due to upward flaring of hyperactive fire of the liver and gallbladder along the course of the related meridians, leading to obstruction of qi of jingluo and stagnation of qi and blood.

DIFFERENTIATION

A congested, swollen and painful eye, with photophobia, lacrimation and profuse eye discharge.

If accompanied by headache, fever, and a superficial and rapid pulse, it is due to *feng* heat.

If accompanied by a bitter taste in the mouth, irritability and feverishness, constipation, and wiry-slippery pulse, it is due to hyperactive fire of the liver and gallbladder.

TREATMENT

Needling and moxibustion

Method. Points are mainly selected from the hand Yangming and foot Jueyin meridians. Use a reducing method of needling.

Prescription. Hegu (LI 4), Taichong (Liv 3), Jingming (UB 1), Taiyang (Extra 5).

Modification.
— *Feng* heat: Shaoshang (Lu 11), Shangxing (Du 23).
— Hyperactive fire of liver and gallbladder: Fengchi (GB 20), Xiaxi (GB 43).

Explanation. This prescription is set to clear *feng* and heat, and relieve swelling and pain. The eye is the external orifice of the liver, and the meridians of the Yangming, Taiyang and Shaoyang all supply the eye region.

Therefore Hegu is used to regulate the qi of the Yangming meridians and clear *feng* and heat.

Fengchi, Xiaxi and Taichong from the liver and gallbladder meridians are selected by combining upper and lower points to conduct down the fire of the liver and gallbladder.

Jingming, the crossing point of Taiyang and Yangming meridians, is used to purge away accumulated heat in the affected areas.

Shaoshang, Taiyang and Shangxing are pricked to cause bleeding, so as to clear heat and relieve swelling.

Pricking and picking method

Prick at the sensitive spots in the scapular region, or points on both sides of, and 0.5 cun lateral to, Dazhui (Du 14), and pick up some tissue fibres at these points. This method is indicated for acute conjunctivitis.

Ear needling

Points. Eye, Eye 1, Eye 2, Liver.

Method. After insertion, retain the needles for 20 minutes and manipulate during retention from time to time. Or else prick the apex of the ear, or the veins at the back of the ear, to cause bleeding.

REMARK

In treating this disease with needling in intraorbital acupoints, strict sterilization of the needles is required. The needle should be inserted and withdrawn slowly, with a slight rotation, but without any lifting-thrusting of the needle to prevent infection and avoid bleeding.

2. HORDEOLUM

A hordeolum, also known as a stye in the eye, refers to the small, acutely inflamed swelling of a sebaceous gland on the rim of the eyelid.

AETIOLOGY AND PATHOGENESIS

This disease is often due to accumulated heat in

the spleen and stomach or upward flaring of the heart-fire, which is then affected by exogenous *feng* and heat. Therefore the accumulated heat combined with the exogenous *feng* heat gives rise to stagnation of qi and blood and accumulation of fire and heat, leading to redness, swelling and even purulent discharge on the eyelid.

DIFFERENTIATION

At the onset, there is limited redness, swelling, a hard nodule, and pain or tenderness at the rim of the eyelid. Then the redness and swelling gradually develop in size, and, several days later, there appears a yellow purulent spot at the top of the hard nodule from which pus discharges after the rupture of the lesion. It can be accompanied by thirst, constipation, and a yellow coating on the tongue.

TREATMENT

Pricking and picking method

Find the eruptive spots, which are slightly red in colour, on both sides of vertebrae C1–C7 between the scapular regions. Then prick these spots with a three-edged needle and squeeze out a small amount of blood, 3–5 times. Alternatively prick and break the subcutaneous fibrous tissues at these spots with an ordinary sewing needle.

Ear needling

Points.   Eye, Liver, Spleen.
Method.   Manipulate the needles from time to time during their retention for 20 minutes. Treatment is given once a day.

REMARKS

1. Never try to squeeze or press the lesion at an early stage when it is not yet purulent. This will force the bacteria into the blood, which may result in especially serious and unfavourable results.

2. The above methods are indicated for relieving the redness and swelling of the hordeolum. If it is already purulent it should be treated by a eye specialist.

3. OTITIS MEDIA

This includes acute and chronic otitis media. Clinically it is marked by purulent ear discharge, and is mostly seen in children.

AETIOLOGY AND PATHOGENESIS

The ear is the external orifice of the kidney, and the Shaoyang meridians circle the auricle. Children have delicate *wei* qi and are susceptible to invasion by pathogenic *feng* and heat via the ear, so pathogenic *feng* heat is accumulated in the collaterals of the Shaoyang meridians, giving rise to stagnation of qi of the gallbladder and Sanjiao meridians which turns into fire forming pus.

If there are repeated attacks, lasting a long time, yin fluid will be consumed leading to syndromes of kidney yin insufficiency.

DIFFERENTIATION

In acute cases, it is marked by chilliness, fever, headache, throbbing pain at the base of the ear, and rupture of the tympanic membrane with purulent discharge coming out from it—this is the excess syndrome due to an upward attack of qi and fire of the Sanjiao associated with the *feng* and yang.

If the case is lingering and marked by vertigo, tinnitus, impaired hearing, and scanty and dilute pus discharged from the ear, it is a deficiency syndrome due to kidney yin deficiency.

TREATMENT

Needling and moxibustion

Method.   To dispel *feng* and clear heat, by selecting points mainly from the Shaoyang meridians, with mainly a reducing method of needling.

Prescription.   Fengchi (GB 20), Tinghui (GB 2), Yifeng (SJ 17), Hegu (LI 4).

Modification.
— Excessive heat: Dazhui (Du 14), Quchi (LI 11).
— Yin deficiency: Shenshu (UB 23), Taixi (K 3).

Explanation. Fengchi from the Shaoyang meridian is used in combination with Hegu to dispel *feng* and clear heat from the Shaoyang meridians.

Tinghui and Yifeng from the hand and foot Shaoyang, and near the auricle, are used with a reducing method to disperse the local accumulated heat.

In excessive heat, Dazhui and Quchi are used to clear and reduce the yang pathogens.

In chronic cases, due to yin deficiency, a reinforcing method is applied in Shenshu and Taixi to replenish the kidney qi. Then the kidney qi can, as usual, supply the ear and the tinnitus and vertigo will be cured spontaneously.

Ear needling

Points.   Kidney, Internal ear, Intertragus, Occiput, External ear.

Method.   2–3 points are used each time, with manipulation of needles from time to time during the 20 minutes of needle retention. Treatment is given once every day or every other day.

REMARKS

1. Clean the purulent discharge from the external auditory canal with a sterilized cotton ball, and wash the external auditory canal with hydrogen peroxide solution. After the canal is dried acupuncture treatment is given.
2. Avoid water getting into the ear, and when blowing one's nose avoid blockage of both nostrils by hand pressure.

4. TINNITUS AND DEAFNESS

Both tinnitus and deafness are auditory distur-

bances which may be caused by various kinds of diseases. Tinnitus is marked by a ringing sound in the ear felt by the patient, while deafness is impaired hearing or loss of hearing. Because of the similarities between these two conditions in aetiology and treatment, they are discussed together.

AETIOLOGY AND PATHOGENESIS

Tinnitus and deafness are due to internal and external causes.

The internal causes are anger, fright and fear, which lead to upward rebellion of *feng* fire of the liver and gallbladder and obstruction of qi in the Shaoyang meridians.

Otherwise it is due to deficiency of kidney essence and qi which fail to go up to nourish the ear.

The external causes are invasion of pathogenic *feng* obstructing the passage of the qi in the auditory orifice, or a violent sound which damages the ear, leading to auditory disturbances.

DIFFERENTIATION

According to the conditions of its onset, accompanying symptoms and pulse, tinnitus and deafness are divided into deficiency and excess syndromes.

Excess syndrome.   Sudden deafness, or a distending sensation and constant ringing in the ear that cannot be alleviated by pressure.

In cases of upward rebellion of pathogenic *feng* fire of the liver and gallbladder, there is distension in the head, flushed face, dry throat, irritability and a hot temper, and wiry pulse.

In cases affected by exogenous pathogenic *feng*, there may be aversion to cold, fever, and a superficial and rapid pulse.

Deficiency syndrome.   Protracted deafness, intermittent tinnitus with a sound like cicadas singing in the ear, which is aggravated by strain or fatigue and can be alleviated by pressure. It is accompanied by dizziness and vertigo, lumbar and knee-joint soreness and weakness, seminal emission, morbid leucorrhoea, and an empty-thready pulse (a pulse of the deficiency type).

TREATMENT

Needling and moxibustion

Method. Points are selected mainly from the hand and foot Shaoyang meridians. Use a reducing method of needling in excess syndromes.

Points are also selected from the foot Shaoyin meridian in addition to the above points, with a reinforcing method, in deficiency syndrome, with moxibustion in small cones applied to points around the affected site.

Prescription. Yifeng (SJ 17), Tinghui (GB 2), Xiaxi (GB 43), Zhongshu (SJ 3).

Modification.
— Hyperactive fire of the liver and gallbladder: Taichong (Liv 3), Qiuxu (GB 40).
— Exogenous affection by pathogenic *feng*: Waiguan (SJ 5), Hegu (LI 4).
— Kidney deficiency: Shenshu (UB 23), Guanyuan (Ren 4).

Explanation. The hand and foot Shaoyang meridians both supply the auricular region, so Zhongshu and Yifeng from the hand Shaoyang and Tinghui and Xiaxi from the foot Shaoyang are used together as the main points of this prescription. These regulate the qi and remove obstruction from the Shaoyang meridians.

In hyperactive fire of the liver and gallbladder, Taichong from the liver meridian and the *yuan* point of the gallbladder meridian, Qiuxu, are used with a reducing method of needling. These purge the fire of the liver and gallbladder, so that the disease above can be relieved by using points below and the excess syndrome can be reduced.

In exogenous affection by pathogenic *feng*, Waiguan and Hegu are used to relieve exterior symptoms and regulate the qi of meridians.

In cases of kidney deficiency, which fails in ascending to nourish the ear, Shenshu and Guanyuan are used to regulate and nourish the vital qi of the kidney meridian so that the essence and qi can ascend to the ear and hearing can be restored.

Point-injection therapy

Points. Tinggong (SI 19), Yifeng (SJ 17), Wangu (GB 12), Qimai (SJ 18).

Method. Vitamin B12 (100 micrograms) is used, 0.2–0.5 ml is injected into each point with the needle being inserted 0.5–1 cun into the point.

Scalp needling

The Vertigo-Auditory Area on both sides is used, with needle retention for 20 minutes during which the needles are manipulated from time to time. The treatment is given once every day or every other day. This method is indicated for nervous tinnitus and impaired hearing.

REMARK

Tinnitus and deafness are due to various causative factors. Needling and moxibustion have a good effect in treating tinnitus and deafness due to nerve conditions.

5. RHINORRHOEA

Rhinorrhoea is marked by a fishy or foul, turbid nasal discharge, nasal obstruction and loss of the sense of smell. Severe cases are referred to as "fluid leaking from the brain". It is often seen in chronic rhinitis, and acute or chronic paranasosinusitis.

AETIOLOGY AND PATHOGENESIS

The nose is the external orifice of the lung, so the occurrence of rhinorrhoea is related to the lung meridian being affected by pathogenic factors.

Acute cases are due to pathogenic *feng* and cold affecting the lung which accumulates and turns into heat, or to *feng* and heat affecting the lung which gives rise to impaired dispersion of the lung qi and the upward disturbance of the nose by these pathogens, leading to nasal obstruction and discharge.

After the *feng* has been relieved, the pathogenic accumulated heat turns into turbid fluid which obstructs the nose, leading to rhinorrhoea with a lingering nasal discharge.

DIFFERENTIATION

The main symptoms are a turbid nasal discharge which is purulent and fishy, and nasal obstruction impairing the sense of smell. In acute cases, it is accompanied by headache, fever, anorexia and a rapid pulse. In chronic cases with repeated attacks, it is accompanied by dizziness, supraorbital distending pain, absence of mind and impaired memory.

TREATMENT

Needling and moxibustion

Method. To clear heat, promote the dispersion of lung qi, remove obstruction from the nose and ease the functioning of the nose. Points are selected mainly from the hand Taiyang and Yangming, using a reducing method of needling.

Prescription. Lieque (Lu 7), Hegu (LI 4), Yingxiang (LI 20), Bitong (Extra 7), Yintang (Extra 2), Fengchi (GB 20).

Explanation. The *luo* point of the lung meridian, Lieque, is used to promote the dispersion of lung qi and dispel pathogenic *feng*.

The hand Yangming and Taiyin are externally-internally related and supply the nose, so Hegu and Yingxiang are used to regulate the qi of, and remove obstruction from, the hand Yangming, and to clear the lung heat. Yingxiang is especially effective in treating an impaired sense of smell.

Yintang on the Du meridian is near the nose, and Bitong is located either side of the nose, and they are both used to disperse the local accumulated heat and remove obstruction.

Fengchi is an effective point for treating disorders of the eye and nose. It is used to dispel *feng* and ease the functioning of the nose.

The above points can be selected according to the syndrome.

Point-injection therapy

Points. Hegu (LI 4), Yingxiang (LI 20).

Method. Injection of Vitamin B complex is used, with 0.2–0.5 ml injected into each point; one point is selected each time. Treatment is given once every other day.

Ear needling

Points. Internal nose, Lower apex of tragus, Forehead, Lung.

Method. 2–3 points are used for each treatment, with 20–30 minutes retention of needle, during which manipulation of the needles from time to time is needed. Otherwise embed the needles for one week. This method is indicated for simple rhinitis.

For allergic rhinitis, points Soothing Asthma and Intertragus can be added.

REMARK

Acupuncture has a definite effect in treating chronic rhinitis, but less effect in treating paranasosinusitis when it can be applied as a supplementary therapy.

6. TOOTHACHE

Toothache is a commonly seen symptom of oral diseases and is often seen in dental caries, pulpitis and pericoronitis. In TCM it is held that toothache is mainly related to accumulated fire in the stomach meridian and insufficient kidney yin. It is divided into deficiency and excess syndromes.

AETIOLOGY AND PATHOGENESIS

The hand and foot Yangming enter into the upper and lower gums respectively, so toothache may be due to the upward flaring of pathogenic fire along the meridians, transformed from accumulated heat in the large intestine and stomach.

Alternatively it results from exogenous pathogenic *feng* affecting and accumulating in the Yangming. The kidney dominates the bones, and the teeth are an extension of the bones, so insufficient kidney yin gives rise to upward flaring up of empty fire, leading to toothache.

Toothache may also be due to dental caries caused by over-intake of sweet or sour foods, or poor oral hygiene.

DIFFERENTIATION

Severe toothache, accompanied by foul breath, a yellow tongue coating, thirst, constipation, and an overflowing pulse, manifests in cases of toothache due to pathogenic fire in the Yangming.

If there is severe pain and swollen gums, accompanied by aversion to cold, general feverishness, and a superficial and rapid pulse, it is toothache due to *feng* fire.

If there is dull pain on and off, absence of foul breath, a thready pulse or loose teeth, it is toothache due to kidney deficiency.

TREATMENT

Needling and moxibustion

Method. Points are selected mainly from the hand and foot Yangming. Use a reducing method of needling. Contralateral puncture can be applied on distal points selected along the course of the meridians.

Prescription. Hegu (LI 4), Jiache (St 6), Neiting (St 44), Xiaguan (St 7).

Modification.
— *Feng* fire: Waiguan (SJ 5), Fengchi (GB 20).
— Yin deficiency: Taixi (K 3), Xingjian (Liv 2).

Explanation. Hegu is used to clear heat from the hand Yangming. Jiache, Neiting and Xiaguan are used to regulate the qi of the foot Yangming.

Waiguan and Fengchi are used to relieve exterior symptoms by eliminating *feng* heat.

Taixi is used to replenish kidney yin, and Xingjian to purge liver fire. They are both used to treat toothache due to yin deficiency.

Ear needling

Points. Maxilla, Mandible, Ear-Shenmen, Superior Apex of Tragus, Toothache point.

Method. 2–3 points are selected and strong stimulation is applied, with retention of needles for 20–30 minutes.

REMARKS

1. Acupuncture has a good effect in treating toothache, except for dental caries in which acupuncture has only a temporary analgesic effect.
2. The treatment of toothache should be differentiated from that of trigeminal neuralgia.
3. Attention should be paid to personal oral hygiene.

7. CONGESTED AND SORE THROAT

A congested or sore throat is a main symptom of oral-pharyngeal and laryngeal-pharyngeal disorders. It includes that which was mentioned in the ancient medical classics as a throat ulcer, throat Bi syndrome, throat pain, etc., and is similar to chronic tonsillitis and sudden hoarseness of voice in aetiology and pathogenesis. Therefore they are all referred to here.

AETIOLOGY AND PATHOGENESIS

The pharynx connects with the oesophagus and stomach; the larynx connects with the trachea and lung.

The excess heat syndrome of this disease is due to exogenous pathogenic *feng* heat that burns and scorches the lung system. Or else it is due to accumulated heat in the lung and stomach meridians disturbing upwards.

The yin deficiency syndrome of this disease is due to exhaustion of kidney yin, failing to flow up to moisten the throat and thus leading to upward flaring of empty fire.

DIFFERENTIATION

The excess heat syndrome manifests as a congested, swollen and sore throat, with dysphagia.

If accompanied by coughing, a dry throat, thirst, constipation and also chills, fever and headache, it is mostly caused by exogenous *feng* heat and excessive heat in the lung and stomach.

If due to a yin deficiency syndrome, there is a slightly swollen throat of a dim red colour and mild pain, or pain on swallowing, slight feverishness, and symptoms aggravated during the night.

TREATMENT

Needling and moxibustion

a) Excess heat syndrome

Method.   Points are selected mainly from the hand Taiyin, and hand and foot Yangming using a reducing method of needling.

Prescription.   Shaoshang (Lu 11), Hegu (LI 4), Chize (Lu 5), Xiangu (St 43), Guanchong (SJ 1).

Explanation.   This prescription is effective in treating various kinds of congested sore throat due to heat.

Shaoshang is the Jing-well point of the hand Taiyin, and is pricked to let out blood in order to clear lung heat. It is the main point in treating syndromes of the throat.

Chize is the He-sea point of the hand Taiyin, and is used to clear heat from the lung meridian by "reducing the son in case of excess". Hegu and Xiangu from the hand and foot Yangming are used to purge accumulated heat in the Yangming.

Guanchong, the Jing-well point of the Sanjiao meridian, is pricked to cause bleeding, so as to potentiate the effect in purging heat from the lung and stomach, so that the congested, swollen and sore throat can be relieved.

b) Yin deficiency syndrome

Method.   Points are selected mainly from the foot Shaoyin. An even method of needling is applied.

Prescription.   Taixi (K 3), Zhaohai (K 6), Yuji (Lu 10).

Explanation.   Taixi is the *yuan* point of the foot Shaoyin. Zhaohai is the crossing point of the foot Shaoyin and the Yinqiao, and both supply the throat. Their points are used to regulate the qi of the meridians.

Yuji, the Ying-spring point of the hand Taiyin, is used to ease the throat and clear lung heat.

These three points are used together to purge the empty fire and prevent the yin fluid from being consumed by it. Therefore they are indicated for a congested or sore throat due to yin deficiency.

Ear needling

Points.   Throat, Heart, Lower apex of tragus.

Method.   Retain needles for 10–20 minutes, during which time manipulation of needles from time to time is needed. This method is indicated for chronic laryngopharyngitis.

In cases of acute tonsillitis, points Heart and "Lower apex of tragus" are removed, but "Tonsil" and "Helix 1–6" are added instead, and are needled with a moderate or strong stimulation by intermittent rotation of the needles for 2–3 minutes. Needles are retained for one hour, and the treatment is given once a day.

REMARKS

1. Acupuncture has a good effect in treating a congested and sore throat. In cases of a peritonsillar abscess with difficulty in food intake, fluid transfusion should be applied, and if pus has been formed surgical management should be resorted to.
2. The patient should avoid smoking, alcohol and a sour or spicy, or irritating diet.

8. MYOPIA

Myopia, in the ancient medical classics, is known as a near sightedness with an inability to see distant objects. Myopia and astigmatism are both eye diseases classified as ametropia.

Myopia is due to a congenital insufficiency or an acquired bad habit of using one's eyes— such as reading or writing at too short a distance, or taking an improper sitting position, or working under too strong or poor light. Clinically it is manifest as normal nearsightedness, but additionally distant objects are not seen distinctly.

TREATMENT

Needling and moxibustion

Principle of treatment.   To regulate the qi of the meridians supplying the eye region, by selecting adjacent and distal points in combination.

Prescription. Chengqi (St 1), Jingming (UB 1), Fengchi (GB 20), Yiming (Extra 11), Hegu (LI 4), Zusanli (St 36).

Method. The above points can be divided into two groups to be used alternately.

A certain slow insertion, gentle rotation, a retreat to the subcutaneous layer, and then a swift withdrawal of the needle followed by pressing the puncture hole with a cotton ball for one minute, is required for points in the eye region.

Hegu, Zusanli, Fengchi and Yiming are stimulated with rotation or lifting-thrusting of the needle, intermittent manipulation, and 20–30 minutes of needle retention.

It is necessary to have the needling sensation in Fengchi and Yiming radiate to the temporal, forehead or eye regions.

REMARKS

1. Acupuncture has a good effect in treating conditions such as myopia.
2. Pay attention to personal hygiene in using the eyes.

E. Emergency diseases

1. SYNCOPE

Syncope refers to sudden and temporary loss of consciousness. Such fainting may be due to deficiency of vital qi, or failure of qi and blood.

It may be due to recovery from illness, or massive blood-loss in labour, or overstrain or sudden change of position from squatting to standing, in which the qi and blood of the jingluo fail to ascend in time to nourish the brain and the yang qi fails to reach the extremities.

Alternatively it may be due to an abnormal emotional disturbance, or severe pain in trauma, which gives rise to temporary rebelling of the passage of the qi, and disturbance of the qi and blood circulation, affecting the brain and leading to sudden syncope.

Symptoms. Subjective weakness and lassitude at the onset, followed by blacking-out before the eyes, nausea and sudden loss of consciousness, accompanied by pallor, profuse sweating, cold limbs, a thready and slowed-down pulse, and lowering of blood pressure.

TREATMENT

Needling and moxibustion

Principle of treatment. Mainly to promote resuscitation or restore consciousness.

Prescription. Renzhong (Du 26), Hegu (LI 4), Zusanli (St 36), Zhongchong (P 9).

Explanation. Renzhong lies at the juncture of the Ren and Du meridians, on the Du meridian which runs up to the vertex and enters the brain. It is used to communicate with the qi of the yin and yang meridians, and is stimulated by rotating the needle in order to promote resuscitation.

Zhongchong is the Jing-well point of the hand Jueyin and is located at the tip of the middle finger. It is punctured to regulate the qi of the yin and yang meridians and is an important point for treating syncope.

Hegu and Zusanli are respectively the *yuan* and He-sea points of the hand and foot Yangming, which are rich in qi and blood. They are stimulated using a reinforcing method of needling in order to promote the qi and blood upwardly along the meridians to promote resuscitation and clear the mind.

In cases with cold limbs, moxibustion can be applied to Baihui (Du 20) and Qihai (Ren 6) to warm the four extremities.

Ear needling

Points. Heart, Brain, Lower apex of tragus, Ear-Shenmen.

Method. After manipulation of the needles for a short while, retain the needles for 20 minutes.

REMARKS

1. In managing such cases, first let the patient lie flat at once; unbutton the clothing yet keep the patient warm.
2. Besides needling and moxibustion, a detailed examination should be given to ascertain the

cause of the syncope so that measures can be adopted accordingly.

3. Needling and moxibustion have a good effect in treating syncope caused by pain in traumatic injury, and can be applied as temporary measures in treating syncope due to other causes.

2. PROSTRATION SYNDROME

Prostration syndrome corresponds to shock in modern medicine, and it is an acute, violent and critical condition in onset and severity.

It is often due to profuse sweating, violent vomiting or diarrhoea, massive loss of blood, or long-term accumulation of epidemic mild-heat or heat, which severely damages the qi, blood and body fluid.

Otherwise it is due to a congenital deficiency of vital yang and being affected by severe pathogenic cold, when the antipathogenic qi fails to fight against the pathogenic qi and yang qi prostration occurs.

Both of the above two causes may lead to collapse of yin and yang, and they are sometimes called "prostration of yin" and "prostration of yang".

DIFFERENTIATION

Pallor, apathy or coma, cold limbs, sweating, and drop in blood pressure.

If accompanied by feeble breathing, cyanosis of the lips, a flabby tongue, and a thready and forceless, or hollow and big pulse, it is a syndrome of prostration of yang.

If accompanied by irritability, thirst, dry and red lips and tongue, and a thready-rapid or thready, rapid and forceless pulse, it is a syndrome of prostration of yin.

In deteriorating cases, the critical condition of prostration of both yin and yang often results.

TREATMENT

Needling and moxibustion

Principle of treatment. To promote resuscitation and restore the collapsed yang.

Prescription. Suliao (Du 25), Neiguan (P 6).

Modification.
— Coma: Renzhong (Du 26), Zhongchong (P 9), Yongquan (K 1).
— Cold limbs and fading pulse: apply moxibustion to Baihui (Du 20), Shenque (Ren 8), Guanyuan (Ren 4).

Explanation. Suliao from the Du meridian, and Neiguan from the pericardium meridian, are connected with the Yinwei meridian. They are stimulated with a continuous manipulation of the needles, and have the effect of raising the blood pressure and improving the cardiac function. They are used as main points.

Renzhong from the Du meridian is used to promote resuscitation and to raise the blood pressure as well. It is mostly indicated for syncope due to qi rebellion, and coma or unconsciousness.

Zhongchong and Yongquan are Jing-well points of the pericardium and kidney meridians respectively. They are used to promote resuscitation and relieve unconsciousness when there are cold limbs, and clear heat.

Baihui, Shenque and Guanyuan from the Ren and Du meridians are used with moxibustion to restore the depleted yang and the pulse.

Ear needling

Points. Lower apex of tragus, Antihypotensive point, Occiput, Heart, Brain.

Method. Points are used alternately, 2–3 points each time, with intermittent needle manipulation during a needle retention of 1–2 hours.

REMARK

Prostration syndrome or shock can be caused by various factors, with a sudden onset and complicated conditions of disease. Different therapies should be applied according to the causative factors. Needling and moxibustion can be employed as one of the emergency measures.

3. HYPERPYREXIA

Hyperpyrexia or high fever refers to a high body

temperature over 39°C tested with an oral thermometer. It is often seen in acute infection, acute contagious diseases, parasitosis, sunstroke, rheumatic fever, tuberculosis and malignant tumour.

Hyperpyrexia is a commonly seen emergency condition, and acupuncture can be employed as one of the measures in treating this disease.

TREATMENT

Principle of treatment. To dispel *feng* and clear heat.

Prescription. Dazhui (Du 14), Quchi (LI 11), Hegu (LI 4), Shaoshang (Lu 11).

Modification.
— Coma: Renzhong (Du 26), Shixuan (Extra 24).
— Irritability: Yintang (Extra 2), Shenmen (H 7).

Explanation. This prescription is set to dispel *feng* and clear heat. A reducing method of needling is applied on Dazhui, Quchi and Hegu, which has a remarkable effect in relieving fever. Dazhui clears heat and replenishes qi and it is indicated in strong fevers and chills. Quchi, being the He-sea point of the Yangming, is indicated for fever and thirst.

Hegu is used to clear heat and dispel *feng*. It is especially good for *feng* heat affecting the head and face.

Shaoshang, the Jing-well point of the lung meridian, is pricked to cause bleeding, so as to clear lung heat and ease the throat. It is indicated for a sore throat due to *feng* heat.

In cases of coma, Renzhong is used with needle rotation for a short while, and the Shixuan are pricked to cause bleeding. Together these points are used to promote resuscitation and purge heat.

Yintang and Shenmen are important points for calming the heart and mind, and can be used to treat irritability.

4. MUSCULAR CONVULSIONS

Convulsions refer to violent, involuntary muscular contractions or spasms of the limbs. Also there are accompanying symptoms of rigidity of the neck (the nape), opisthotonos, or loss of consciousness during the attacks, or coma after the attack.

This disease is clinically divided into pyretic convulsions and apyretic convulsions. The former are often due to epidemic mild-heat and heat affecting the *ying* and blood systems, or else pathogenic heat affecting the pericardium along with excessive heat stirring up internal *feng*; while the latter are due to a deficiency in the spleen with impaired transportation giving rise to an accumulation of body fluid, which is then condensed into *tan*, or else spleen yang deficiency and chronic diarrhoea consuming body fluid, which gives rise to stirring of liver *feng* and *tan* misting the collaterals and mind, finally resulting in convulsions and perhaps coma.

This disease is often seen in infantile convulsions, epidemic febrile diseases in which the *ying* and blood systems are affected by pathogens, tetanus, epilepsy, craniocerebral traumatic injuries and hysteria.

TREATMENT

Principle of treatment. To subdue *feng*, tranquillize the convulsions, clear heat and restore consciousness. Select points mainly from the Du meridian.

Prescription. Yintang (Extra 2), Baihui (Du 20), Dazhui (Du 14), Jinsuo (Du 8), Hegu (LI 4), Houxi (SI 3), Taichong (Liv 3), Shenmai (UB 62).

Modification.
— Fever: Dazhui (Du 14), Quchi (LI 11).
— Coma: Renzhong (Du 26), Shixuan (Extra 24).
— Excessive *tan*: Neiguan (P 6), Fenglong (St 40).

Method. Points in the above prescription can be used by selecting only some of them, or using them alternately in groups.

Transverse insertion with an intermittent manipulation of the needles is used on Yintang, Baihui and Renzhong. Pricking to cause bleeding is applied onto the Shixuan.

REMARK

Acupuncture can be employed as a temporary

treatment for this emergency. The causative factors should be identified so as to give appropriate treatment according to the concrete conditions.

5. ACUTE PAIN

Various analgesic effects of acupuncture have been proven through long-term practice by the ancient physicians, and large numbers of clinical trials and experiments during modern times.

The acupuncture treatment of headache, toothache, trigeminal neuralgia and sciatica has been introduced in previous sections. Now the treatment of other commonly seen diseases which involve acute pain is discussed.

ANGINA PECTORIS

Angina pectoris is due to insufficient blood supply to the heart muscle, leading to cardiac muscular anoxia. It is marked by a sudden onset of severe pain in the left chest behind the sternum, which may radiate to the left neck, shoulder and medial aspect of the left upper arm, accompanied by a contracting sensation in the chest, sweating and fear.

Treatment

Prescription. Neiguan (P 6), Tiantu (Ren 22), Shanzhong (Ren 17), Xinshu (UB 15), Jueyinshu (UB 14).
Method. 2–3 points are selected each time. Manipulate the needles for 30 seconds or several minutes by rotating them, then retain them for 15–20 minutes.

ACUTE CHOLECYSTITIS AND CHOLELITHIASIS

Cholecystitis and cholelithiasis can appear at the same time. The attack is marked by sudden pain in the right hypochondrium and upper right abdomen which is persistently and paroxysmally aggravated and radiates to the right scapular region. It is accompanied by nausea and vomiting. There is an obvious tenderness and muscular tension in the right upper abdomen where the gallbladder is located, and the enlarged gallbladder can sometimes be palpated.

If it is complicated by cholangitis, jaundice and high fever may appear.

Treatment

Prescription. Yanglingquan (GB 34), Zhongwan (Ren 12), Danshu (UB 19).

Modification.
— Vomiting: Neiguan (P 6), Zusanli (St 36).
— Flank pain: Riyue (GB 24), Taichong (Liv 3).

Method. 2–4 points are used each time. A reducing method is applied to all the points, with intermittent manipulation of the needles during the retention period of 30 minutes to one hour.

BILIARY ASCARIASIS

Marked by a sudden onset of paroxysmal violent colic-type pain in the middle and upper right abdomen, and a kind of boring, penetrating sensation at the xiphoid process of the sternum. It is accompanied by vomiting, sometimes with roundworms vomited out, profuse sweating and cold limbs which occurs with the pain. The pain may last several minutes or hours, and several attacks of pain may occur in one day; during the intervals there is stuffiness and a distending sensation.

Palpation of the abdomen shows no muscular tension, only slight tenderness in the deep region.

Treatment

Needling and moxibustion

Prescription. Yingxiang (LI 20), Dannangxue (Extra 46), Renzhong (Du 26), Yanglingquan (GB 34).

Modification.
— Vomiting: Neiguan (P 6), Zusanli (St 36).
— Expelling roundworms: Sifeng (Extra 23), Daheng (Sp 15).

Method. 2–4 points are used each time. Use all of them with a reducing method of needling, with a retention of 30 minutes. A rotation of the needle is applied, with the needle inserted from Yingxiang towards Sibai.

Ear needling

Points. Gallbladder, tip of inferior antihelix crus, Liver, Duodenum.

Method. Each time 2–3 points are punctured with a reducing method by rotating the needles, with needle retention for 20–30 minutes.

RENAL COLIC

Marked by a sudden onset of colic-type pain which radiates from the kidney area in the lower back to the abdomen and scrotum on the same side, and medial aspect of the thigh. It is accompanied by cold sweating, nausea and vomiting. There is percussive pain in the renal region.

Treatment

Needling and moxibustion

Prescription. Shenshu (UB 23), Sanyinjiao (Sp 6), Zhishi (UB 52), Taixi (K 3), Jingmen (GB 25), Yinlingquan (Sp 9).

Method. One point is selected from the lumbar region and the lower limb (points can be used alternately). Apply a reducing method of needling, with continuous manipulation of needles for 3–5 minutes. Otherwise, apply electroneedling onto Shenshu and Sanyinjiao for 5–10 minutes.

Ear needling

Points. Kidney, Ureter, Brain, tip of inferior antihelix crus.

Method. Manipulate the needles for 3–5 minutes.

REMARKS

1. Comprehensive measures should be applied in case of persistent attacks of angina pectoris due to suspected myocardial infarction. In some cases the renal colic cannot be relieved even after the acupuncture treatment has been applied.

2. In cases of empyema of the gallbladder, purulent cholangitis and obstruction by a large biliary stone, strict observation is needed and an operation should be resorted to as early as possible.

6. HAEMORRHAGE

Haemorrhage includes various diseases which involve bleeding in different parts of the body, such as haemoptysis, haematemesis, epistaxis and haematuria. It can be seen in various kinds of diseases of different organs.

It is divided into two types. The excessive syndrome is due to excessive heat in the stomach, dryness in the lung and excessive fire of the heart and liver, which propels the blood into circulation in an abnormal manner, leading to extravasation of blood.

The deficiency syndrome is mainly due to yin deficiency of the lung and kidney, which causes stirring of empty fire. This injures the collaterals and results in extravasation of blood. Otherwise it is due to qi deficiency of the spleen and stomach, failing to control blood.

HAEMOPTYSIS

Haemoptysis refers to blood discharged from the mouth owing to bleeding of the trachea, bronchi and pulmonary tissues.

In mild cases of haemoptysis, there is only blood-tinged sputum; in severe cases there is haemoptysis in large amounts, and after the bleeding has been checked, persistent bloody sputum can be seen.

Treatment

Prescription. Chize (Lu 5), Kongzui (Lu 6), Yuji (Lu 10), Feishu (UB 13), Zusanli (St 36), Taixi (K 3).

Method. 3–4 points are selected each time,

with an even method of needling. Retain the needles for 20–30 minutes.

HAEMATEMESIS

Haematemesis is vomiting blood, and is a clinical manifestation of bleeding of the upper digestive tract. It is often seen in bleeding due to gastric or duodenal ulcers, and with the complication of cirrhosis of the liver. The blood of haematemesis is fresh red or brown in colour and mixed with food. This disease is accompanied by a tarry stool which may be either formed or else like paste.

Treatment

Prescription.   Shangwan (Ren 13), Daling (E 7), Ximen (P 4), Shenmen (H 7), Yuji (Lu 10).
Method.   3–5 points are selected, and a reinforcing or reducing method is applied according to the condition of deficiency or excess. Retain the needle for 20–30 minutes.

EPISTAXIS

This is a commonly seen clinical symptom; it can be seen in febrile diseases, haemopathy, hypertension, hepatocirrhosis, uraemia and disorders of the nose cavity itself. In mild cases there is nasal discharge tinged with blood, in severe cases incessant nasal bleeding.

Treatment

Prescription. Dazhui (Du 14), Shangxing (Du 23), Yingxiang (LI 20), Hegu (LI 4), Shaoshang (Lu 11).
Method.   2–4 points are selected with an even method of needling. Retain the needles for 20–30 minutes. Bloodletting can be applied to Dazhui and Shaoshang, and moxibustion can be used on Shangxing.

HAEMATOCHEZIA

Blood discharged from the anus is known as haematochezia. The amount of blood may vary and the blood be fresh red or dim red in colour. It is often seen in haemorrhoids, prolapse of the rectum, anal fissure, intestinal ulcers or inflammation, tumour or polyp of the rectum or colon.

Treatment

Prescription. Pishu (UB 20), Dachangshu (UB 25), Zhongliao (UB 33), Changqiang (Du 1), Guanyuan (Ren 4), Sanyinjiao (Sp 6).
Method.   3–4 points are selected and a reinforcing or even method is applied. Retain the needles for 20–30 minutes.

HAEMATURIA

This is urine tinged with blood. In mild cases, haematuria can be observed only under microscopic examination of the urine, hence it is known as microscopic haematuria. It is often due to renal tuberculosis, urinary calculi, nephritis and tumours.

Treatment

Prescription. Mingmen (Du 4), Shenshu (UB 23), Guanyuan (Ren 4), Zusanli (St 36), Liangqiu (St 34), Sanyinjiao (Sp 6).
Method.   3–4 points are selected, each of which is stimulated with an even or reinforcing method of needling. Retain the needles for 20–30 minutes. Moxibustion can be applied on Liangqiu.

REMARKS

1. In the above haemorrhagic diseases, a careful examination and diagnostic observation should be given and thus treatment given accordingly.
2. In cases of haematemesis accompanied by sweating, cold limbs, thready pulse and a drop in the blood pressure, acupuncture should be combined with other methods at once.
3. Needling and moxibustion have a decided effect in treating haemorrhage.

NOTES

1. *Plain Questions*, Ch. 43, "Discussion on Bi Syndrome".

2. *Miraculous Pivot*, Ch. 20, "The 5 Evil Pathogens".
3. *Plain Questions*, Ch. 44.
4. *Miraculous Pivot*, Ch. 24, "Discussion on Jue Disease".

APPENDICES

Appendix 1
Abstracts from classical literature on acupuncture and moxibustion

The Nine Needles, and 12 Yuan-source Points[1]

The Yellow Emperor asked Yu Qibo, "I love and cherish my people. I tax them and I always show sympathy towards them, as they often fall ill. Now I intend to treat them not with poisonous medicines or *bian* stone needles, but with filiform needles; by needling, the obstruction in the meridians can be removed and the qi and blood regulated.

At the same time I want this therapy to pass on from one generation to another. So we must set out the theory and principle of acupuncture to make it clear and easy to master. The theory should be described in different chapters, with a clear differentiation of exterior and interior, the starting and terminating points, and every aspect of it made clear and discussed. I think a Classic on acupuncture should be published. Now I want to listen to your opinion."

Qibo said: "Let me talk about this matter from beginning to the end. First the general rules for treating diseases with acupuncture, which are easy to say, but difficult to follow perfectly. An inferior practitioner only knows how to carry on the rules mechanically without adapting them, while a superior physician can manipulate the needle with reinforcing and reducing techniques, according to the conditions of the vital qi and the patient. This is because qi and blood circulate in meridians through openings, and it is just by these openings that the pathogenic factors invade the body. If the physician doesn't study the conditions, how can he decide on the treatment for each different patient?

As for the acupuncture effect, it lies not only in the "rapid-slow" reinforcing and reducing method, but also in the perfect selection of points, i.e. an inferior doctor only treats disease by puncturing the points around the four joints; while a superior doctor selects points according to the conditions of pathogenic factors and antipathogenic qi, which can be known by observing the meridional qi through the points, because it flows in the meridians through points. When pathogenic factors affect the body they will circulate in the meridians together with the meridional qi, and thus some change will take place in the meridional qi which can be observed at the points.

But this change is so delicate that it can't be discovered unless enough care is taken. If the pathogen is vigorous, puncturing with reinforcing is not allowed to avoid keeping the pathogen in; and if the pathogen has gone and the patient is in a weak state, puncturing with reducing is not permitted so as not to damage the vital qi.

Understanding this relation between the two, the practitioner will treat the patient with a perfect manipulation; otherwise he will have the feeling of holding a dart in his hand without knowing when to release it.

But how to perform these reinforcing and reducing methods? First we should know the course of the meridian, then we can direct the needle either against the meridian to dispel the pathogen or along the meridian to strengthen the body's resistance. This is the method of reinforcing and reducing achieved by directing the needle tip along the meridian, and actually the main reason for treating disease with acupuncture.

What a pity that the inferior doctor does not know the indications for reinforcing and reducing! Usually reinforcing is used to treat deficiency syndromes, and reducing is used to treat excess syndromes or blood stasis. But the sequence of the reinforcing and reducing depends on the emergence of the illness, the conditions of vital qi and time of needling.

If all these are considered, then, when reinforcing is performed the patient will feel as he is being given something, and when reducing is performed he will feel that he has lost something.

Among all the kinds of needles, the nine kinds of needles are the most suitable for performing the reinforcing and reducing method. When reducing is applied, the needle is inserted swiftly into the point; after the qi arrives, the needle is withdrawn slowly and shaken to enlarge the hole in order to expel the pathogenic factors. When reinforcing is applied, the needle is inserted gently as if a mosquito pierced the skin, and the needle thrust in with the tip directed along the meridian; after the qi arrives, the needle is removed as swift as an arrow leaving a bow. All these must be done with two hands: the right hand holds the needle while the left hand presses the hole to keep the meridional qi inside the body and invigorate the *zong* qi, or pectoral qi. If there is bleeding, remove the needle at once.

The result of the acupuncture is also related to many other aspects, such as holding the needle firmly, inserting the needle without deviation, observing the patient's complexion and reaction, and avoiding needling the blood vessels.

Concerning the needles themselves, they are nine kinds in all, which are named differently according to their shape. The first is called the "sagittal needle" and it is about 1.6 cun long; the second is called the "ovoid-tipped needle", and is about 1.6 cun long; the third is the "grain-tipped" needle, about 3.5 cun long; the fourth is the "ensiform needle", about 1.6 cun long; the fifth is the "sword-shaped needle", about 4 cun long and 2.5 fen in diameter; the 6th is the "round-sharp needle", about 1.6 cun long; the seventh is the "filiform needle", about 3.6 cun long; the eighth is the "long needle", about 7 cun long; and the ninth is the "large needle", about 4 cun long.

Because they are different in length their functions are various, i.e. the sagittal needle is suitable for puncturing superficially to dispel pathogenic heat from the exterior; the ovoid-tip needle is used to massage muscular disorders to expel pathogens from the meridian, but care should be taken not to injure the muscles; the grain-tipped needle is advised for massage along the meridian to promote qi circulation, but it can't be thrust deeply into the muscles otherwise the body resistance is weakened; the three-edged ensiform needle is suitable for treating intractable diseases; the sword-shaped needle is used to needle large carbuncles to remove pus; the round-sharp needle, shaped like a horse's tail with a round-sharp tip and thick body, is advised when treating acute diseases; the filiform needle is suitable for numbness and pain for it has a thin tip and a long body, which can be retained for the arrival of qi; the long needle with a sharp tip and long thin body can be applied to treat prolonged arthralgia; the large needle, whose tip is sharp and whose body is thick like a walking-stick, can be used to remove fluid from the joints. Such are the shapes and functions of the nine kinds of needles.

Knowing the above is not enough; other things are also very important, such as the condition of the patient, indications for reinforcing and reducing, etc.

Usually pathogenic factors obey the following rules when they invade the body: *feng* and heat invade the upper portion, food accumulates in the middle portion and cold and damp invade below. So the treatment should be adapted according to the conditions: that is, to puncture the points on the upper portion to dispel *feng* and heat, and to needle the He-sea point of the Yangming (St 36) to relieve food retained in the stomach and intestines. But be careful not to insert the needle too deeply, otherwise the pathogen will be led in deeper and the disease aggravated. Therefore the depth of insertion should be well considered—usually this is decided on the basis of the anatomy and the conditions of the pathogenic factor.

Now how about indications for reinforcing and reducing? First let's see some examples. If a patient is suffering from insufficient vital essence, then reducing while the Shu points are needled must result in death due to yin deficiency; but if a patient is suffering from insufficient yang qi, then reducing the points of yang meridians must lead to mental disorder due to deficiency of vital essence. Generally speaking, needling the points of yin meridians with reducing, by mistake, exhausts the zang qi, resulting in death; whilst needling the points of yang meridians with reducing, by mistake, wastes the yang qi, resulting in madness. Such is the harm done by mistakenly reinforcing and reducing!

The arrival of the qi is rather significant in the treatment of disease with acupuncture, as it is the sign of effect. So if the qi fails to arrive during treatment, wait for it, by manipulating the needle, without caring how often this is done. When the qi arrives, the needle can be removed. But all this can be done only with the proper needles, thus the practitioner must select the needle according to the conditions."

Yellow Emperor went on to say: "I want to know something about where the qi of the zangfu organs emerges".

Qibo answered: "This is connected with the Shu points of the meridians. Among the meridians there are 5 Shu points for each of the 5 meridians of the zang organs, 25 Shu points in all. But for the meridians of the 6 fu organs, there are 6 Shu points, making 36 Shu points in all. As for the jingluo, there are 12 regular meridians (jing) and 15 large collaterals (luo). So there are 27 kinds of meridional qi running through the body.

The point where the meridional qi starts to bubble up is called the Jing-well point, the point where the meridional qi starts to gush is called the Ying-spring point, where the qi is flushing through is the Shu-stream point, the point where the qi is pouring in abundantly is the Jing-river point, and the point where the qi is most flourishing is the He-sea point: it is just through these Shu points that the qi of the 27 meridians circulates. Besides, there are another 365 covering points in the spaces between the joints of the human body. If one understands this, he will feel it easy to grasp the points.

Before treating the disease, the practitioner must try to differentiate the conditions of the pathogenic factors and antipathogenic factors by observing the patient's complexion, eyes, movement, voice and by feeling the pulse; otherwise, the wrong treatment may be adopted.

For example, in treating enfeebled qi of the 5 zang organs due to yin deficiency, if the practitioner applies reinforcing while puncturing the points of yang meridians on the axillary and pectoral regions, the treatment may cause the yang qi to be more vigorous and the yin qi more insufficient, leading to further exhaustion, which must end in a "quiet" death.

Another example is in treating insufficient yang in disorders of the 5 zang organs. If the practitioner employs reinforcing on the points of the yin meridians on the four limbs, this treatment may cause the yin qi to become vigorous and the yang qi to sink, resulting in prostration with cold limbs, which must lead to a restless death. All these result from misusing reinforcing and reducing on the meridians.

Besides this, an improper withdrawal of the needle is also the cause of accidents. For instance, a mistake made in retaining the needle after the arrival of qi may induce the essential qi out, resulting in an aggravation of the disease; or else, withdrawing the needle before the arrival of qi may fail to dispel the pathogen, giving rise to carbuncles.

The 5 zang organs are connected with the 6 fu organs, and on the 12 meridians of the zangfu organs there are 12 *yuan* points, which are located at the joints and can be used to treat disorders of the zangfu. This is because they are nourished by the essential qi of the zangfu and have a close relationship with them. When the zangfu organs are affected, signs may show in these 12 *yuan* points. So by observing these points, one can judge the conditions of the zangfu.

The following are the 12 *yuan* points of the zang organs: the lung's *yuan* point is Taiyuan (Lu 9), one on either hand; the heart's *yuan* point is Daling (P 7), one on either hand; the liver's is Taichong (Liv 3); the spleen's is Taibai (Sp 3); the kidney's is Taixi (K 3); the *Gao's* (膏) is Jiuwei (Ren 15) and the *Huang's* (肓) is Qihai (Ren 6); these two points plus the two *yuan* points of each zang organ are the 12 *yuan* points. They are dominant in treating disorders of the zangfu, i.e. abdominal distension is treated by needling the *yuan* points on the three yang meridians of foot, and lienteric diarrhoea is stopped by puncturing the *yuan* points on the three yin meridians.

When the zangfu organs are disturbed by the pathogenic factors, it is as if someone has a thorn thrust into them, or an object is dirtied, an overhand knot is made in a rope or a river is blocked off. Although this condition may remain for a long time, yet the thorn can be removed, the dirt can be washed away, the knot can be untied, and the blockage removed. So it is with the human body, a physician well versed in acupuncture can treat disease just like solving these problems. There is no disease that cannot be cured unless a poor manipulation is performed.

For example, to treat febrile disease, the points should be punctured superficially and rapidly as if the hand touched boiling water, but to treat a disease of a cold nature, the points should be inserted into deeply and the needle retained in the point as if it were a lingering visitor, forgetting to return home.

For diseases due to heat pathogens in the yin

system, Zusanli (St 36) is selected and the needle manipulated and withdrawn after the pathogen is expelled. If there is no response, the point is punctured again. If the affected site is in the upper portion or related to zang organs, the He-sea point of the foot Taiyin, Yinlingquan (SP 9), is needled; if the disease is located in the upper portion or related to fu organs, the He-sea point, Yanglingquan (GB 34), is punctured."

Explaining the Filiform Needle[2]

This article is specially written to explain the filiform needle mentioned above in the chapter "On the Nine Needles, and 12 Yuan-source Points".

The filiform needle is something easier to talk about than manipulate. An inferior doctor only knows how to follow the needling rules mechanically and the points he selects are just limited to those on the four limbs. This is because he does not consider the condition of the qi and blood, the pathogenic and antipathogenic factors. But a superior doctor knows the importance of differentiating the condition of the qi and blood, the pathogenic and anti-pathogenic factors; so when he treats diseases, he always makes these conditions quite clear, and then analyses which meridian the disease pertains to and selects the acupoints for treatment.

As a superior doctor, he must understand the condition of the patient and master the technique of "rapid-slow" manipulation of the needle. When a point is punctured, the needling sensation must be obtained. When the pathogenic factors are vigorous, reducing must be adopted instead of reinforcing, and when the antipathogenic qi is weakened, reinforcing must be employed instead of reducing. A feeble pulse felt at the qikou (气口), the radial pulse at the wrist, pertains to a deficiency syndrome, so reinforcing is applicable; a forceful pulse at the qikou pertains to an excess syndrome, so reducing is applicable. Reducing is also suitable for removing blood stasis and pathogenic factors.

But since the pathogenic factors affect the body at differing sites, treatment should also be varied. For example, pathogenic factors in-

vading the body from the upper portion are simply termed pathogenic qi—which should be treated by needling points on the upper portion. The middle portion is the place where the turbid qi stays, and if this is portion is disturbed, disease may result. Thus "turbid" is the way the pathogenic factor in the middle portion is described, and it should be treated by selecting points in the middle portion. Cold or damp pathogens often invade the body from the feet, giving rise to disease, so this pathogen is called the "clear" pathogenic factor.

As for the reinforcing and reducing methods, they are performed differently. Reinforcing is applied by pointing the needle-tip along the meridian, and inserting the needle slowly yet withdrawing it rapidly; the patient may feel a warmth under the needle and as if he were given something. Reducing is employed by pointing the needle-tip against the meridian, and inserting the needle swiftly yet removing it gently; the patient may feel a coolness and hollowness under the needle, as if he had lost something.

Besides this, attention should be paid to the insertion of the needle. A superficially located disease cannot be treated by inserting the needle deeply, otherwise an aggravation of the disease may appear, causing death due to exhaustion of the kidney yin or yang qi.

To be a superior doctor, just knowing the things mentioned above is not enough. He must also know how to differentiate the cause and condition of the illness by observing the complexion, feeling the pulse, and applying auscultation and olfaction. At the same time he concentrates his mind on manipulating the needle.

The Source of the Shu Points[3]

The Yellow Emperor said to Qibo: "A doctor who practises acupuncture must know the course of the 12 regular jingluo, the location of the 5 Shu points of the zangfu organs, the variation of the qi and blood at the different seasons, and the diameter, location and distribution of the meridians. Now I want to have you explain to me all these subjects."

Qibo answered: "Let me first say something about the Shu points of the zangfu.

The meridional qi of the lung starts to bubble in Shaoshang (Lu 11) on the medial aspect of the thumb, which is the Jing-well point pertaining to wood; then the qi starts to gush in Yuji (Lu 10) on the midpoint of the first metacarpal bone, which is the Shu-stream point; later it is pouring abundantly in Jingqu (Lu 8) at the *cunkou* (寸口) where the pulse is felt, which is the Jing-river point; and lastly the qi is most flourishing in Chize (Lu 5) near the artery of the elbow, which is the He-sea point. These are the 5 Shu points of the hand Taiyin.

Then the Jing-well point of the heart meridian is Zhongchong (P 9) on the end of the middle finger, which pertains to wood; the Ying-spring point is Laogong (P 8) on the centre of the palm; the Shu-stream point is Daling (P 7) on the centre of the transverse crease of the palmar side; the Jing-river point is Jianshi (P 5), 3 cun posterior to the transverse crease, where the pulse can be felt only when the meridian is affected; then the He-sea point is Quze (P 3) on the interior aspect of the elbow, and located with the arm flexed. These are the 5 Shu points of the hand Shaoyin meridian.

As for the liver meridian, the Jing-well point is Dadun (Liv 1) on the end of the big toe, pertaining to wood; and Xingjian (Liv 2) on the big toe is the Ying-spring point; Taichong (Liv 3) in the depression 2 cun above Xingjian is the Shu-stream point; then Zhongfeng (Liv 4) in the depression 1.5 cun anterior to the medial malleolus is the Jing-river point; and Ququan (Liv 8) on the medial end of the transverse crease of the knee is the He-sea point. Those are the 5 Shu points of the foot Jueyin.

Next, Yinbai (Sp 1) on the medial end of the big toe is the Jing-well point of the spleen meridian, which pertains to wood; Dadu (Sp 2) in the depression posterior to the basic joint is the Ying-spring point; and Taibai (Sp 3) inferior to the bony nodule is the Shu-stream point; Shangqiu (Sp 5) in the depression inferior to the medial malleolus is the Jing-river point; then Yinlingquan (Sp 9) in the depression on the medial border of the tibia is the He-sea point; those are the 5 Shu points of the foot Taiyin.

Yongquan (K 1) in the centre of the sole is the Jing-well point of the kidney meridian, which pertains to wood; Rangu (K 2) in the depression on the lower border of the tuberosity of the navicular bone is the Ying-spring point, and Taixi (K 3) in the depression between the medial malleolus and tendo calcaneus is the Shu-stream point; Fuliu (K 7) 2 cun superior to the medial malleolus is the Jing-river point; and Yingu (K 10) on the medial side of the popliteal fossa is the He-sea point; those are the 5 Shu points of the foot Shaoyin.

Then the yang meridians. Zhiyin (UB 67) on the end of the small toe is the Jing-well point of the bladder meridian, which pertains to metal; Zutonggu (UB 66) on the lateral side of the small toe is the Ying-spring point; Shugu (UB 65) in the depression posterior to the basal joint is the Shu-stream point; and Jinggu (UB 64) below the tuberosity of the fifth metatarsal bone is the *yuan* point, where the source qi is retained; then Kunlun (UB 60) in the depression between the external malleolus and tendo calcaneus is the Jing-river point; Weizhong (UB 40) on the midpoint of the transverse crease of the popliteal fossa is the He-sea point; these are the Shu points of the foot Taiyang.

Then Zuqiaoyin (GB 44) on the end of the fourth toe is the Jing-well point of the gallbladder meridian, which pertains to metal; Xiaxi (GB 43) between the fifth and fourth toes is the Ying-spring point; Zulinqi (GB 41) in the depression 1.5 cun superior to Xiaxi is the Shu-stream point; Qiuxu (GB 40) in the depression anterior and inferior to the external malleolus is the *yuan* point; Yanglingquan (GB 34) in the depression lateral to the knee joint is the He-sea point; these are the Shu points of the foot Shaoyang.

Lidui (St 45) on the end of the second toe is the Jing-well point of the stomach meridian which pertains to metal; Neiting (St 44) on the exterior side of the second toe is the Ying-spring point, and the *yuan* point is Chongyang (St 42) in the depression between the second and third metatarsal bones; Jiexi (St 41) in the depression 2 cun above Chongyang is the Jing-river point; and Zusanli (St 36) 3 cun inferior to the knee is the He-Sea point; besides this, Shangjuxu (St 37) 3 cun inferior to Zusanli and Xiajuxu (St 39)

3 cun inferior to Shangjuxu are the lower He-Sea points of the large intestine and small intestine respectively, for they connect with the stomach inside the body.

The qi of the Sanjiao coming up to the hand Shaoyang starts to bubble in Guanchong (SJ 1) on the end of the ring finger, which is known as the Jing-well point, pertaining to metal; Yemen (SJ 2) between the small finger and fourth finger is the Ying-spring point; Zhongzhu (SJ 3) in the depression posterior to the basal joint of the ring finger is the Shu-stream point; Yangchi (SJ 4) in the depression within the transverse crease of the wrist is the *yuan* point; Zhigou (SJ 6) 3 cun posterior to the transverse crease is the Jing-river point; and Jianjing (SJ 10) in the depression 1 cun superior to the olecranon is the He-sea point.

The meridional qi of the Sanjiao also goes down between the meridians of the foot Taiyang and the foot Shaoyang to the lower part of the body and emerges from Weiyang (UB 40). The meridian here is still called the Shaoyang but, at the same time, it is the collateral of the foot Taiyang, for it is supported both by the foot Shaoyang and Taiyang. It diverges from the foot Taiyang at a place 5 cun superior to the external malleolus, passing through the belly of the leg and emerging from Weiyang (UB 40), combining itself with the meridional qi of the foot Taiyang, which runs up to the abdomen to connect with the bladder. It functions in controlling the lower-jiao. When its qi is excessive, oliguria takes place, which should be treated with reducing; and when its qi is insufficient, anuria occurs, which should be treated with reinforcing.

The qi of the small intestine comes up to the meridian of the hand Shaoyang. Shaoze (SI 1) on the end of the small finger is the Jing-well point of the Small Intestine meridian, which pertains to metal; Qiangu (SI 2) in the depression anterior to the basal joint on the exterior side is the Ying-spring point; Houxi (SI 3) posterior to the basal joint of the small finger is the Shu-stream point; the *yuan* point is Wangu (SI 4) anterior to the carpal bone on the exterior side; the Jing-river point is Yanggu (SI 5) in the depression posterior to the wrist; the last is the He-sea point, Xiaohai (SI 8), in the depression 0.5 cun away from the tip of the large elbow-bone; these are the Shu points of the hand Taiyang meridian.

Now comes the last fu organ, the large intestine, whose qi comes up to the hand Yangming and starts to bubble in Shangyang (LI 1) on the end of the index finger, which is the Jing-well point, pertaining to metal; and Erjian (LI 2) anterior to the basal joint of the index finger is the Ying-spring point; the *yuan* point is Hegu (LI 4) between the first and second metacarpal bones; and the Jing-river point is Yingxi (LI 5) in the depression on the transverse crease near the thumb; then the He-Sea point is Quchi (LI 11) in the depression of the radius lateral to the elbow; such are the Shu points of the hand Yangming.

The above mentioned are all the important points of the 5 zang and 6 fu organs, 25 points for the zang organs and 36 points for the fu organs, among which the qi of the three fu organs goes up to the hand and emerges from the yang meridians of the hand.

Concerning the course of the meridians, let's see how the yang meridians are located around the neck. Between the left and right supra-clavicular fossa runs the Ren meridian, whose point is Tiantu (Ren 22). Then at regular intervals from the artery backwards, the meridians are located in the following order: firstly, the foot Yangming, whose point is Renying (St 9); the hand Yangming, whose point is Futu (LI 18); the hand Taiyang, Tianchuang (SI 16); the foot Shaoyang, Tianrong (SI 17); the hand Shaoyang, Tianyou (SJ 16); the foot Taiyang, Tianzhu (UB 10); then in the centre of the nape is the Du meridian, whose point is Fengfu (Du 16).

In addition to these, let's see the location of the two yin meridians; one is the hand Taiyin, which goes along the artery on the medial aspect of the arm under the axilla and whose point is Tianfu (Lu 3); the other is the Pericardium meridian of the hand Jueyin, which goes along the lateral side of the chest 5 cun below the axilla and whose point is Tianchi (P 1).

Knowing the location of the yang meridians around the neck, we'll see how they are distributed on the head. The foot Yangming meridian travels along the artery of the throat, some of the points are on the chest; the hand Yangming runs through the place which is 1 cun away from the cheek, and the hand Taiyang meridian goes through the cheek; next is the foot Shaoyang meridian, which goes beside the cheek, then the hand Shaoyang meridian which goes behind the ear, and the foot Taiyang which goes along the big tendon of the nape of the neck.

The meridians of the zangfu organs are connected with each other, so are the zangfu organs themselves. For instance, the lung is connected with the large intestine which is the organ transporting the digested food from the small intestine; the heart is connected with the small intestine, which receives food from the stomach; the liver is connected with the gallbladder, which is situated in the centre of the body to receive the clear liquid bile; the spleen is connected with the stomach, which digests food; the kidney is connected with the bladder, which functions to store urine; however the Sanjiao is like a water channel, transporting water to the bladder, thus the Sanjiao pertains to the bladder and both are controlled by the kidney. These are the connections between the zangfu organs.

There is another thing I want to mention—that is the variation of the needling method along with the four seasons. It is based on the depth of the meridional qi, the location of the pathogenic factors and the relation between the weather, the meridian and the zangfu organs. Usually the *luo* point and Ying-spring points are chosen in spring, with superficial insertion employed in mild cases and deep insertion in severe ones. In summer, the Shu-stream points and small luo (collaterals) are selected; and in autumn the He-sea points are chosen while other methods are the same as those in spring. The Jing-well points or Back-Shu points are punctured in winter and deep insertion and retention of the needle is employed.

When some points are needled, care should be taken, i.e. Shangguan (GB 3) should be needled with the mouth open, yet Xiaguan (St 7) with the mouth closed; also Dubi (St 35) is punctured with the knee flexed, Neiguan (P 6) and Waiguan (SJ 5) with the hand stretched. Besides this, spasm should be treated while the patient is standing, but flaccidity should be treated with the four limbs relaxed."

The Just Choice of the Needle[4]

"The key to acupuncture lies in selecting from the nine kinds of needles according to the conditions. Because they are shaped differently, they have differing functions and are selected to treat differing diseases. Otherwise no effect will be obtained.

For example, deep insertion with a long needle for a superficially located disease may injure the healthy muscle, resulting in carbuncles; while superficial insertion with a small needle for a deeply located disease cannot dispel the pathogen—on the contrary, it leads to the presence of lesions with pus. A large needle for a mild case may weaken the body resistance, aggravating the disease by too much reducing. A small needle for a severe case cannot eliminate the pathogen and may lead to other disorders. These are the mistakes made in selecting needles.

Now for the correct methods. If the disease is located superficially and erratically, a sagittal needle is selected. But if the local skin is pale or white, acupuncture is contraindicated. A round-sharp needle may be selected to treat a disease located in the muscles. An ensiform needle can be used to treat prolonged obstruction in the jingluo. If the disease is located in the meridians and caused by insufficient meridional qi, a grained-tip needle is used with the reinforcing method to massage the Jing-well, Ying-spring, Shu-stream, Jing-river and He-sea points of each meridian. A sword-shaped needle is selected to treat large swellings with pus. If an arthralgia-like syndrome suddenly occurs, puncture with a round-sharp needle. A filiform needle can be used to treat chronic painful joints. A long needle can be used to treat deeply located diseases.

If the patient is suffering from oedema in the joints, puncture the points with a large needle. If a chronic disease is caused by disorders of the 5 zang organs, use an ensiform needle to puncture the 5 Shu points of each meridian with the reducing method, selecting the points according to the four seasons.

There are nine types of needling for nine kinds of syndromes. The first is called "Shu point needling", when points are selected from the 5 Shu points of each meridian, and the Back-Shu points pertaining to the zangfu organs on the foot Taiyang. The second is called "remote needling" in which the points on the lower portion are selected to treat a disease located on the upper portion, mainly the points of the three yang foot meridians pertaining to the 6 fu organs. The third is called "jing needling" in which points on the connection between the jing (meridian) and the luo (collateral) are needled, because they are obstructed. The fourth is called "luo needling" in which small superficial luo are needled. The fifth is called "inter-muscular needling", in which meridional points deeply located in the muscles are needled. The sixth is called "drainage needling", in which a sword-shaped needle is used to treat large swellings with pus. The seventh is "filiform and cutaneous needling", in which points are selected on the right aspect to treat diseases on the left and vice versa. The ninth is "quenching needling", in which points are needled with a heated needle in order to treat numbness.

Besides this, there are 12 needling methods which are especially for treating the disorders of the 12 meridians. The first one is known as "paired needling", which is indicated in angina pectoris. The method is performed in this way—first try to find the tender spot on the chest, then one needle is inserted on the chest, the other on the back; the insertion should be oblique to avoid injuring the viscera. The second is known as "trigger needling", which is used for treating unlocalized pains by inserting a needle directly and retaining it till another painful trigger point is found with the left hand, then removing the needle and puncturing the second point. The third is known as "relaxing needling", which is to insert the needle around the muscle and manipulate the needle forward and backward, or up and down, to enlarge the hole and relax a spasm so as to treat muscular aching or spasm. The fourth is known as "triple needling", indicated in painful syndromes due to cold, where the affected site is small yet deeply located. The method is performed by inserting one needle in the centre of the affected site and two needles on either side. The method is also known as "punc-

turing by three needles". The fifth is known as "centre square needling", which is the method of inserting one needle superficially at the centre of the affected area and another four around it in a square shape. Indications are painful syndromes due to cold pathogens where the affected site is relatively large and superficially located.

The sixth is called "straight insertion", a method of inserting the needle with the skin pinched up, thrusting the needle along the skin, to treat disease due to superficial retention of cold. The seventh is called "rapid thrusting and lifting", indicated in heat syndromes with excessive qi, in which only a few points should be selected and the needle lifted and thrust rapidly. The eighth is called "short thrust needling" which is used to treat osseous rheumatism by inserting the needle gently, thrusting the needle slowly to the bone then thrusting and lifting the needle as if rubbing the bone. The ninth is called "superficial needling", which is to puncture the points lateral to the affected part to treat muscular spasms due to cold. The tenth is called "yin needling", which is for the treatment of cold syncope by puncturing bilaterally the points of the Shaoyin. The eleventh is called "jingluo needling", which is used to treat rheumatoid arthritis by inserting needles in pairs, one point on the jing (meridian) and the other on the luo (collateral). The twelfth is "repeated shallow needling", which is to insert and withdraw the needle perpendicularly, rapidly, superficially and repeatedly, to cause bleeding so as to treat carbuncles.

The points of the meridian located in a deep region should be punctured gently and the needle retained for a long time so as to promote the circulation of the meridional qi. The points of the meridian in a superficial region should be inserted by pressing the meridian with the finger nail, in order to achieve the aim of only expelling the pathogen and not letting out the vital essence. The method of obtaining needling sensation by thrusting the needle three times is performed thus—firstly insert the needle just under the skin to dispel the pathogen from the exterior, secondly thrust the needle to the muscle to expel the pathogen from the interior, thirdly thrust the needle deeply to obtain needling sensation. Thus a good physician must master a knowledge of the relationship between the weather and man, the conditions of the pathogenic qi and antipathogenic factors, and the formation of a deficiency and an excess.

There are another 5 needling techniques for treating disorders of the 5 zang organs. The first is called "shallow needling", which is to insert the needle very superficially and withdraw it swiftly as if plucking out a hair, so as not to injure the muscles. It is indicated in pulmonary tuberculosis. The second is called "leopard spot needling", which is to insert the needle around the affected area and prick to cause bleeding. This is for treating heart diseases. The third is called "joint needling", which is used to treat rheumatoid arthritis by inserting the needles on the end of the tendons near the joints, but bleeding is forbidden. This method is related to the liver. The fourth is called "joining valleys needling", which is to insert the needle first deeply then lift the needle to just under the skin and at the same time thrust another two needles obliquely, one to the right of the first and the other to the left, like the claws of a chicken. This is used for treating numbness and pain in the muscles, which is related to the spleen. The fifth is called "deep straight thrusting and lifting needling" which is used for treating numbness and pain in the bones. The method is related to the kidney."

Contralateral Needling[5]

Yellow Emperor said: "I have known about contralateral insertion but I don't know the meaning of it. What is it like?"

Qibo answered "Well, this needling method is created by recognizing the way in which pathogenic factors invade the body. Usually there are three steps—first they affect the skin; if they are not expelled there, they will go on to affect the minute luo (collaterals), then other luo, and then go into the jing (meridians), there they invade zang organs, and stop in the stomach and intestines. If both the yin and yang meridians are affected, the 5 zang organs will be disturbed. That is how the exogenous pathogen invades the body from the skin to the zang organs. Under such conditions, "jing needling" therapy is selected, that is to puncture the points of the affected jing.

Now if the exogenous pathogen invades the minute luo through the skin and stays there, an obstruction in the luo may form, blocking the way of the pathogen in its entry into the jing. Then the pathogen goes into the large luo, causing disease. When the pathogen invades the large luo from the left, it will go on further to the right and if it invades the large luo from the right, it will go on to affect the right. Sometimes it invades the upper portion, without having a fixed situation, and it doesn't affect the jing but only follows on to the large luo to the four limbs. When the pathogen localizes on the right of the body, the manifestation will appear on the left, and when it invades the left part of the body, the manifestation appears on the right. So "contralateral needling" is adopted, that is, to puncture the luo on the left part of the body to stop pain on the right and to puncture the luo on the right to stop pain on the left."

The Yellow Emperor asked: "I want to hear you explain the reason for contralateral needling. And tell me how to distinguish "contralateral needling" from "opposite needling"."

Qibo said: "After the pathogen enters the jing, the patient will feel pain on the right part of the body if the pathogen on the left is exuberant; and if the pathogen on the right is exuberant, the patient may feel pain on the left. Sometimes the patient may feel pain on both sides. Under such conditions, the "opposite needling" method is applied. But it is only suitable for expelling the pathogen from the jing; contralateral needling is used to dispel the pathogen in the luo. The two kinds of pain are different in places."

Yellow Emperor said: "I would like to know how to perform "contralateral needling"."

Qibo said: "For example, if the pathogen affects the luo of the kidney foot Shaoyin, the patient feels epigastric pain, abdominal distension, and a full sensation in the hypochondriacal region; so then puncture Rangu (K 2) to cause bleeding. If there is no food accumulation, the patient may feel relieved in 20 minutes. If the symptoms still remain, puncture the points on the right to stop the pain on the left, and points on the left to relieve the symptoms on the right. The patient will recover in 5 days.

If the pathogen invades the luo of the Sanjiao hand Shaoyang, manifestations such as a sore throat, obstructed nose, curled-up tongue, dry mouth, restless and suffocating feeling in the chest, and pain along the exterior aspect of the arm with inability to lift it may occur. Then puncture Guanchong (SJ 1) at the juncture of the skin and nail on the ulnar side of the fourth finger, once on each side. The patient with a strong body resistance may feel relieved at once, and even the elderly may feel well in a few minutes. The method is the same, namely puncturing the points on the left to treat disorders on the right and points on the right to treat disorders on the left; even if the patient is newly affected, he will recover in a few days.

When the pathogen invades the luo of the liver foot Jueyin, the patient may feel the sudden pain of a hernia; puncture Dadun (Liv 1) at the juncture between the nail and skin of the big toe, once each side. A male will feel well at once and a female will be well in a minute. The method is the same, the left point for a right disorder and vice versa.

When the pathogen invades the luo of the bladder foot Taiyang, the patient feels pain in the head, neck and shoulder. Puncture Zhiyin (UB 67) at the juncture between the nail and the skin of the small toe, once each side. The pain will disappear at once. If this fails, puncture Jinmen (UB 63) inferior to the external malleolus thrice for each foot; if contralateral insertion is adopted, the pain will be checked in about 20 minutes.

When the pathogen affects the luo of the large intestine hand Yangming, the patient feels fullness and a hot sensation in the chest and difficulty in breathing. Needle Shangyang (LI 1) at the juncture between the nail and skin of the index finger near the thumb, once each side; contralateral insertion is used. The patient will feel relieved in about 20 minutes.

When the pathogen affects the luo of the pericardium hand Jueyin, manifestations such as pain around the arm, palm, and the wrist occur. The treatment is to feel for the tender spot before puncturing the points behind the wrist. The number of needles used is decided according to the waxing and waning of the moon. That is, to add needles according to the Chinese calendar, one needle on the first day when the moon tends to wax, two needles on the second day. The number of needles is thus increased with each day until it reaches 15 needles on the fifteenth day. The sixteenth is the day when the moon tends to wane, so then the number of the needles is reduce. That is 14 needles on the sixteenth, 13 needles on the seventeenth.

If the pathogen invades the Yangqiao meridian beginning at the foot, pain of the eyes will occur from the inner canthi. This is treated by puncturing Shenmai 0.5 cun inferior to the exterior malleolus twice on each side and contralateral insertion is applied. The pain will be checked in one or two hours.

If there is abdominal distension caused by blood stasis due to falling, or traumatic injury, the patient should first be treated with drugs to relax the bowels and remove blood stasis, then by pricking the blood vessels anterior to the navicular bone and inferior to the medial malleolus to cause bleeding, and puncturing Chongyang (St 42) on the dorsal artery of the foot; for falling may injure the Jueyin and the luo of the Shaoyang. If the treatment doesn't work, needle Dadun (Liv 1) on the exterior aspect near the nail of the big toe, once for each foot, selecting the point according to contralateral needling. The patient will feel well after blood letting. And this treatment is also effective for a patient in a panic.

If the pathogen affects the luo of the large intestine hand Yangming, the patient will suffer from deafness, though some can still hear. Puncture Shangyang (LI 1) on the radial side of the index finger about 0.1 cun posterior to the corner of the nail, once each side. The ability to listen will reappear. Otherwise puncture Zhongchong (P 9) on the radial side of the middle finger near the corner of the nail. If the listening ability is completely lost due to exhaustion of the luo qi, then acupuncture is not allowed. If the patient has tinnitus like "blowing wind", the treatment is the same as the above—the left point for the right disorder, and vice versa.

Usually the pain of arthralgia has the character of migrating without a fixed place. So tender spots should be found at first, then punctured by needles, which had best be thrust deep into the muscles. The number of needles used in treatment is often decided according to the waxing and waning of the moon; but the practitioner has the right to decide the number of needles on the basis of both this rule and the conditions of illness and the patient. If the number of needles is larger than that required, the antipathogenic qi will be wasted, but if it is smaller then the pathogen can't be expelled. As for choosing the acupoints, contralateral insertion is employed. If the manifestations remain unchanged after the treatment, the same treatment is again applied.

If the pathogen affects the luo of the stomach foot Yangming, manifestations such as nasal discharge, epistaxis, and a cold sensation of the upper teeth occur. Puncture Lidui (St 45) about 0.1 cun posterior to the nail on the exterior side of the second toe, once for each toe. The left point is needled to treat the symptoms on the right and vice versa,

If the pathogen invades the luo of the gallbladder foot Shaoyang, the patient may feel hypochondriacal pain, difficulty in breathing and sweating on coughing. Puncture Qiaoyin (GB 44) about 0.1 cun from the corner of the nail, on the exterior side of the fourth toe, once for each point. The dyspnoea and sweating will disappear at once. If the cough continues, pay attention to diet and clothing—it will be cured in a day. Still use the left point for the right disorder and the right point for the left disorder. If there is no improvement, treat it with the same method again.

When the pathogen invades the luo of the kidney foot Shaoyin, the patient feels soreness in the throat, difficulty in swallowing, angry without any reason and ascending qi up to the cardiac region. This is treated by puncturing Yongquan (K 1) at the centre of the sole, three needles for each foot. If there is no response, puncture the left point to treat disease on the right and vice versa. If the swelling of the throat makes one unable to swallow even a drop of water or spit, then puncture Rangu (K 2) anterior

to the navicular bone at once to cause bleeding. The same method is adopted.

When the pathogen invades the luo of the spleen foot Taiyin, the patient will feel pain in the lumbar region which refers to the lower abdomen and hypochondrium, and affects the breathing. Puncture Xialiao (UB 34) superior to the muscles beside the spinal column in the lumbosacral region. The number of needles used is decided by the waxing of the moon. Manifestations on the left should be treated by puncturing points on the right and vice versa.

When the pathogen affects the luo of the bladder foot Taiyang, contracture and a dragging pain of the hypochondriacal region may occur. Insert three needles in the places along both sides of the spinal bones near the nape where the patient feels pain on pressing. The pain will be checked at once.

If the pathogen invades the luo of the gallbladder, the patient may feel pain around Huantiao (GB 30) and be unable to lift the leg. Puncture Huantiao with a thin filiform needle, and retain the needle for a relatively long time if cold is dominant in the syndrome. The waxing and waning of the moon decide the number of needles used in the treatment.

The treatment of the diseases in the jing means puncturing the jing. But if the manifestations do not appear in the course of the jing but in the luo, contralateral insertion is then employed. Puncture Shangyang (LI 1) of the hand Yangming to treat deafness. If there is no response, puncture Tinggong (SI 19) pertaining to the hand Yangming which runs towards the ear. If puncturing Shangyang doesn't cure decayed teeth, needle the jing passing through to the tooth. The result will be seen at once.

When the pathogen invades the 5 zang organs, disorders may occur and be accompanied by dragging pain and an intermittent pain in the jing. Contralateral insertion is applied on the finger tips according to the conditions, pricking the luo with blood stasis to cause bleeding, once every other day. If the manifestations continue, treat in the same way 5 times. If the hand Yangming is affected, the pathogen may go up to invade the upper teeth, causing cold and a painful sensation in the teeth. Prick the jing with the blood stasis to cause bleeding and expel the pathogen, and also Neiting (St 44) of the foot Yangming on the middle toe, and Shangyang (LI 1) on the radial side of the index finger, once for each point. Contralateral needling is applied.

The luo of the hand and foot Shaoyin, hand Taiyin, foot Taiyin and Yangming meridians all converge into the ear and circle the frontal angle above the left ear. If the pathogen causes total exhaustion of the meridional qi of these 5 jing, the jing all over the body are stimulated, giving rise to unconsciousness when you lie like a dead body, or a cold corpse-like syndrome.

In such cases, first puncture Yinbai (Sp 1) about 0.1 cun posterior to the nail on the medial side of the big toe, then Yongquan (K 1) at the centre of the sole and Lidui (St 45) near the nail of the middle toe, one needle for each point. Then Shaoshang (LI 1) about 0.1 cun posterior to the nail on the medial side of the thumb, Zhongchong (P 9) of the hand Jueyin and Shenmen (H 7) of the hand Shaoyin located on the ulnar side posterior to the palm, one needle for each point.

If this treatment doesn't work, blow at the two ears of the patient through a bamboo pipe. Then cut the hair in an area about 1 cun square, judging it from the ear's left frontal angle. Roast the hair, grind it into powder and mix it with some fine wine. After this is done get the patient to drink it. If the patient has completely lost consciousness, put it into the patient's mouth. He will soon come to himself.

Generally all acupuncture techniques are based on the jing, on feeling for the pulse, on observing the deficiency and excess and regulating them. If they are irregular they should be treated with needling, yet if there is simply pain without the accompanying symptoms or disorders of the jing, it should be treated with contralateral needling. What is also important is cutaneous bleeding and pricking the luo which have blood stasis to cause bleeding. This is the contralateral needling which we have now described."

NOTE

1. Chapter 1 of the *Miraculous Pivot*, "On the Nine Needles, and 12 Yuan-source Points".
2. Chapter 8 of the *Miraculous Pivot*, "Explaining the Filiform Needle".
3. Chapter 2 of the *Miraculous Pivot*, "The Source of the Shu Points".
4. Chapter 7 of the *Miraculous Pivot*, "The Just Choice of the Needle".
5. Chapter 63 of the *Plain Questions*, "Contralateral Needling".

Appendix 2
Abstracts from ancient rhymes on acupuncture and moxibustion

The Lyric of Standard Profundities[1]

The secret of acupuncture in saving people's lives is in the perfect use of needling,

In which the factors of the seasons, the weather and the patient's condition are considered;

For example, superficial insertion in spring and summer, deep insertion in autumn and winter.

Without a comprehensive knowledge of the meridians, zangfu organs, and yin and yang,

One would always meet the contraindications of needling during the treatment of disease.

After having detected the condition of deficiency or excess of the zang-fu organs,

Needling is applied according to the theory of meridians.

The meridional qi originates from the middle-jiao,

The Taiyin emerging from Point Yunmen (Lu 2),

It circulates around reaching the Jueyin,

And ending at Qimen (Liv 14).

There are 12 regular jing (meridians),

With more than 300 luo (collaterals),

And over 600 sites which manifest qi and blood all over the body.

The three yin meridians of the hand travel from the chest down to the hands,

While the three yang meridians of the hand run from the hands up to the head;

The three yang meridians of the foot from the head to the feet

And the three yin meridians of the foot from the feet to the abdomen.

On the basis of the above, reinforcing is applied by directing the needle along the meridian,

Whilst reducing by directing the needle against the meridian.

And different meridians have different volumes of qi and blood:

The meridians of the hand and foot Taiyang and Jueyin

Are characterized by less qi and more blood,

The meridians of the hand and foot Shaoyang, Taiyin and Shaoyin

Are characterized by more qi and less blood,

While the meridians of the hand and foot Yangming

Are rich both in qi and blood.

As for the arrival of the qi:

Usually a gentle, smooth and slow motion suggests qi absence,

Which gives the operator a kind of feeling as if walking on wild and empty ground;

But a sinking, uneven and tense motion under the operator's fingers

Is the sign of arrival of the qi, which feels as if a fish is biting the hook and pulling the line downward.

The arrival of the qi is of great importance in acupuncture,

Usually a quick arrival of qi shows a good effect

But a slow arrival of qi shows a slow qi, which may even be without effect.

Thus in the clinic, if the qi fails to arrive,

Methods should be taken to promote it

According to the condition of deficiency or excess;

While if the qi has arrived,

The needle can be retained or withdrawn

According to the condition, either cold or heat.

Concerning the needle itself, there are nine kinds of needles in all,

Among which the filiform needle is the best.

It is suitable for needling all the points on the body.

The needling process can be explained by the five elements,

That is, the needle is considered as pertaining to "metal"—

Both in the material it is made from

And in its function of expelling the pathogenic factors and strengthening the body resistance;

The jingluo pertain to "water"—

Both in their distribution and in their function of supplying the body with nutrition;

The needle also pertains to "wood"—

Because it stands erect as tree and can be inserted into the body perpendicularly, obliquely and horizontally;

At the same time it also pertains to "fire"—

Because it is often warmed before being inserted in, in order to expel the pathogen;

And lastly a cotton ball is applied to press the hole after removal of the needle

As if "earth" is being used to fill up the hole.

Though the needle is fine and only 3.6 cun long,

It can harmonize the zangfu organs

And, through its use, spasm and obstruction can be removed by expelling the exogenous pathogenic factors;

And furthermore cold or heat syndromes, and arthralgia, can be stopped by puncturing points at the joints.

As for the acupuncturist, he should remember to insert the needle

Only when the patient is relaxed

And to observe the patient's complexion and reaction during treatment.

Before the points are prescribed,

The meridians should be related to the main symptoms

And their volume of qi and blood taken into consideration.

The following are some points for reference:

Baihui (Du 20), Xuanji (Ren 21) and Yongquan (K 1).

Although they are located respectively on the "three portions"— (Heaven=head, Man=trunk, and Earth=foot),

They can be used as well to treat corresponding disorders in other regions.

For example Baihui is chosen for the trunk,

And Yongquan is selected for the head, because they are connected by meridians;

Likewise with Dabao (Sp 21), Tianshu (St 25) and Diji (Sp 8),

Which are located respectively in the Sanjiao.

Also note the following:

The Yangqiao, Yangwei, Du and Dai are indicated

In treating exterior syndromes manifesting on the shoulders, back, legs and lumbar region;

Whilst the two Yinqiao, two Yinwei, Ren and Chong are indicated

In treating interior syndromes manifesting on the chest, abdominal and hypochondriacal regions.

Yanglingquan (GB 34) and Yinlingquan (Sp 9),

Shenmai (UB 62) and Zhaohai (K 6),

Yangjiao (GB 35) and Sanyinjiao (Sp 6)

Can be punctured to treat disorders of the head, hands and feet;

Erjian (LI 2) and Sanjian (LI 3),

Shaoshang (Lu 11) and Shangyang (LI 1),

Tianjing (SJ 10) and Jianjing (GB 21)

Are connected respectively by two meridians.

Besides these, the location of the points is also important.

The correct location depends on many aspects,

Such as the use of bone-length measurement, the operator's experience,

The patient's constitution and a proper position.

The points of the yang meridians are usually on the exterior aspect of the body

And those of the yin meridians on the interior aspects,

They are often located between the tendons and bones in a depression, and by joints and along arteries.

A good way of locating points is to fix one point by finding another four points around it for reference,

And to locate one meridian with the help of another two.

Now for indications of different points:

The *luo* points are often used to stop pain,

The Back-Shu, Front-Mu points and those named *men* (gate) and *hai* (sea),

Such as Yunmen (Lu 2), Shenmen (H 7), Qihai (Ren 6), etc.

Are effective in treating disorders of the zangfu organs.

The *yuan*, connecting, converging and influential points

Are dominant in removing obstruction and blood stasis.

Points of the four limbs can be used to treat local problems

As well as disorders of the head, chest and abdomen.

The 5 Shu points are punctured to dispel pathogens and strengthen the body resistance.

The 8 Confluent points are connected with the extra meridians,

The 12 *yuan* points are often employed in treating disorders of the zangfu organs.

Besides this, there are also some other methods for selecting points

Such as the Ziwu Liuzhu (Midnight-Midday-Ebbing-Flowing) Method,[2]

The Exterior-Interior Point-Association Method,

Contralateral Needling, Remote Needling, and so on.

Before needling, the needle should be inspected carefully,

Then it is warmed in the mouth before the insertion, which is performed with two hands,

The left hand pressing around the point to disperse the qi,

While the right hand inserts the needle gently.

The patient should be either sitting or lying to avoid fainting.

The treatment of diseases should be decided according to the zangfu organs,

The theory of the Five Elements and the theory of Root and Branch, Origin and Termination

And the points to puncture chosen according to the methods

Of using 66 points each and every day,

And 12 *yuan* points during each and every time period,

And the Eight Methods of the "intelligent turtle".[3]

The following are treatments for some diseases:

Uterine bleeding is checked by needling Yinjiao (Ren 7), Sanyinjiao (Sp 6) and Yangchi (SJ 4).

Retention of placenta in difficult labour

Is removed by puncturing Zhaohai (K 6) and Waiguan (SJ 5),

Numbness, cold limbs and hemiplegia are treated

By needling with reinforcing or reducing methods to remove obstruction from the meridians.

Metrorrhagia, metrostaxis and leucorrhoea are stopped

By puncturing with warming and reinforcing methods to invigorate the qi and blood.

Cold syndromes are treated by retaining the needle.

Disorders of the throat are removed by Zhaohai (K 6),

Mental depression is treated by Dazhong (K 4).

Pain pertaining to excess-type symptoms is often stopped by reducing,

Itching and excess numbness pertaining to deficiency-type symptoms are treated by reinforcing.

Lassitude and painful joints are relieved by Shu-stream points,

Abdominal distension is removed by the Jing-well points.

A sore throat or hypochondriacal fullness is alleviated by Taichong (Liv 3),

Belching, vomiting and stomach-ache are treated by Gongsun (Sp 4) with reducing.

Neiguan (P 6) is indicated in fullness of the chest and abdominal pain,

Zhigou (SJ 6) is used for hypochondriacal pain due to various reasons.

Hunmen (UB 47) is employed for spasm and pain of the bones,

Pohu (UB 43) is applied to treat fever and constipation.

Shenmai (UB 62) and Jinmen (UB 63) are selected to check headaches and *feng* syndromes of the head,

For ophthalmalgia and itching of the eyes, Guangming (GB 37) and Diwuhui (GB 42) are chosen.

For night-sweats and a hectic fever in children, Yinxi (H 6) is adopted,

For retention of urine and ascites in adults, Pianli (LI 6) is employed.

For apoplexy, Huantiao (GB 30) is used,

For consumptive diseases, Tianshu (S 25) is chosen.

Now for the reinforcing and reducing methods.

Usually reinforcing is performed in the morning, or during days when the moon is waxing,

And by pressing the skin along the meridian, flicking the needle,

Then retaining the needle and removing the needle whilst inhaling,

Or else by puncturing the mother-point with reinforcing,

Or applying the method of "setting the mountain on fire".

On the other hand, reducing is performed in the afternoon, or on days when the moon is waning,

And by pressing the point with the finger nail,

Lifting and thrusting with reducing, then removing the needle whilst exhaling,

Or by needling the son-point with reducing,

Or adopting the method of "penetrating the heaven's coolness".

Contraindications in acupuncture should also be noticed.

No needling is allowed in critical cases or in any one of the following conditions:

Disagreement of pulse and symptoms,

Extremely hot or cold weather, hunger, drunkenness, or fatigue,

As this may cause fainting during needling.

Besides this, reinforcing can't be used whilst the tide is coming in,

And reducing is forbidden whilst the tide is going out.

As for forbidden points, there are 49 points (in addition to those on the extremities)

Which are contraindicated to moxibustion;

And 22 points (besides the six points named by "shu", that is, the Xinshu, Feishu, Geshu, Ganshu, Pishu and Shenshu)

Which are contraindicated to needling.

Generally speaking, acupuncture was used and developed by ancient physicians.

It was by using the needle that they saved many people's lives and cured many an intractable disease.

For example, a doctor whose surname was Li relieved an intractable disease of the *Gao* Emperor by puncturing Juque (Ren 14).

Bianque woke the prince by needling Zhongji (Ren 3).

Zhenquan chose Jianjing (GB 21) and Quchi (LI 11) to stop pain in the arms.

Huatuo selected Xuanzhong (GB 39) and Huantiao (GB 30) to treat lameness.

Ganshu (UB 18) and Neiting (Du 4) could be employed to treat blindness,

And Tinghui (GB 2) and Yangchi (SJ 4) could be adopted to treat deafness, and so on.

The ancient physicians have left us a rather profuse and complicated theory of acupuncture.

Which can't be understood and grasped unless enough study and work have been done.

The Lyric of the Hundred Diseases[4]

One should study the meridians seriously and select the acupoints. The following are points indicated for different diseases:

Points	Indications
Xinhui (Du 22) and Yuzhen (UB 9)	*feng* syndromes of the head
Xuanlu (GB 5) and Hanyan (GB 4)	migraine
Qiangjian (Du 18) and Fenglong (St 40)	intolerable headache
Shuigou (Du 26) and Qianding (Du 21)	*feng* oedema
Tinghui (GB 2) and Yifeng (SJ 17)	deafness
Yingxiang (LI 20)	itching of the face
Tinghui (GB 2)	tinnitus like a cicada chirping
Zhizheng (SI 7) and Feiyang (UB 58)	blurred vision
Yanggang (UB 48) and Feiyang (UB 58)	yellow sclera
Shaoze (SI 1) and Ganshu (UB 18)	disorders of the eyeball
Zulinqi (GB 41) and Touwei (St 58)	lacrimation
Zanzhu (UB 2) and Sanjian (LI 13)	blurred vision
Yanglao (SI 6) and Tianzhu (UB 10)	visual hallucination
Jingming (UB 1) and Xingjian (Liv 2)	night blindess due to a liver problem
Fuliu (K 7) and Qimen (Liv 14)	neck rigidity due to cold
Lianquan (Ren 23) and Zhongchong (P 9)	swelling under the tongue
Tianfu (Lu 3) and Hegu (LI 4)	haemorrhage from the nose
Ermen (SJ 21) and Sizhukong (SJ 23)	toothache
Jiache (St 6) and Dicang (St 4)	deviation of the mouth
Yemen (SJ 2) and Yuji (Lu 10)	sore throat
Jingmen (GB 25) and Qiuxu (GB 40)	spasm
Yanggu (SI 5) and Xiaxi (GB 43)	submandibular swelling and lockjaw
Shaoshang (Lu 11) and Quze (P 3)	thirst, and blood deficiency
Tongtian (UB 7)	absence of smell
Fuliu (K 7)	dryness of mouth and tongue
Yamen (Du 15) and Guanchong (SJ 1)	flaccid tongue with aphasia
Tianding (LI 17) and Jianshi (P 5)	sudden aphonia
Taichong (Liv 3) with reducing	deviation of the mouth
Chengjiang (Ren 24) with reducing	toothache
Shugu (UB 65) and Tianzhu (UB 10)	neck rigidity with aversion to wind
Dadu (Sp 2) and Jingqu (Lu 8)	febrile disease without sweating
Shaohai (H 3) and Shousanli (LI 10)	numbness of the arms

Points	Indications
Yanglingquan (GB 34) and Quchi (LI 11)	hemiplegia
Jianli (Ren 11) and Neiguan (P 6)	fullness of the chest
Tinggong (SI 19) and Pishu (UB 20)	mental depression
Qihu (St 13) and Huagai (Ren 20)	pain in the hypochondriacal region
Xiawan (Ren 19) and Xiangu (St 43)	borborygmus
Zhangmen (Liv 13)	fullness in the chest
Shanzhong (Ren 17) and Juque (Ren 14)	fluid retention above the diaphragm
Zhongfu (Lu 1) and Yishe (UB 49)	distension of the chest and dysphagia
Shenshu (UB 23) and Juliao (St 3)	blood stasis in the chest
Shencang (K 25) and Xuanji (Ren 21)	distension of the chest and neck rigidity
Baihuanshu (UB 30) and Weizhong (UB 40)	dragging pain in the lumbar region from the back
Shuidao (St 28) and Jinsuo (Du 8)	back rigidity
Quanliao (SI 18) and Daying (St 5)	flickering eyelid
Luxi (SJ 19)	convulsive disease
Rangu (K 2)	tetanus in the new-born
Weiyang (UB 39) and Tianchi (P 1)	swelling of the axilla
Houxi (SI 3) and Huantiao (GB 30)	pain in the legs
Lidui (St 45) and Yinbai (Sp 1)	dream-disturbed sleep
Shangwan (Ren 13) and Shenmen (H 7)	manic psychosis
Yangjiao (GB 35) and Jiexi (St 41)	palpitations
Tianchong (GB 9) and Daheng (Sp 15)	infantile convulsions
Shenzhu (Du 12) and Benshen (GB 13)	epilepsy
Shaochong (H 9) and Quchi (LI 11)	fever
Taodao (Du 13) and Feishu (UB 13)	epidemic febrile disease
Shendao (Du 11) and Xinshu (UB 15)	*feng* epilepsy
Xialiao (UB 34)	cold dampness or damp-heat
Yongquan (K 1)	cold limbs
Erjian (LI 2) and Yinxi (Ren 18)	vomiting and restlessness
Xingjian (Liv 2) and Yongquan (K 1)	diabetes
Yinlingquan (Sp 9) and Shuifen (Ren 9)	oedema around the umbilicus
Pohu (UB 42) and Gaohuang (UB 43)	consumptive disease
Yingu (K 10) and Zusanli (St 36)	cholera morbus
Houxi (SI 3) and Laogong (P 8)	jaundice
Tongli (H 5) and Dazhong (K 4)	lassitude

Points	Indications
Feishu (UB 13) and Tiantu (Ren 22)	cough
Lidui (St 45) and Xiaohai (SI 8)	dark urine
Changqiang (Du 1) and Chengshan (UB 57)	haemofaecia and enterorrhagia
Sanyinjiao (Sp 6) and Qihai (Ren 6)	gonorrhoea and emission
Huangshu (K 16) and Henggu (K 11)	five types of stranguria
Yinxi (H 6) and Houxi (SI 3)	night sweats
Pishu (UB 20) and Pangguangshu (UB 28)	anorexia
Huangmen (UB 15) and Weishu (UB 21)	indigestion
Yinjiao (Ren 7)	nasal polyps
Fubai (GB 10)	goitre
Dadun (Liv 1) and Zhaohai (K 6)	peri-umbilical colic
Shouwuli (LI 13) and Binao (LI 14)	scrofula
Zhiyin (UB 67) and Wuyi (St 15)	itching and pain
Jianyu (LI 15) and Yangxi (LI 5)	German measles
Diji (Sp 8) and Xuehai (Sp 10)	irregular menstruation
Jiaoxin (K 8) and Heyang (UB 55)	uterine bleeding
Chongmen (Sp 12) and Qichong (St 30)	leuchorrhoea and menorrhagia
Tianshu (St 25) and Shuiquan (K 5)	irregular menstrual cycle
Jianjing (GB 21)	necrotic mass of breast
Shangqiu (Sp 5)	nasal fistula
Baihui (Du 20) and Jiuwei (Ren 15)	prolapse of the rectum
Yinjiao (Du 28) and Shiguan (K 18)	sterility
Zhongwan (Ren 12)	chronic dysentery
Waiqiu (GB 36)	prolapse of the rectum
Shangyang (LI 1) and Taixi (K 3)	algid malaria
Chongmen (Sp 12)	a mass in the abdomen

Ode to the Jade Dragon[5]

The points and their indications mentioned in the book are listed below:

Points	Indications
Xinhui (Du 22) and Baihui (Du 20)	apoplexy
Shangxing (Du 23)	nasal discharge, pain of the eye and *feng* syndrome of the head

Points	Indications
Shenting (Du 24)	vomiting, blurred vision and *feng* syndrome of head
Yintang (Extra 2) with moxibustion	chronic infantile convulsions
Chengjiang (Ren 24) Fengfu (Du 16)	headache and toothache
Sizhukong (SJ 23) and Shuaigu (GB 8)	migratory aching all over the head
Fengchi (GB 20)	*feng* syndromes of the head with *tan*
Hegu (LI 4)	*feng* syndromes of the head without *tan*
Dicang (St 4) with reducing method	deviation of mouth and eye
Yingxiang (LI 20)	no sense of smell
Yifeng (SJ 17) with reducing method	deafness and goitre
Tinghui (GB 2) with reducing method	deafness, tinnitus as a chirping cicada, skin disease
Yamen (Du 15)	aphonia
Zanzhu (UB 2) and Touwei (St 8)	pain between the eyebrows and blurred vision
Jingming (UB 1) Yuwei (SJ 23) and pricking Taiyang (Extra 5) to cause bleeding	congestion and swelling of the eyes
Yingxiang (LI 20), pricking to cause bleeding	congestion of the eyes due to heart-fire
Shuigou (Du 26) with reducing and Weizhong (UB 40)	back rigidity and traumatic injury of the waist
Shenshu (UB 23) with moxibustion	soreness of the lumbar region due to deficiency of the kidney
Huantiao (GB 30), Juliao (St 3) and Weizhong (UB 40) to cause bleeding	pain of the legs
Fengshi (GB 31) and Yinshi (St 33)	weakness of legs due to invasion by *feng* dampness
Kuangu (hip bone)	pain of the two legs
Xiyan (Extra 39) and Xiguan (Liv 7)	swelling of the knee joint
Zusanli (St 36), Yinjiao (Ren 7) and Xuanzhong (GB 39)	beriberi due to a cold-damp pathogen
Kunlun (UB 60), Shenmai (UB 62) and Taixi (K 3)	swelling of legs and feet
Qiuxu (GB 40), Jiexi (St 41) and Shangqiu (p 5)	pain of the dorsum of foot
Taichong (Liv 3), Zusanli (St 36) and Zhongfeng (Liv 4)	difficulty in walking
Yinlingquan (Sp 9) and Yanglingquan (GB 34)	arthritis of knee
Wangu (GB 12)	weakness of wrist
Jianjing (GB 21) with reinforcing	pain of the arms
Beifeng (Extra)	pain of the shoulder referring to the arms
Wushu (GB 27)	soreness of the lumbar region
Quchi (LI 11) with reducing and Chize (Lu 5)	spasm of the elbows referring to the wrist
Jianyu (LI 15) with moxibustion	swelling and pain of the shoulder due to cold and damp pathogen

Points	Indications
Chize (Lu 5)	spasm of the arm
Hegu (LI 4)	disorders of the head
Neiguan (P 6)	mass in the abdomen and abdominal disorder
Daling (P 7) and Waiguan (SJ 5)	abdominal pain
Zhigou (SJ 6)	hypochondriacal pain and constipation
Jianshi (P 5)	disease of the spleen
Shangwan (Ren 13) and Zhongwan (Ren 12)	pain of pericardium and spleen
Erbai (Extra 31)	haemorrhoids
Guanchong (SJ 1) to cause bleeding	bitter taste, and dryness of the mouth due to heat in the upper-jiao
Yemen (SJ 2) and Zhongdu (Liv 9)	swelling of arms and dragging pain of wrist
Zhongchong (P 9) and Shuigou (Du 26)	*feng* syndrome
Shaochong (H 9)	timidity due to deficiency of the heart
Houxi (SI 3) with moxibustion	epidemic malaria
Erjian (LI 2)	toothache
Zhongkui (Extra 26)	regurgitation and vomiting
Shaoshang (Lu 11) to cause bleeding	tonsillitis
Tianjing (SJ 10) with moxibustion	urticaria and goitre
Lieque (Lu 7) and Taiyuan (Lu 9) with moxibustion	cough with sputum due to *feng* cold
Shaoze (SI 1)	acute mastitis and thick sputum mixed with blood
Dazhui (Du 14)	fever and night sweating
Shenzhu (Du 12) with moxibustion	cough and low back pain
Zhiyang (Du 9)	jaundice
Mingmen (Du 4) and Shenshu (UB 23) with moxibustion	frequent urination due to deficiency of the kidney
Chengshan (UB 57) and Changqiang (Du 1)	haemorrhoids
Feishu (UB 13)	chronic cough
Fenglong (St 40)	profuse sputum
Gaohuang (UB 43) only with moxibustion	many kinds of diseases
Fengmen (UB 12) with moxibustion	sneezing, cough, and nasal discharge
Xinshu (UB 15) and Baihuanshu (UB 30)	timidity, emission and gonorrhoea
Ganshu (UB 18) and Zusanli (St 36)	blurred vision due to the liver problem
Wangu (GB 12) and Zhongwan (Ren 12)	regurgitation, vomiting and jaundice due to the spleen disorder
Fuliu (K 7) with reducing	febrile disease without sweating
Hegu (LI 4)	febrile disease with sweating
Zhaohai (K 6) and Zhigou (SJ 6)	constipation
Neiting (St 44)	abdominal distension
Zulinqi (GB 41)	oedema of the feet

Points	Indications
Dadun (Liv 1)	hernia
Guanyuan (Ren 4) and Daimai (GB 26)	reversed flow of kidney qi
Yongquan (K 1) to cause bleeding	consumptive disease
Fenglong (St 40) with reducing	profuse sputum
Guanyuan (Ren 4)	asthma
tender spots	pain all over the body
Laogong (P 8)	skin and external disease over the hand
Daling (Sp 15) with reducing	disorders of the heart and chest
Tiantu (Ren 22) and Shanzhong (Ren 17) with moxibustion	asthma
Jiuwei (Ren 15) with 7 cones of moxibustion	five types of epilepsy
Xuanji (Ren 21) and Qihai (Ren 6)	asthma
Guanyuan (Ren 4) and Dadun (Liv 1)	hernia and reversed flow of qi
First Shuifen (Ren 9) and Shuidao (St 28) with moxibustion, then Zusanli (St 36) and Yinjiao (Ren 7)	oedema and abdominal distension
Zhongji (Ren 3) with reducing	leucorrhoea
Shufu (K 27) and Rugen (St 18)	asthma, cough and sputum
Qimen (Liv 14)	transmission of febrile disease to the Taiyang
Zusanli (St 36) with reducing	asthma and fullness of the chest
Tianshu (St 25) with moxibustion	diarrhoea due to deficiency of spleen
Daling (P 7) and Shuigou (Du 26) with reducing	foul breath

A Handbook of Ballads for Emergencies[6]

The following is the list of some useful points and their indications mentioned in the book:

Points	Indications
Zhiyin (UB 67)	disorder of face and head
Fengfu (Du 16)	diseases of legs and feet
Shaofu (H 8)	troubles of heart and chest
Ququan (Liv 8)	affection of abdomen
Jiaoxin (K 8)	rigidity and soreness of lumbar region and knee
Houxi (SI 3)	pain of legs and hypochondrium
Taichong (Liv 3)	swelling of thigh and knee joints

Points	Indications
Baihui (Du 20)	goitre
Yongquan (K 1)	pain of vertex
Chize (Lu 5), Quchi (LI 11) and Fengfu (Du 16)	arthritis of knee
Chize (Lu 5)	contraction of arm
Quchi (LI 11)	back spasm
Chengshan (UB 57)	five kinds of hernia
Fenglong (St 40)	asthma
Jianshi (P 5)	manic mental disorder, and night sweating
Lingdao (H 4)	heat syndrome due to extreme cold
Jianshi (P 5) penetrating Zhigou (SJ 6) and Dazhui (Du 14) with 7 cones of moxa	malaria
Jingmen (GB 25)	continuous fever and chills due to malaria
Fuliu (K 7)	chills due to malaria
Jianshi (P 5)	fever due to malaria
Lieque (Lu 7)	convulsive diseases due to fever caused by febrile disease
Fuliu (K 7)	cold limbs and feeble pulse due to febrile disease
Xuanzhong (GB 39) with reinforcing method	cold symptoms and deep thready pulse due to febrile disease
Xuanzhong (GB 39) with reducing method	heat symptoms and a superficial, full pulse due to febrile disease
Hegu (LI 4) Dicang (St 4)	"lily" disease and lockjaw parasites
Zhongwan (Ren 12)	vomiting, ascariasis and abdominal pain due to febrile disease
Yongquan (K 1)	fullness of the chest and fever without sweating
Qimen (Liv 14)	fullness of the chest and hypochondriacal pain due to febrile disease
Hegu (LI 4)	no sweating in a febrile disease
Fuliu (K 7)	spontaneous sweating and oliguria
Zhigou (SJ 6)	epigastric distension
Shaoshang (Lu 11)	convulsive disease and malar flushing
Yinbao (Liv 9)	fullness of epigastric region
tender spots and and Chengshan (UB 57)	tetanus due to traumatic injury
Dadu (Sp 2)	chronic pain of legs and the lumbar region
Kunlun (UB 60) and Taxi (K 3)	intractable pain of knee joints and feet
Dashu (UB 11) and Ququan (Liv 8)	migratory arthralgia and flaccidity
Zhigou (SJ 6)	hypochondriacal pain, and limited movement of feet
Weizhong (UB 40)	weakness of the lumbar region.

The Guide to the Secret of Qi Flow (Extract)[7]

In the treatment of diseases the needle is the best instrument, which can expel pathogenic factors, invigorate the body resistance and regulate yin and yang by puncturing different points. Thus the selection of acupoints is of great importance.

The following are some points appearing in the classics which are effective in treating different diseases:

Taichong (Liv 3) is used for treating difficulty in walking,

Shuigou (Du 26) is chosen for treating epilepsy and spasm.

Shenmen (H 7) is selected for treating dementia due to a heart problem,

Fengfu (Du 16) is adopted for treating tetanus causing neck rigidity.

To treat vertigo and blurred vision, Fengchi (GB 20) is punctured,

To treat deafness, Tinghui (GB 2) is needled.

To check pain of the eyes, Hegu (LI 4) is employed,

To remove jaundice and fullness of the chest, Yongquan (K 1) is applied.

Dizziness and congestion of the eyes are relieved by puncturing Zanzhu (UB 2),

Spasm of the elbow is relaxed by needling Quchi (LI 11).

Weakness of the limbs is treated by puncturing Zhaohai (K 6),

Toothache is stopped by needling Taxi (K 3).

Chengshan (Ren 24) is used to relax rigidity of the neck,

Qichong (St 30) or Taibai (Sp 3) is selected to subdue the rushing of the qi.

Shuidao (St 28) or Yinlingquan (Sp 9) is chosen to remove retention of urine,

Neiting (St 44) is employed to relieve abdominal distension.

Spasm of lower leg is smoothed by Chengshan (UB 57),

Pain of the ankle is checked by Kunlun (UB 60).

Pain of the femur is stopped by Yinshi (St 33),

Epilepsy is alleviated by Houxi (SI 3).

For malaria, Jianshi (P 5) is punctured,

For blood stasis in the chest, Qimen (Liv 14) is needled.

For heat syndromes of the heart, Laogong (P 8) is chosen,

For the seven kinds of hernias, Dadun (Liv 1) is selected.

Zusanli (St 36) is employed for various stomach troubles,

Wangu (GB 12) is applied for jaundice.

Rangu (K 2) is adopted for heat in the kidney,

Xingjian (Liv 2) is selected for oedema of the knee joints and congestion of the eyes.

To treat pain and spasm of the elbow, Chize (Lu 5) is needled,

To treat blurred vision, Erjian (LI 2) is punctured.

To remove nasal obstruction, Yingxiang (LI 20) is chosen,

To eliminate flaccidity from the shoulders Jianjing (GB 21) is selected.

Severe headache is stopped by Sizhukong (SJ 23),

A cough with clear sputum is checked by Lieque (Lu 7).

Disorders related to the eyes are removed by Toulinqi (GB 15),

Pain of the legs is stopped by Huantiao (GB 30).

Shenshu (UB 23) is used for pain in the lumbar region,

Daling (P 7) is punctured for all heart troubles.

Shousanli (LI 10) is needled for the disorders of the shoulder and back,

The He-sea point of the foot Yangming is punctured for arthralgia due to cold-dampness,

The He-sea point of the foot Shaoyin is employed for periumbilical colic due to cold retention.

For pain of the chest and back, Zhongdu (Liv 9) is applied,

For hypochondriacal pain, Yanglingquan (GB 34) is adopted.

For pain of the vertex, Houxi (SI 3) is employed,

For pain of the leg and lumbar region, Weizhong (UB 40) is punctured.

Besides this, pain and exogenous pathogens pertain to excess syndromes, while numbness and internal consumption pertain to deficiency syndromes, and so their treatment is different.

Usually deficiency syndromes are treated by puncturing the mother-point with a reinforcing method, while excess syndromes are treated by puncturing the son-point with a reducing method.

The Ode to the Golden Needle[8]

In the treatment of diseases, acupuncture has quick results,

But the effects depend on the perfect manipulation of the methods of reinforcing and reducing,

Selecting the proper time for needling,

The correct selection of points,

And a knowledge about the course of the jingluo and the patient's condition.

Firstly the location of the disease should be known so as to choose the needling method,

For example, "remote needling", "opposed needling", etc.

Secondly the time for needling—

Usually the qi of a man is in the upper portion of the body in the morning and the lower portion in the afternoon,

While the qi of a woman is just the opposite.

Thirdly, the course of the meridians—

The yang meridians of hand start from the hands to the head,

The yang meridians of foot from head to feet,

The yin meridians of foot start from the feet and end at the chest,

From where start the yin meridians of hand to travel to the hands.

Knowing this, the reinforcing method can be performed by pointing the needle tip along the meridian

And the reducing performed by pointing the needle tip against the meridian.

Fourthly, there is the relation between the seasons, the patient's condition and the insertion of the needle—

Generally superficial insertion is applied on a thin patient or during spring and summer,

Whilst deep insertion is employed on a fat patient or during autumn and winter.

As for reinforcing and reducing technique,

Their key lies in the manipulation with fingers and the cooperation of the respiration.

For example when reinforcing is performed, the needle is rotated to the left with the thumb going forward

And the rotation is accompanied by exhaling;

When reducing is performed, the needle is rotated to the right with the thumb going backward

And the rotation is accompanied by inhaling.

Lifting the needle is considered reinforcing (for heat)

While thrusting the needle is reducing (for cold).

This is the reinforcing and reducing method performed for a man, during the morning;

For a woman, the reinforcing and reducing should be performed in the opposite way and in the afternoon.

Another reinforcing and reducing method is like this:

Reinforcing is performed when the needle is rotated forward once

And the fingers scrape the handle thrice,

Whilst reducing is performed when the needle is rotated backward thrice

And the fingers scrape the handle once.

Usually reinforcing is indicated by itching, numbness and deficiency syndromes,

And reducing by swelling, pain and excess syndromes.

The therapeutic effect depends on the arrival of qi,

A quick qi arrival brings rapid effects,

A slow qi arrival suggests a retarded result.

As for inserting the needle,

It is completed with both hands,

The left hand presses the skin around the point with the finger nail

Whilst the right hand inserts the needle,

At the same time the patient is asked to cough so that his attention may be diverted.

If reinforcing is applied, then the needle is inserted while exhaling,

First to the superficial region just beneath the skin (imagined as Heaven)

Then to the middle region (imagined as Man),

And lastly to the deep region (Earth), where the needle is manipulated with a reinforcing method.

After the needle is retained, it is lifted back to the middle region,

Where the needle is retained again until the qi arrives;

Then the needle is directed towards the affected site,

And manipulated by lifting, thrusting and rotating to cause the meridional qi to become active through the meridians.

If reducing is performed, the needle is inserted while inhaling, first to the superficial region (Heaven),

Then directed to the deep region (Earth),

Where the needle is manipulated with the reducing method.

Then, after the needle is retained, it is lifted back to the middle region and retained for the arrival of qi,

Then the needle is directed towards the affected site and manipulated.

In case of fainting during acupuncture,

The patient should be tonified by needling and given something warm to drink.

Now the method of regulating qi.

If one intends to induce the meridional qi upward,

The needle is twirled to the right after the needle is withdrawn to the middle region (Man);

If one intends to induce the qi downward,

The needle is twirled to the left.

When reinforcing is performed the patient should first exhale then inhale,

While with reducing it is just the opposite.

If the qi fails to arrive, it can be promoted by massaging along the meridian,

Shaking, twirling, twisting and flicking the needle.

When the patient is treated with the "dragon and tiger, ascending and descending" method,

One can press at the front to induce the qi backward

And press at the back to induce the qi forward,

Anyhow the qi should be induced to the location of the pain,

Then the needle is thrust directly in to keep the qi going on to the site.

If the qi is stopped by obstruction,

Descent and ascent by the "dragon and tiger", "tortoise" methods,

And detecting the point by the "phoenix spreading its wings" method

Can be used with the help of pressing and massage,

To remove obstruction and induce the qi from one meridian to another.

Now something about the withdrawal of the needle.

The needle can only be removed when the operator feels it loose under his fingers.

If the operator feels it tight instead of loose,

It shows that the pathogen is still vigorous

And the genuine qi hasn't arrived yet at this time,

And the needle should be manipulated with reinforcing or reducing methods to promote the arrival of the qi.

When a loose sensation appears, the needle can be lifted a little and shaken.

Also the reinforcing method is performed by the swift withdrawal of the needle

Whilst inhaling and with the hole pressed quickly;

The reducing method is performed by a gentle withdrawal of the needle

Whilst exhaling, with the hole left open.

Thus from this we can see that regulating the qi can only be done in a close and intimate situation,

It is said that, "slow insertion is better than quick insertion, which consumes blood,

And gentle withdrawal is better than swift withdrawal which injures the qi".

As for the therapeutic methods with acupuncture, there are eight.

The first is called "setting the mountain on fire",

Which is often used to treat intractable numbness and cold arthralgia.

It is performed first with superficial then deep insertion,

The needle is gently lifted thrice and heavily thrust thrice

With the nine manipulations of the reinforcing method, called "nine yang".

When the patient feels warm at the punctured part, the needle is quickly removed and the hole is pressed.

The second is called "penetrating the heavens coolness",

And it is indicated in treating heat of the muscles and hectic fever.

The method is performed first with deep then superficial insertion,

Then the needle is gently thrust thrice and rapidly lifted thrice,

With six manipulations of the reducing method called "six yin".

When the patient feels coolness at the punctured part,

The needle is removed gently.

The third is called Yang Harbouring Yin,

And it is employed firstly with superficial then deep insertion,

Then the needle is manipulated first with reinforcing then reducing methods.

The fourth is known as Yin Harbouring Yang,

Which is applied firstly with deep then superficial insertion,

Then the needle is manipulated first with reducing, then reinforcing methods.

The four methods mentioned above should be applied perfectly,

That is to say, the reducing method should bring a cool sensation under the needle

While the reinforcing method should allow the patient to feel warm around the needle.

Furthermore, superficial insertion and deep insertion must not be confused with each other,

And the depth of the insertion should be well controlled, this will guarantee the effect.

The fifth is known as Pounding the Meridian Mortar,

Which is indicated in ascites and diaphragmic *tan*.

It is performed by rotating, lifting and thrusting the needle evenly,

According to the reinforcing of nine yang and reducing of six yin,

And one treatment is composed of performing it ten times.

The sixth is known as the Secret of Inducing the Qi,

Which is indicated in treating soreness of the lumbar region, back, knee, elbow or migratory pain all over the body.

The needle is inserted 0.9 cun deep and manipulated with the reinforcements of "nine yang",

Then it is retained for a period of time

While the person breathes five to seven times until the qi travels to the affected part.

Otherwise the Dragon and Tiger Contending Method is used,

In which the needle is rotated to the left nine times and then to the right six times;

This is indicated for stopping pain.

The seventh is known as the Secret of Maintaining the Qi,

Which is indicated for masses in the abdomen.

It is performed by inserting the needle 0.7 cun deep with the "pure yang" reinforcing method,

Then it is thrust while erect and inserted deeply after the needling sensation is achieved,

Then the needle is lifted and retained.

The eighth is known as the Secret of Balancing (removing or adding) the Qi,

Which is indicated in paralysis and skin diseases.

First the main points are selected and then the reinforcing method is adopted.

The needle is lifted and thrust to make the qi circulate all over the body,

Then it is thrust while erect to keep the qi going.

The needle manipulated with the fingers can regulate yin and yang.

But this can be done only on the basis of combining theory and practice.

There are also some other methods of inducing qi through the meridians by removing obstructions.

The first is called "wagging the tail of the dragon",

In which the needle is moved to the left and right gently without being lifted or thrust.

The second is called "the white tiger shaking his head",

In which the needle is moved to the left and right as if a bell was being shaken

And at the same time, the needle is lifted and thrust.

The third is known as the "tortoise searching for his hole",

In which the needle is lifted and thrust and pointed in all directions.

The fourth is known as "the red phoenix spreading his wings to welcome the spring",

In which the needle is inserted to a deep region and then lifted to a superficial region

Where the needle is shaken, lifted and thrust.

If the disorder is in the upper portion, the needle is lifted while inhaling;

If it is in the lower portion, the needle is thrust while exhaling.

As for hemiplegia, the method of promoting the qi through meridians is used

In which the qi travels about 6 cun within the time-unit of one breath.

As it is known, the length of the yang meridians of hand is 50 cun,

That of the yang meridians of foot is 80 cun,

Of the yin meridians of hand 35 cun

And of the yin meridians of foot 65 cun.

Thus when the points on these meridians are punctured

The needle should be kept in for a time period of nine breaths, fourteen breaths,

Seven breaths or twelve breaths respectively.

But the time of the breaths is more than the time taken by the meridional qi to travel the whole course,

The extra time is allowed for the qi to continue to go onto another meridian.

During the whole time, the needle is shaken, lifted and thrust in coordination with the breathing,

To induce qi from one meridian to another

And at last through the whole body.

Thus the patient being punctured for cold syndrome may feel warm,

And the patient with heat syndrome may feel cool,

Pain can be stopped and distension removed,

As if the obstruction (in a ditch, stream and river) was removed,

And the water again flowed smoothly along to irrigate the fields.

The jingluo are like ditches and rivers,

The qi and blood are like water.

When the jingluo are unobstructed,

The qi and blood can nourish the body like water.

But when they are obstructed, illness may ensue.

So though there are three categories of aetiology for illness,

They all lead to the obstruction in the jing or the luo

And the treatment is always the same,

Namely, to remove obstruction from the meridians, regulate qi and blood,

Expel the pathogen and strengthen the body resistance.

The needle is the best instrument to complete these tasks.

The theory of acupuncture is so complicated and profound that it can't be explained in a few words.

The best way is to study and use it seriously and carefully for a long time,

Only in this way can all the many diseases be cured.

The Ballad of the Twelve Points' Indications[9]

Among more than 300 points, there are 12 points which are the most important. Here are the points and their indications.

Points	Indications
1. Zusanli (St 36)	epigastric distension, cold sensation in the stomach, borborygmus and diarrhoea, numbness and oedema of legs and knee-joints, febrile disease, consumptive disease, tympanites.

Note: applying moxibustion to Zusanli after 30 years of age can keep the eyes from invasion by heat.

Points	Indications
2. Neiting (St 44)	cold limbs, preference for quiet, urticaria, sore throat, frequent yawning, toothache and malaria.
3. Quchi (LI 11)	pain of elbow, limited movement of the arm due to hemiplegia, spasm and flaccidity of the arm, inflammation of the throat, shortness of breath, prolonged fever, skin and external diseases characterized by itching.

Points	Indications	Points	Indications
4. Hegu (LI 4)	headache, facial oedema, malaria, dental caries, epistaxis, and lockjaw.	8. Kunlun (UB 60)	spasm, lumbosacral pain, shortness of breath, palpitations and difficulty in walking.
5. Weizhong (UB 40)	soreness of the lumbar region and dragging pain of the back, limited movement of the knee joints, and migratory arthralgia.	9. Huantiao (GB 30)	failure to bend the waist due to soreness, arthralgia of *feng* dampness, and pain over the leg which is severe at night.
6. Chengshan (UB 57)	soreness of the lumbar region, hernia, beriberi, swelling of the knee joints, cramp of gastrocnemius muscle in cholera morbus.	10. Yinlingquan (GB 34)	numbness and swelling of the knee joints, arthralgia, hemiplegia, foot paralysis and inability to sit erect.
7. Taichong (Liv 3)	infantile convulsions, epilepsy, swelling of the throat, hypochondriacal distension, flaccidity of the feet, hernia, blurred vision and soreness of the lumbar region.	11. Tongli (H 5)	voicelessness due to tongue trouble, restlessness, palpitations, heaviness of the body, flushed face, poor appetite, sudden aphonia and pallor.
Note: the artery palpation at the point can show the prognosis of a disease.		12. Lieque (Lu 7)	migraine, migratory arthralgia, numbness, retention of *tan*, and lockjaw.

NOTES

1. The *Biaoyou Fu*, contained in Dou Hanqing's *Guide to Acupuncture and Moxibustion*, probably written around AD 1234.
2. For a discussion in detail, see Appendix 3.
3. Based upon the *Yi Jing*, or *Book of Change*, see Appendix 4.
4. The *Baizheng Fu*, from Gao Wu's *Gathering of Outstanding Acupuncturists* (1529).
5. The *Yulong Ge*, written in the Yuan Dynasty by Wang Guorui, probably around AD 1329.
6. The *Zhouhou Ge*, contained in the *Gathering of Outstanding Acupuncturists* (1529).
7. The *Tongxuan Zhiyao Fu*, by Dou Hanqing, written around AD 1230.
8. The *Jinzhen Fu*, first appeared in 1439, authorship unknown.
9. The *Shier Xue Zhuzhi Zabing Ge*, by Ma Tanyang, Song Dynasty.

Appendix 3
The "Ziwu Liuzhu" acupuncture therapy

Ziwu Liuzhu acupuncture therapy is one method underlining the selection of "open-points" for acupuncture treatment; the foundation of this method lies in the use of the 66 Shu (输) points located along the jingluo, below the elbow and the knee.[1]

It incorporates the concept of the circulation of qi in the meridians, its variations in intensity, and phases of growth and decline, and the opening and closure of the meridians and points. It is in accordance with the idea of the qi circulation from the Jing-well points where it emerges, to the Ying-spring points where it bubbles up, to the Shu-stream points where it pours forth and flourishes, to the Jing-river points where it flows along easily, finally to the He-sea points where it converges together like the confluence of rivers at the sea.

Furthermore, these concepts are combined together with the theories of yin and yang, the 5 Elements (wood, fire, earth, metal, water), the zangfu organs and the Heavenly Stems and Earthly Branches in order to synthesize a method for calculating the "open-point" for a specific time of day, each and every day, with regards to its use in treatment.

The external variations in climate and weather conditions exert a direct influence on the circulation of qi and blood in the human body; and man in nature adapts as an integrated whole to this surrounding environment.

As stated in the *Miraculous Pivot*, "generation in spring, growth in summer, collection in autumn and storage in winter, are the normal variation and evolution of the seasons to which man in nature adapts. With regard to the day as it corresponds to the four seasons: dawn—spring, noon—summer, evening—autumn, and midnight—winter."[2]

Therefore, when one falls sick, owing to the vicissitudes of time and space, one can often observe the following characteristic pattern of and progression of symptoms: morning—mildness, noon—ease, sunset—aggravation, late night—worsening. The method of Ziwu Liuzhu calculates the flourishing and decline of the circulation of qi and blood, and the opening and closure of the meridians and acupoints of each day, according to the influences of the immediate environment upon the human body, in order thereby to apply treatment.

The theory of this method in its embryonic stage can be dated back to as early as the *Yellow Emperor's Book of Medicine*: "Knowing or not knowing the mechanism by which the qi passes, determines the presence or absence of needling effect. Knowing the coming and going of the flowing qi, one can wait for, and expect, an effective treatment at a certain time."[3] And again, "to relieve symptoms of "wood", wait for the time and puncture the Jing-well point of the foot Jueyin (liver), to relieve symptoms of "fire", wait for the time and especially for the monarch-fire (heart) and minister-fire (kidney), and puncture the Ying-spring point of the pericardium meridian; to relieve symptoms of "earth", wait for the time and then puncture the Shu-stream point of the foot Taiyin (spleen), to relieve symptoms of "metal", wait for the time and then puncture the Jing-river point of the hand Taiyin (lung), to relieve symptoms of "water", wait for the time and then puncture the He-sea point of the foot Shaoyin (kidney)".[4]

These summarize the experience of the earliest application of the therapeutic method of waiting for, and selecting, "open-points". The *Miraculous Pivot* states that "the lung meridian starts from Shaoshang (Lu 11), located at the medial aspect of the thumb which is a Jing-well point pertaining to wood" and "the large intestine meridian goes up and links with the hand Yangming, it starts from Shangyang (LI 1) located at the tip of the index finger which is a Jing-well point pertaining to metal".[5] This is the earliest evidence for the harmonization of softness and hardness (yin and yang) among the 5 Elements, also manifest in the statement, "in yin meridians the Jing-well points pertaining to wood come first; in yang meridians the Jing-well points pertaining to metal come first", as is later further explained in the *Classic of Difficult Problems*.[6]

The therapeutic method of Ziwu Liuzhu has been perfected since the Jin (AD 1115–1234) and Yuan (AD 1271–1368) dynasties. The method adopting the Earthly Branches was put forward in the *Lyric of Standard Profundities*[7] (AD 1234) written by Dou Hanqing. In this poem it states that, "one who can treat disease by selecting from among the 66 points at differing times of the day has got the real medical secret".

The method adopting the Heavenly Stems was put forward by Xu Feng (fl. AD 1400) who described the methods of calculation in his *Rhymes on Selecting Open-Points at Differing Times of Each and Every Day, According to Ziwu Liuzhu Acupuncture Therapy*.

Below are outlined the three major aspects of Ziwu Liuzhu acupuncture therapy: the meaning of Ziwu Liuzhu, the composition of the Ziwu Liuzhu method, and its clinical application.

The meaning of Ziwu Liuzhu

Zi-wu (子午) refers to time-period, yin-yang and orientation.

Time-period. One day is divided into 12 time-periods: *zi* (子) corresponds to midnight while *wu* (午) corresponds to midday; in the lunar calendar, *zi* corresponds to the 11th month and the Winter Solstice representing winter, while *wu* corresponds to the 5th month in the lunar calendar, and the Summer Solstice representing summer.

Yin-yang. *Zi* corresponds to the time-period of midnight and extreme yin, and also as extreme yin generates yang it indicates the starting-point of yang. *Wu* corresponds to the time-period of midday and extreme yang, and also as extreme yang generates yin it indicates the starting-point of yin.

Orientation. It is stated in the *Miraculous Pivot* that "there are twelve months in a year and twelve time-periods in a day. *Zi-wu* serves as longitude while *mao-you* serves as latitude."[8] Longitude here refers to south and north (above and below), while latitude refers to east and west (left and right).

Therefore, in these broad aspects, Ziwu involves a very wide concept of time and space.

The two remaining words, *liu* (流) and *zhu* (注), in a narrow sense, both refer to the circulation, with *liu* meaning the flowing current of water and *zhu* referring to water's function of pouring into and transporting things. This is described in the *Book of Odes* when it states, "the river water flows onwards, pouring eastwards into the sea!" In a broad sense, Ziwu concerns the changes within all matter in the universe.

Therefore Ziwu Liuzhu is built upon a scientific theory which involves the synchronicity of time and space according to the cyclical change within all matter in the universe. It sets forth new tasks for scientific research, and, in the sphere of acupuncture, applies itself to explaining how the qi and blood within the human body have a circulatory, cyclical, and synchronous relationship with all natural phenomena.

The composition of the Ziwu Liuzhu method

The Ziwu Liuzhu method is composed of two parts: firstly, combining the 5 Shu points with yin-yang and the 5 Elements, and secondly, combining the Heavenly Stems and Earthly Branches with the zangfu organs and the time-periods.

COMBINING THE 5 SHU POINTS WITH YIN-YANG AND THE 5 ELEMENTS

The 5 Shu points are of great significance in clinical practice and much importance has been attached to them by physicians throughout the generations. The *Miraculous Pivot* set forth the location of the 5 Shu points and pointed out how they combine with yin-yang and the 5 Elements: "in yin meridians the Jing-well point pertaining to Wood comes first while in yang meridians the Jing-well point pertaining to Metal comes first".[9] And the *Classic on Medical Problems*[10] built upon and perfected the above description.

Among the 10 important points set forth in the *Prescriptions Worth A Thousand Gold Coin*, 8 are Shu points. Also there are 35 Shu points among the 126 points described in the *Jade Dragon Rhymes*. Among the 66 points described in the *Superior To Jade Rhymes*, 23 are Shu points, and among the 12 favourite points of the famous Daoist doctor, Ma Danyang, 8 are Shu points.

The combination of the 5 Shu points of the 12 Regular meridians with the 5 Elements is shown in the table below (see Table App. 1).

THE HEAVENLY STEMS AND EARTHLY BRANCHES

The Heavenly Stems start with *jia* and end with *gui*, they are: *jia* (甲), *yi* (乙), *bing* (丙), *ding* (丁), *wu* (戊), *ji* (己), *geng* (庚), *xin* (辛), *ren* (壬), *gui* (癸). The Earthly Branches start with *zi* and end with *hai*, they are *zi* (子), *chou* (丑), *yin* (寅), *mao*

Table App. 1 The five shu points combined with the zangfu, yin-yang and the five Elements (the 66 points)

The 6 Shu points of the yang meridians

Meridian	Well (metal)	Spring (water)	Stream (wood)	Yuan-source	River (fire)	Sea (earth)
Gallbladder (wood)	Foot-Qiaoyin (GB 44)	Xiaxi (GB 43)	Linqi (GB 41)	Qiuxu (GB 40)	Yangfu (GB 38)	Yanglingquan (GB 34)
Small intestine (fire)	Shaoze (SI 1)	Qiangu (SI 2)	Houxi (SI 3)	Hand-Wangu (SI 4)	Yanggu (SI 5)	Xiaohai (SI 8)
Stomach (earth)	Lidui (St 45)	Neiting (St 44)	Xiangu (St 43)	Chongyang (St 42)	Jiexi (St 41)	Zusanli (St 36)
Large intestine (metal)	Shangyang (LI 1)	Erjian (LI 2)	Sanjian (LI 3)	Hegu (LI 4)	Yangxi (LI 5)	Quchi (LI 11)
Urinary bladder (water)	Zhiyin (UB 67)	Tonggu (UB 66)	Shugu (UB 65)	Jinggu (UB 64)	Kunlun (UB 60)	Weizhong (UB 40)
Sanjiao (fire)	Guanchong (SJ 1)	Yemen (SJ 2)	Zhongzhu (SJ 3)	Yangchi (SJ 4)	Zhigou (SJ 6)	Tianjing (SJ 10)

The 5 Shu points of the yin meridians

Meridian	Well (wood)	Spring (fire)	Stream (earth)	River (metal)	Sea (water)
Liver (wood)	Dadun (Liv 1)	Xingjian (Liv 2)	Taichong (Liv 3)	Zhongfeng (Liv 4)	Ququan (Liv 8)
Heart (fire)	Shaochong (H 9)	Shaofu (H 8)	Shenmen (H 7)	Lingdao (H 4)	Shaohai (H 3)
Spleen (earth)	Yinbai (Sp 1)	Dadu (Sp 2)	Taibai (Sp 3)	Shangqiu (Sp 5)	Yinlingquan (Sp 9)
Lung (metal)	Shaoshang (Lu 11)	Yuji (Lu 10)	Taiyuan (Lu 9)	Jingqu (Lu 8)	Chize (Lu 5)
Kidney (water)	Yongquan (K 1)	Rangu (K 2)	Taixi (K 3)	Fuliu (K 7)	Yingu (K 10)
Pericardium (fire)	Zhongchong (P 9)	Laogong (P 8)	Daling (P 7)	Jianshi (P 5)	Quze (P 3)

(卯), *chen* (辰), *si* (巳), *wu* (午), *wei* (未), *shen* (申), *you* (酉), *xu* (戌), *hai* (亥).

The first of the Heavenly Stems is *jia*, the first of the Earthly Branches is *zi*, the stems and branches combined together produce the couplets *jia-zi*, *yi-chou*, *bing-yin*, *ding-mao*, and so on.

As there are 10 Heavenly Stems and 12 Earthly Branches, 6 cycles of stems and 5 cycles of Earthly Branches combined together form the Sexagenary Cycle. This Cycle consists of a permutation of a decimal cycle with a duodecimal cycle, in which 6 of the decimal cycle or 5 of the duodecimal cycle make up a complete cycle of 60, the Sexagenary Cycle, indicating cyclical circulation.

As to the use of the stems and branches in Ziwu Liuzhu acupuncture, a knowledge of the following 5 aspects is essential for its calculation and application:

THE STEMS AND BRANCHES COMBINED TOGETHER FORMING THE SEXAGENARY CYCLE OF 60 AS USED BY THE ANCIENT CHINESE AS SYMBOLS TO RECORD THE YEAR, MONTH, DATE, AND TIME-PERIOD (see Table App. 2)

THE CLASSIFICATION OF HEAVENLY STEMS AND EARTHLY BRANCHES INTO YIN AND YANG

The classification of stems and branches into yin

Table App. 2   The cycle of 60 formed by combining the stems and branches

Jia-Zi	Yi-Chou	Bing-Yin	Ding-Mao	Wu-Chen	Ji-Si	Geng-Wu	Xin-Wei	Ren-Shen	Gui-You
Jia-Xu	Yi-Hai	Bing-Zi	Ding-Chou	Wu-Yin	Ji-Mao	Geng-Chen	Xin-Si	Ren-Wu	Gui-Wei
Jia-Shen	Yi-You	Bing-Xu	Ding-Hai	Wu-Zi	Ji-Chou	Geng-Yin	Xin-Mao	Ren-Chen	Gui-Si
Jia-Wu	Yi-Wei	Bing-Shen	Ding-You	Wu-Xu	Ji-Hai	Geng-Zi	Xin-Chou	Ren-Yin	Gui-Mao
Jia-Chen	Yi-Si	Bing-Wu	Ding-Wei	Wu-Shen	Ji-You	Geng-Xu	Xin-Hai	Ren-Zi	Gui-Chou
Jia-Yin	Yi-Mao	Bing-Chen	Ding-Si	Wu-Wu	Ji-Wei	Geng-Shen	Xin-You	Ren-Xu	Gui-Hai

Table App. 3   The classification of Heavenly Stems and Earthly Branches into yin and yang

Representative numbers:	1	2	3	4	5	6	7	8	9	10	11	12
Heavenly Stems:	Jia	Yi	Bing	Ding	Wu	Ji	Geng	Xin	Ren	Gui	Jia	Yi
Earthly Branches:	Zi	Chou	Yin	Mao	Chen	Si	Wu	Wei	Shen	You	Xu	Hai
	Yang	Yin	Yang	Yin	Yang	Yin	Yang	Yin	Yang	Yin	Yang	Yin

Yang   Yin

and yang, according to their use in different conditions, has a meaning in two aspects.

Firstly, it concerns the rule—"yang advances, yin retreats" (阳进阴退) applied when opening the Jing-well points of the 12 regular meridians. By this rule the stems are taken as the yang while the branches are the yin. A second rule concerns the division into yin and yang according to the odd and even numbers of the stems and branches.

The former rule can be referred to in the section on the clinical application of Ziwu Liuzhu (by "adopting the stems" method), the latter rule is discussed here as follows:

The stems are 10: odd numbers 1, 3, 5, 7, 9 are yang, even numbers 2, 4, 6, 8, 10 are yin.

The branches are 12: odd numbers 1, 3, 5, 7, 9, 11 are yang, even numbers 2, 4, 6, 8, 10, 12 are yin. (Refer to Table App. 3.) In the above chart, the relationship between the representative numbers and the stems and branches is very important, because when calculating the stems and branches of the date, the stems and branches—especially the stems—are decided according to the representative numbers by the remainder of the calculation formula. For example, if after the calculation the remainder is 1, then it represents *jia*, if the remainder is 2 it represents *yi*, if the remainder is 3 it represents *bing*, 4 represents *ding*, 5 represents *wu*, 6 represents *ji*, 7 represents *geng*, 8 represents *xin*, 9 represents *ren*, and 10 represents *gui*.

COMBINING THE HEAVENLY STEMS WITH THE 5 ELEMENTS

The combination of the stems and the 5 Elements is based on harmonization and balance between hardness and softness (yang and yin), and the interpromotion of the 5 Elements, which forms the foundation for the "mutual use of points on paired days" within the "adopting the stems" method. (Refer to Fig. 179.)

THE 12 TIME-PERIODS AND THE 24 HOURS IN THE DAY

In a day, there are 24 hours. In ancient China, the 12 Earthly Branches were used as periods to define the day, with two hours in each time-period. (Refer to Table App. 4.)

The hours here are with reference to the standard time, or the official civil time, for any given region; the international congress held in 1884 divided the earth into 24 time zones extending from pole to pole, by distance east or west of

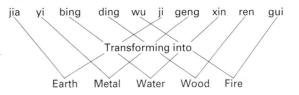

Fig. 179

Table App. 4   The relationship between time-periods and time

Time-branch:	Zi	Chou	Yin	Mao	Chen	Si	Wu	Wei	Shen	You	Xu	Hai
Time-period:	23–1	1–3	3–5	5–7	7–9	9–11	11–13	13–15	15–17	17–19	19–21	21–23

Greenwich, England (Standard/Prime Meridian). Throughout the world, adjacent time zones are one hour (15 degrees) apart; the 7.5 degrees west meridian to 7.5 degrees east meridian is taken as the central time zone, from which 12 time zones both eastwards and westwards are defined.

The longitude is the distance east or west on the earth's surface measured by the difference in time. One rotation (360 degrees) of the earth takes 24 hours and therefore, in each hour, the earth rotates 15 degrees ($360 \div 24 = 15$); and the time difference between each individual adjacent degree of longitude is 4 minutes ($60 \div 15 = 4$) which is taken as the basis for calculating regional time differences.

For example, in China, Beijing (Peking) time is the official standard time. The exact time in any particular region should consider the time difference on the basis of Beijing Time. To take one instance, Beijing is located 116 degrees east while Harbin is 126 degrees east, so the time difference between the two places is 40 minutes $[(126 - 116) \times 4 = 40]$; again, Chengdu is 104 degrees east and the time difference between Beijing and Chengdu is 48 minutes $[(116 - 104) \times 4 = 48]$.

THE CALCULATION OF THE YEAR, MONTH, DATE AND TIME-PERIOD IN HEAVENLY STEMS AND EARTHLY BRANCHES

For selecting the open-point(s) according to the method of Ziwu Liuzhu, it is necessary, first of all, to work out the year, month, date and time-period in stems and branches of the patient's visit for treatment. Among these the calculation of the date and time-period is especially important

1. Calculation of the year in stems and branches

Refer to Table App. 2. The couplet defines the stem and branch for the year, following a orderly sequence; for example, 1983 is a *gui-hai* year, the following (1984) year's stem and branch is *jia-zi*, the next (1985) is *yi-chou*, and so on, calculating the stems and branches of the following years accordingly.

2. Calculation of the month in stems and branches

This will be discussed through the two aspects of month-stem and month-branch. Both calculations are based on the lunar calendar.

Month-branch

Each year the 1st Month = *yin* month-branch
          —5th Month = *wu* month-branch
        —11th Month = *zi* month-branch.
    This rule remains constant without ever changing, and regardless of the year-branch. Generally, as the *yin* (1st month) is fixed, the following months can be calculated accordingly.

Month-stem

This follows a rule and is defined by the year-stem of that particular year.

A *jia* or *ji* year-stem,

The first month's stem is always *bing*,

A *yi* or *geng* year-stem,

The first month's stem is always *wu*,

A *bing* or *xin* year-stem,

The first month's stem is always *geng*,

A *ding* or *ren* year-stem,

The first month's stem is always *ren*,

A *wu* or *gui* year-stem,

The first month's stem is always *jia*.

Therefore, by combining the month-stem and month-branch together according to the above "5-Tigers Escape" method (五虎遁编), the stem and branch of any month is calculated.

For example, for either a *jia* year-stem or a *ji* year-stem, the stem and branch of the first month is always *bing-yin*; for either a *yi* or *geng* year-stem, the stem and branch of the first month is always *wu-yin*; a *bing* or *xin* year, the first month's stem-branch is always *geng-yin*; a *ding* or *ren* year, the first month's stem-branch is always *ren-yin* and, for a *wu* or *gui* year, the first month's stem-branch is always *jia-yin*.

The stem-branch of the other months can be calculated and worked out in the same way by analogy.

3. Calculation of the date stem-branch

Since the duration of the longest and shortest month and the incidence of the leap month are not fixed in the lunar calendar, the calculation of the stem and branch of the date of each month would be rather complicated, and it is much more convenient to calculate the stem-branch of the lunar date from the solar calendar. In practice, the following four aspects are required; with them, the stem-branch of any date can be worked out:

— the representative number of the stem-branch of New Year's Day of that particular year;
— the necessary numbers to add or subtract for the calculation of the stem-branch of the month;
— during a leap year, considering the one extra

day at the end of the 2nd month, the number "1" is added from the 3rd month onwards for calculation;
— the date number of that particular day.

As for the representative number of the stem-branch of New Year's Day, Table App. 3 can be referred to. Additionally the stem-branch of New Year's Day for 60 successive years from 1980–2039 are listed in Table App. 5.

As for the necessary numbers to add or subtract for the calculation of stem-branch of the month, they are calculated and worked out according to the relationship between the date numbers and the "Cycle of 60".

For example, the 1st and 5th month, subtract 1 from both the stem and branch; for the 2nd and 6th month, add zero to the stem and add 6 to the branch; the 3rd month, subtract 2 from the stem and add 10 to the branch; the 4th month, subtract 1 from the stem and add 5 to the branch; the 7th month add zero to both stem and branch and the 8th month, add 1 to the stem and 7 to the branch; the 9th month add 2 to both stem and branch; the 10th month, add 2 to the stem and 8 to the branch; the 11th month, add 3 to both stem and branch; and the 12th month, add 3 to the stem and 9 to the branch.

The above rules are for calculations made during normal years. In the case of a leap year, add 1 onto the answer, from the 3rd month onwards. (Refer to Table App. 6.)

Table App. 5   Stem and branch of New Year's Day, the years 1980–2039

Leap years		Normal years					
Year	New Year's Day	Year	New Year's Day	Year	New Year's Day	Year	New Year's Day
1980	Gui-You	1981	Ji-Mao	1982	Jia-Shen	1983	Ji-Chou
1984	Jia-Wu	1985	Geng-Zi	1986	Yi-Si	1987	Geng-Xu
1988	Yi-Mao	1989	Xiao-Yuo	1990	Bing-Yin	1991	Xin-Wei
1992	Bing-Zi	1993	Ren-Wu	1994	Ding-Hai	1995	Ren-Chen
1996	Ding-You	1997	Gui-Mao	1998	Wu-Shen	1999	Gui-Chou
2000	Wu-Wu	2001	Jia-Zi	2002	Ji-Si	2003	Jia-Xu
2004	Ji-Mao	2005	Yi-You	2006	Geng-Xin	2007	Yi-Wei
2008	Geng-Zi	2009	Bing-Wu	2010	Xin-Hai	2011	Bing-Chen
2012	Xia-You	2013	Ding-Mao	2014	Ren-Kun	2015	Ding-Chou
2016	Ren-Zi	2017	Wu-Zi	2018	Gui-Si	2019	Wu-Xu
2020	Gui-Mao	2021	Ji-You	2022	Jia-Yin	2023	Ji-Wei
2024	Jia-Zi	2025	Geng-Wu	2026	Yi-Hai	2027	Geng-Chen
2028	Bing-Xu	2029	Xin-Mao	2030	Bing-Shen	2031	Xin-Chou
2032	Ding-Wei	2033	Ren-Zi	2034	Ding-Si	2035	Ren-Wu
2036	Ding-Mao	2037	Gui-You	2038	Wu-Yin	2039	Gui-Hai

Table App. 6 Rule for (+) or (−) for the stem and branch of each month

Month	Jan		Feb		Mar		April		May		June		July		Aug		Sept		Oct		Nov		Dec	
	S	B	S	B	S	B	S	B	S	B	S	B	S	B	S	B	S	B	S	B	S	B	S	B
Normal year (+)or(−)	−1	−1	+0	+6	−2	+10	−1	+5	−1	−1	+0	+6	+0	+0	+1	+7	+2	+2	+2	+8	+3	+3	+3	+9
Leap year	For Leap Year add '1' (+1) to the remainder, for all months except January and February																							

For example, New Year's Day in 1984 is found to be *jia-wu* by referring to Table App. 5, and the representative number of *jia* is found to be 1 and that of *wu* is 7 by referring to Table App. 3. Furthermore 1984 is a leap year. Therefore the stem and branch of the 1st days of all 12 months of 1984 can be worked out through the following formulae.

Formula for calculating the date-stem

[(representative number of stem of New Year's Day) + (number of date) + (added/subtracted numbers for calculating stem & branch of each month; add "1" from 3rd month onwards in leap years)] divided by 10 = quotient plus remainder

Formula for calculating the date-branch

[(representative number of branch of New

Table App. 7 Calculation of the stem and branch of the first of each month for 1984 (a leap year, the stem-branch of New Year's Day is jia-wu)

Month and date	Calculating formula		Stem-branch of date
Feb 1st	Stem	1 + 1 + 0 = 2	Yi-Chou
	Branch	7 + 1 + 6 = 14	
Mar 1st	Stem	1 + 1 + 1 − 2 = 1	Jia-Wu
	Branch	7 + 1 + 1 + 10 = 19	
April 1st	Stem	1 + 1 + 1 − 1 = 2	Yi-Chou
	Branch	7 + 1 + 1 + 5 = 14	
May 1st	Stem	1 + 1 + 1 − 1 = 2	Yi-Wei
	Branch	7 + 1 + 1 − 1 = 8	
June 1st	Stem	1 + 1 + 1 − 0 = 3	Bing-Yin
	Branch	7 + 1 + 1 + 6 = 15	
July 1st	Stem	1 + 1 + 1 + 0 = 3	Bing-Shen
	Branch	7 + 1 + 1 + 0 = 9	
Aug 1st	Stem	1 + 1 + 1 + 1 = 4	Ding-Mao
	Branch	7 + 1 + 1 + 7 = 16	
Sept 1st	Stem	1 + 1 + 1 + 2 = 5	Wu-Xu
	Branch	7 + 1 + 1 + 2 = 11	
Oct 1st	Stem	1 + 1 + 1 + 2 = 5	Wu-Chen
	Branch	7 + 1 + 1 + 8 = 17	
Nov 1st	Stem	1 + 1 + 1 + 3 = 6	Si-Hai
	Branch	7 + 1 + 1 + 3 = 12	
Dec 1st	Stem	1 + 1 + 1 + 3 = 6	Si-Ji
	Branch	7 + 1 + 1 + 9 = 18	

Year's Day) + (number of date) + (added/subtracted numbers for calculating stem & branch of each month; add "1" from 3rd month onwards in leap years)] divided by 12 = quotient plus remainder

4. Calculation of stems and branches of the time-period

By utilizing the theory of the "5 Elements and Ten Transformations" in combination and transformation, among the Heavenly Stems and 5 Elements, and based upon a "5-Mice Escape" method, the calculation of the stem and branch of the time-period proceeds according to the following rule:

The stem and branch of the 12 time-periods of

a *jia* or *ji* Date, starts with *jia-zi*;

a *yi* or *geng* Date, starts with *bing-zi*;

a *bing* or *xin* Date, starts with *wu-zi*;

a *ding* or *ren* Date, starts with *geng-zi*;

a *wu* or *gui* Date, starts with *ren-zi*.

5. Combining the heavenly stems with the zangfu

In the *Plain Questions* it states that "the liver dominates spring, with indications of the foot Jueyin and Shaoyang, its date is *jia-yi*; the heart dominates summer, with indications of the hand Shaoyin and Taiyang, its date is *bing-ding*; the spleen dominates late summer, with indications of the foot Taiyin and Yangming, its date is *wu-ji*; the lung dominates autumn, with indications of the hand Taiyin and Yangming, its date is *geng-xin*; the kidney dominates winter, with indications of the foot Shaoyin and Taiyang, its date is *ren-gui*...".[11]

The combining of the Heavenly Stems with the zangfu organs is one of the foundations of the method of "adopting the stems". When applying the Ziwu Liuzhu method for the selection of open-points for everyday use, points on the meridians pertaining to their zangfu organs are selected sequentially according to the order of qi circulation through the Jing-well, Ying-spring, Shu-stream, Jing-river and He-sea points, according to the Heavenly Stem of the time-period at that time. It follows the rule:

Yang		Yin	
Stem	Fu	Stem	Zang
jia	GB	yi	Liv
bing	SI (SJ)	ding	H (P)
wu	St	ji	Sp
geng	LI	xin	Lu
ren	UB	gui	Kid

6. Combining the earthly branches with the zangfu

The combination of Earthly Branches with the zangfu organs indicates that the 12 Earthly Branches of a day are paired together with the zangfu. This is one of the foundations of the method "adopting the branches" in which the 12 time-periods are used as codes representing the 12 meridians, for the selection of points.

The circulation of qi and blood in the human body starts from the middle-jiao, and pours upward into the lung meridian, then to the large intestine, stomach, spleen, heart, small intestine, urinary bladder, kidney, pericardium, Sanjiao, gallbladder, and liver meridians, and then back to the lung. The circulation runs in an orderly fashion from the time-periods *yin, mao, ...* back to *yin*, and the branches of the time-periods are paired with zangfu as follows:

Lung—*yin*, large intestine—*mao*, stomach—*chen*,

Spleen—*si*, heart—*wu*, small intestine—*wei*;

Bladder—*shen*, kidney—*you*, pericardium—*xu*,

Sanjiao—*hai*, gallbladder—*zi*, liver—*chou*.

The clinical application of Ziwu Liuzhu acupuncture therapy

Ziwu Liuzhu acupuncture therapy is applied clinically in two separate ways: the method of "adopting the stems" and the method of "adopting the branches".

THE METHOD OF ADOPTING THE STEMS

This method is a method of selecting open-point(s) by combining or pairing the Heavenly Stems with the zangfu organs; for the application of this method it is necessary to study the following aspects.

1. Get familiar with the previously mentioned idea of combining the Heavenly Stems with the zangfu. Then follow the rule "the yang advances, the yin retreats" (阳进阴退); here the "yang" refers to the Heavenly Stems and the "yin" refers to the Earthly Branches. That is to say, in opening the Jing-well points, the "yang" (Heavenly Stems) advance forwards in the natural order of the stems: *jia–yi–bing–ding–wu–ji–geng–xin–ren–gui*; but the "yin" (Earthly Branches) retreat backwards in an order *opposite* to the natural order of branches, so "the yin retreats" in the order: *xu–you–shen–wei–wu–si–chen–mao–yin–chou–zi–hai*, in combination with the stems, opening the Jing-well points of the various meridians. (Refer to Table App. 8.)

2. "On a yang date, at a yang time-period, open the Jing-well point of a yang meridian (of a fu organ)" is the rule to follow. And when the qi circulation passes on into a yin date, continue opening points at yang time-periods according to the order of progression of the Jing-well, Ying-spring, Shu-stream, Jing-river and He-sea points.

For example, on a *jia* date, at a *jia-xu* time-period, open the Jing-well point, Foot-Qiaoyin (GB 44) of the gallbladder meridian; the next time-period *yi-hai* is a yin stem-branch and thus has no "open-point". Now the 12 time-periods of the *jia* date have finished, and the qi circulation passes on into a *yi* date, so at the yang time-period *bing-zi*, continue opening the Ying-spring point Qiangu (SI 2) of the small intestine meridian (of a fu organ, yang).

3. "On a yin date, at a yin time-period, open the Jing-well point of a yin meridian (of a zang organ)" is the rule to follow. And when the qi

Table App. 8 Opening the Jing-well points according to the method of Ziwu Liuzhu at differing times for each and every day

Heavenly Stem	Jia	Yi	Bing	Ding	Wu	Ji	Geng	Xin	Ren	Gui
Time-period	Jia → Xu -->	Yi → You -->	Bing → Shen -->	Ding → Wei -->	Wu → Wu -->	Ji → Si -->	Geng → Chen -->	Xin → Mao -->	Ren → Yin -->	Gui → Hai -->
Meridian	GB	Liv	SI	H	St	Sp	LI	Lu	UB	Kid
Jing-well point	Foot Qiaoyin	Dadun	Shaoze	Shaochong	Lidui	Yinbai	Shangyang	Shaoshang	Zhiyin	Yongquan

Note: → = yang advances, --> = yin retreats.

circulation passes on into a yang date, continue opening points at yin time-periods according to the order in progression of the 5 Shu points.

For example, on a *yi* date, at a *yi-you* time-period, open the Jing-well point Dadun (Liv 1) of the liver meridian; the next yin time-period is *ding-hai*, so open the Ying-spring point Shaofu (H 8) of the heart meridian, ..., and when the 12 time-periods of the *yi* date have finished, the qi circulation passes on into the *bing* date and, on the *bing* date, at the *ji-chou* time-period, continue opening the Shu-stream point Taibai (Sp 3) of the spleen meridian (of a zang organ, yin).

4. At the same time as opening the Shu-stream point, open also the *yuan* point of the meridian to which the open Jing-well point pertains.

For example, as mentioned above, on a *bing* date, at a *ji-chou* time-period, you open the Shu-stream point of the spleen meridian Taibai (Sp 3); but also, because on the *yi* date, at the *yi-you* time-period, the Jing-well point of the governing meridian—Dadun (Liv 1) on the liver meridian—has been opened, so, at the same time as opening the Shu-stream point Taibai, the *yuan* point Taichong (Liv 3) of the liver meridian (to which the open Jing-well point Dadun pertains) should also be opened. (In the case of yin meridians, the *yuan* point is included in, or replaced by, the Shu-stream point.)

This is what is meant by the saying, "returning to the original governing meridian, is returning to the source".

5. "The qi adopts the Sanjiao, it gives rise to me". As the Sanjiao dominates the qi, and qi pertains to yang, after having passed through all 5 Shu points, for every yang meridian, (after the He-sea point), at the next yang time-period the

principle "the qi adopts Sanjiao, it gives rise to me" should be applied.

Here "me" refers to the meridian on duty, or governing meridian, i.e. the meridian to which the open Jing-well point pertains; and "it" refers to one of the 5 Shu points of the Sanjiao meridian, which is then used.

For example, on a *jia* date, at a *xu* time-period, open Foot Qiaoyin (GB 44) of the gallbladder meridian, and as the qi passes on into the *yi* date the opening of points is continued at yang time-periods, and at the *ren-wu* time-period the He-sea point is opened; then, the next yang time-period is *jia-shen*, and the Ying-spring point Yemen (SJ 2) which is the "water" point on the Sanjiao meridian is opened or selected. This is because the gallbladder pertains to "wood", and "water gives birth or rise to wood", hence the rule "it gives rise to me".

The selection of open-point(s) on other yang meridians can also be calculated according to this principle, by analogy.

6. "The blood returns to the pericardium, I give rise to it". The pericardium dominates blood and blood belongs to yin, so after having passed through opening the He-sea point, at the next yin time-period, one should apply the principle "the blood returns to the pericardium, I give rise to it".

For example, on a *yi* date, at a *you* time-period, you open the Jing-well point Dadun (Liv 1) of the liver meridian. The next yin time-period *ding-hai*, open the Ying-spring point Shaofu (H 8) of the heart meridian. After passing on into the *bing* date, the opening of points is continued at yin time-periods, until at the *gui-si* time-period the He-sea point of the kidney meridian Yingu (K 10) is opened. So what about the next yin time-period *yi-wei*?

Then the principle "the blood returns to the pericardium, I give rise to it" should be applied to open the "I-give-rise-to-it" point, which is the Ying-spring point of the pericardium meridian. This is because the liver pertains to "wood" and "wood gives birth or rise to fire". The liver is referred to as "I" or the meridian on duty, and the "fire" point is "it", one of the 5 Shu points of the pericardium meridian which is to be opened.

The selection of open-point(s) on other yin meridians can also be calculated according to this principle, by analogy.

Based on the above mentioned 6 rules and in combination with the previously discussed substance of the previous section, "The Composition of the Ziwu Liuzhu Method" (see above), you are now ready and able to perform the calculations, and carry out the application of the Ziwu Liuzhu acupuncture therapy.

In applying the method of "adopting the stems" according to Ziwu Liuzhu, the following two methods of calculation are worth introducing:

1. Selecting open-points at differing times for each and every day according to the Ziwu Liuzhu method

1. On a *jia* date, at a *xu* time, the Jing-well, Foot-Qiaoyin of gallbladder,

At a *bing-zi* time, open the Ying-spring, Qiangu of the small intestine,

At a *wu-yin* time, open the Shu-stream, Xiangu of the stomach,

At a yin time, return to the source, Qiuxu of gallbladder.

At a *geng-chen* time, open the Jing-river, Yangxi of the large intestine.

At a *ren-wu* time, open the He-sea, Weizhong of the bladder.

At a jia-shen time, "adopting water from the Sanjiao" and combining with the Heavenly Stems,

Open the Ying-spring and Water point, Yemen of the Sanjiao.

2. On a *yi* date, at a *you* time, open the Jing-well, Dadun of the liver,

At a *ding-hai* time, open the Ying-spring, Shaofu of the heart,

At a *ji-chou* time, open the Shu-stream, Taibai of the spleen and the *yuan* point, Taichong of the liver,

At a *xin-mao* time, open the Jing-river, Jingqu of the lung,

At a *gui-si* time, open the He-sea, Yingu of the kidney,

At a *yi-wei* time, open the Ying-spring, the fire point, Laogong, according to "blood returns to the pericardium".

3. On a *bing* date, at a *shen* time, open the Jing-well, Shaoze of the small intestine,

At a *wu-xu* time, open the Ying-spring, Neiting of the stomach,

At a *geng-zi* time, open the Shu-stream, Sanjian of the large intestine, and Hand-Wangu, returning to the source.

At a *ren-yin* time, open the Jing-river, the fire point, Kunlun of the bladder,

At a *jia-chen* time, open the He-sea, Yanglingquan of the gallbladder,

At a *bing-wu* time, open the Shu-stream, Zhongzhu, according to "the qi adopts the Sanjiao".

4. On a *ding* date, at a *wei* time, open the Jing-well, Shaochong of the heart,

At a *ji-you* time, open the Ying-spring, Dadu of the spleen,

At a *xin-hai* time, open the Shu-stream, the earth point, Taiyuan of the lung,

And Shenmen of the heart, according to the principle of "returning to the source".

At a *gui-chou* time, open the Jing-river, Fuliu, of the kidney,

At a *yi-mao* time, open the He-sea, Ququan of the Liver,

At a *ding-si* time, open the Shu-stream, the earth point, Daling, according to "blood returning to the pericardium".

5. On a *wu* date, at a *wu* time, open the Jing-well, Lidui of the stomach,

At a *geng-shen* time, open the Ying-spring, Erjian, of the large intestine,

At a *ren-xu* time, open the Shu-stream, Shugu, of the bladder and "returning to the source", Chongyang of the stomach.

At a *jia-zi* time, open the Jing-river, Yangfu of the gallbladder,

At a *bing-yin* time, open the He-sea, Xiaohai of the small intestine,

At a *wu-chen* time, open the Jing-river, the fire point, Zhigou, according to "the qi adopts the Sanjiao".

6. On a *ji* date, at a *si* time, open the Jing-well, Yinbai of the spleen,

At a *xin-wei* time, open the Ying-spring, Yuji of the lung,

At a *gui-you* time, open the Shu-stream, earth, Taixi of the kidney,

And Taibai of the spleen, according to the principle of "returning to the source".

At a *yi-hai* time, open the Jing-river, Zhongfeng of the liver,

At a *ding-chou* time, open the He-sea, Shaohai of the heart,

At a mao time, open the Jing-river, Jianshi, according to the principle "blood returns to the pericardium".

7. On a *geng* date, at a *chen* time, open the Jing-well, Shangyang of the large intestine,

At a *ren-wu* time, open the Ying-spring, Tonggu of the bladder,

At a *jia-shen* time, open the Shu-stream, the earth point, Foot-Linqi of the gallbladder,

And Hegu of the large intestine, returning to the source.

At a *bing-xu* time, open the Jing-river, the fire point, Yanggu of the small intestine,

At a *wu-zi* time, open the He-sea, Zusanli of the stomach,

At a *geng-yin* time, open the He-sea, the earth point, Tianjing, according to the principle "the qi adopts the Sanjiao".

8. On a *xin* date, at a *mao* time, open the Jing-well point, Shaoshang of the lung,

At a *gui-si* time, open the Ying-spring, Rangu of the kidney,

At a *yi-wei* time, open the Shu-stream, the earth point, Taichong of the liver,

And Taiyuan of the lung, returning to the source.

At a *ding-you* time, open the Jing-river, Lingdao of the heart,

At a *ji-hai* time, open the He-sea, Yinlingquan of the spleen,

At a *xin-chou* time, open the He-sea, the water point, Quze, according to the principle "blood returns to the pericardium".

9. On a *ren* date, at a *yin* time, open the Jing-well point, Zhiyin of the bladder,

At a *jia-chen* time, open the Ying-spring, Xiaxi of the gallbladder,

At a *bing-wu* time, open the Shu-stream, Houxi of the small intestine,

And Jinggu (on the bladder) and Yangchi (on the Sanjiao)

According to the principle "returning to the original is returning to the source".

At a *wu-shen* time, open the Jing-river, Jiexi of the stomach,

At a *geng-xu* time, open the He-sea, Quchi of the large intestine,

At a *ren-zi* time, open the Jing-well, the metal point, Guanchong,

According to the principle "the qi adopts the Sanjiao",

By which Metal (Guanchong), and Water (*ren*) are in the relation of "a mother giving birth to a son".

10. On a *gui* date, at a *hai* time, open the Jing-well, Yongquan of the kidney,

At a *chou* time, open the Ying-spring, Xingjian of the large intestine,

At a *ding-mao* time, open the Shu-stream, Shenmen of the heart,

And Taixi (on the kidney) and Daling (on the pericardium)

According to the principle "returning to the original is returning to the source".

At a *ji-si* time, open the Jing-river, Shangqiu of the spleen,

At a *xin-wei* time, open the He-sea, Chize of the lung,

At a *gui-you* time, open the Jing-well, the wood point, Zhongchong,

According to the principle "the blood returning to the pericardium".

On the basis of the above principles and rules,

Carry out the calculation according to sequential order of the ten Heavenly Stems.

2. The 1, 4, 2, 5, 3, 0, counter-acting calculation method

This method means carrying out calculations on the basis of the "6 *jia* cycle", "the yang advances, the yin retreats, open Jing-well points" along with "on a yang date, at a yang time-period, open a yang meridian", and "on a yin date, at a yin time-period, open a yin meridian" along with the "progression of Earthly Branches along with time". By these means you solve the problem, and inadequacy, of having no open-points at 10 time-periods for a *gui* date". (Refer to Table App. 9.)

THE METHOD OF ADOPTING THE BRANCHES

The method "adopting the branches" is a method of opening points at differing times of the day on the basis of combining the 12 time-periods within each day with the zangfu organs (refer to the previous description of the Earthly Branches paired with the zangfu organs, above).

This method is applied in two ways in clinic. One is "tonifying the mother and reducing the son" and the other is "the selection of 66 points at differing time-periods of the day".

THE SELECTION OF POINTS ACCORDING TO "TONIFYING THE MOTHER AND REDUCING THE SON"

Based on the classification of the involved meridians with the 5 Elements, and the classification of the 5 Shu points with the 5 Elements, calculate the relationship of mother and son.

Table App. 9   The 1, 4, 2, 5, 3, 0 counter-acting calculation method

Routine 5 Shu points		1 Jing-well	4 Jing-river	2 Ying-spring	5 He-sea	3 Shu-stream	0 Qi adopts the Sanjiao, blood returns to the pericardium
6 Jia	Stem-branch: point:	Jia day Jia-Xu Qiaoyin	Ji day Jia-Zi Yangfu	Wu day Jia-Yin Xiaxi	Ding day Jia-Chen Yanglingquan	Bing day Jia-Wu Linqi	Yi day Jia-Shen Yemen
6 Yi	Stem-branch: point:	Yi day Yi-You Dadun	Ji day Yi-Hai Zhongfeng	Ji day Yi-Chou Xingjian	Wu day Yi-Mao Ququan	Ding day Yi-Si Taichong	Bing day Yi-Wei Laogong
6 Bing	Stem-branch: point:	Bing day Bing-Shen Shaoze	Geng day Bing-Xu Yanggu	Geng day Bing-Zi Qiangu	Ji day Bing-Yin Xiaohai	Wu day Bing-Chen Houxi	Ding day Bing-Wu Zhongzhu
6 Ding	Stem-branch: point:	Ding day Ding-Wei Shaochong	Xin day Ding-You Lingdao	Geng day Ding-Hai Shaofu	Geng day Ding-Chou Shaohai	Ji day Ding-Mao Shenmen	Wu day Ding-Si Daling
6 Wu	Stem-branch: point:	Wu day Wu-Wu Lidui	Ren day Wu-Shen Jiexi	Xin day Wu-Xu Neiting	Xin day Wu-Zi Zusanli	Geng day Wu-Yin Xiangu	Ji day Wu-Chen Zhigou
6 Ji	Stem-branch: point:	Ji day Ji-Si Yinbai	Gui day Ji-Wei Shangqiu	Ren day Ji-You Dadu	Xin day Ji-Hai Yinlingquan	Xin day Ji-Chou Taibai	Geng day Ji-Mao Jianshi
6 Geng	Stem-branch: point:	Geng day Geng-Chen Shangyang	Jia day Geng-Wu Yangxi	Gui day Geng-Shen Erjian	Ren day Geng-Xu Quchi	Ren day Geng-Zi Sanjian	Xin day Geng-Yin Tianjing
6 Xin	Stem-branch: point:	Xin day Xin-Mao Shaoshang	Yi day Xin-Si Jingqu	Jia day Xin-Wei Yuji	Gui day Xin-You Chize	Ren day Xin-Hai Taiyuan	Ren day Xin-Chou Quze
6 Ren	Stem-branch: point:	Ren day Ren-Yin Zhiyin	Bing day Ren-Chen Kunlun	Yi day Ren-Wu Tonggu	Jia day Ren-Shen Weizhong	Gui day Ren-Xu Shugu	Gui day Ren-Zi Guanchong
6 Gui	Stem-branch: point:	Gui day Gui-Hai Yongquan	Wu day Gui-Chou Fuliu	Ding day Gui-Mao Rangu	Bing day Gui-Si Yingu	Yi day Gui-Wei Taixi	Jia day Gui-You Zhongchong

Then, according to the principle of "in case of deficiency tonify the mother, in case of excess reduce the son", carry out the selection of open-points at differing time-periods of the day.

For example, for disease of the lung meridian of the hand Taiyin, in conditions of an excess of pathogenic qi, the Lung pertains to metal, its mother-point is Taiyuan (earth) and son-point is Chize (water). Select Chize with a reducing needling method at the *yin* time-period, when qi of the lung meridian is flourishing. In conditions of deficiency of the antipathogenic qi, then select the mother-point, Taiyuan, with a tonification needling technique at the *mao* time-period when the lung meridian qi is in deficiency.

If the "open-point time" of the involved meridian has passed when the patient comes for the treatment, or in cases which are neither deficient nor excess, one can select the "origin" (本) point from the involved meridian, which is the point with the same classification within the 5 Elements as the involved meridian; or else select the *yuan* point of the involved meridian for treatment.

For example, the "origin" point of the lung meridian (with the same classification within the 5 Elements) is Jingqu (Lu 8), and the *yuan* point of lung meridian is Taiyuan (Lu 9).

The selection of points according to "tonifying the mother and reducing the son" is shown in Table App. 10.

THE SELECTION OF THE 66 POINTS AT DIFFERING TIME-PERIODS OF THE DAY

The method of "adopting the branches" can be applied with a certain flexibility and is therefore of great importance in the clinic.

However, the selection of open-points according to "in case of deficiency tonify the mother, in case of excess reduce the son" is not comprehen-

Table App. 10 Selection of points according to "tonifying the mother and reducing the son", the "root-origin" points and yuan-source points

Meridian	5 Elements	Opening time	Chief symptom	Tonification mother-point	Time	Reducing son-point	Time	Origin point	Yuan point
Lung	Xin Metal	Yin	cough, restlessness, fullness in chest	Taiyuan	Mao	Chize	Yin	Jingqu	Taiyuan
Large intestine	Geng Metal	Mao	toothache, sore throat	Quchi	Chen	Erjian	Mao	Shangyang	Hegu
Stomach	Wu Earth	Chen	abdominal distension, pain	Jiexi	Si	Lidui	Chen	Zusanli	Chongyang
Spleen	Ji Earth	Si	abdominal fullness, distension, diarrhoea	Dadu	Wu	Shangqiu	Si	Taibai	Taibai
Heart	Ding Fire	Wu	dry throat, tongue pain, feverish palm	Shaochong	Wei	Shenmen	Wu	Shaofu	Shenmen
Small intestine	Bing Fire	Wei	stiff nape, neck swelling	Houxi	Shen	Xiaohai	Wei	Yanggu	Wangu
Urinary bladder	Ren Water	Shen	headache, blurred vision, epilepsy	Zhiyin	You	Shugu	Shen	Tonggu	Jinggu
Kidney	Gui Water	You	palpitations, lumbar pain	Fuliu	Xu	Yongquan	You	Yingu	Taixi
Pericardium	Ding Fire	Xu	spasms, a restless mind, hypochondriacal pain	Zhongchong	Hai	Daling	Xu	Laogong	Daling
Sanjiao	Bing Fire	Hai	deafness and pain of the eyes	Zhongzhu	Zi	Tianjing	Hai	Zhigou	Yangchi
Gallbladder	Jia Wood	Zi	headache and hypochondriacal pain	Xiaxi	Chou	Yangfu	Zi	Linqi	Qiuxu
Liver	Yi Wood	Chou	hypochondriacal pain, hernia	Ququan	Yin	Xingjian	Chou	Dadun	Taichong

sive enough (only 20 points may be selected from the yin meridians and 24 points from the yang meridians in any one day), and there remain 22 points unused. Therefore Dou Hanqing, in his *Lyrics of Standard Profundities* (see Appendix 2) stated that "one who can treat disease by selecting from the 66 points at differing times of the day, has got the medical secret".

This precisely describes responding according to the 12 time-periods of the day combined with the zangfu organs to which they pertain, in order to select from the 5 open-points (Jing-well, Ying-spring, Shu-stream, Jing-river and He-sea) of the yin meridians and the 6 open-points (Jing-well, Ying-spring, Shu-stream, *yuan* points, Jing-river and He-Sea) of the yang meridians, for treatment.

In the clinical application of this method, treatment may be given according to the aetiology, nature and conditions of the disease, by flexibly selecting from the 5 Shu points of the involved meridian(s) and their inter-relationships with the open time-period(s) when the qi circulation of related meridians is flourishing.

NOTES

1. See Ch. 2 on this category of points.
2. *Miraculous Pivot*, Ch. 44, "Yielding to the Qi of a Single Day as Divided among the Four Seasons".
3. *Miraculous Pivot*, Ch. 1, "On the 9 Needles and 12 Yuan-sources".
4. *Plain Questions*, Ch. 72, "Discussion of Needling Methods".
5. Both selections from the *Miraculous Pivot*, Ch. 2, "Source of the Shu Points".
6. The *Classic on Difficult Medical Problems*, 64th problem.
7. See Appendix 2.
8. *Miraculous Pivot*, Ch. 52, "Wei Qi Circulation".
9. *Miraculous Pivot*, Ch. 2, "Source of the Shu Points".
10. The Classic on *Difficult Medical Problems*, 64th problem.
11. *Plain Questions*, Ch. 22, "Discussion on the Seasonal Rules of the Qi of the Zangfu".

Appendix 4
The Eight Methods of the Mystic Turtle and The Eight Methods of Flying and Soaring

The Eight Methods of the Mystic Turtle

The *Linggui Ba Fa* (灵龟八法), or Eight Methods of the Mystic Turtle, are also known as the "Methods of the Extra Meridians by Adopting the Eight Trigrams" or *Qijing Nagua Fa* (奇经纳卦法). It is a method of acupuncture therapy which selects points during differing times of the day. Again, the Mystic Turtle method and the Ziwu Liuzhu method (described in Appendix 3, above) complement each other in the treatment of disease.

The Eight Methods of the Mystic Turtle combines the theories of the *jiugong* (九宫) or "9 Palaces" and the *ba gua* (八卦) or "8 Trigrams" from ancient Chinese philosophy, with the circulation and confluence of the qi and blood of the 8 extra meridians within the human body.

It selects the 8 Confluent points (see Ch. 2) which communicate with the 8 extra meridians, according to a time worked out through calculating the change in the representative numbers of the Heavenly Stems and Earthly Branches of that particular date and time-period.

THE COMPOSITION OF THE METHOD OF THE MYSTIC TURTLE

NINE PALACES AND EIGHT TRIGRAMS

The 8 Trigrams

The trigrams are symbols derived from the ancient classic of the *Book of Change*, consisting of broken and unbroken lines, the shapes of yin and yang, which the ancient sages in China combined to symbolize Heaven, Earth, water, fire, the wind, the thunder, the mountain and the marsh, all represented in nature. They are named as follows:

Qian (Heaven)	☰
Kun (Earth)	☷
Kan (water)	☵
Li (fire)	☲
Sun (the wind)	☴
Zhen (the thunder)	☳
Gen (the mountain)	☶
Dui (the marsh)	☱

The names and diagram of the 8 Trigrams are further combined with the four directions forming the so-called "9 Palaces". Each of the trigrams has its own position and orientation; they are then combined with the 9 Palaces according to an arrangement of numbers.

$$4\text{—}Sun \quad 9\text{—}Li \quad 2\text{—}Kun$$
$$3\text{—}Zhen \quad 5\text{—}Kun \quad 7\text{—}Dui$$
$$8\text{—}Gen \quad 1\text{—}Kan \quad 6\text{—}Qian$$

9 in the upper of the chart, 1 in the lower,

3 on the left and 7 on the right.

2 and 4 on both sides (right and left) above like the "shoulders of man", and

8 and 6 on both sides (left and right) below like the "feet of man".

5 and 10 in the middle of the chart

Then each "palace" is further combined with an extra meridian point which communicates with it, thus forming the arrangement and the representative numbers of their 8 points:

Kan 1 = Shenmai (UB 62),

Kun 2 & 5 = Zhaohai (K 6),

Zhen 3 = Waiguan (SJ 5),

Sun 4 = Foot-Linqi (GB 41),

Qian 6 = Gongsun (Sp 4),

Dui 7 = Houxi (SI 3),

Gen 8 = Neiguan (P 6),

Li 9 = Lieque (Lu 7).

The representative numbers of these 8 points are very important in the calculation of the Mystic Turtle method, so it is advisable to keep them firmly in mind when applying this method.

THE 8 EXTRA MERIDIANS AND THE 8 CONFLUENT POINTS

The 8 extra meridians are the Ren, Du, Chong, Dai, Yinwei, Yangwei, Yinqiao and Yangqiao meridians, which command and regulate the 12 regular meridians.

Also, the 12 regular meridians, owing to their

own circulation, inter-crossing and connection, have 8 points, known as the 8 Confluent points, which are located at the extremities, communicating with the 8 extra meridians.

These are: Houxi of the small intestine meridian which communicates with the Du meridian, Lieque of the lung meridian which communicates with the Ren meridian, Gongsun of the spleen meridian which communicates with the Chong meridian, Foot-Linqi of the gallbladder meridian which communicates with the Dai meridian, Zhaohai of the kidney meridian which communicates with the Yinqiao meridian, Shenmai of the bladder meridian which communicates with the Yangqiao meridian, Neiguan of the pericardium meridian which communicates with the Yinwei meridian, and Waiguan of the Sanjiao meridian which communicates with the Yangwei meridian.

In addition, the 8 points have a close relationship and connection among themselves.

For instance: Gongsun and Neiguan communicate with each other and converge at the heart, chest and stomach; Houxi and Shenmai communicate and converge at the inner canthus, neck, nape, ear, shoulder, small intestine and urinary bladder; Foot-Linqi and Waiguan communicate and converge at the outer canthus, retroauricular region, neck, nape, and shoulder; Lieque and Zhaohai communicate and converge at the lung system, throat, chest and diaphragm.

This combines and classifies the 8 Extra meridians and 8 Confluent points into four groups which each have similar therapeutic properties and indications.

THE REPRESENTATIVE NUMBERS OF THE HEAVENLY STEMS AND EARTHLY BRANCHES OF THE DATE AND TIME-PERIOD BY THE METHOD OF THE MYSTIC TURTLE

As for the composition of the Mystic Turtle method, in addition to the 8 Extra meridians, 8 Points and 8 Trigrams, the representative numbers of the stems and branches of the date and time-period also act as a basis in selecting points.

The representative numbers of the stems and branches of the particular date and time-period are determined according to the stems and branches method of transforming into the 5 Elements, and according to the yin-yang classification of the stems and branches, in sequential order.

These representative numbers are the basis for calculating and selecting points by the Mystic Turtle method (refer to Table App. 11).

THE REPRESENTATIVE NUMBERS OF THE TIME-PERIODS ACCORDING TO THE MYSTIC TURTLE METHOD

The stems and branches of the time-periods of each day also have their representative numbers, which are as important as those of the stems and branches of the date, in the calculation and application of this method. These numbers should also be memorized well (refer to Table App. 12).

THE APPLICATION OF THE METHOD OF THE MYSTIC TURTLE

The calculation and the application of this method is guided by the following procedure.

The calculation is fairly straightforward. Add the representative numbers of the stems and branches of the date and the time-period together; the answer is then divided by 9 for a yang date or 6 for a yin date.

Then the quotient and the remainder are worked out, and, according to the "remainder", the representative number of a point as arranged in the 8 Trigrams is obtained. That point is the open-point during that time-period.

The formula is as follows:

Table App. 11 The representative numbers of the stems and branches of the date for selecting points according to the Linggui Ba Fa method

Representative numbers	10	9	8	7
Heavenly Stems	Jia Ji	Yi Geng	Ding Ren	Wu Gui Bing Xin
Earthly Branches	Chen Chou Xu Wei	Shen You	Yin Mao	Si Wu Hai Zi

Table App. 12 The representative numbers of the stems and branches of the time-period for selecting points according to the Ling-Gui Ba-Fa method

Representative numbers	9	8	7	6	5	4
Heavenly Stems	Jia Ji	Yi Geng	Bing Xin	Ding Ren	Wu Gui	
Earthly Branches	Zi Wu	Chou Wei	Yin Shen	Mao You	Chen Xu	Si Hai

[(Represent Number of Date-Stem) + (Represent Number of Date-Branch) + (Represent Number of Time-Stem) + (Represent Number of Time-Branch)] divided by 9 for a yang date or 6 for a yin date = Quotient plus Remainder.

If one wants the open points during the *zi* and *chou* time-periods of a *jia-zi* date, one has to first of all find out the time-stem by a "Five Tigers Method" (see Appendix 3). This method initiates the time-stem from the date, in this case *jia-zi*. Then, according to the sequential order of the "Cycle of 60", the next time-period should be *yi-chou*.

According to the representative numbers of the stems and branches of the date (see above, Table App. 11), *jia*=10, *zi*=7; and according to the representative numbers of stems and branches of the time-period (by Table App. 12), *jia*=9 and also *zi*=9. Put these four numbers together, 10+7+9+9 = 35. Then, since the *jia* Heavenly Stem pertains to yang, 35 is divided by 9 = 3 and remainder 8.

The remainder 8 is simply the representative number of the point Neiguan, therefore the open-point which should be selected during the *jia-zi* time-period of a *jia-zi* date is Neiguan.

If there is no "remainder" from the division for a yang date, take the number 9 into account—thus the point Lieque should be opened; e.g. during the *wu-chen* time-period on a *jia-zi* date, the representative numbers of the date stem-branch are *jia*=10, and *zi*=7, and the representative numbers of the time stem-branch are *wu*=5, *chen*=5. Put these four numbers together and it makes 10+7+5+5 = 27.

Jia is a yang date, and so 27 divided by 9=3, without a "remainder". In such a case, select point according to the number 9 as it is a yang date, i.e. point Lieque.

Another example: during the *xin-si* time-period of a *yi-chou* date, *yi*=9, *chou*=10, *xin*=7, *si*=4, and 9+10+7+4=30. The *yi* date pertains to yin, so 30 divided by 6=5, without a "remainder". Then take the number 6 into account and thus select the point Gongsun.

The above is an application according to the calculation formula of point selection. Clinically, another method which combines points in applying the Mystic Turtle method can also be adopted. In this, Gongsun is paired with Neiguan, Waiguan is paired with Foot-Linqi, Lieque is paired with Zhaohai, and Houxi is paired with Shenmai, to enhance their therapeutic effect.

The Eight Methods of Flying and Soaring

The Eight Methods of Flying and Soaring, or *Feitang Ba Fa* (飞腾八法), is also a method of selecting the point during differing time-periods of the day, on the basis of the 8 Extra meridians tand their 8 points. Its application is slightly different from that of the method of the Mystic Turtle.

The Flying and Soaring Method does not use a formula with remainder, that is to say, it focuses mainly on the Heavenly Stem for either the stems and branches of the date, or the stems and branches of the time-period.

For its application, the rules shown in Table App. 13 should be remembered well.

For example, on a *jia* or *ji* date (the date-stem), according to a "Five-Tigers Escape", then "on *jia* or *ji* date it starts from *bing-yin*". So during a *bing-yin* time-period point Neiguan should be selected because *bing* corresponds to the *Gen*

Table App. 13   The combination of 8 points, 8 Trigrams and Heavenly Stems

Stems:	Ren/Jia	Bing	Wu	Geng	Xin	Yi/Gui	Ji	Ding
Points:	Gongsun	Neiguan	Linqi	Waiguan	Houxi	Shenmai	Leique	Zhaohai
Trigrams:	Qian	Gen	Kan	Zhen	Sun	Kun	Li	Dui

trigram and Neiguan. And it would be the same for *bing-shen, bing-xu, bing-zi, bing-chen, bing-wu,* etc., as they all have the same stem.

According to the same rule, Foot-Linqi should be selected during a *wu-chen* time-period and Lieque be selected during a *ji-si* time-period.

Note. In applying the Mystic Turtle method and the Flying and Soaring method, basing it on selecting open-points during differing time-periods of the day, the reinforcing and reducing needling methods as described in this book should also be applied, according to the nature and conditions of the disease.

Glossary of Chinese
terms and phrases

yin 阴	"female, passive, inner"
yang 阳	"male, active, outer"
qi 气	"vital energy, breath"
jing 经	"meridians, channels"
luo 络	"collaterals, sub-channels"
jingluo 经络	generic for "meridians"
shuxue 输穴	"acupoints"
yi tong wei shu 以痛为输	"tender spots can be used as acupoints"
zang 脏	"solid organs, viscera"
fu 腑	"hollow organs, bowels"
zangfu 脏腑	generic for "organs"
yi yuan sanqi 一源三岐	"three branches from the same origin"
si gen 四根	"four origins"
san jie 三结	"three terminations"
ben 本	"root"
biao 标	"branch"
qi jie 气街	"major passages for the qi"
zong qi 宗气	"pectoral qi"
zhen qi 真气	"true qi"
yuan qi 原气	"source qi"
ying qi 营气	"nutrient qi"
wei qi 卫气	"defensive qi"
jing qi 经气	"meridional qi"
cun 寸	"anatomical Chinese inch"
cunkou 寸口	"inch of pulse at the radial wrist"
qikou 气口	"qi pulse at the radial wrist"
Shu points 输穴	"transportation" points (distinguish "Back-Shu points")
Jing-well 井	"well" points
Ying-spring 荥	"spring" points
Shu-stream 俞	"stream" points
Jing-river 经	"river" points
He-sea 合	"sea" points (distinguish Lower *He*-Sea points)
yuan points 原穴	"source" points
luo points 络穴	"connecting" points
Xi-Cleft points 郄穴	"cleft" points
Lower *He*-Sea points 下合穴	lower "sea" points
Front-*Mu* points 募穴	front "reactive" points
Back-*Shu* points 俞穴	back "transportation" points
bu 补	"reinforce, tonify"
xie 泻	"reduce, drain"
qing long bai wei 青龙摆尾	"the green dragon shaking its tail"
de qi 得气	"arrival of qi, getting the qi"
feng zhen 锋针	"sharp-edged needle"
wai zhi 外治	"external treatment"
fu zheng 扶正	"strengthen the antipathogenic qi"
qu xie 祛邪	"eliminate the pathogenic qi"
zhen jiu 针灸	"acupuncture and moxibustion"
qi 艾	"moxa"
feng stroke 中风	"cerebral stroke"
zu zhong 卒中	"sudden inner attack"
jue syndrome 厥	"collapse, syncope"
pian ku 偏枯	"hemiplegia"
bi syndrome 痹	"rheumatism, arthritis"
wei syndrome 痿	"flaccidity, muscular weakness"
mingmen 命门	"gate of life"
zang zao 脏躁	"hysteria"
jing ji 惊悸	"mild palpitations"
zheng zhong 怔忡	"serious palpitations"
shangfeng 伤风	"common cold"
chuan 哮	"dyspnoea"
xiao 喘	"wheezing"
gu zhen 骨蒸	"bone-steaming disease"
chuan shi 传尸	"infectious disease"
si zhen 四诊	"four diagnostic methods"
bian zheng 辨证	"differentiation of syndromes"
ba gang 八纲	"eight principles"
yin/yang 阴/阳	"yin/yang"
biao/li 表/里	"exterior/interior"
xu/shi 虚/实	"deficiency/excess"
han/re 寒/热	"cold/heat"
jun 君	"monarch" points or remedies

chen 臣   "minister" points or remedies

zuo 佐   "assistant" points or remedies

shi 使   "guide" points or remedies

ziwu 子午   "midnight/midday, winter/summer, yin/yang, north/south, etc."

liuzhu 流注   "circulating and flowing"

linggui Ba Fa 灵龟八法   The "Eight Methods of the Mystic Turtle"

Qijing Nagua Fa 奇经纳卦法   The "Methods of the Extra Meridians by Adopting the Eight Trigrams"

jiu gong 九宫   the "Nine Palaces"

ba gua 八卦   the "Eight Trigrams"

Bibliography

Book of Odes (Shi Jing), ascribed to Confucius, (9–5th centuries BC).

Book of Change (Yi Jing), ascribed to Confucius, (c. 300 BC).

Moxibustion Classic on the Eleven Meridians of the Foot and Hand, Han.

Moxibustion Classic on the Eleven Meridians of Yin and Yang, Han.

Book of the Fifty-two Prescriptions, Han.

Ming Tang Charts of Acupuncture and Moxibustion, now lost, probably Han.

Ming Tang Essentials of Points, now lost, probably Han.

Yellow Emperor's Book of Medicine (Huangdi Neijing) including the two volumes, the *Plain Questions* and the *Miraculous Pivot*, Han, (c. 100 BC).

Classic on Medical Problems (Nan Jing), Han.

Systematic Classic of Acupuncture and Moxibustion (Zhen Jiu Jia Yi Jing), Huangfu Mi, Jin (c. AD 260).

Prescriptions for Emergencies (Zhou Hou Be Ji Fan), Ge Hong, Eastern Jin (c. AD 340).

Other Records by Famous Physicians (Ming Yi Bie Lu), Tao Hongjing, Liang (c. AD 510).

General Treatise on the Causes and Symptoms of Diseases (Zhu Bing Yuan Hou Lun), Chao Yuanfang, Sui (AD 610)

Prescriptions Worth A Thousand Gold Coin (Qian Jin Yao Fang), Sun Simiao, Tang (AD 659).

The Medical Secrets of An Official (Wai Tai Bi Yao), Wang Tao, Tang (AD 952).

An Illustrated Manual on Points for Acupuncture and Moxibustion on the New Bronze Figure (Tong Ren Zhen Jiu Shu Xue Tu Jing), Wang Weiyi, Song (1026).

Bianque's Medical Experiences (Bian Que Xin Shu), Dou Cai, Song (1146).

Guide to Acupuncture and Moxibustion (Zhen Jing Zhi Nan), Dou Hanqing, Jin-Yuan (1241).

Twelve Points Corresponding to the Stars Above (Tian Xing Shi Er Xue), also named *The Ballad of the Twelve Points and their Indications* (She Er Xue Zhu Zhi Za Bing Ge), Ma Danyang, Jin.

The Lyric of Standard Profundities (Biao You Fu), Dou Hanqing, Jin (1234).

Prescriptions for Relieving the Sick (Ji Sheng Fang), Du Sijing, Yuan (1315).

An Exposition of the Fourteen Meridians (Shi Si Jing Fa Hui), Hua Shou, Yuan (1341).

Classic of Magical Effective Treatment (Shen Ying Jing), Chen Hui, Ming (1425)

A Complete Collection of Acupuncture and Moxibustion, (Zhen Jiu Da Quan) Xu Feng, Ming (1439).

An Exemplary Collection of Acupuncture and Moxibustion (Zhen Jiu Ju Ying), Gao Wu, Ming (1529).

Jade Dragon Rhymes (Yu Long Ge), found in the *Exemplary Collection*.

A Handbook of Ballads for Emergencies (Zhou Hou Ge), author unknown, found in the *Exemplary Collection*.

The Lyric of the Hundred Diseases (Bai Zheng Fu), Gao Wu, Ming (1529).

Questions and Answers Concerning Acupuncture and Moxibustion (Zhen Jiu Wen Dui), Wang Ji, Ming (1532).

Introduction to Medicine or *Elementary Medicine* (Yi Xue Ru Men), Li Ting, Ming (1575).

Research on the Eight Extra Meridians (Qijing Bamai Kao), Li Shizhen, Ming (1578).

A Plumbline for Treatment (Zhen Zhi Zhun Sheng), Wang Kentang, Ming (1582).

Supplement with Diagnosis to the Systematic Compilation of the Internal Classic (Lie Jing Tu Yi), Zhang Jiebin, Ming (1624).

Secrets of Acupuncture And Moxibustion for Health Care, later called the *Great Compendium of Acupuncture and Moxibustion* (Zhen Jiu Da Cheng), Yang Jizhou, Ming (1601).

Superior-To-Jade Rhymes (Sheng Yu Ge), found in the *Great Compendium*.

The Guide to the Secret of Qi Flow (Tong Xuan Zhi Yao Fu), He Ruoyu, found in the *Great Compendium*.

The Ode to the Golden Needle (Jin Zhen Fu), author unknown, found in the *Great Compendium*.

The Rhymes of Grand Number One (Tian Yuan Tai Yi Ge), author unknown, contained in the *Great Compendium*.

A Golden Mirror of Medicine (Yi Zong Jin Jian) by Wu Qian, Qing (1742).

A Collection of Acupuncture and Moxibustion (Zhen Jiu Ji Cheng), Liao Runhong, Qing (1874).

Subject index

Points index